Progress in
Cancer Research and Therapy
Volume 31

HORMONES AND CANCER 2
PROCEEDINGS OF THE
SECOND INTERNATIONAL CONGRESS ON
HORMONES AND CANCER

Progress in Cancer Research and Therapy

Progress in
Cancer Research and Therapy
Volume 31

Hormones and Cancer 2

Proceedings of the
Second International Congress on
Hormones and Cancer

Editors

Francesco Bresciani, Ph.D.
Institute of General Pathology and Oncology
First Faculty of Medicine and Surgery
University of Naples
Naples, Italy

Roger J.B. King, Ph.D.
Hormone Biochemistry Department
Imperial Cancer Research Fund
London, England

Marc E. Lippman, M.D.
Medicine Branch
National Cancer Institute
National Institutes of Health
Bethesda, Maryland

Moïse Namer, M.D.
Centre Antoine Lacassagne
Nice, France

Jean-Pierre Raynaud, Ph.D.
Roussel-Uclaf
Paris, France

Raven Press ■ New York

Raven Press, 1140 Avenue of the Americas, New York, New York 10036

Made in the United States of America

Library of Congress Cataloging in Publication Data

International Congress on Hormones and Cancer (2nd :
    1983 : Monte Carlo, Monaco)
    Hormones and cancer 2.

    (Progress in cancer research and therapy ; v. 31)
    Includes bibliographies and index.
    1. Cancer—Endocrine aspects—Congresses.
I. Bresciani, Francesco.   II. Title.   III. Series.
[DNLM: 1. Cell Transformation, Neoplastic—congresses.
2. Breast Neoplasms—congresses.   3. Genital Neoplasms,
Female—congresses.   4. Hormones—pharmacodynamics—
congresses.   5. Molecular biology—congresses.   6. Neo-
plasms—congresses.   W1 PR667M v.31 / QZ 200 I608 1983h]
RC268.2.I58   1983   616.99′4071   84-11722
ISBN 0-88167-031-6

Preface

Confronted by the question of defining the major research areas encompassed by the expression "Hormones and Cancer," most people would respond: hormone action at a cellular level, hormonal abnormalities either causing cancers or vice-versa, clinical use of hormones, and the development of hormone-resistant tumors from previously sensitive counterparts.

This volume covers these areas in varying degrees. Since we are in the era of molecular biology, that discipline assumes prominence with respect to topics such as oncogenes, gene cloning, and molecular structure of receptors. Cellular biology is well represented, especially in the chapters dealing with hormonal control of cell proliferation. The seemingly inevitable progression from the responsible to autonomous state exhibited by the major endocrine-sensitive tumors of humans remains a baffling phenomenon, but we are beginning to recognize that such autonomy can be attained via different mechanisms, not all of which involve the classical target cell itself.

Inevitably in books on the subject of hormones and cancer, leukemia and cancers of the breast, female reproductive tract, and prostate receive the most attention, and this treatise is no exception. In addition, the novel peptide hormone production by tumors previously considered to be nonhormone producing receives consideration. The clinical aspects discussed in these sections are supplemented by a review of the interrelationship of hormone and chemotherapy in the treatment of breast cancer.

This volume contains research-type chapters interspersed with chapters of a more general appeal; basic science predominates but clinical practice is not neglected.

This volume will be of interest to both scientists and clinicians interested in the pathogenesis and therapy of endocrine related cancers.

The Editors

Acknowledgments

This volume presents the proceedings of the Second International Congress on Hormones and Cancer, held in Monte Carlo in September 1983.

The scientific advisory committee deserves credit for selecting topics and speakers for the meeting and thanks also go to Dr. Namer and his local organizing committee for getting participants to the right place at the right time. Major credit for the appearance of this book goes to Tiiu Ojasoo who coped with the voluminous correspondence and members of the editorial board with equal efficiency. The facilities provided by Roussel-Uclaf, Paris, are gratefully acknowledged.

Contents

Section I: Steroid Hormone Action

Section IV: Gynecological Cancer

Section V: Prostate Cancer

Section IX: Tumor Markers

Section X: Quality Control of Receptor Assay

Contributors

F. Aghini-Lombardi
Patologia Medica 2
University of Pisa
Via Roma, 67
56100 Pisa, Italy

Sigrid Aliau
U 58 INSERM
60, rue de Navacelles
34100 Montpellier, France

Joseph Charles Allegra
Department of Medicine
University of Louisville
Ambulatory Care Building
Louisville, Kentucky 40292

D. Amroch
Department of Surgery A
Kaplan Hospital
Rehovot, Israel

Diane Anderson
Department of Obstetrics and Gynecology
University of Chicago
Pritzker School of Medicine
5841 South Maryland Avenue
Chicago, Illinois 60637

Ferdinando Auricchio
Istituto di Patologia Generale e Oncologia
Universita di Napoli
Via S. Andrea delle Dame, 2
80138 Naples, Italy

Giovanni Bambini
Patologia Medica 2
University of Pisa
Via Roma, 67
56100 Pisa, Italy

Mozenna Bano
Laboratory of Pathophysiology
Cell Cycle Regulation Section
National Cancer Institute
Bethesda, Maryland 20205

Wilfried Bartsch
Department of Clinical Chemistry
Medical Clinic
University of Hamburg
Martinistrasse 52
D-2000 Hamburg 20, Federal Republic of Germany

Lidio Baschieri
Patologia Medica 2
University of Pisa
Via Roma, 67
56100 Pisa, Italy

Miguel Beato
Institute of Physiological Chemistry
University of Marburg
Deutschhausstrasse 2
D-3550 Marburg, Federal Republic of Germany

A. Bélanger
Department of Molecular Endocrinology and
*   Medicine*
Le Centre Hospitalier de L'Université Laval
Québec, G1V 4G2 Canada

Philip Alan Bell
Tenovus Institute for Cancer Research
Welsh National School of Medicine
Heath Park
Cardiff CF4 4XX, Wales, United Kingdom

Th. Benraad
Department of Experimental and Chemical
*   Endocrinology*
Geert Grooteplein Zuid 8
6525 GA Nijmegen, The Netherlands

Chris Benz
Cancer Research Institute
University of California
San Francisco, California 94143

Constance Benz
Department of Medicine
Yale University School of Medicine
New Haven, Connecticut 06510

Paul A. Beranek
Department of Chemical Pathology
St. Mary's Hospital Medical School
London W2 1PG, United Kingdom

Christine D. Berg
Medicine Branch
National Cancer Institute
National Institutes of Health
Building 10, Room 12N226
Bethesda, Maryland 20205

Els M.J.J. Berns
Department of Biochemistry II
Erasmus University Rotterdam
P.O. Box 1738
3000 DR Rotterdam, The Netherlands

Eric Bignon
U 58 INSERM
60, rue de Navacelles
34100 Montpellier, France

R.W. Blamey
Department of Surgery
City Hospital
Nottingham, United Kingdom

Rien A. Blankenstein
Department of Biochemistry
Rotterdam Radio-Therapeutic Institute
Dr. Daniel den Hoed Clinic
P.O. Box 5201
3008 AE Rotterdam, The Netherlands

Clara Derber Bloomfield
Section of Medical Oncology
Department of Medicine
University of Minnesota
Box 277, University Hospitals
Minneapolis, Minnesota 55455

H. Bojar
Onkologische Chemie
Universität Düsseldorf
Universitätsstrasse 1
D-4000 Düsseldorf, Federal Republic of Germany

Johannes M.G. Bonfrèr
The Netherlands Cancer Institute
121 Plesmanlaan
1066 CX Amsterdam, The Netherlands

Jean-Louis Borgna
Centre National de la Recherche Scientifique
  (CNRS)
U 148 INSERM
60, rue de Navacelles
34100 Montpellier, France

C. Bossé
Hôtel-Dieu Hospital
Chicoutimi, Canada

Zsuzsanna Bösze
Institute of Genetics
Biological Research Center
Hungarian Academy of Sciences
P.O. Box 521
H-6701 Szeged, Hungary

J.L. Boublil
Centre Antoine-Lacassagne
36 Voie Romaine
06054 Nice Cedex, France

Diane A. Bronzert
Medical Breast Cancer Section
Medicine Branch
National Cancer Institute
National Institutes of Health
Building 10, Room 12N226
Bethesda, Maryland 20205

Jerry R. Brooks
Merck Sharp & Dohme Research Laboratories
P.O. Box 2000
Rahway, New Jersey 07065

Nicholas Bruchovsky
Department of Cancer Endocrinology
Cancer Control Agency of British Columbia
2656 Heather Street
Vancouver, British Columbia, V5Z 3J3 Canada

Peter F. Bruning
The Netherlands Cancer Institute
121 Plesmanlaan
1066 CX Amsterdam, The Netherlands

Nelson A. Burstein
Department of Pathology
St. Elizabeth's Hospital
736 Cambridge Street
Boston, Massachusetts 02135

Françoise Capony
U 148 INSERM
60, rue de Navacelles
34100 Montpellier, France

Simone Casteels
Université Libre de Bruxelles
Hôpital Brugmann
4 Place Van Gehuchten
1020 Brussels, Belgium

Gabriella Castoria
Istituto di Patologia Generale e Oncologia
Università di Napoli
Via S. Andrea delle Dame 2
80138 Naples, Italy

Dany Chalbos
U 148 INSERM
60, rue de Navacelles
34100 Montpellier, France

S. Chatsubi
Department of Hormone Research
The Weizmann Institute of Science
Rehovot, 76100 Israel

Helen Cheng
Department of Cancer Endocrinology
Cancer Control Agency of British Columbia
2656 Heather Street
Vancouver, British Columbia, V5Z 3J3 Canada

Anne Cheung
Merck Sharp & Dohme Research Laboratories
P.O. Box 2000
Rahway, New Jersey 07065

Piergiorgio G. Chiodini
Division of Endocrinology
Ente Ospedaliero Niguarda Ca' Granda
Piazza Ospedale Maggiore, 3
20162 Milan, Italy

Charles Donald Christian
Department of Obstetrics and Gynecology
University of Arizona Health Sciences Center
1501 North Campbell Avenue
Tucson, Arizona 85724

K. Chrumka
Cancer Control Agency of British Columbia
Vancouver, V5Z 3J3 Canada

Geoffrey M. Cooper
Laboratory of Molecular Carcinogenesis
Dana Farber Cancer Institute
44 Binney Street
Boston, Massachusetts 02115

Maureen Costello
Department of Pharmacology
Stanford University
Stanford, California 94305

Marie-Pierre Cotard
Centre de Recherches Roussel-UCLAF
102 Route de Noisy
93230 Romainville, France

S. Cox
Tissue Cell Relationship Laboratory
Imperial Cancer Research Fund
London WC2A 3PX, United Kingdom

Pierre Crabbé
UNESCO
Division of Scientific Research and Higher
  Education
5 Rue François Bonvin
75700 Paris, France

Andre Crastes de Paulet
Department of Biochemistry
U 58 INSERM
60, rue de Navacelles
34100 Montpellier, France

Gerald R. Cunha
Department of Anatomy
University of California
Third and Parnassus Street
San Francisco, California 94143

Sally Ann Curtis
Hormone Biochemistry Department
Imperial Cancer Research Fund
P.O. Box 123
Lincoln's Inn Fields
London WC2A 3PX, United Kingdom

Benoit Cypriani
U 58 INSERM
60, rue de Navacelles
34100 Montpellier, France

Daniela Dallabonzana
Division of Endocrinology
Ente Ospedaliero Niguarda Ca' Granda
Piazza Ospedale Maggiore, 3
20162 Milan, Italy

David Danielpour
Department of Biochemistry and Molecular Biology
The University of Texas Medical School
P.O. Box 20708
Houston, Texas 77225

Philippa Denise Darbre
Hormone Biochemistry Department
Imperial Cancer Research Fund
P.O. Box 123
Lincoln's Inn Fields
London WC2A 3PX, United Kingdom

Peter Davies
Hormone Action Group
Tenovus Institute for Cancer Research
Welsh National School of Medicine
Heath Park
Cardiff, CF4 4XX, United Kingdom

John Robert Davis
Department of Pathology
University of Arizona Health Sciences Center
1501 North Campbell Avenue
Tucson, Arizona 85724

Maartje de Jong-Bakker
The Netherlands Cancer Institute
121 Plesmanlaan
1066 CX Amsterdam, The Netherlands

R. Delisle
Hôtel-Dieu Hospital
Roberval, Canada

Yu Ding
Institute of Organic Chemistry
Academia Sinica
Shanghai, Peoples Republic of China

Deborah Dobson
Department of Pharmacology
Stanford University
Stanford, California 94305

A. Dupont
Department of Molecular Endocrinology and
*   Medicine*
Le Centre Hospitalier de L'Université Laval
Québec, G1V 4G2 Canada

Jeff Dyas
Tenovus Institute for Cancer Research
Welsh National School of Medicine
Heath Park
Cardiff, CF4 4XX, United Kingdom

Colby Lancaster Eaton
Tenovus Institute for Cancer Research
Welsh National School of Medicine
Heath Park
Cardiff, CF4 4XX United Kingdom

Howard J. Eisen
Laboratory of Developmental Pharmacology
National Institute of Child Health and Human
*   Development*
National Institutes of Health
Building 10, Room 8C-416
Bethesda, Maryland 20205

J. Emond
Hôtel-Dieu Hospital
Lévis, Québec, Canada

Elaine Evans
U 148 INSERM
60, rue de Navacelles
34100 Montpellier, France

Sture Falkmer
Department of Pathology
University of Lund
Malmö General Hospital
S-214 01 Malmö, Sweden

Joël Fauque
University of Sciences
U 148 INSERM
60, rue de Navacelles
34100 Montpellier, France

Arpad G. Fazekas
The Montreal General Hospital
University Surgical Clinic
1650 Cedar Avenue
Montreal, Quebec, H3G 1A4 Canada

John Albert Foekens
Department of Cancer Endocrinology
Cancer Control Agency of British Columbia
2656 Heather Street
Vancouver, British Columbia, V5Z 3J3 Canada

J.L. Formento
Centre Antoine-Lacassagne
36 Voie Romaine
06054 Nice Cedex, France

Carol M. Foster
Laboratory of Developmental Pharmacology
National Institute of Child Health and Human
*   Development*
National Institutes of Health
Building 10, Room 8C-416
Bethesda, Maryland 20205

G. Francini
Institute of Medical Semeiotics
University of Siena
53100 Siena, Italy

M. Francoual
Centre Antoine-Lacassagne
36 Voie Romaine
06054 Nice Cedex, France

Fred Frankel
Department of Microbiology
University of Pennsylvania
Philadelphia, Pennsylvania 19174

Marcel Garcia
U 148 INSERM
60, rue de Navacelles
34100 Montpellier, France

Ulrich Gehring
Institut für Biologische Chemie
Universität Heidelberg
1m Neunenheimer Feld 501
D-6900 Heidelberg, Federal Republic of Germany

C. Gennari
Institute of Medical Semeiotics
University of Siena
53100 Siena, Italy

Margaret W. Ghilchik
Department of Surgery
St. Charles Hospital
Exmoor Street
London W10, United Kingdom

Jacques Gilbert
CERCOA-CNRS
2 rue Henri Dunant
94320 Thiais, France

J.G. Girard
Asbestos Medical Center
Québec, Canada

S. Gonnelli
Institute of Medical Semeiotics
University of Siena
53100 Siena, Italy

Lars Granholm
Department of Neurosurgery
Karolinska Institute
P.O. Box 60500
S-104 01 Stockholm, Sweden

Flora Hull Grantham
Laboratory of Pathophysiology
Cell Cycle Regulation Section
National Cancer Institute
Bethesda, Maryland 20205

Keith Griffiths
Tenovus Institute for Cancer Research
Welsh National School of Medicine
Heath Park
Cardiff, CF4 4XX, United Kingdom

David Spencer Grosso
Department of Obstetrics and Gynecology
University of Arizona Health Sciences Center
1501 North Campbell Avenue
Tucson, Arizona 85724

Jan-Åke Gustafsson
Department of Medical Nutrition
Huddinge University Hospital (F69)
S-141 86 Huddinge, Sweden

Carol Hall
DNAX Research Institute
Palo Alto, California 94302

Rosemary E. Hall
Ludwig Institute for Cancer Research
University of Sydney
Blackburn Building
Sydney, New South Wales 2006, Australia

R. Hallowes
Tissue Cell Relationship Laboratory
Imperial Cancer Research Fund
London WC2A 3PX, United Kingdom

Stephen D. Halmo
Department of Obstetrics and Gynecology
University of Western Ontario
London, Ontario, Canada N6A 5C1

Augustinus A.M. Hart
The Netherlands Cancer Institute
121 Plesmanlaan
1066 CX Amsterdam, The Netherlands

Arthur Lee Herbst
Department of Obstetrics and Gynecology
University of Chicago
Pritzker School of Medicine
5841 South Maryland Avenue
Chicago, Illinois 60637

Nikki J. Holbrook
Laboratory of Pathology
National Institutes of Health
Building 10, Room 2N-113
Bethesda, Maryland 20205

Michel Hospital
CNRS
Université de Bordeaux 1
Laboratoire de Cristallographie et de Physique
 Cristalline
351 Cours de la Libération
33405 Talence, France

J.G. Houle
Hôtel-Dieu Hospital
Lévis, Québec, Canada

Marian Munroe Hubby
Department of Obstetrics and Gynecology
University of Chicago
Pritzker School of Medicine
5841 South Maryland Avenue
Chicago, Illinois 60637

Helen Hurst
Imperial Cancer Research Fund
P.O. Box 123
Lincoln's Inn Fields
London WC2A 3PX, United Kingdom

J.M. Husson
Centre de Recherches Roussel-UCLAF
Romainville, France

T. William Hutchens
Department of Biochemistry and James Graham
 Brown Cancer Center
University of Louisville
Louisville, Kentucky 40292

Stefano Iacobelli
Laboratory of Molecular Endocrinology
Department of Obstetrics and Gynecology
Catholic University
Largo Gemelli, 8
00168 Rome, Italy

Tatsuhiko Ikeda
Faculty of Nutrition
Kobe-Gakuin University
Igawadani-cho Arise
Nishi-ku, Kobe, 673 Japan

Julianne Imperato-McGinley
Department of Medicine
New York Hospital—Cornell University Medical
* Center*
1300 York Avenue
New York, New York 10021

H. Imura
Second Division
Departments of Internal Medicine and Clinical
* Nutrition*
Kyoto University Faculty of Medicine
54 Kawaharacho
Shogoin, Sakyo-ku, Kyoto 606, Japan

Hannu Ensio Isotalo
Department of Clinical Chemistry
University of Oulu
SF-90220 Oulu 22, Finland

G.C. Jackson
Cancer Control Agency of British Columbia
Vancouver, V5Z 3J3 Canada

C. Rolin Jacquemyns
Hormone and Metabolic Research Unit
International Institute of Cellular and Molecular
* Pathology*
B-1200 Brussels, Belgium

Vivian H.T. James
Department of Chemical Pathology
St. Mary's Hospital Medical School
London W2 1PG, United Kingdom

Ivy E. Johnson
Department of Surgery
University of Toronto
Medical Sciences Building, Room 7336
Toronto, M5S 1A8 Canada

Christopher Nicholas Jones
Tenovus Institute for Cancer Research
Welsh National School of Medicine
Heath Park
Cardiff CF4 4XX, Wales, United Kingdom

Nobuyuki Kadohama
Roswell Park Memorial Institute
Buffalo, New York 14263

Nadim Kassem
Department of Clinical Research
Schering Corporation
2000 Galloping Hill Road
Kenilworth, New Jersey 07033

Antti Jaakko Kauppila
Department of Obstetrics and Gynecology
University of Oulu
SF-90220 Oulu 22, Finland

Alvin M. Kaye
Department of Hormone Research
The Weizmann Institute of Science
Rehovot, 76100 Israel

Thomas M. Kelly
Department of Internal Medicine
Division of Endocrinology and Metabolism
University of Utah
School of Medicine
50 North Medical Drive
Salt Lake City, Utah 84132

William Robert Kidwell
Laboratory of Pathophysiology
Cell Cycle Regulation Section
National Cancer Institute
Bethesda, Maryland 20205

Roger J.B. King
Hormone Biochemistry Department
Imperial Cancer Research Fund
P.O. Box 123
Lincoln's Inn Fields
London WC2A 3PX, United Kingdom

Mary Ellen Kirk
Department of Obstetrics and Gynecology
University of Western Ontario
London, Ontario, Canada N6A 5C1

Seppo Tapio Kivinen
Department of Obstetrics and Gynecology
University of Oulu
SF-90220 Oulu 22, Finland

Hartmut Klein
Department of Clinical Chemistry
Medical Clinic
University of Hamburg
Martinistrasse 52
D-2000 Hamburg 20, Federal Republic of Germany

A. Maria Koenders
Department of Experimental and Chemical
  Endocrinology
St. Radbpud Hospital
Geert Grooteplein Zuid 8
6525 GA Nijmegen, The Netherlands

Krisztina Kovács
Institute of Genetics
Biological Research Center
Hungarian Academy of Sciences
P.O. Box 521
H-6701 Szeged, Hungary

Paul Krauter
Institute of Physiological Chemistry
University of Marburg
Deutschausstrasse 2
D-3550 Marburg, Federal Republic of Germany

B.P. Krebs
Centre Antoine-Lacassagne
36 Voie Romaine
06054 Nice Cedex, France

Micheal Krieg
Department of Clinical Chemistry
Medical Clinic
University of Hamburg
Martinistrasse 52
D-2000 Hamburg 20, Federal Republic of Germany

Thomas Tomi Kubota
Division of Medical Oncology and James Graham
  Brown Cancer Center
Department of Medicine
University of Louisville
Louisville, Kentucky 40292

H. Giok Kwa
The Netherlands Cancer Institute
121 Plesmanlaan
1066 CX Amsterdam, The Netherlands

C. Labrie
Department of Molecular Endocrinology and
  Medicine
Le Centre Hospitalier de L'Université Laval
Québec, G1V 4G2 Canada

F. Labrie
Department of Molecular Endocrinology and
  Medicine
Le Centre Hospitalier de L'Université Laval
Québec, G1V 4G2 Canada

Y. Lacourcière
Department of Molecular Endocrinology and
  Medicine
Le Centre Hospitalier de L'Université Laval
Québec, G1V 4G2 Canada

C.M. Lalanne
Centre Antoine-Lacassagne
36 Voie Romaine
06054 Nice Cedex, France

R. Lari
Patologia Medica 2
University of Pisa
Via Roma, 67
56100 Pisa, Italy

Secondo Lastoria
Istituto di Patologia Generale e Oncologia
Università di Napoli
Via S. Andrea delle Dame, 2
80138 Naples, Italy

Leslie Lazarus
The Garvan Institute of Medical Research
St. Vincent's Hospital
Sydney, New South Wales 2010, Australia

Frank Lee
DNAX Research Institute
Palo Alto, California 94302

Marc L'Hermite
Department of Gynecologie-Obstetrique
Université Libre de Bruxelles
Hôpital Brugmann
4 Place Van Gehuchten
1020 Brussels, Belgium

Mireille L'Hermite-Balériaux
Université Libre de Bruxelles
Hôpital Brugmann
4 Place Van Gehuchten
1020 Brussels, Belgium

Tehming Liang
Merck Sharp & Dohme Research Laboratories
P.O. Box 2000
Rahway, New Jersey 07065

Marc E. Lippman
Medical Breast Cancer Section
Medicine Branch
National Cancer Institute
National Institutes of Health
Building 10, Room 12N226
Bethesda, Maryland 20205

Antonio Liuzzi
Division of Endocrinology
Ente Ospedaliero Niguarda Ca' Granda
Piazza Ospedale Maggiore, 3
20162 Milan, Italy

Claude Loriaux
Department de Senologie
Universitè Libre de Bruxelles
Hôpital Brugmann
4 Place Van Gehuchten
1020 Brussels, Belgium

John K. MacFarlane
The Montreal General Hospital
University Surgical Clinic
1650 Cedar Avenue
Montreal, Quebec, H3G 1A4 Canada

Henri Magdelenat
Laboratoire de Radiopathologie
Institut Curie
26, rue d'Ulm
75231 Paris, Cedex 5, France

S. Malnick
Department of Hormone Research
The Weizmann Institute of Science
Rehovot, 76100 Israel

Paolo Marchetti
Laboratory of Molecular Endocrinology
Department of Obstetrics and Gynecology
Catholic University
Largo Gemelli, 8
00168 Rome, Italy

Hans Mårtensson
Department of Surgery
University of Lund
University Hospital
S-221 85 Lund, Sweden

Pierre-Marie Martin
Cancérologie Expérimentale
Faculté de Médecine Nord
Blvd. Pierre Dramard
13326 Marseille, Cedex 3, France

E. Martino
Patologia Medica 2
University of Pisa
Via Roma, 67
56100 Pisa, Italy

S. Matsukura
Second Division
Departments of Internal Medicine and Clinical
  Nutrition
Kyoto University Faculty of Medicine
54 Kawaharacho
Shogoin, Sakyo-ku, Kyoto 606, Japan

Robynne McGinley
The Garvan Institute of Medical Research
St. Vincent's Hospital
Sydney, New South Wales 2010, Australia

P.J. Meunier
U 234 INSERM
Pathologie des Tissus Calcifiés
Faculté A. Carrel
Rue G. Paradin
69008 Lyon, France

Jean Paul Mialot
Ecole Nationale Véterinaire
7 Avenue de General de Gaulle
94704 Maisons Alfort, Cedex, France

Francoise Michel
U 58 INSERM
60, rue de Navacelles
34100 Montpellier, France

Antimo Migliaccio
Istituto di Patologia Generale e Oncologia
Via S. Andrea delle Dame, 2
80138 Naples, Italy

G. Milano
Centre Antoine-Lacassagne
36 Voie Romaine
06054 Nice Cedex, France

Jean-Francois Miquel
CNRS
15 Quai Anatole France
75700 Paris, France

Betty G. Mobbs
Department of Surgery
University of Toronto
Medical Sciences Building, Room 7336
Toronto, M5S 1A8 Canada

Martine Moguilewsky
Centre de Recherches Roussel-UCLAF
111 Route De Noisy
93230 Romainville, France

J.L. Moll
Centre Antoine-Lacassagne
36 Voie Romaine
06054 Nice Cedex, France

G. Monfette
Hôtel-Dieu Hospital
St. Jérôme, Québec, Canada

M. Montagnani
Institute of Medical Semeiotics
University of Siena
53100 Siena, Italy

E. Motz
Patologia Medica 2
University of Pisa
Via Roma, 67
56100 Pisa, Italy

Henning T. Mouridsen
Department of Oncology I
Finseninstitute
49 Strandboulevarden
DK-2100 Copenhagen, Denmark

Eppo Mulder
Department of Biochemistry II
Erasmus University Rotterdam
P.O. Box 1738
3000 DR Rotterdam, The Netherlands

Allan U. Munck
Department of Pathology
Dartmouth Medical School
Hanover, New Hampshire 03755

Leigh C. Murphy
Ludwig Institute for Cancer Research
University of Sydney
Blackburn Building
Sydney, New South Wales 2006, Australia

Liam Joseph Murphy
The Garvan Institute of Medical Research
St. Vincent's Hospital
Sydney, New South Wales 2010, Australia

Darrell K. Murray
Department of Internal Medicine
Division of Endocrinology and Metabolism
University of Utah
School of Medicine
50 North Medical Drive
Salt Lake City, Utah 84132

Y. Nakai
Second Division
Departments of Internal Medicine and Clinical
*   Nutrition*
Kyoto University Faculty of Medicine
54 Kawaharacho
Shogoin, Sakyo-ku, Kyoto 606, Japan

K. Nakao
Second Division
Departments of Internal Medicine and Clinical
*   Nutrition*
Kyoto University Faculty of Medicine
54 Kawaharacho
Shogoin, Sakyo-ku, Kyoto 606, Japan

M. Namer
Centre Antoine-Lacassagne
36 Voie Romaine
06054 Nice Cedex, France

R. Nami
Institute of Medical Semeiotics
University of Siena
53100 Siena, Italy

Bahman Nassim
Department of Chemistry
University of Missouri
Columbia, Missouri 65211

Vittoria Natoli
Laboratory of Molecular Endocrinology
Department of Obstetrics and Gynecology
Catholic University
Largo Gemelli, 8
00168 Rome, Italy

Hajime Nawata
Yayoi 1-5-24
Sawara-ku, Fukuoka City, 814 Japan

Günter Nehse
Department of Clinical Chemistry
Medical Clinic
University of Hamburg
Martinistrasse 52
D-2000 Hamburg 20, Federal Republic of Germany

D.H. Nelson
Department of Internal Medicine
Division of Endocrinology and Metabolism
University of Utah
School of Medicine
50 North Medical Drive
Salt Lake City, Utah 84132

Rudolph Neri
Department of Clinical Research
Schering Corporation
2000 Galloping Hill Road
Kenilworth, New Jersey 07033

Robert Ian Nicholson
Tenovus Institute for Cancer Research
Welsh National School of Medicine
Heath Park
Cardiff, CF4 4XX, United Kingdom

Jeffrey A. Nisker
Department of Obstetrics and Gynecology
University of Western Ontario
London, Ontario, Canada N6A 5C1

Anders Nobin
Department of Surgery
University of Lund
University Hospital
S-221 85 Lund, Sweden

Guy Nöel
Laboratory of Senobiochemistry
University of Louvain
P.O. U.C.L. 5369
1200 Brussels, Belgium

Willem Nooyen
The Netherlands Cancer Institute
121 Plesmanlaan
1066 CX Amsterdam, The Netherlands

Tiiu Ojasoo
Roussel-UCLAF
35 Blvd. des Invalides
75007 Paris, France

S. Oki
Second Division
Departments of Internal Medicine and Clinical
* Nutrition*
Kyoto University Faculty of Medicine
54 Kawaharacho
Shogoin, Sakyo-ku, Kyoto 606, Japan

Giuseppe Oppizzi
Division of Endocrinology
Ente Ospedaliero Niguarda Ca' Granda
Piazza Ospedale Maggiore, 3
20162 Milan, Italy

C. Kent Osborne
Department of Medicine/Oncology
University of Texas Health Science Center at San
* Antonio*
7703 Floyd Curl Drive
San Antonio, Texas 78284

Furio Pacini
Patologia Medica 2
University of Pisa
Via Roma, 67
56100 Pisa, Italy

Martin Page
Imperial Cancer Research Fund
P.O. Box 123
Lincoln's Inn Fields
London WC2A 3PX, United Kingdom

J.P. Paquet
Enfant-Jesus Hospital
Québec, Canada

Malcolm Parker
Imperial Cancer Research Fund
P.O. Box 123
Lincoln's Inn Fields
London WC2A 3PX, United Kingdom

André-Laurent Parodi
Ecole Nationale Vétérinaire
7 Avenue du General de Gaulle
94704 Alfort, Cedex, France

A.H.G. Paterson
Provincial Cancer Hospitals Board of Alberta
Edmonton, T6G 1Z2 Canada

James Pellegrini
Department of Medicine
University of Massachusetts Medical School/
* Worcester*
Student Box 273
55 Lake Avenue North
Worcester, Massachusetts 01605

Bertrand F. Pertuiset
Clinique Neurologique
Hôpital de la Salpétrière
47 Boulevard de l'Hôpital
75651 Paris, Cedex 13, France

Daniel Philibert
Centre de Recherches Roussel-UCLAF
111 Coute de Noisy
93230 Romainville, France

Colin Geoffrey Pierrepoint
Tenovus Institute for Cancer Research
Welsh National School of Medicine
Heath Park
Cardiff, CF4 4XX United Kingdom

Aldo Pinchera
Cattedra di Endocrinologia e Medicina
* Costituzionale*
University of Pisa
Via Roma, 67
56100 Pisa, Italy

M. Poisson
Clinique Neurologique (Pr. A. Buge)
Pitié-Salpétrière
75651 Paris, France

Michel Pons
U 58 INSERM
60, rue de Navacelles
34100 Montpellier, France

Martin Posner
Department of Physics
University of Massachusetts/Boston
Boston, Massachusetts 02125

Gilles Precigoux
CNRS
Université de Bordeaux 1
Laboratoire de Cristallographie et de Physique
 Cristalline
351 Cours de la Libération
33405 Talence, France

Robert H. Purdy
Department of Organic Chemistry
Southwest Foundation for Research and Education
P.O. Box 28147
San Antonio, Texas 78284

Jacques Irénée Charles Quivy
Unite Hormones et Metabolisme
Institute of Cellular and Molecular Pathology
ICP/Horm, UCL 7529
Avenue Hippocrate, 75
1200 Brussels, Belgium

Gary H. Rasmusson
Merck Sharp & Dohme Research Laboratories
P.O. Box 2000
Rahway, New Jersey 07065

Jean-Pierre Raynaud
Roussel-UCLAF
35 Blvd. des Invalides
75007 Paris, France

Roger R. Reddel
Ludwig Institute for Cancer Research
University of Sydney
Blackburn Building
Sydney, New South Wales 2006, Australia

Michael J. Reed
Department of Chemical Pathology
St. Mary's Hospital Medical School
London W2 1PG, United Kingdom

Paul Stephen Rennie
Department of Cancer Endocrinology
Cancer Control Agency of British Columbia
2656 Heather Street
Vancouver, British Columbia, V5Z 3J3 Canada

Glenn F. Reynolds
Merck Sharp & Dohme Research Laboratories
P.O. Box 2000
Rahway, New Jersey 07065

Gordon Ringold
Department of Pharmacology
Stanford University
Stanford, California 94305

M.R.G. Robinson
Department of Urology
Pontefract General Infirmary
Southgate
Pontefract, West Yorkshire, United Kingdom

Henri Rochefort
U 148 INSERM
60, rue de Navacelles
34100 Montpellier, France

Focko F.G. Rommerts
Department of Biochemistry II
Erasmus University Rotterdam
P.O. Box 1738
3000 DR Rotterdam, The Netherlands

Carsten Rose
Department of Oncology I
Finseninstitute
49 Strandboulevarden
DK-2100 Copenhagen, Denmark

Anthony L. Rosner
New England Pathology Services
330 Cummings Park
Woburn, Massachusetts 01801

Andrea Rotondi
Istituto di Patologia Generale e Oncologia
Università di Napoli
Via S. Andrea delle Dame, 2
80138 Naples, Italy

Guy G. Rousseau
Unite Hormones et Metabolisme
Institute of Cellular and Molecular Pathology
ICP/Horm, UCL 7529
Avenue Hippocrate, 75
1200 Brussels, Belgium

Avery A. Sandberg
Roswell Park Memorial Institute
Buffalo, New York 14263

Giovanni Scambia
Laboratory of Molecular Endocrinology
Department of Obstetrics and Gynecology
Catholic University
Largo Gemelli, 8
00168 Rome, Italy

Claus Scheidereit
Institute of Physiological Chemistry
University of Marburg
Deutschhausstrasse 2
D-3550 Marburg, Federal Republic of Germany

F.H. Schroeder
Department of Urology
Erasmus University Rotterdam
P.O. Box 1738
3000 DR Rotterdam, The Netherlands

A. Shaer
Department of Hormone Research
The Weizmann Institute of Science
Rehovot, 76100 Israel

Nahid A. Shahabi
Department of Biochemistry and James Graham
  Brown Cancer Center
University of Louisville
Louisville, Kentucky 40292

G. Shyamala
Lady Davis Institute for Medical Research
Sir Mortimer B. Davis Jewish General Hospital
3755 Cote Saint Catherine Road
Montreal, Quebec, H3T 1E2 Canada

David A. Sirbasku
Department of Biochemistry and Molecular Biology
The University of Texas Medical School
P.O. Box 20708
Houston, Texas 77225

David Alan Nigel Sirett
Unite Hormones et Metabolisme
Institute of Cellular and Molecular Pathology
I.C.P./Horm. U.C.L. 7529
Avenue Hippocrate, 75
1200 Brussels, Belgium

Kendall A. Smith
Department of Hematology Research
Dartmouth Medical School
Remsen 323
Hanover, New Hampshire 03755

W. Staib
Physiologische Chemie II
Universität Düsseldorf
Universitätsstrasse 1
D-4000 Düsseldorf, Federal Republic of Germany

M. Stuschke
Onkologische Chemie
Universität Düsseldorf
Universitätsstrasse 1
D-4000 Düsseldorf, Federal Republic of Germany

Frank Sundler
Department of Histology
University of Lund
Biskopsgatan 5
S-223 62 Lund, Sweden

Earl Allan Surwit
Department of Obstetrics and Gynecology
University of Arizona Health Sciences Center
1501 North Campbell Avenue
Tucson, Arizona 85724

Robert L. Sutherland
Ludwig Institute for Cancer Research
University of Sydney
Blackburn Building
Sydney, New South Wales 2006, Australia

K.D. Swenerton
Cancer Control Agency of British Columbia
Vancouver, V5Z 3J3 Canada

Christiane Julia Tabacik
U 58 INSERM
60, rue de Navacelles
34100 Montpellier, France

I. Tanaka
Second Division
Departments of Internal Medicine and Clinical
  Nutrition
Kyoto University Faculty of Medicine
54 Kawaharacho
Shogoin, Sakyo-ku, Kyoto 606, Japan

Ian W. Taylor
Ludwig Institute for Cancer Research
University of Sydney
Blackburn Building
Sydney, New South Wales 2006, Australia

Susan Jane Taylor
Laboratory of Pathophysiology
Cell Cycle Regulation Section
National Cancer Institute
Bethesda, Maryland 20205

Sharon Elaine Thomas
Tenovus Institute for Cancer Research
Welsh National School of Medicine
Heath Park
Cardiff, CF4 4XX United Kingdom

T. Tsukada
Second Division
Departments of Internal Medicine and Clinical
  Nutrition
Kyoto University Faculty of Medicine
54 Kawaharacho
Shogoin, Sakyo-ku, Kyoto 606, Japan

Aslihan Turkes
Tenovus Institute for Cancer Research
Welsh National School of Medicine
Heath Park
Cardiff, CF4 4XX, United Kingdom

Atilla Turkes
Tenovus Institute for Cancer Research
Welsh National School of Medicine
Heath Park
Cardiff, CF4 4XX, United Kingdom

A. Valentin-Opran
U 234 INSERM
Pathologie des Tissus Calcifiés
Faculté A. Carrel
Rue G. Paradin
69008 Lyon, France

A. Vallières
Saint Sacrament Hospital
Québec, Canada

Henk J. van der Molen
Department of Biochemisty II
Erasmus University Rotterdam
P.O. Box 1738
3000 DR Rotterdam, The Netherlands

G.J. van Steenbrugge
Department of Urology
Erasmus University Rotterdam
P.O. Box 1738
3000 DR Rotterdam, The Netherlands

Frédéric Veith
U 148 INSERM
60, rue de Navacelles
34100 Montpellier, France

Anikó Venetianer
Institute of Genetics
Biological Research Center
Hungarian Academy of Sciences
P.O. Box 521
H-6701 Szeged, Hungary

Giuseppe Verde
Division of Endocrinology
Ente Ospedaliero Niguarda Ca' Granda
Piazza Ospedale Maggiore, 3
20162 Milan, Italy

Albertus A. Verstraeten
The Netherlands Cancer Institute
121 Plesmanlaan
1066 CX Amsterdam, The Netherlands

Pirkko Katri Vierikko
Department of Clinical Chemistry
University of Oulu
SF-90220 Oulu 22, Finland

Françoise Vignon
U 148 INSERM
60, rue de Navacelles
34100 Montpellier, France

Reijo Kalevi Vihko
Department of Clinical Chemistry
University of Oulu
SF-90220 Oulu 22, Finland

Klaus-Dieter Voigt
Department of Clinical Chemistry
Medical Clinic
University of Hamburg
Martinistrasse 52
D-2000 Hamburg 20, Federal Republic of Germany

Alain Vokaer
Université Libre de Bruxelles
Hôpital Brugmann
4 Place Van Gehuchten
1020 Brussels, Belgium

Elizabeth Vrhovsek
The Garvan Institute of Medical Research
St. Vincent's Hospital
Sydney, New South Wales 2010, Australia

Kerry Jane Walker
Tenovus Institute for Cancer Research
Welsh National School of Medicine
Heath Park
Cardiff, CF4 4XX, United Kingdom

Colin K.W. Watts
Ludwig Institute for Cancer Research
University of Sydney
Blackburn Building
Sydney, New South Wales 2006, Australia

Bruce Westley
U 148 INSERM
60, rue de Navacelles
34100 Montpellier, France

Hannes M. Westphal
Institute of Physiological Chemistry
University of Marburg
Deutschhausstrasse 1-2
D-3550 Marburg, Federal Republic of Germany

Mike Williams
Department of Surgery
City Hospital
Nottingham, United Kingdom

James L. Wittliff
Department of Biochemistry and James Graham
Brown Cancer Center
University of Louisville
Louisville, Kentucky 40292

Israel Wiznitzer
Department of Medicine
Yale University School of Medicine
New Haven, Connecticut 06510

Örjan Wrange
Department of Medical Nutrition
Huddinge University Hospital (F69)
S-141 86 Huddinge, Sweden

T. Yoshimasa
Second Division
Departments of Internal Medicine and Clinical
Nutrition
Kyoto University Faculty of Medicine
54 Kawaharacho
Shogoin, Sakyo-ku, Kyoto 606, Japan

Zhao-Ying Yu
Departments of Medical Nutrition and
Neurosurgery
Huddinge University Hospital (F69)
S-141 86 Huddinge, Sweden

David T. Zava
Ludwig Institute for Cancer Research
Inselspital
3010 Bern, Switzerland

Progress in Cancer Research and Therapy,
Vol. 31, edited by F. Bresciani, et al.
Raven Press, New York © 1984.

Activation of Cellular Transforming Genes in Neoplasms

Geoffrey M. Cooper

Laboratory of Molecular Carcinogenesis, Dana-Farber Cancer Institute,
and Department of Pathology, Harvard Medical School,
Boston, Massachusetts 02115

Many neoplasms contain transforming genes which efficiently induce transformation of NIH 3T3 mouse cells upon transfection (see Cooper, 1982 for review). Since DNAs of normal cells lack efficient transforming activity, these results indicate that the development of neoplasms can involve dominant genetic alterations resulting in the activation of cellular transforming genes which are then detectable by their biological activity in transfection assays. Activated transforming genes have been identified in a wide variety of neoplasms including carcinomas, sarcomas, neuroblastomas, lymphomas and leukemias of human, rodent and chicken origin. These neoplasms include spontaneously-occurring tumors, chemically-induced tumors and virally-induced tumors. In addition, transforming genes have been detected by transfection of DNAs from primary neoplasms as well as tumor-derived cell lines.

At present several distinct cellular transforming genes have been identified in different types of neoplasms. The biochemical properties and distribution of these genes in tumors is discussed below.

ras genes:

Blot-hybridization analysis initially identified the transforming genes activated in a human bladder and lung carcinoma cell line as cellular homologs of the transforming genes of Harvey (ras^H) and Kirsten (ras^K) sarcoma viruses, respectively (Der et al, 1982; Parada et al, 1982; Santos et al, 1982). Activation of ras^H has been reported in only one additional human tumor (Yuasa et al, 1983), so it is not a commonly occurring transforming gene in human neoplasms. However, activation of ras^K has been reported in a variety of different human tumors, including carcinomas of the bladder, colon, lung, gall bladder and pancreas, a rhabdomyosarcoma, and a T cell leukemia (Pulciani et al, 1982; Der and Cooper, 1983; McCoy et al, 1983; Shimizu et al, 1983c; Eva et al, 1983). Another member of the ras gene family, ras^N, has also been detected as an activated transforming gene in several human neoplasms including a neuroblastoma, a colon carcinoma, fibrosarcomas, a Burkitt's lymphoma, and myeloid and T cell leukemias (Shimizu et al, 1983 b and c; Hall et al, 1983; Murray et al, 1983; Eva et al, 1983).

These three different members of the ras gene family are thus activated in a variety of neoplasms without apparent specificity in relation to cell type. However, they are activated in a relatively small fraction (10-20%) of human neoplasms. It is possible that ras genes can contribute to development of neoplasia in a wide variety of different cells but are not essential for development of any particular type of neoplasm. Alternatively, further studies may reveal a common underlying biological property of neoplasms specifically correlated with ras gene activation.

The ras genes encode proteins of approximately 21,000 daltons (designated p21) which are localized in the plasma membrane and bind guanine nucleotides (Ellis et al, 1981; Willingham et al, 1980; Papageorge et al, 1982). These proteins are expressed at high levels in cells transformed by Harvey (rasH) or Kirsten (rasK) sarcoma viruses and at lower levels in normal cells (Langbeheim et al, 1980). Ligation of normal rat or human rasH genes to viral transcriptional regulatory sequences results in activation of transforming activity, indicating that abnormally high expression of normal cell rasH is sufficient to induce transformation (DeFeo et al, 1981; Chang et al, 1982).

Comparisons of ras gene expression in normal and malignant human cells have indicated that the level of p21 expression in neoplasms which contain activated ras genes is elevated only about 5-fold compared to normal bladder epithelial cells and is not different from the level of p21 in human carcinoma cell lines which do not contain activated ras genes detectable by transfection (Der and Cooper, 1983). In several cases, it has now been found that activation of transforming activity of rasH (Tabin et al, 1982; Reddy et al, 1982) and rasK (Der and Cooper, 1983; Shimizu et al, 1983a; Capon et al, 1983) genes is a consequence of mutations which affect the structure of ras gene products rather than the level of ras gene expression. In addition, different mutations can activate the same ras gene in different individual neoplasms. How these alterations affect the biochemical activities of ras gene products remains to be elucidated.

Blym-1

The Blym-1 transforming gene was initially identified by transfection of DNAs of chicken B cell lymphomas (Cooper and Neiman, 1980). Activation of Blym-1 was detected in DNAs of six out of six chicken lymphomas analyzed, but not in DNAs of normal tissues of the same individual birds, indicating that in contrast to ras genes, activation of this gene is a highly reproducible event in lymphomagenesis.

The isolated chicken Blym-1 transforming gene is unusually small (approximately 0.6 kb) and its nucleotide sequence indicates that it encodes a predicted protein product of 65 amino acids (7,800 daltons) (Goubin et al, 1983). Comparison of the amino acid sequence of the predicted chicken Blym-1 gene product with amino acid sequences of known cellular proteins revealed partial homology (36%) between the chicken Blym-1 transforming protein and the amino-terminal region of transferrin family proteins (Goubin et al, 1983). This homology is concentrated in regions which are conserved between legitimate members of the transferrin family, suggesting a common ancestry for the chicken Blym-1 transforming protein and the amino terminal sequences of transferrins. Since transferrin has been implicated as a lymphocyte growth factor, it is intriguing to speculate that this homology may also suggest a functional relationship.

Blot hybridization analysis indicated that the chicken Blym-1 transforming gene was a member of a family of 6-8 related genes in both chicken and human DNAs (Goubin et al, 1983). The detection of human genes homologous to Blym-1 suggested the possibility that the transforming genes detected by transfection of some human lymphocyte neoplasm

DNAs might be members of this Blym gene family. This was initially approached by analysis of a transforming gene detected by transfection of DNAs of Burkitt's lymphomas, which are human B-cell lymphomas representing the same stage of B cell differentiation (surface immunoglobulin-positive) as the chicken B-cell lymphomas from which chicken Blym-1 was isolated. These experiments (Diamond et al, 1983) indicated that a human homolog of chicken Blym-1 was activated in DNAs of six out of six Burkitt's lymphomas investigated. Characterization of the isolated human Blym-1 transforming gene indicates that, like chicken Blym-1, it is less than 1 kb and is not homologous to retroviral transforming genes (Diamond et al, 1983).

Blot hybridization analysis indicated that Blym-1 is not rearranged in either chicken or human lymphomas (Goubin et al, 1983; Diamond et al, 1983). In addition, activation of Blym-1 in Burkitt's lymphomas is not associated with an increased level of gene expression (J. Devine, A. Diamond, M.-A. Lane and G.M. Cooper, unpublished observations). It therefore appears likely that activation of Blym-1, like ras genes, is a consequence of structural mutations.

The finding that Blym-1 is activated with a high degree of reproducibility in B cell lymphomas of both chicken and man provides strong support for the role of this gene in lymphomagenesis.

Transforming Genes of Other Lymphoid Neoplasms

Distinct transforming genes have been identified by transfection of DNAs of human and mouse neoplasms representing other stages of B- and T-lymphocyte differentiation (Lane et al, 1982a and b). Like Blym-1, these genes are activated in a high fraction (80-100%) of the neoplasms which have been investigated. Analysis of the susceptibility of these transforming genes to cleavage with a series of restriction endonucleases indicates that they include a gene common to human and mouse pre B cell neoplasms, a different gene common to human myelomas and mouse plasmacytomas, a third gene common to human and mouse neoplasms of intermediate T lymphocytes and a fourth gene common to human and mouse neoplasms of mature T lymphocytes (Lane et al, 1982a and b).

The transforming genes activated in lymphocyte neoplasms thus appear to be specifically related to the stage of normal cell differentiation exhibited by those neoplasms. This suggests the possibility that transformation may result from alterations in genes that are normally involved in differentiation-specific control of cell proliferation. In addition, the specificity of the transforming genes activated in these neoplasms further supports the role of these genes in the disease process.

Mammary Carcinoma Transforming Gene

Restriction endonuclease analysis of transforming activity of DNAs of the human mammary carcinoma cell line MCF-7 and of mouse mammary carcinomas induced by either dimethylbenzanthracene or mouse mammary tumor virus indicated that a common transforming gene was activated in these neoplasms (Lane et al, 1981). This gene is not homologous to ras^H, ras^K or other retroviral transforming genes and can be distinguished from Blym-1 and the other lymphoid neoplasm transforming genes by its pattern of sensitivity to restriction endonuclease cleavage (Lane et al, 1981).

Sera from mice bearing tumors induced by NIH cells transformed by human mammary carcinoma DNA immunoprecipitate four proteins which are specifically expressed in these transformants (Becker et al, 1982).

These proteins include two glycoproteins of 72 and 86 kd and two non-glycosylated proteins of 19 and 70 kd. Sera from mice bearing primary mammary carcinomas, or from mice bearing tumors induced by NIH cells transformed by mouse mammary carcinoma DNA, immunoprecipitate the same four proteins from NIH cells transformed by human mammary carcinoma DNA, indicating that expression of these antigens is specifically associated with expression of a transforming gene common to human and mouse mammary carcinomas.

Transforming Genes and Pathogenesis of Neoplasms

The development of neoplastic disease is classically considered a multi-step process involving a series of progressive changes, rather than a single-step conversion of a normal cell to a neoplastic cell. Thus, most neoplasms develop with long latent periods and through a series of progressive pre-neoplastic and neoplastic pathological stages. It is therefore expected that oncogenesis will involve more than simply the activation of a single transforming gene. In this regard, it should be noted that NIH 3T3 cells have been used as recipients in transfection assays because they integrate exogenous DNAs with relatively high efficiency. However, NIH 3T3 cells are not normal mouse cells: they are an established cell line with the capacity for continuous proliferation in culture and thus already appear to have undergone some of the alterations required for transformation of normal cells. If this is the case, transfection of NIH 3T3 cells might be expected to identify genes involved in relatively advanced stages of the neoplastic process whereas naturally-occurring tumorigenesis would involve additional alterations at earlier stages of disease.

Candidates for such events have been identified in both chicken and human B cell lymphomas. Induction of chicken B cell lymphomas by retroviruses involves transcriptional activation of c-myc as a consequence of adjacent integration of viral regulatory sequences (Hayward et al, 198₁). Burkitt's lymphomas are closely associated with chromosomal translocations (Klein, 1981; Rowley, 1981) which have recently been found to occur in the region of c-myc (Dalla-Favera et al, 1982; Taub et al, 1982). Since c-myc is not homologous to Blym-1 (Cooper and Neiman, 1981; Goubin et al, 1983; Diamond et al, 1983), these observations suggest that at least two distinct transforming genes are involved in pathogenesis of B cell lymphomas of both chicken and man. In addition, Burkitt's lymphoma in some regions of Africa is strongly associated with EBV infection. Infection of normal lymphocytes with EBV leads to the outgrowth of immortalized B lymphocyte cell lines which are capable of continuous growth in culture (Nilsson, 1979). Since these immortalized B cell lines are not tumorigenic in nude mice, they are thought to represent an early pre-neoplastic stage of lymphomagenesis (Nilsson, 1979). The pathogenesis of EBV-induced lymphomas may therefore involve at least three identifiable events: (1) EBV stimuation of cell proliferation, (2) activation of c-myc and (3) activation of Blym-1.

Activation of multiple transforming genes has also been observed in neoplasms other than B-cell lymphomas. Virus-induced mouse mammary carcinomas have been found to contain a transforming gene, detectable by transfection, which is not linked to viral DNA (Lane et al, 1981), as well as a candidate transforming gene whose expression is induced by regional integration of viral DNA (Nusse and Varmus, 1982). Abelson virus-induced moure pre-B-cell lymphomas contain a non-viral transforming gene detected by transfection (Lane et al, 1982a), in addition to the transforming gene (v-abl) of Abelson virus. Finally, mouse plasmacytomas also appear in some cases to involve both rearrangement of c-myc (Shen-Ong et al, 1982), and activation of a distinct transforming gene detected by transfection (Lane et al, 1982b). Although the role of these genes in carcinogenesis remains to be established, it is an attractive hypothesis that the reproducible activation of multiple transforming genes in neoplasms identifies genes which function at different stages of oncogenesis.

REFERENCES

1. Becker, D., Lane, M.-A., and Cooper, G.M. (1982): Proc. Natl. Acad. Sci. USA 79:3315-3319.

2. Capon, D.J., Seeburg, P.H., McGrath, J.P., Hayflick, J.S., Edman, U., Levinson, A.D., and Goeddel, D.V. (1983): Nature 304:507-513.

3. Chang, E.H., Furth, M.E., Scolnick, E.M., and Lowy, D.R. (1982): Nature 297:479-483.

4. Cooper, G.M. (1982): Science 217:801-806.

5. Cooper, G.M., and Neiman, P.E. (1980): Nature 287:656-659.

6. Cooper, G.M., and Neiman, P.E. (1981): Nature 292:857-858.

7. Dalla-Favera, R., Gregni, M., Erikson, J., Patterson, D., Gallo, R.C., and Croce, C.M. (1982): Proc. Natl. Acad. Sci. USA 79: 7824-7827.

8. DeFeo, D., Gonda, M.A., Young, H.A., Chang, E.H., Lowy, D.R., Scolnick, E.M., and Ellis, R.W. (1981): Proc. Natl. Acad. Sci. USA 78:3328-3332.

9. Der, C.J., and Cooper, G.M. (1983): Cell 32:201-208.

10. Der, C.J., Krontiris, T.G., and Cooper, G.M. (1982): Proc. Natl. Acad. Sci. USA 79:3637-3640.

11. Diamond, A., Cooper, G.M., Ritz, J., and Lane, M.-A. (1983): Nature, in press.

12. Ellis, R.W., DeFeo, D., Shih, T.Y., Gonda, M.A., Young, H.A., Tsuchida, N., Lowy, D.R., and Scolnick, E.M. (1981): Nature 292: 506-511.

13. Eva, A., Tronick, S.R., Gol, R.A., Pierce, J.H., and Aaronson, S.A. (1983): Proc. Natl. Acad. Sci. USA 80:4926-4930.

14. Goubin, G., Goldman, D.S., Luce, J., Neiman, P.E., and Cooper, G.M. (1983): Nature 302:114-119.

15. Hall, A., Marshall, C.J., Spurr, N.K., and Weiss, R.A. (1983): Nature 303:396-400.

16. Hayward, W.S., Neel, B.G., and Astrin, S.M. (1981): Nature 290: 475-480.

17. Klein, G. (1981): Nature 294:313-318.

18. Lane, M.-A., Sainten, A., and Cooper, G.M. (1981): Proc. Natl. Acad. Sci. USA 78:5185-5189.

19. Lane, M.-A., Neary, D., and Cooper, G.M. (1982a): Nature 300:659-661.

20. Lane, M.-A., Sainten, A., and Cooper, G.M. (1982b): Cell 28:873-880.

21. Langbeheim, H., Shih, T.Y., and Scolnick, E.M. (1980): Virology 106:292-300.

22. McCoy, M.S., Toole, J.J., Cunningham, J.M., Chang, E.H., Lowy, D. R., and Weinberg, R.A. (1983): Nature 302:79-81.

23. Murray, M.J., Cunningham, J.M., Parada, L.F., Dautry, F., Lebowitz, P., and Weinberg, R.A. (1983): Cell 33:749-757.

24. Nilsson, D.K. (1979): In: The Epstein-Barr Virus, edited by M.A. Epstein, and B.G. Achong, pp. 225-281. Springer-Verlag, New York.

25. Nusse, R., and Varmus, H.E. (1982): Cell 31:99-109.

26. Papageorge, A., Lowy, D., and Scolnick, E.M. (1982): J. Virol. 44: 509-519.

27. Parada, L.F., Tabin, C.J., Shih, C., and Weinberg, R.A. (1982): Nature 297:474-478.

28. Pulciani, S., Santos, E., Lauver, A.V., Long, L.K., Aaronson, S.A., and Barbacid, M. (1982): Nature 300:539-542.

29. Reddy, E.P., Reynolds, R.K., Santos, E., and Barbacid, M. (1982): Nature 300:149-152.

30. Rowley, J. (1982): Science 216:749-751.

31. Santos, E., Tronick, S.R., Aaronson, S.A., Pulciani, S., and Barbacid, M. (1982): Nature 298:343-347.

32. Shen-Ong, G.L.C., Keath, E.J., Piccoli, S.P., and Cole, M.D. (1982): Cell 31:443-452.

33. Shimizu, K., Birnbaum, D., Ruley, M.A., Fasano, O., Suard, Y., Edlund, L., Taparowsky, E., Goldfarb, M., and Wigler, M. (1983a): Nature 304:497-500.

34. Shimizu, K., Goldfarb, M., Perucho, M., and Wigler, M. (1983b): Proc. Natl. Acad. Sci. USA 80:383-387.

35. Shimizu, K., Goldfarb, M., Suard, Y., Perucho, M., Li, Y., Kamata, T., Feramisco, J., Stavnezer, E., Fogh, J., and Wigler, M. (1983c): Proc. Natl. Acad. Sci. USA 80:2112-2116.

36. Tabin, C.J., Bradley, S.M., Bargmann, C.I., Weinberg, R.A., Papageorge, A.G., Scolnick, E.M., Dhar, R., Lowy, D.R., and Chang, E.H. (1982): Nature 300:143-149.

37. Taub, R., Kirsch, I., Morton, C., Lenoir, G., Swarz, D., Tronick, G., Aaronson, S., and Leder, P. (1982): Proc. Natl. Acad. Sci. USA 79:7837-7841.

38. Willingham, M.C., Pastan, I., Shih, T.Y., and Scolnick, E.M. (1980): Cell 19:1005-1014.

39. Yuasa, Y., Srivastava, S.K., Dunn, C.Y., Rhim, J.S., Reddy, E.P., and Aaronson, S.A. (1983): Nature 303:775-779.

Progress in Cancer Research and Therapy,
Vol. 31, edited by F. Bresciani, et al.
Raven Press, New York © 1984.

Glucocorticoid Regulation of Gene Expression

*Gordon Ringold, *Maureen Costello, *Deborah Dobson,
**Fred Frankel, † Carol Hall, and † Frank Lee

*Department of Pharmacology, Stanford University, Stanford, California 94305;
**Department of Microbiology, University of Pennsylvania, Philadelphia,
Pennsylvania 19174; and †DNAX Research Institute, Palo Alto, California 94302

Glucocorticoids, as well as other classes of steroid hormones, appear to function via the "two-step" model originally proposed by Jensen and his colleagues (15). It is generally accepted that steroids interact with a soluble receptor protein inducing a structural alteration that increases the receptor's affinity for DNA or chromatin. This so-called "activated" form of the steroid-receptor complex accumulates within the nucleus of the cell leading to increased (and perhaps in some cases, decreased) transcription of specific genes. In this view, the primary role of the steroid is to act as an allosteric effector that unmasks a DNA-binding site on the receptor protein. The detailed molecular mechanisms by which the steroid-receptor complex stimulates transcription of specific genes are poorly understood.

We have previously documented the utility of glucocorticoid inducible mouse mammary tumor virus (MMTV) as a model system to study the mechanisms of steroid hormone action. (25,27). In this report we briefly summarize some of these studies and present a detailed account of the use of MMTV in furthering our understanding of the mechanisms by which glucocorticoids regulate gene expression.

MOUSE MAMMARY TUMOR VIRUS

As is true of all retroviruses, MMTV is an enveloped virus containing a single-stranded RNA genome (3). During infection of a cell, MMTV binds to a surface receptor, becomes internalized and the nucleoprotein core becomes enzymatically functional. Within the cytoplasm of the infected cell, a linear double-stranded DNA copy of the viral RNA is synthesized by the viral reverse transcriptase (2,22,24,26,34). Later, MMTV DNA becomes covalently linked to the host DNA where it resides as a stable Mendelian locus in the progeny of the infected cell. Once the DNA is integrated in the host cell's genome (in this state the DNA is referred to as a provirus) it is controlled in large part by the normal cellular machinery. Several species of RNA, including genomic-sized RNA for encapsidation into progeny virus and smaller RNAs for use as messenger RNAs are synthesized by cellular RNA polymerase II (12,28,30). As has been alluded to earlier, and is the major focus of our work, it is the production of these RNAs that is under glucocorticoid control. The viral life cycle is completed by assembling the appropriate RNAs into a virion precursor which buds from the cell membrane, thereby releasing an intact virus particle.

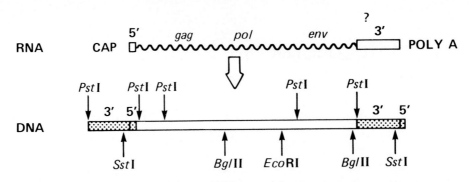

FIG. 1. The structure of the DNA and RNA forms of the MMTV genome. The RNA is approximately 9000 bases in length and encodes the genes for coat proteins or group-specific antigens (gag), envelope glycoproteins (env), reverse transcriptase (pol), and a postulated, but as yet unidentified, gene product (?). The linear form of MMTV DNA is the direct product of reverse transcription. At each end is a long terminal repeat (LTR) consisting of sequences derived from both the 5' and 3' ends of viral RNA; these are shown as the boxes denoted 3' (~ 1200 base pairs)/5' (~130 base pairs). The PstI fragment (stippled) containing the left-hand LTR plus 135 base pairs coding for RNA beyond the 5' boxed region, was used in construction of the recombinant plasmids as shown in Fig. 2.

The synthesis of retroviral DNA by reverse transcription is a fascinating and remarkably complex process (32,35). An important feature of such DNAs is that they are longer than the parental RNA; this extra length arises by duplication of sequences present at the extreme 5' and 3' ends of the viral RNA. These duplications exist at the ends of the linear viral DNA and are thus commonly referred to as the long terminal repeats or LTR's (35). In the case of MMTV DNA, the LTR's are approximately 1350 base-pairs (b.p.) in length, 130 of these arising from the 5' end (8,17,23). The structures of MMTV RNA and DNA are depicted in Fig. 1. For the purposes of this discussion, it is only of primary importance to note that the beginning (5') end of the viral RNA resides within the left-hand LTR; indeed, as will be discussed later, the promoter and the glucocorticoid regulatory region of the viral genome reside within the LTR.

Glucocorticoid Induction of MMTV

We have previously documented that induction of MMTV RNA is a primary response to the glucocorticoid-receptor complex (25,27). The evidence supporting this statement includes: 1) induction of viral RNA does not require protein synthesis; 2) the effect of the hormone is to increase the rate of synthesis of RNA within 5-15 minutes; 3) induction requires functional glucocorticoid receptors (13). Based on these findings, it seems likely that the glucocorticoid-receptor complex itself, interacting with viral DNA (and perhaps other chromosomal proteins), is sufficient to stimulate transcription at the MMTV promoter.

MMTV LTR-Fusion Plasmids

The results of our previous studies on integration and transcription of MMTV and our genetic studies provide strong circum-

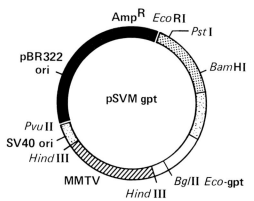

FIG. 2. Structure of the fusion plasmid containing E. coli gpt DNA linked to the MMTV LTR. The solid black segment is a 2.3 Kb fragment of the plasmid pBR322 (from the EcoRI site to the PvuII site) containing the ampicillin-resistance gene and the origin of replication. The stippled regions are derived from SV40 virus and provide signals for processing of mRNA transcripts. The hatched region represents the MMTV LTR, derived from the Pst fragment shown in Fig. 1. The open region is the Eco gpt DNA. Transcription from the MMTV promoter is in the counterclockwise direction as is the coding region for gpt. See Refs. 5 and 16 for further description of the construction of this plasmid.

stantial evidence that MMTV encodes its own glucocorticoid regulatory region. To test this directly, we first constructed hybrid genes containing the putative promoter and regulatory region from MMTV fused to the coding region for mouse dihydrofolate reductase (dhfr) (16). When such plasmids were introduced into dhfr⁻ CHO cells, mouse dhfr was produced under the control of the MMTV promoter. Moreover, addition of glucocorticoids resulted in a 5-fold stimulation of enzyme production (16).

Similar experiments have recently been performed using an analogous plasmid (Figure 2) containing the E. coli gene encoding xanthine guanine phosphoribosyl transferase (XGPRT) (5). This plasmid designated pSVMgpt was used to transform mouse 3T6 cells using the dominant selection scheme described by Mulligan and Berg (18). We have quantitated the amount of XGPRT RNA and determined that the message initiates at the known start site of MMTV transcription using the procedure of Berk and Sharp (1). The hybrid band detected by autoradiography is ~400 b.p. in length (Figure 3) indicating that the predominant 5' end of the XGPRT RNA maps to a site within the MMTV LTR, ~275 bases upstream of the XGPRT insert; this corresponds to the 3'-5' border of the LTR (i.e. the start site for MMTV transcription). Moreover, the production of this RNA is increased in dexamethasone-treated cells 5-15 fold.

As described in the dhfr and XGPRT experiments, expression of foreign genes encoded on plasmids has generally been studied in stable transformants arising either from direct selection for the functional gene or from co-transfection with another selectable marker (20). A general shortcoming of this approach is the length of time required to grow sufficient numbers of cells from individual clones for analysis. A very useful alternative is provided by experiments in which expression of plasmid genes is assayed within the first few days following DNA infection. These so-called "transient-expression assays" offer

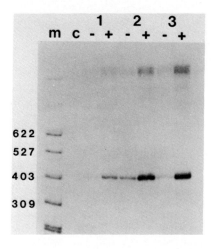

FIG. 3. Glucocorticoid induction and mapping of gpt RNA in 3T6 cells transformed with pSVM gpt. Mouse 3T6 cells were transfected with plasmid DNA using $CaPO_4$; transformants expressing gpt were selected by their ability to grow in the presence of mycophenolic acid and xanthine (18). Three such transformants were grown in the presence (48 hours) or absence of dexamethasone (10^{-6}M) and cytoplasmic RNA was isolated. Poly(A)-containing RNA was prepared by chromatography on oligo dT-cellulose and approximately 1 µg was hybridized with a probe end labeled with [^{32}P] ATP at the BglII site within the gpt gene (see Fig. 2). Hybridization was performed at 50°C for ~ 16 hours in 80% formamide according to the procedure of Berk and Sharp (1). RNA-DNA hybrids were treated with S_1 nuclease and run on a 6% acrylamide gel which was autoradiographed for 4 days. Left lane: size marker of [^{32}P] pBR322 DNA digested with Hinf I. RNA from cells grown in the absence (-) or presence (+) of dexamethasone. The band migrating at a size of ~ 410 base pairs corresponds to a gpt RNA that is initiated at the proper MMTV promoter.

not only a time advantage, but since the average level of gene expression from the transfected population is measured, the considerable variability typically observed among individual clones can be avoided.

The gene we have utilized for this series of experiments is the E. coli lac Z gene, which encodes the enzyme β-galactosidase. Quantitation of the enzyme is performed by a very simple, reproducible, and extremely sensitive colorimetric assay. The plasmid we have constructed, pCH105 (14), is again a derivative of the pSVMgpt plasmid (Figure 2) in which the XGPRT gene has been replaced by the E. coli lac Z gene obtained originally as a fusion gene product (4). A similar plasmid, pCH110, containing the SV40 promoter, rather than the MMTV promoter, was also constructed (14). As shown in Table I, when these plasmids are introduced into mouse L cells using the DEAE-dextran procedure (29), the levels of β-galactosidase detected in cell extracts three days after DNA infection was approximately the same as mock infected cells. However, when dexamethasone (10^{-6}M) was added to the transfected cells 24 hours prior to assaying the enzyme, the levels were at least 25 times above background when pCH105 was used. In contrast, β-galactosidase production from the SV40 promoter is not glucocorticoid inducible.

TABLE I.   Glucocorticoid Induction of β-galactosidase in
Transient Expression Experiments

β-galactosidase Specific Activity

Plasmid		-DEX	+DEX	Fold Induction
mock		0.67 (4)	0.95 (4)	1.4
pCH110 (SV40-	gal)	11.8 (2)	8.6 (2)	0
pCH105 (MMTV-	gal)	0.7 (4)	18.3 (4)	26

Infections with DNA were performed by incubating mouse L Tk⁻ cells with
10-20 μg plasmid in the presence of 200 μg/ml DEAE-dextran for
4 hours.   Cells were washed and then incubated for 2 days in growth
medium.   Dexamethasone (10^{-6}M) was added for 1 day and cells were
collected, pelleted, and resuspended in 0.25 M sucrose, 10 mM Tris-HCl
pH 7.4 and 10 mM EDTA.   Cells were lysed by freeze-thawing and debris
was removed by a 5 minute centrifugation in a microfuge.   β-galactosidase activity is expressed as nmoles ONPG cleaved per minute per mg
protein.

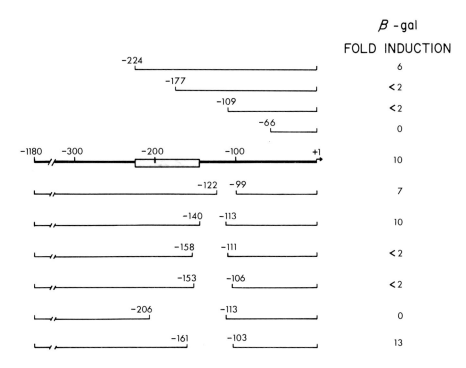

FIG. 4.   Mapping the glucocorticoid regulatory region of the MMTV
LTR by deletion analysis.   Construction of the indicated molecules was
accomplished either by removal of specific redistribution endonuclease
fragments or by digestion with Bal 31 exonuclease.   In some cases the
deletions were reconstructed so as to replace sequences between -110
and +1 as shown in the diagram.   Analysis of β-galactosidase activity
was as described in Table I.   The end points of the deletions were
determined by direct sequencing analysis of the DNA.

Deletion Mapping Studies of the MMTV LTR

The results of our gene fusion experiments clearly demonstrate that
the MMTV LTR contains a region that confers glucocorticoid responsiveness on the expression of any linked gene. To further delineate the
sequences of importance for hormonal regulation, we have constructed
deletion mutants that remove portions of the LTR in either the XGPRT
plasmid (PSVMgpt) or the β-galactosidase plasmid (pCH 105). Data
from the XGPRT deletions were obtained by RNA mapping studies in transformed 3T6 cells as described above; from the β-gal plasmids, data was
obtained using the transient expression assay. A summary of a large
set of such studies is presented in Figure 4.

The results of these experiments allow three major conclusions to
be made. The first is that one can eliminate inducible expression
without interfering with basal promoter function; moreover, the
sequences important for regulation must reside (at least in part)
upstream of nucleotide -109, since deletion of such sequences
abolishes hormonal responsiveness. Second, the left hand (upstream)
border of the glucocorticoid regulatory region must be downstream of
nucleotide -224, since plasmids in which the entire left end of the LTR
has been removed up to residue -224 respond to hormone. Third, the
right hand boundary of the regulatory region must be upstream of
nucleotide -141, since plasmids in which the sequence between -109 and
-141 is deleted retain inducibility. Deletion of the nucleotides
between -210 and -109 eliminates glucocorticoid responsiveness cor-
roborating these points. In the aggregate, these studies strongly
suggest that the major region of the MMTV LTR responsible for glucocorticoid sensitivity resides between nucleotides -210 and -141 relative to the start of transcription.

A further, and perhaps subtle, point that can be made from analysis
of some of the internal deletions is that the absolute spacing between
the promoter and regulatory region need not be constant. In fact, we
have also found that insertion of 4 nucleotides at position -109 does
not interfere with induction by dexamethasone. Since this is a minor
alteration, we are currently determining the maximum distance by which
the promoter and regulatory region can be separated by inserting
larger fragment at position -109.

A point must be made of the anomalous behavior of a deletion mutant
in which the sequence between -103 and -161 have been removed. Although we currently have no explanation for the ability of this mutant
to respond normally to hormone, we hypothesize that a fortuitous regulatory region may have been reconstructed in this molecule.

The Hormone Regulatory Region Confers Glucocorticoid
Responsiveness on a Heterologous Promoter

Analysis of a deletion mutant that removes all but 66 nucleotides
upstream of the start of MMTV transcription revealed that such a mutant
contains the DNA sequences required for appropriate basal level of
expression (7). We have recently asked whether these so-called promoter sequences can be replaced with similar regions from a non-gluco-
corticoid regulated promoter. The constructions entailed fusing a
portion of the MMTV LTR containing the regulatory region to a series of
fragments containing all or part of the SV40 early promoter region.
Results of two such constructions are depicted in Figure 5 and document
that the glucocorticoid regulatory region will indeed confer hormonal
responsiveness on a heterologous promoter. Moreover, as indicated

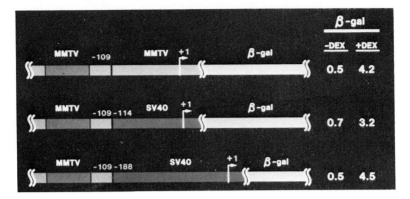

FIG. 5. Glucocorticoid induction from SV40 promoters fused to the hormone regulatory region. The sequences in the MMTV LTR upstream of residue -109 were fused to portions of the SV40 early promoter provided by M. Fromm and P. Berg (9). These molecules were then inserted into a plasmid of the type described in Fig. 2; in this case, as in Table I and Fig. 4, the gene assayed was E. coli β -galactosidase as described (14).

above, the absolute spacing between the regulatory region and the start of transcription does not need to be constant.

Induction from Extrachromosomal, Replicating Plasmids

In an attempt to assess the role of chromatin structure in glucocorticoid control of MMTV gene expression, we have constructed a derivative of the plasmid pMTVdhfr (16) containing the entire early region of Polyoma virus (Fig. 6). This plasmid, pMDPY, should therefore be able to replicate in transfected mouse cells and thus provide a source of

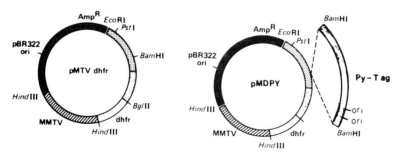

FIG. 6. Structure of the fusion plasmids pMTV dhfr and pMDPY. The basic format of these plasmids is detailed in the legend to Figure 2. The polyoma fragment used in construction of pMDPY contains a duplication of the origin of replication of polyoma virus and the entire early region of the virus. It was derived from the pSV5 vectors described by Subramani et al. (31) and was inserted at the Bam HI site of pMTV dhfr (16).

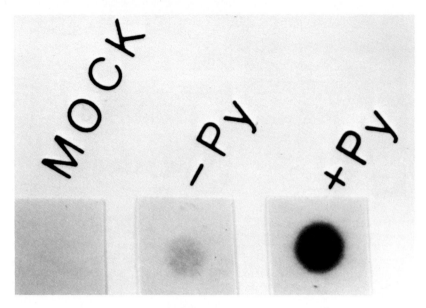

FIG. 7. Analysis of dhfr RNA produced in transfections with pMTV
dhfr and pMDPY. Mouse L cells were infected with approximately 10 µg
of the corresponding DNAs using DEAE-dextran as described (14).
Forty-eight hours later total cell RNA was harvested using guanidine
thiocyanate as described by Chirgwin et al. (6). Three µg of RNA from
each preparation were applied to a nitrocellulose filter using a "dot-
blot" matrix, baked, and hybridized with a nick-translated pMTV dhfr
probe (specific activity ~ 1 x 10^8 cpm/µg) to detect dhfr-specific
RNA.

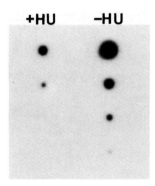

FIG. 8. Effect of hydroxyurea on production of dhfr RNA in pMDPY
infected L cells. Mouse L cells were infected with 15 µg of pMDPY DNA
using DEAE-dextran. Twelve hours after DNA infection, one half of the
cells were treated with hydroxyurea (10 µg/ml) to inhibit DNA synthesis. After an additional 48 hours, total RNA was harvested from the
infected cells. Samples of each were spotted on nitrocellulose using a
dot-blot matrix and probed with nick-translated pMTV dhfr. In each
case, 1:3 dilutions of the RNA were analyzed using 3 µg of RNA in the
most concentrated sample.

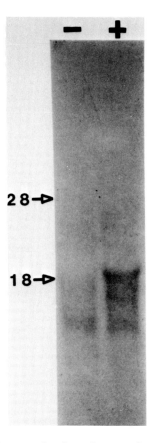

FIG. 9. Northern blot analysis of RNAs from control and glucocorticoid treated L cells transfected with pMDPY. Cells were infected with 10-20 μ g of pMDPY using DEAE-dextran. Twenty-four hours later, one half of the cells were incubated with 10^{-6} M dexamethasone. After an additional 36 hours, total cell RNA was harvested using guanidine thiocyanate and 15 μ g of each were electrophoresed on an agarose (1.5%) gel. The RNA was transferred to nitrocellulose and probed with nick-translated pMTV dhfr (sp. act. ~ 1 x 10^{-8} cpm/ μg).

minichromosomes that contain an MMTV transcription unit. Moreover, the high DNA copy number resulting from replication should increase the yield of RNA transcripts thereby facilitating the identification and characterization of gene products in transfected cells.

To test these assumptions, RNA was isolated from L cells transfected with both pMTV dhfr and pMDPY and the amount of dhfr RNA produced was determined using nick-translated pMTV dhfr. The results shown in Figure 7 clearly document that about 20 times more RNA is produced in the cells transfected with pMDPY. That this is indeed due to replication, treatment of pMDPY infected cells with hydroxyurea, an inhibitor of DNA synthesis, dramatically reduces the amount of RNA produced (Figure 8).

Despite the fact that more RNA is made in pMDPY infected L cells, we were concerned that replicating plasmids present at high copy number might not retain hormonal sensitivity. To test whether dhfr RNA is indeed glucocorticoid inducible we isolated total RNA from control and

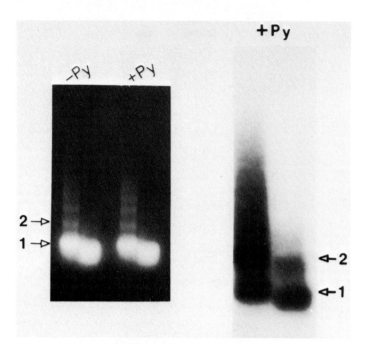

FIG. 10. Micrococcal nuclease digestion of nuclei from pMTV dhfr and pMDPY infected L cells. Forty-eight hours after infection with 15 µg of plasmid DNA, nuclei were prepared and incubated with varying amounts of micrococcal nuclease. The left panel represents the ethidium bromide stained pattern of micrococcal nuclease digested DNA electrophoresed on a 1.5% agarose gel; the characteristic pattern of nucleosome monomers and multimers is apparent. The left lane of each digest represents incubation with a low concentration of enzyme whereas the right lane represents incubation with sufficient enzyme to trim the inter-nucleosomal DNA. The gel was transferred to nitro-cellulose and probed with nick-translated pMTV dhfr. The right panel is the hybridization to the DNA from pMDPY-infected nuclei; indicated are the positions of mono and di-nucleosomes. The lanes containing DNA from pMTV dhfr transfected nuclei were barely visible after a twenty-fold longer exposure time (not shown).

dexamethasone-treated cells (after infection with pMDPY) and analyzed them by "Northern" - blot analysis (33). The results shown in Figure 9 clearly indicate the presence of a major glucocorticoid inducible RNA of approximately 2 Kb in these cells. There are also additional RNAs produced that seem to be unaffected by hormonal treatment; the origin of these dhfr-containing RNAs is unclear. Thus active replication does not interfere with glucocorticoid inducibility from unintegrated pMDPY plasmids. We presume therefore that active glucocorticoid-receptor complexes remain associated with pMDPY minichromosomes.

We have succeeded in isolating small amounts of minichromosomes by homogenizing the infected cells and sedimenting this material on glycerol gradients. Relative to a size marker of whole SV40 virions the pMDPY minichromosomes sediment at a value of approximately 150S (data not shown). Lastly, we have begun to assess the configuration of these minichromosomes using partial nuclease digestions. Figure 10 demonstrates that nuclei treated with micrococcal nuclease yield a typical nucleosome-like pattern of DNA sizes when electrophoresed on an agarose gel. When probed with pMTV dhfr it is clear that the bulk of the plasmid sequences are in the monomer and dimer region of the gel suggesting that the pMDPY DNA is in a typical chromatin-like configuration. More recent experiments (not shown) indicate that the nucleosomes may in fact be phased along the LTR region of the DNA. Future studies using these minichromosomes should allow us to investigate in detail the effects of glucocorticoid receptor interactions on the chromatin configuration of an MMTV transcription unit.

SUMMARY

We have analyzed the glucocorticoid responsive transcription of MMTV DNA using genetic and molecular techniques. The major conclusions we can draw are: 1) induction is at the transcription level and is dependent on functional glucocorticoid receptors; 2) sequences within MMTV DNA are required for hormone responsiveness; 3) at least one glucocorticoid regulatory domain resides within a 50-60 nucleotide region of the MMTV LTR. It is noteworthy that this region has been shown by other groups to contain a high affinity binding site for the glucocorticoid-receptor complex (10,11,19,21); speculations on the function of receptor binding to the regulatory region must take into account the facts that the position of these sequences need not be fixed with respect to the start of transcription and that heterologous promoters are suitable substrates for activation of transcription by this regulatory machinery. Lastly, it is clear that inducible expression of a fusion gene is retained on replicating minichromosomes. Further analysis of the changes imparted by binding of glucocorticoid-receptor complexes to such minichromosomes may shed further light on the processes involved in hormonal stimulation of transcription.

ACKNOWLEDGMENT

Dr. G. Ringold's work was supported by NIH Grant GM 25821 and a Basil O'Connor Grant from the March of Dimes.

REFERENCES

1. Berk, A. and Sharp, P. Cell 12: 721 (1977).
2. Bishop, J.M. Ann. Rev. Biochem. 47: 35 (1978).
3. Cardiff, R. and Duesberg, P. Virology 36: 696 (1968).
4. Casadaban, M. and Cohen, S. J. Mol. Biol. 138: 179 (1980).
5. Chapman, A.B., Costello, M.A., Lee, F., and Ringold, G.M. Mol. Cell Biol. 3: 1421-1429 (1983).
6. Chirgwin, J.M., Przybyla, A.E., MacDonald, R.J., and Rutter, W.J. Biochemistry 18: 5294-5299 (1979).
7. Dobson, D.E., Lee, F., and Ringold, G.M. In Gene Expression, UCLA-CETUS Symposium (Homer, D., ed.), in press.
8. Donehower, L., Huang, A., and Hager, G. J. Virol. 37: 226 (1981).
9. Fromm, M. and Berg, P. J. Mol. Appl. Genet. 1: 457 (1982).
10. Geisse, S., Scheiderist, C., Westphal, H.M., Hynes, N.E., Groner, B., and Beato, M. EMBO J. 1: 1613 (1982).
11. Govindan, M.V., Spiess, E., and Majors, Proc. Natl. Acad. Sci. 79: 5757 (1982).

12. Groner, B., Hynes, N., and Diggelman, H. J. Virol. <u>30</u>: 417 (1979).

13. Grove, J.R., Dieckmann, B., Schroer, K., and Ringold, G.M. Cell 21: 47 (1980).

14. Hall, C.V., Jacob, P.E., Ringold, G.M., and Lee, F. J. Mol. Appl. Genet. 2: 101 (1982).

15. Jensen, E.V., Suzuki, T., Kawashima, T., Strumpf, W.E., Jungblut, P.W., and DeSombre, E.R. Proc. Natl. Acad. Sci. 59: 632 (1968).

16. Lee, F., Mulligan, R., Berg, P., and Ringold, G. Nature 294: 228 (1981).

17. Majors, J. and Varmus, H. Nature 289: 253 (1981).

18. Mulligan, R. and Berg, P. Proc. Natl. Acad. Sci. 78: 2072 (1981).

19. Payvar, F., Firestone, G.L., Ress, S.R., Chandler, V.C., Wrange, O., Carlstedt-Duke, J., Gustafson, J.-A., and Yamamoto, K.R. J. Cell. Biochem. 19: 241 (1982).

20. Perucho, M., Hanahan, D., Wigler, M. Cell 22: 309 (1980).

21. Pfahl, M. Cell 31: 475 (1982).

22. Ringold, G., Cardiff, R., Varmus, H., and Yamamoto, K. Cell 10: 11 (1977).

23. Ringold, G., Shank, P., Varmus, H., Ring, J., and Yamamoto, K. Proc. Natl. Acad. Sci. 76: 665 (1979).

24. Ringold, G., Shank, P., and Yamamoto, K. J. Virol. 26: 93 (1978).

25. Ringold, G., Yamamoto, K., Bishop, J.M., and Varmus, H. Proc. Natl. Acad. Sci. 74: 2879 (1977).

26. Ringold, G., Yamamoto, K., Shank, P., and Varmus, H. Cell 10: 19 (1977).

27. Ringold, G., Yamamoto, K., Tomkins, G., Bishop, J.M., and Varmus, H. Cell 6: 299 (1975).

28. Robertson, D. and Varmus, H. J. Virol. 30: 576 (1979).

29. Sompayrac, L. and Danna, K. Proc. Natl. Acad. Sci. 78: 7575 (1981).

30. Stallcup, M., Ring, J., and Yamamoto, K. Biochemistry 17: 1515 (1978).

31. Subramani, S., Mulligan, R., and Berg, P. Molec. Cell. Biol. 1: 854 (1981).

32. Temin, H. Cell 27: 1 (1981).

33. Thomas, P.S. Proc. Natl. Acad. Sci., USA 77: 5201-5205 (1980).

34. Vaidya, A. Lasfargues, E., Henkel, G., Lasfargues, J., and Moore, D. J. Virol. 18: 911 (1976).

35. Varmus, H. Science 216: 812 (1982).

Progress in Cancer Research and Therapy,
Vol. 31, edited by F. Bresciani, et al.
Raven Press, New York © 1984.

New Steroidal and Nonsteroidal Inhibitors of Aromatase Activity

*D.A.N. Sirett, *J.I. Quivy, *C. Rolin Jacquemyns, **Y. Ding, **B. Nassim, **P. Crabbé, and *G.G. Rousseau

*Hormone and Metabolic Research Unit, International Institute of Cellular and Molecular Pathology, B-1200 Brussels, Belgium; and **Department of Chemistry, University of Missouri, Columbia, Missouri 65211*

While investigating the effects of synthetic dicyclohexane steroid analogues on aspects of the male reproductive system, we noted that some of the compounds were capable of inhibiting the aromatization of testosterone to estradiol-17β, both in primary culture of Sertoli cells from immature rats and in a microsome preparation from human placenta (15). Inhibitors of aromatase activity are of interest to us in our own work, but may be of more significant importance in the treatment of estrogen-dependent tumours. Brodie et al. (1,2) have demonstrated that the potent aromatase inhibitor 4-hydroxy-4-androstene-3,17-dione (4-OHA) is able to promote the regression of dimethylbenz(a)anthracene-induced estrogen-dependent breast tumours in rats in vivo. We have carried out further experiments to examine the nature of the inhibition of aromatase by the dicyclohexane compounds, and have also tested some novel A-nor and A-hetero steroid derivatives for aromatase inhibition.

MATERIALS AND METHODS
Chemicals

$[1,2,6,7-^{3}H]$Testosterone, $[4-^{14}C]$estradiol-17β and $[4-^{14}C]$estrone were obtained from Amersham International PLC. Testosterone, androstenedione, estradiol-17β, estrone, diethylstilbestrol (DES) and meso-hexestrol (HEX) were supplied by Sigma, and 1,4,6-androstatriene-3,17-dione (ATD) by Steraloids. Glucose-6-phosphate, NADP and glucose-6-phosphate dehydrogenase were from Boehringer Mannheim. Precoated plates for thin-layer chromatography (TLC; silica gel 60_{F254} on plastic sheet) were obtained from Merck. Solvents were analytical grade, from Carlo Erba, UCB, and Merck.

The syntheses of the dicyclohexane compounds used in this study have been described previously (4,15). The syntheses of the A-nor and A-hetero steroids will be published elsewhere (5,7,8).

Preparation of Human Placental Microsome Fraction

This preparation is based on the method of Ryan (12). Tissue from human full-term placenta was homogenized (Waring Blendor, 1 min) in 1 vol 0.05 M sodium phosphate buffer, pH 7.6, containing 0.25 M sucrose and 0.04 M nicotinamide. The homogenate was centrifuged at 15000 rpm (gmax = 20,400) for 20 min in a Beckman 50 Ti rotor. The supernatant was decanted

and retained. The pellet was resuspended in buffer, and the centrifugation was repeated. The pooled supernatants were centrifuged at 50000 rpm
(gmax = 226,400) for 25 min in the same rotor. The supernatant was
discarded, and the pellet was washed twice by resuspension in buffer and
centrifugation. The final pellet was resuspended in a small volume of
buffer, treated briefly with a teflon-glass homogenizer to ensure full
dispersion, and divided into aliquots (250 µl) for storage at -80° C.
Protein concentration of this suspension was 35 mg/ml.

Measurement of Aromatase Activity

This procedure was based on the incubation of tritiated testosterone
with placental microsome fraction in the presence of an NADPH-generating
system. After extraction into organic solvent, the products were
separated from the substrate by thin layer chromatography. Appropriate
regions of the TLC plate were removed for quantitation of radioactivity.
Product recovery was monitored by the addition of [14C]estrogens to the
incubation mixtures prior to extraction. No correction was made for the
loss of 1β- and 2β-^{3}H during the reaction.

Single substrate concentration assay for screening of potential inhibitors.

Each incubation mixture contained 0.05 µCi or 0.1 µCi [^{3}H]testosterone,
0.5 µM testosterone, 10 µM test compound, 5 U glucose-6-phosphate
dehydrogenase, 1 mM NADP and 10 mM glucose-6-phosphate in 0.05 mM sodium
phosphate buffer, pH 7.6, in a final volume of 0.5 ml. Reaction was
initiated by the addition of the enzyme (15 or 20 µg microsomal protein),
and continued at 37° C for 40 or 45 min. The incubation was terminated
by chilling the tubes in ice-water.[14C]estradiol-17β and [14C]estrone
(each approximately 10000 dpm in 10 µl ethanol) were added to each tube.
The contents of each tube were extracted with 3 ml cyclohexane: ethyl
acetate 1:1 (v/v) (16), vortexing 2 x 30 s. Following centrifugation for
5 min at 3000 rpm (gmax = 800), the aqueous phase was frozen by immersing
the tubes to the interface in an acetone-dry ice freezing mixture; the
organic phase was decanted and evaporated under nitrogen. Residues were
transferred, in 20 µl ethyl acetate containing 5 µg each of estradiol-17β
and estrone, to TLC plates, which were developed (2 x 15 cm) in diethyl
ether: n-hexane 3:1 (v/v). Carrier steroids were located by I$_2$ vapour;
the corresponding areas of the plates were cut out, and placed in vials
with scintillation fluid. All vials were counted for 10 min at channel
settings suitable for double-labelled (^{3}H, ^{14}C) samples. The amounts of
estradiol-17β and estrone formed were calculated using the specific
activity of the substrate and the [14C]estrogen recovery values, and the
results expressed in pmoles.

Characterization of aromatase inhibition.

The procedure used was similar to that described in the previous
section. Five or six different concentrations of nonradioactive testosterone in the range 0.025 - 0.5 µM, and a single concentration of test
compound, chosen with reference to the degree of inhibition of aromatase
activity demonstrated in the single substrate concentration assay, were
incubated in duplicate in the same reaction medium at 37° C for 7.5 min.
The rate of aromatization was calculated as the sum of estradiol-17β and
estrone formation, expressed in pmol per mg of protein per min. Results
were examined using double reciprocal plots; unweighted linear regression
analysis was used to determine values for Km in the presence and absence

of test compound, facilitating the calculation of an estimated Ki value for the latter.

RESULTS

Preliminary experiments showed that both estrone and estradiol-17β were formed from testosterone as substrate, indicating that the microsomal preparation used in this study contained 17β -hydroxysteroid dehydrogenase activity as well as aromatase. No other metabolites were detected following extraction and separation as described. After extended incubation in the absence of NADP as substrate for the NADPH-generating system, a small amount of estrone (less than 1 % conversion of the substrate) was the only metabolite detected. The amount of estrogen formed was related linearly to the amount of microsomal protein in the incubation mixture, up to the point where substrate depletion became apparent during the incubation time used. The initial rate of reaction was constant for at least 10 min, with a slightly lower rate being maintained for a further 35 min. The Km for testosterone in our system was 0.103 ± 0.008 μM (mean $\pm$ S.E.M., n = 29), and the Vmax for aromatization was within the range 100–300 pmol per mg of protein per min.

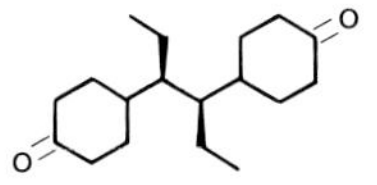

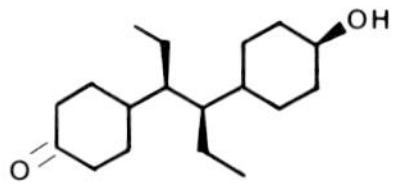

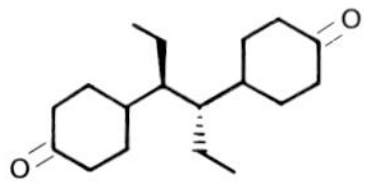

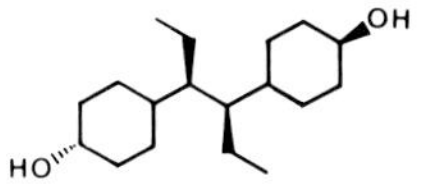

FIG. 1. Dicyclohexane derivatives tested for the inhibition of aromatase. PRDX: d,l-3,4-bis(4-oxocyclohexyl)-hexane; PRXL: d,l-3-(4-oxocyclohexyl)-4-(cis-4-hydroxycyclohexyl)-hexane; PMDX: meso-3,4-bis(4-oxocyclohexyl)-hexane; PRCL: d,l-3-(cis-4-hydroxycyclohexyl)-4-(trans-4-hydroxycyclo-hexyl)-hexane; PRTL: d,l-3,4-bis(trans-4-hydroxycyclohexyl)-hexane.

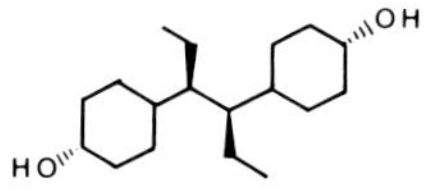

Effect of Dicyclohexane Derivatives on Aromatase Activity

The compounds used in this study are illustrated in Fig. 1. Each compound, with the exception of PRCL, was tested for its ability, at a concentration of $10\,\mu M$, to inhibit the aromatization of testosterone, at a concentration of $0.5\,\mu M$, by human placental microsomes. Extended incubation times were used, giving 20-25 % conversion of the substrate in the absence of test compound. Results are given in Table 1; also included are data for DES and HEX, the starting compounds for the synthesis of the dicyclohexane derivatives, and ATD, a steroid known to be a potent inhibitor of aromatase activity (13).

TABLE 1. <u>Inhibition by dicyclohexane derivatives of the aromatization of testosterone</u>

Compounds	Aromatase activity [a] (% of control)	Ki [b] (μM)
PRDX	48	0.60 ± 0.12 (6)
PMDX	61	0.99 ± 0.26 (4)
PRXL	66	1.08 ± 0.29 (4)
PRCL	n.d.	5.00 ± 1.96 (6)
PRTL	93	9.12 ± 2.10 (3)
DES	96, 94	n.d.
HEX	91, 93	n.d.
ATD	8, 5	n.d.

[a] Activity in presence of $10\,\mu M$ test compound as percentage of activity in absence of test compound. 40 min incubation at 37° C.
[b] Incubation for 7.5 min at 37° C. Results are given as means $\pm$ S.E.M. (number of experiments).
n.d. = not determined.

The inhibitory capacity of ATD was confirmed, and three of the dicyclohexane compounds inhibited aromatase activity to a significant extent. In these conditions PRTL, DES and HEX showed little or no ability to inhibit the enzyme.

Subsequent experiments were carried out to elucidate the type of inhibition involved, using a range of substrate concentrations in the presence and absence of test compound at a single concentration chosen with reference to the results in Table 1. A short incubation time was used in order to approximate initial rate conditions. Data were examined using double reciprocal plots; an example is given in Fig. 2., showing inhibition by PRDX. For all five dicyclohexane derivatives tested inhibition was competitive; Ki values are summarized in Table 1.

Effect of A-Modified Steroid Derivatives on Aromatase Activity

A selection of novel A-nor and A-hetero estrene derivatives was examined using the same approach as for the dicyclohexane derivatives. These compounds are illustrated in Fig. 3. The preliminary screening at a single substrate concentration revealed a wide range of ability to inhibit aromatase activity (Table 2).

Some compounds which displayed a significant capability for inhibition in this type of experiment were examined further, and shown to be competitive inhibitors; an example, compound III, is given in Fig. 4. Ki values are summarized in Table 2.

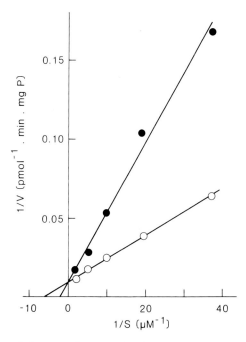

FIG. 2. Inhibition of human placental microsome aromatase activity by
PRDX. o–o, no inhibitor; o–o, with PRDX (1.6 μM). Points are mean values
for duplicate incubations. Lines are the result of simple linear
regression using the individual data points. In this experiment, Km
(testosterone) = 0.15 μM; Ki (PRDX) = 0.89 μM.

DISCUSSION

The dicyclohexane derivatives examined in this study have been shown
to be capable of competitive inhibition of human placental microsome
aromatase activity. We have not yet investigated whether they also lead
to a time-dependent inactivation of the enzyme, as has been reported for
4-OHA (1) and ATD (3). The most potent inhibitor, PRDX, has an affinity
for the enzyme about six-fold lower than that of the substrate testosterone; it is thus a much weaker inhibitor than some known steroidal
aromatase inhibitors such as ATD, which in our hands has a Ki value of
about 0.02 μM (14). However, PRDX lacks almost completely the ability to
bind to receptors for androgens (11), estrogens (9) and glucocorticoids
(9); it may therefore be possible to use this compound at sufficiently
high doses to be effective in inhibiting peripheral aromatase activity _in
vivo_ without provoking serious endocrine effects. Comparison with the
other dicyclohexane derivatives suggests that the substitution of hydroxyl groups for the ketone groups leads to a reduction in the potency of
inhibition. This parallels the situation observed with the natural
substrates, in which androstenedione is a more effective substrate
(having a lower Km value) than testosterone (6,10). The _meso_ configuration of PMDX appears to reduce the potency of inhibition slightly by
comparison with the racemic mixture PRDX, but, as the difference is small
and only one _meso_ derivative has been studied, no general conclusion can
be drawn on this effect.

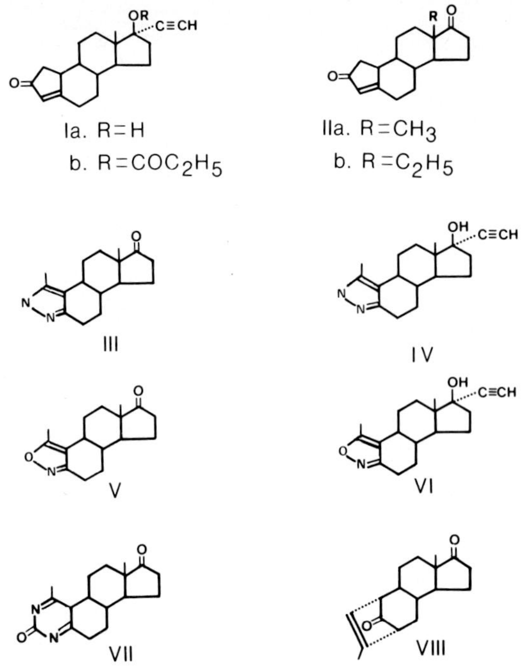

FIG. 3. A-nor and A-hetero estrene derivatives tested for the inhibition of aromatase. Ia: (-)-17 -ethynyl-17 -hydroxy-4-norestr-3(5)-ene-2-one; Ib: (-)-17 -ethynyl-17 -hydroxy-4-norestr-3(5)-ene-2-one proprianate; IIa: (+)-4-norestr-3(5)-ene-2,17-dione; IIb: (-)-4-nor-18-homo-estr-3(5)-ene-2,17-dione; III: 4-nor-1-methyl-2,3-diaza-estr-1(10),3(5)-dien-17-one; IV: 4-nor-1-methyl-2,3-diaza-17 -ethynyl-estr-1(10),3(5)-dien-17-ol; V: 4-nor-1-methyl-2-oxa-3-aza-estr-1(10),3(5)-dien-17-one; VI: 4-nor-1-methyl- 2-oxa-3-aza-17 -ethynyl-estr-1(10),3(5)-dien-17 -ol; VII: 1-methyl-2,4-diaza-estr-1,4-dien-3,17-dione; VIII: 4-nor-A-seco-2-methyl-2,6 -cyclo-estr-1(2)-ene-5,17-dione.

TABLE 2. Inhibition by A-modified steroid derivatives of the aromatisation of testosterone

Compound	Aromatase Activity[a] (% of control)	Ki[b] (μM)
Ia	98	n.d.
Ib	87	n.d.
IIa	89	n.d.
IIb	83	4.05 + 0.92 (3)
III	36, 34	0.20 + 0.07 (5)
IV	94	n.d.
V	51, 53	1.07 + 0.39 (4)
VI	76, 81	4.16 (2)
VII	82	n.d.
VIII	7	0.08 + 0.03 (4)

[a] Activity in the presence of 10 μM test compound as a percentage of activity in the absence of test compound. 45 min incubation at 37° C.
[b] Incubation for 7.5 min at 37° C. Results are given as means + S.E.M. (number of experiments); n.d. = not determined.

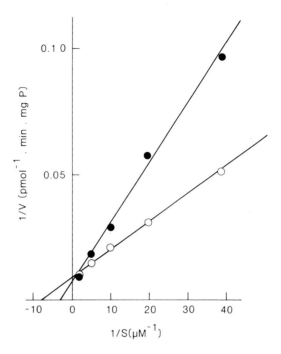

FIG. 4. Inhibition of human placental microsome aromatase activity by compound III (FIG. 3). o-o, no inhibitor; o-o, with III (0.72 µM). Points are mean values for duplicate incubations. Lines are derived by simple linear regression using the individual data points. In this experiment, Km (testosterone) = 0.13 µ M; Ki (III) = 0.42 µ M.

Two members of the series of steroids with modifications of ring A demonstrated particularly effective inhibition of aromatase activity. Compound III, with a five-membered ring A including two nitrogen atoms, has a Ki value only two-fold greater than the Km for testosterone. Compound VIII, however, was the most potent aromatase inhibitor in this series, perhaps surprisingly when its probable conformation is compared to the near-planar structure of other potent inhibitors such as ATD. Compound VIII is only about five-fold less potent than ATD in the placental microsome system. Both III and VIII have very low affinity for androgen and glucocorticoid receptors (9), but have not yet been tested for association with estrogen receptor.

None of the compounds examined in this study has yet been tested for its ability to reduce the aromatization of androgens in vivo. Nevertheless, the results of experiments in vitro reported here may provide a basis for the design and synthesis of a wider repertoire of effective aromatase inhibitors for therapeutic use.

ACKNOWLEDGEMENTS

We are grateful for support by the Ford, Mellon and Rockefeller Foundations (grant n° 820-0444), and by the World Health Organisation Special Programme for Research in Human Reproduction. We thank Mrs Th. Lambert for secretarial help.

REFERENCES

1. Brodie, A.M.H., Garrett, W.M., Hendrickson, J.R., Tsai-Morris, C.-H., Marcotte, P.A. and Robinson, C.H. (1981): Steroids, 38:693-702.
2. Brodie, A.M.H., Schwarzel, W.C., Shaikh, A.A. and Brodie, H.J. (1977): Endocrinology, 100:1684-1695.
3. Covey, D.F. and Hood, W.F. (1981): Endocrinology, 108:1597-1599.
4. Devis, R. and Bui, X.H. (1979): Bull. Soc. Chim. Fr., 2:1-8.
5. Ding, Y., Nassim, B. and Crabbé, P. (1983): J. Chem. Soc. (Perkin Transcations I), in press.
6. Gibb, W. and Lavoie, J.C. (1980): Steroids, 36:507-519.
7. Li, Y., Nassim, B. and Crabbé, P. (1983): J. Chem. Soc. (Perkin Transactions I), in press.
8. Nassim, B., Schlemper, E.O. and Crabbé, P. (1983): J. Chem. Soc. (Perkin Transactions I), in press.
9. Quivy, J., unpublished observations.
10. Reed, K.C. and Ohno, S. (1976): J. Biol. Chem., 251:1625-1631.
11. Rousseau, G.G., Quivy, J.I., Kirchhoff, J., Bui, X.H. and Devis, R. (1980): Nature, 284:458-459.
12. Ryan, K.J. (1959): J. Biol. Chem., 234: 268-272.
13. Schwarzel, W.C., Kruggel, W. and Brodie, H.J. (1973): Endocrinology, 92:866-880.
14. Sirett, D.A.N., unpublished observations.
15. Verhoeven, G., Cailleau, J., Quivy, J.I. and Rousseau, G.G. (1983): J. Steroid Biochem., 18:127-133.
16. Verhoeven, G., Dierickx, P. and De Moor, P. (1979): Mol. Cell. Endocrinol., 13:241-253.

Progress in Cancer Research and Therapy,
Vol. 31, edited by F. Bresciani, et al.
Raven Press, New York © 1984.

A Rational Approach to the Design of Anti-Estrogens: The Case of Hydroxylated Triphenylethylene Derivatives

*M. Pons, *F. Michel, *E. Bignon, *A. Crastes de Paulet,
**J. Gilbert, **J.F. Miquel, † G. Precigoux, † M. Hospital,
‡ T. Ojasoo, and ‡ J.P. Raynaud

*INSERM U. 58, 34100 Montpellier; **CERCOA-CNRS, 94320 Thiais; † CNRS,
University Bordeaux I, 33405 Talence; and ‡ ROUSSEL-UCLAF,
75007 Paris, France*

The estrogenic and anti-estrogenic activities of several triphenyl-ethylene (TPE) derivatives have been widely reported (for reviews see 1, 36,37). These compounds are reputed to compete for estradiol binding to the estrogen receptor (ER). The presence of a p-hydroxy group, as in monohydroxy tamoxifen, enhances this binding but also the anti-estrogen activity (2-4,7,15,19-21,25,26,31,32) in which the alkylaminoethoxy side-chain has been suggested to play an important role (23). Moreover, this side-chain is essential (29) in binding to the "anti-estrogen" specific binding sites recently described in estrogen target organs (14,17,22,38, 39), non-target organs (24,35) and in an ER-free cell-line (33).

In order to optimize the biological activity of these molecules and to obtain pure agonists or pure antagonists, we have undertaken a systematic study to determine the nature and localisation of the substituents on the phenyl rings responsible for biological activity. This paper describes the first results of studies on structure-affinity and structure-activity relationships performed on a series of mono-, di- and tri-hydroxylated 2,3,3-triphenyl-acrylonitriles with the general formula shown in Fig. 1A. Affinities of some derivatives of the diphenylethylene series (Fig. 1 B & C) were also measured for comparison.

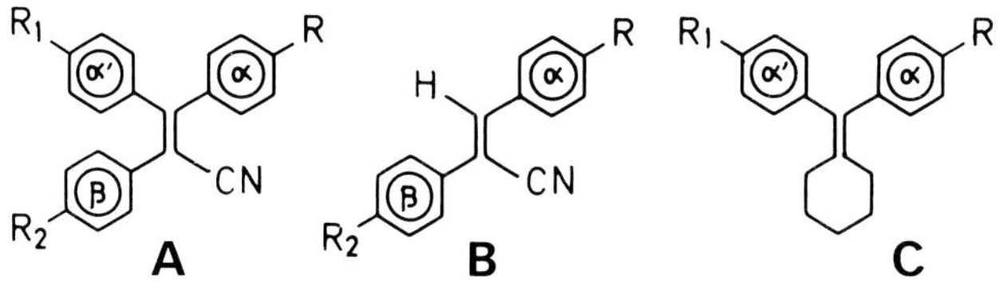

FIG. 1. General chemical structures. (A) 2,3,3-Triphenyl-acrylonitriles : α, α' and β correspond to the three phenyl rings substituted in positions R, R_1, or R_2 by H and/or OH. (B) 2,3-Diphenyl-acrylonitriles hydroxylated in R or R_2. (C) Cyclofenil (R = R_1 = OAc) or deacetylated cyclofenil (R = R_1 = OH).

It has been suggested that the variations in biological activity of derivatives of this type in different species might be due to differences in their kinetics and metabolism. In order to determine whether differences could arise from the interaction with the receptor, we compared affinities in two species, the rat and the mouse, known to have differing sensitivities to estrogen. In a first series of experiments, biological activity was assayed on an in vitro system, MCF_7 cells, minimizing metabolic activity. A significant and reproducible estrogen-specific endpoint, the induction of progesterone receptor (PR), was chosen.

EXPERIMENTAL METHODS

The triphenyl-acrylonitrile derivatives were synthetized as previously described (28,30).

The competition experiments against 5 nM tritiated estradiol (CEA, 50 Ci/mmole) for the cytosolic estrogen receptor were performed at 0°C for 2 hr and 25°C for 5 hr with increasing competitor concentrations. The 180 000 g, 1 hr cytosol from immature rat or mouse uterus was prepared in 10 mM Tris buffer pH 7.4 containing 10 mM sodium molybdate and 0.25 M sucrose. The free radioactive estradiol was removed by a dextran-coated charcoal (DCC) adsorption technique. Relative binding affinities (RBAs) deduced from the competition curves are the geometrical means of several determinations.

The competition experiments for the "anti-estrogen" specific binding site were performed according to Sudo et al. (35). The 12 000 g immature rat kidney supernatant was preincubated for 30 min at 0°C with 10^{-6}M estradiol, then incubated for 2 hr at 0°C with 1.5 nM tritiated tamoxifen (NEN, 81 Ci/mmole) in the presence of increasing concentrations of competitor. Specific binding was measured by the DCC technique and RBAs were calculated from the competition curves as above.

Progesterone receptor (PR) induction in the MCF_7 cell-line was assayed according to Eckert and Katzenellenbogen (13). Cells were grown for four days in T 75 flasks in MEM (F17 Gibco) supplemented with 1 % non-essential amino-acids, 10^{-9}M insulin, 2 mM glutamine, penicillin 100 units/ml, streptomycin 100 µg/ml and 5 % charcoal-treated fetal calf serum. The medium was replaced by fresh medium on day 2. The cells were then incubated for 5 days in the same supplemented medium containing 10^{-10}, 10^{-9} or 10^{-8}M estradiol or test-compound ; the estradiol and the test-compounds were added in ethanol (final concentration 0.1 %). The medium was renewed every 2 days. For the assays, the cells from three T 75 flasks were suspended by a 15 min incubation at 37°C in 2 mM EDTA containing PBS. After a 800 g centrifugation the cell pellets were resuspended in buffer (10 mM Tris pH 7.4, 2 mM EDTA, 1 mM DTT), then sonicated. Cytosols were obtained by centrifugation at 180 000 g for 30 min. These cytosols containing 10 % glycerol were used immediately or stored at −70°C until assay (within 3 days). The PR level was given by the specific binding after 4 hr incubation at 0°C of 10^{-8}M $[6,7^3H]$-promegestone (Roussel-Uclaf, 50 Ci/mmole) measured in the presence or in the absence of 10^{-5}M unlabelled promegestone. The values are the means of 4 independent determinations (two experiments in duplicate).

Protein assay was performed by the Lowry method (27). The DNA content was determined according to Burton (5).

STRUCTURE OF THE TRIPHENYL-ACRYLONITRILE DERIVATIVES

The structure of eight molecules of the TPE series, including tamoxifen, enclomiphene and broparestrol, have been analyzed by X-ray crystal-
lography (16) to determine the spatial orientation of the three phenyl
rings and the absolute configuration of the Z and E isomers. The angles
($\hat{\alpha}$, $\hat{\alpha}'$ and $\hat{\beta}$) between the phenyl rings and the plane of the central
double bond lie in the 40° to 64° range (Fig. 2A). These molecules thus
look like a propeller with a shaft perpendicular to the plane in the middle of the central double bond.

To establish whether this configuration in the solid state corresponds
to the intrinsically most stable conformation of the molecule, molecular
energy calculations on the unsubstituted molecule were performed by the
Script program (8) (Fig. 2B). Values of 51.1°, 51.1° and 49.7° were re-
corded for the $\hat{\alpha}$, $\hat{\alpha}'$ and $\hat{\beta}$ angles, respectively. These values are close to
the mean values obtained by X-ray analysis of substituted compounds (16)
and correspond to the same propeller shape conformation.

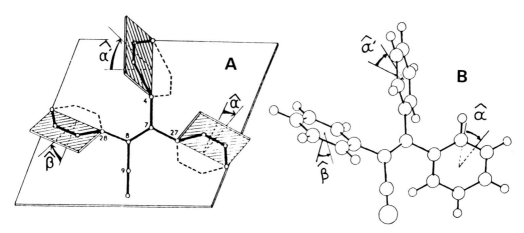

FIG. 2. Propeller-like configuration of TPEs drawn from crystallographic
data (A) and by the Script program (B). $\hat{\alpha}$, $\hat{\alpha}'$ and $\hat{\beta}$ are the angles between the phenyl rings and the plane of the central double bond.

In solution, the phenyl rings can rotate around the bond linking them
to the double bond to give two equally stable but inseparable atropo-
isomers (the orientations of the rings are symmetrical with reference to
the plane of the central double bond). Possibly only one atropo-isomer is
active.

AFFINITY FOR THE ESTROGEN RECEPTOR

Mouse Uterus Cytosol

The unsubstituted compound I had no affinity for the estrogen receptor
(ER) (Table 1), whereas the monohydroxylated derivative with the hydroxy
group in position R (II Z) had a relative binding affinity (RBA) at 0°C
as high as estradiol. It is worth noting that the poor competitor tamoxifen Z can be hydroxylated in this position in vivo to give high affinity 4-hydroxy tamoxifen Z. Similarly II E, with a hydroxyl group in

position R_1 and an almost 10 times lower RBA than II Z, is comparable to 4-hydroxy tamoxifen E with regard to the position of the OH-group and the RBA value.

TABLE 1. Relative binding affinities (RBA) for the estrogen receptor of mouse uterus cytosol

STRUCTURE	COMPOUNDS	R	R_1	R_2	RBA 0°C 2 H	RBA 25°C 5 H
	I	H	H	H	<0.1	<0.1
	II Z	OH	H	H	100	65
	II E	H	OH	H	7	14
	III	H	H	OH	5	3
	IV	OH	OH	H	100	470
	V Z	OH	H	OH	75	200
	V E	H	OH	OH	21	37
	VI	OH	OH	OH	57	200
	VII	OH	–	H	0.1	0.1
	III	H	–	OH	0.1	0.1
	CYCLOFENIL	OAc	OAc	–	3.7	0.7
	DEACETYLATED CYCLOFENIL	OH	OH	–	11	10
	TAM[a] TRANS(Z)	H	X[b]	H	1.0	0.4
	TAM CIS (E)	X[b]	H	H	0.05	0.06
	4-OH-TAM TRANS(Z)	OH	X[b]	H	25.6	47
	4-OH-TAM CIS (E)	X[b]	OH	H	1.7	9

[a] TAM : TAMOXIFEN   [b] $X = O-CH_2-CH_2-N(Me)_2$

The RBAs of the three dihydroxylated compounds IV, V Z and V E were relatively high at 0°C and even higher at 25°C. IV and V Z with a hydroxyl group in position R were better ligands than V E. The higher RBAs recorded at 25°C compared to 0°C suggest that the presence of two hydroxyl groups is important for the stability of the complex formed with the receptor. Another dihydroxylated compound, deacetylated cyclofenil, had a relatively high RBA (10 %) compared to the parent compound, cyclofenil, with no free hydroxyl groups.

The trihydroxylated compound VI also had a fairly high RBA for ER and formed a stable complex as shown by the increased RBA at 25°C.

The RBAs of two derivatives of the 2,3-diphenyl-acrylonitrile series were also measured : 3-(hydroxyphenyl)-2-phenyl-acrylonitrile (VII) and 2-(hydroxyphenyl)-3-phenyl-acrylonitrile (VIII). Neither compound has an α'-phenyl ring and the hydroxy groups are in positions R and R_2 for VII and VIII respectively. Neither had any appreciable affinity (0.1) for ER.

On the basis of the above data on p-substituted TPEs the following conclusions can be drawn : high affinities are obtained only when position R is hydroxylated. The α-phenol ring thus plays a critical role and might interact with a subsite (S_1) of the receptor as illustrated in Fig.3. Since 3-methoxy or deoxy estradiol have lower affinity for ER than 17 β -methoxy or deoxy derivatives (6,18), it can be reasonably assumed, as suggested by others (9-12), that the α-phenol ring of TPEs takes the place of the estradiol A ring in the receptor site.

Interaction with this S_1 subsite is not sufficient to induce high affinity or a stable complex. A comparison of the RBAs of II Z and VII emphasizes the importance of the α'-phenyl ring which might need to interact with another subsite (S_2) of the receptor. Subsite S_2 interacts even better with an α'-phenol ring as shown by the high RBA of compound IV which is the best competitor of the series. Superimposition of the TPEs and estradiol (Fig. 3) indicates that this subsite could be in the vicinity of the C-11 or C-7,8 atoms of estradiol.

Furthermore, a striking difference in RBA (470 vs 10 at 25°C) was noted when comparing compound IV and deacetylated cyclofenil, compounds with α , α'-phenol rings. Thus the β-phenyl ring might contribute towards the affinity of IV for ER and to complex stability. This contribution can be materialized by a third subsite (S_3) which could interact either with a phenyl ring (compound IV) or, better still, with a phenol ring (compare the pairs I-III, II Z-V Z, II E-V E).

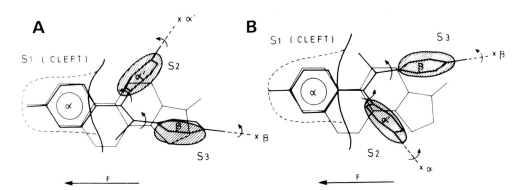

FIG. 3. Model for the binding of TPEs to the estrogen receptor site and superposition of estradiol and TPEs (superposition of estradiol A-ring and TPE α-phenol ring). In both superpositions ("A" and "B"), the phenol rings interact with subsite S_1. "A" differs from "B" by a 180° rotation around the bond linking the α-phenyl ring to the central double bond. In "A", the α'-phenyl ring is close to position C-11 of estradiol, in "B", close to positions C-7,8.

The following model could take account both of the hydrogen bonding of the phenol rings and the hydrophobic interactions of the phenyl rings. Since binding of the α-phenol ring with the receptor is probably at the origin of the high affinity of the α-p-hydroxylated derivatives we suggest that these TPEs enter the binding site along F (Fig. 3). In so doing, the α-phenol ring sinks deeply into the cleft of the S_1 subsite to form a strong interaction, while the α' and β rings which can rotate to some extent around their $x_{\alpha'}$ and x_{β} axes, interact with subsites S_2 and S_3 and confer to the molecule an affinity similar to that of estradiol. The overall conformation of the receptor binding site may, however, be different when complexed with TPEs which, like a wedge, keep the site wide open than with estradiol or diethylstilbestrol which are flatter molecules. This could explain differences in the physicochemical and biological properties of the complexes.

The flexibility of the receptor protein may furthermore enable TPEs without an α-phenol ring to rotate within the binding site. Another phenol ring (α' or β) might then interact with the main site of anchorage, the S_1 subsite. This interaction could explain, at least in part, the low but not zero affinity of compounds such as II E and III.

Rat Uterus Cytosol

The RBAs of these test-compounds, for the estrogen receptor of rat uterus cytosol were also measured and paralleled those for mouse uterus receptor (30). Plotting the logs of the RBAs recorded at 25°C for the rat versus those for the mouse gave a straight line with a coefficient of correlation of 0.92 (Fig. 4) and a slope of 1 indicating that there is a linear relationship between RBAs in these species. According to the intercept on the ordinate, the RBA for mouse receptor was about twice that for rat receptor, suggesting that it is easier for the TPEs to prise open the estrogen binding site in the mouse than in the rat.

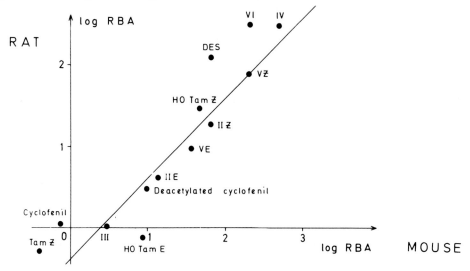

FIG. 4. Correlation between relative binding affinities of TPEs for the estrogen receptor at 25°C in mouse and rat uterus cytosol (y = − 0.3 + x, r = 0.92).

AFFINITY FOR THE ANTI-ESTROGEN BINDING SITE

TPEs with an alkyl-aminoether side-chain can bind to an "anti-estrogen" binding site (AEBS) in several tissues of the rat (35) and human (24,33). None of our test-compounds (I-VI) ever showed more than 20% competition for $[^3H]$-tamoxifen in 12 000 g supernatant from rat kidney at the concentrations used (2.5 10^{-6}M and 10^{-5}M). Cyclofenil and deacetylated cyclofenil did not compete either, whereas tamoxifen E and 4-hydroxy-tamoxifens E and Z competed with RBAs of 76, 32 and 25 respectively compared to tamoxifen Z (RBA = 100). These results for reference compounds are in agreement with those recorded by Sudo et al. (35) in immature rat uterus cytosol.

BIOLOGICAL ACTIVITY OF TPEs : PR INDUCTION IN THE MCF$_7$ CELL-LINE

All the test-compounds induced progesterone receptor (PR) in the MCF$_7$ cell-line at concentrations below 10^{-8}M (Fig. 5). The best ligand, compound IV, was also the best inducer and the least effective ligand, compound III, the least effective inducer. Similar results were obtained if the specific induction was calculated on the basis of DNA content (data not shown).

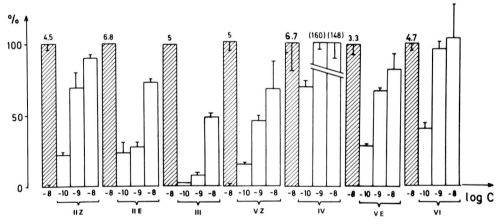

FIG. 5. Progesterone receptor (PR) induction in the MCF$_7$ cell-line expressed as a percentage of the specific induction per mg of protein obtained with 10^{-8}M estradiol (hatched column = 100%). In all these experiments, the basal level of PR induction was in the range 50-100 fmoles/mg protein. The number above the columns corresponds to the induction factor obtained in each experiment with 10^{-8}M estradiol.

To discover whether the PR inducer effect in MCF$_7$ cells was correlated with RBAs for mouse uterus ER, we plotted the log C_{50} for induction versus the log of the inverse of the RBA (Fig. 6). These C_{50} values corresponding to an induction equal to 50% of the maximum induction given by 10^{-8}M estradiol were obtained by interpolation of the experimental values in Fig. 5. For RBAs at 25°C, six of the seven tested compounds fell on a straight line of slope close to 1 suggesting that

these RBAs correspond to functional ER complexes. The correlation disappears for RBA values measured after only 2 hr at 0°C since these may not
reflect the RBA of a compound in a functional receptor complex, but rather the relative formation rate of this complex. The out-of-line position of compound V Z suggests that this compound might undergo isomerisation during incubation to the lower affinity compound V E.

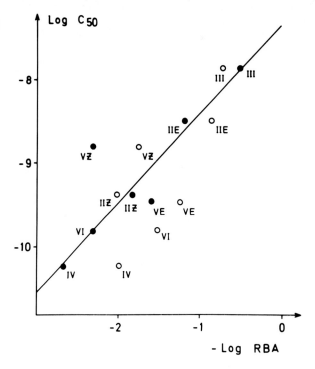

FIG. 6. Correlation bet-
ween RBAs of TPEs at
25°C (●) and at 0°C (o)
for mouse uterus cytosol
ER and PR induction in
MCF$_7$ cells (expressed as
the concentration giving
50% of the maximum speci-
fic induction obtained
with 10^{8}M estradiol).

DISCUSSION

The p-hydroxylated triphenyl-acrylonitrile derivatives we have studied
form a complete and novel series of compounds with a wide range of affinities for the cytosol estrogen receptor of mouse and rat uterus. These
affinities have been related to the position of the hydroxy group. When
this group is in position R (Fig. 1), the affinity is highest, suggesting
that the α-phenol ring interacts with the main anchorage point of the
binding site, subsite S$_1$ (Fig. 3). Hydroxy groups in positions R$_1$ and
R$_2$ contribute less towards affinity but nevertheless enhance binding
and the stability of the complex.

None of the derivatives competed to any appreciable extent for binding
to the "anti-estrogen binding site" probably because they lack an alkyl-
amino ethoxy type side-chain as in tamoxifen.

The study of structure/activity relationships in this series is ham-
pered by the non-availability of a convenient assay of estrogenic activity where metabolic transformation of the ligands is minimal. One of the
most suitable models presently at our disposal is the induction of progesterone receptor (PR) in a cell-line such as MCF$_7$. In this system,
all our test-compounds induced PR. Their C$_{50}$s for induction were linearly related to the relative binding affinity measured at 25°C, indicating that this affinity corresponds to the formation of an equally functional complex whatever the orientation of the TPE derivative within the

binding site. This conclusion obviously applies for the moment only to the derivatives we have studied and only in relation to the biological end-point we have assayed. Recently, 1,1,2-triphenyl-but-1-ene derivatives substituted by acetoxy groups in the meta or para positions have been tested for ER binding affinity in calf uterus cytosol and for mammary tumor inhibiting properties (34). Rather similar results to ours were obtained with respect to the relative importance of the E/Z isomers but no clear correlation could be deduced between binding and activity since, as stated by the authors, the compounds are deacetylated in vivo.

In our TPE series, the presence of a single hydroxy group in position R induced high affinity for the estrogen receptor and high biological activity. Such a compound can be considered an archetype for the further study of structure-function relationships : in future investigations, the steric and electronic effects of the introduction of various substituents on binding and activity will be analyzed in other biological models able to discriminate between estrogenic and anti-estrogenic action.

ACKNOWLEDGEMENTS

We thank S. Saez for the gift of the MCF$_7$ cell-line and for helpful discussions and G. Moreau and G. Lemoine for performing the molecular energy calculations with their Script programm.
Financial support from the Fondation de la Recherche Médicale is gratefully acknowledged.

REFERENCES

1. Agarwal, M.K., editor (1982) : Hormone Antagonists, Walter de Gruyter and Co, Berlin.
2. Binart, N., Catelli, M.G., Geynet, C., Puri, V., Hähnel, R., Mester, J., and Baulieu, E.E. (1979) : Biochem. Biophys. Res. Commun., 91:812-818.
3. Borgna, J.L., Coezy, E., and Rochefort, H. (1982) : Biochem. Pharmacol., 31:3187-3191.
4. Borgna, J.L. and Rochefort, H. (1981) : J. Biol. Chem., 256:859-868.
5. Burton, K. (1956) : Biochem. J., 62:315-323.
6. Chernayev, G.A., Barkova, T.I., Egovora, V.V., Sorokiria, I.B., Ananchenko, S.N., Mataradze, G.D., Sokolova, N.A., and Rozen, V.B. (1975) : J. steroid Biochem., 6:1483-1488.
7. Coesy, E., Borgna, J.L., and Rochefort, H. (1982) : Cancer Res., 42:317-323.
8. Cohen, N.C., Colin, P., and Lemoine, G. (1981) : Tetrahedron, 37:1711-1721.
9. Duax, W.L., Griffin, J.F., Rohrer, D.C., Swenson, D.C., and Weeks C.M. (1981) : J. steroid Biochem., 15:41-47.
10. Duax, W.L., Griffin, J.F., Rohrer, D.C., and Weeks, C.M. (1982) : In : Hormone Antagonists, edited by M.K. Agarwal, pp. 3-24, Walter de Gruyter and Co, Berlin.
11. Durani, S., Agarwal, M.K., Saxena, R., Setty, B.S., Gupta, R.C., Kole, P.L., Ray, S., and Anand, N. (1979) : J. steroid Biochem., 11:67-77.

12. Durani, S. and Anand, N. (1981) : Intl. J. Quantum Chem., XX:71–83.
13. Eckert, R.L. and Katzenellenbogen, B.S. (1982) : Cancer Res., 42: 139–144.
14. Faye, J.C., Lasserre, B., and Bayard, F. (1980) : Biochem. Biophys. Res. Commun., 93:1225–1231.
15. Ferguson, E.R. and Katzenellenbogen, B.S. (1977) : Endocrinology, 100:1242–1251.
16. Gilbert, J., Miquel, J.F., Précigoux, G., Hospital, M., Raynaud, J.P., Michel, F., and Crastes de Paulet, A. (1983) : J. Med. Chem., 26:693–699.
17. Gulino, A. and Pasqualini, J.R. (1980) : Cancer Res., 40:3821–3826.
18. Hähnel, R., Twaddle, E., and Ratajczak, T. (1973) : J. steroid Biochem., 4:21–31.
19. Haye, J.R., Rorke, E.A., Robertson, D.W., Katzenellenbogen, B.S., and Katzenellenbogen, J.A. (1981) : Endocrinology, 108:164–172.
20. Jordan, V.C., Collins, M.M., Rowsby, L., and Prestwich, G. (1977) : J. Endocr., 75:305–316.
21. Jordan, V.C., Dix, C.J., Naylor, K.E., Prestwitch, G., and Rowsby, L. (1978): J. Tox. Environ. Hlth., 4:363–390.
22. Jordan, V.C., Fisher, A.H., and Rose, D.P. (1981) : Eur. J. Cancer, 17:121–122.
23. Jordan, V.C. and Gosden, B. (1982) : Mol. Cell. Endo., 27:291–306.
24. Kon, O.L. (1983) : J. Biol. Chem., 258:3173–3177.
25. Leclercq, G., Devleeschouwer, N., and Heuson, J.C. (1983) : J. steroid Biochem., 19:75–83.
26. Lieberman, M.E., Jordan, V.C., Fritsch, M., Santos, M.A., and Gorski, J. (1983) : J. Biol. Chem., 258:4734–4740.
27. Lowry, O.H., Rosenbrough, N.J., Farr, A.L., and Randall, R.J. (1951) : J. Biol. Chem., 193:265–275.
28. Miquel, J.F., Sekera, A., and Chaudron, T. (1978) : C.R. Acad. Sci. Ser. C, 286:151–154.
29. Murphy, L.C., Sutherland, R.L. (1981) : Biochem. Biophys. Res. Commun., 100:1353–1361.
30. Pons, M., Michel, F., Crastes de Paulet, A. Gilbert, G., Miquel, J.F., Précigoux, G., Hospital, M., Ojasoo, T., and Raynaud, J.P. (1984) : J. steroid Biochem., in press.
31. Ruenitz, P.C., Bagley, J.R., and Mokler, C.M. (1982) : J. Med. Chem., 25:1056–1060.
32. Ruenitz, P.C., Bagley, J.R., and Mokler, C.M. (1983) : Biochem. Pharmacol., 32:2941–2947.
33. Saez, S. and Chouvet, C. (1983) : Ann. Endocr., 44:181.
34. Schneider, M.R., von Angerer, E., Schönenberger, H., Michel, R.T., and Fortmeyer, H.P. (1982) : J. Med. Chem., 25:1070–1077.
35. Sudo, K., Monsma, Jr, F.J., and Katzenellenbogen, B.S. (1983) : Endocrinology, 112:425–434.
36. Sutherland, R.L. and Jordan, V.C., editors (1978) : Non-steroidal Antiestrogens, Academic Press, Sidney.
37. Sutherland, R.L. and Murphy, L.C. (1982) : Mol. Cell. Endo., 25:5–23.
38. Sutherland, R.L., Murphy, L.C., Foo, M.S., Green, M.D., Whybourne, A.M., and Krozowski, Z.S. (1980) : Nature, 288:273–275.
39. Sutherland, R.L., Watts, C.K.W., and Murphy, L.C. (1982) : In : Hormone Antagonists, edited by M.K. Agarwal, pp. 147–161, Walter de Gruyter and Co, Berlin.

Progress in Cancer Research and Therapy,
Vol. 31, edited by F. Bresciani, et al.
Raven Press, New York © 1984.

Defective Activation of the Estrogen Receptor by Triphenylethylene Antiestrogens

Jean-Louis Borgna, Elaine Evans, Joël Fauque, and Henri Rochefort

Unité d'Endocrinologie Cellulaire et Moléculaire, U 148 INSERM, 34100 Montpellier, France

The mechanism of action of non-steroidal antiestrogens is of great interest since : 1. the non-productive interaction of these compounds with the estrogen receptor could help to understand, by comparison, the mechanism of action of estrogens ; 2. tamoxifen one of these triphenylethylene derivatives is now currently used to treat post-menopausal breast cancer (10). The structures of triphenylethylene antiestrogens are related to that of the synthetic estrogen diethylstilbestrol. This similarity becomes more evident with the 4-hydroxylated metabolites which result from either hydroxylation (4-unsubstituted compounds) (9) or 0-demethylation (4-methoxylated compounds) (14). These 4-hydroxylated metabolites probably play an important role in the antiestrogenic activity of classical antiestrogens since in various species, following the administration of the parent compounds, they were found to be retained and concentrated in estrogen target tissues and bound to the estrogen receptor (2,14). Metabolism of the parent compound is, however, not a prerequisite for antiestrogenic activity since in vitro non-metabolized parent antiestrogens themselves display antiestrogenic activity. However, this activity is markedly lower than that of their 4-hydroxylated metabolites (6,21).

The biological activity of non-steroidal antiestrogens varies according to species, and also according to the estrogenic responses considered. For instance, in MCF_7 cells, tamoxifen and 4-hydroxytamoxifen are partial estrogen agonists for the induction of the progesterone receptor (12) whereas they are full estrogen antagonists for the induction of the secreted 52 K glycoprotein, since they are incapable of inducing this protein and they totally prevent its induction by estradiol (21).

Since these antiestrogens interact with the estrogen receptor and translocate it into the nucleus (5,18), the main difficulty is in understanding their relative ineffi-ciency at inducing estrogenic effects. In contrast, their antiestrogenic activity is easier to understand, since by a simple competition mechanism, antiestrogens prevent the binding of estrogens to the estrogen receptor.

Schematically two kinds of alterations could explain the low agonistic activity of antiestrogens. The first concerns the parameters relative to the estrogen receptor/ligand interaction (Chapter 1). Specifically, it has been proposed that antiestrogens are low affinity ligands of the estrogen receptor (3). Another explanation for the low agonistic activity is an altered activation or transconformational change in the receptor, induced by antiestrogens (Chapter 2).

To test these hypotheses we first compared the interaction of estrogens and antiestrogens with the estrogen receptor. We then studied the biochemical properties of both types of complexes and especially their ability to undergo the activation process. We chose 4-hydroxytamoxifen as the antiestrogen instead of tamoxifen since : 1. this hydroxylated metabolite is a more potent antiestrogen in MCF_7 cells than tamoxifen (6,21) ; 2. it is accumulated at the nuclear estrogen receptor level in the rat and lamb uterus and in the chicken oviduct (2), and 3. the estrogen receptor-4-hydroxytamoxifen complex is more stable than the receptor-tamoxifen complex and is therefore more suitable for biochemical studies (1).

INTERACTION OF ESTRADIOL, TAMOXIFEN AND 4-HYDROXYTAMOXIFEN WITH THE CALF UTERINE ESTROGEN RECEPTOR

Recent syntheses of radiolabeled antiestrogens allowed us to demonstrate the direct interaction of these compounds with the estrogen receptor and to determine the binding parameters relative to this interaction (1,4). Table 1 gives the relative kinetic association- (k+) and dissociation- (k-) rate constants and the relative equilibrium dissociation constants (K_D or k-/k+) of estradiol, 4-hydroxytamoxifen and tamoxifen for the calf uterine estrogen receptor. All values are very similar for estradiol and 4-hydroxytamoxifen. For tamoxifen the values calculated for k- and, from competition experiments, for K_D are much higher than the corresponding values calculated for the two other ligands. These results invalidate the general assumption which attributes the antiestrogenic activity of antiestrogens to their high rate of dissociation from the receptor, since 4-hydroxytamoxifen, which dissociates much more slowly than tamoxifen, is a more potent antiestrogen in vitro (6,21). In other species, the relative dissociation rates of estradiol and 4-hydroxytamoxifen from the receptor are slightly different. However, these differences cannot account for the estrogenic or antiestrogenic activity of triphenylethylene derivatives since in both the chick oviduct (where tamoxifen is purely an estrogen antagonist) and in the mouse uterus (were it behaves as a full estrogen) 4-hydroxytamoxifen dissociates more slowly from the receptor than does estradiol (1). We conclude that the estrogen

TABLE 1. Relative Binding Characteristics to the Calf Uterine Estrogen Receptor*

	Estradiol[a]	4-Hydroxy-tamoxifen[a]	Tamoxifen[a][b]
k_+^o	1	1.2	0.4
k_-^o	1	0.9	220
k_-^o/k_+^o	1	0.8	520
K_D^o (Scatchard)	1	0.7	4.3
K_D^{2o} (Competition)	1	1.1	400

*The association rate (k_+^o) and dissociation rate (k_-^o) constants were determined at 0°C. The equilibrium dissociation constants (K_D) were determined either at 0°C from Scatchard analysis using the labeled ligands or at 20°C from competition experiments using (^3H)estradiol and the unlabeled ligands. All values were standardized by taking the estradiol constants as 1. The absolute mean values determined for estradiol were : $k_+^o = 1.7 \times 10^5 \times S^{-1} \times M^{-1}$; $k_-^o = 5.0 \times 10^{-7} \times S^{-1}$; $k_-^o/k_+^o = 2.9$ pM ; K_D^o (Scatchard) = 0.41 nM.
(a) From Borgna and Rochefort (1) and Rochefort et al (17) ; (b) From Capony and Rochefort (4).

agonistic or antagonistic properties of non-steroidal anti-estrogens cannot be interpreted from the relative values of their binding parameters with the estrogen receptor.

ACTIVATION OF THE ESTROGEN RECEPTOR BY ESTRADIOL AND 4-HYDROXYTAMOXIFEN

Activation of the estrogen receptor can be defined as the hormone-dependent process which transforms the inactive estrogen receptor into a biologically active state. In cell-free systems this time- and temperature-dependent process is currently obtained by warming the cytosol containing the estrogen receptor-estradiol complex at 25°C for 30 minutes. The presence of molybdate in the cytosol totally prevents the activation process and is thought to stabilize the receptor complex in the non-activated state (19). In the cell-free system, the criteria used to specify the activation of the estrogen receptor-estradiol complex are : the 4 to 5S receptor transformation (13), the binding of the receptor to nuclei or to DNA (22), and the decrease in the dissociation rate of the receptor-estradiol complex (20). Using these criteria we compared the activation induced by estradiol and 4-hydroxytamoxifen.

Sedimentation in Sucrose Gradients

The sedimentation constants of the cytosolic receptor-
estradiol and receptor-4-hydroxytamoxifen complexes were
very similar in all species studied (rat, lamb, calf). The
sedimentation constants were ~ 4 S and ~ 8 S in high and low
salt sucrose gradients, respectively. No marked changes
were observed upon activation of the complexes, except for
the rat complexes, where the 4S to 5S transformation was
similarly observed with both ligands (16).

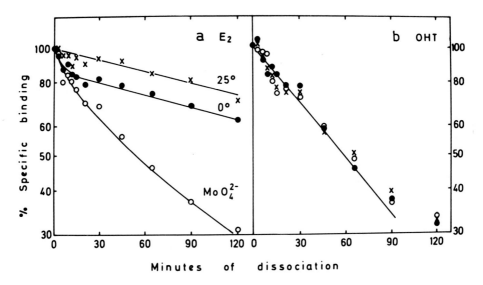

FIG. 1. Dissociation Rate of Estradiol and 4-hydroxy-
tamoxifen from the Estrogen Receptor before and after Heat
Activation. Lamb uterine cytosol with (o) or without ($\bullet$,x)
10 mM MoO_4^{2-} was incubated for 2 h at 0°C with 5 nM (^{3}H)
estradiol (E_2) or (^{3}H) 4-hydroxytamoxifen (OHT) in the
presence (to determine non-specific binding) or absence of
1 µM unlabeled estradiol. One part of the cytosol without
molybdate was heated for 30 min at 25°C, the other part
was maintained at 0°C. The dissociation rate was then
determined at 25°C following the addition of 1 µM
unlabeled estradiol. Specific and non-specific binding was
determined after charcoal treatment. The percentages of
specific binding of a) estradiol, and b) 4-hydroxytamo-
xifen according to the dissociation time are represented
for (x,25°) preactivated receptor ; ($\bullet$,0°) non-
preactivated receptor ; (o, MoO_4^{2-}) molybdate-stabilized
receptor (from Rochefort and Borgna (15), by permission of
editors).

Dissociation Rate from the Estrogen Receptor

The dissociation rate of the receptor-estradiol complex varies according to the state of the complex (20). As illustrated in Fig. 1a with the lamb uterine receptor : the dissociation of the preactivated complex is a first-order process ; the dissociation of the molybdate-stabilized complex, which cannot undergo the activation, is a more rapid quasi-first-order process ; finally, the dissociation of the non-preactivated complex is biphasic, the first slope corresponding to the dissociation of the unactivated complex while the second slope corresponds to that of the residual complex activated during the disso-ciation. Conversely, under similar conditions, no marked variation was observed in the dissociation of the receptor-antiestrogen complex, whatever the pretreatment of the complex (Fig. 1b). In all cases, similar quasi-first-order processes were observed. Thus, we conclude that the dissociation rate of estradiol is decreased by the receptor activation process while that of 4-hydroxy-tamoxifen is not modified. The same results were observed with both complexes in all other species studied : rat, mouse, calf, chicken, and MCF_7 cells (Fig. 2). With the lamb uterine estrogen receptor, the other steroidal estro-gens tested (estrone, estriol, androsta-5-ene-3β,17β-diol) behaved like estradiol while other triphenylethylene anti-estrogens (tamoxifen and CI 628) behaved like 4-hydroxy-tamoxifen (Fig. 2). Therefore, the decrease in the dissociation rate of steroidal estrogen ligands and the absence of variation in the dissociation rate of triphenyl-ethylenic antiestrogen ligands following the activation of the estrogen receptor appear to be general properties.

Interaction of Complexes with Non-Specific DNA

We then compared the apparent affinity of both complexes for double stranded non-specific DNA using the DNA-cellulose batch assay, the receptor activation taking place in the presence of DNA. At 0°C, the time course of binding to DNA was similar for both complexes, with an optimal binding at 18 h (8). Saturation analysis, using a constant concentration of cytosolic complexes and increasing concentrations of DNA, showed that the estrogen receptor displayed an apparently higher affinity for DNA when it was activated by estradiol than by 4-hydroxy-tamoxifen, while the maximal concentrations of the complexes bound to DNA appeared to be similar (8). In a series of similar experiments, the mean value for the equilibrium association constant for the receptor-estradiol/DNA interaction was 2.3 times higher than that for the receptor-4-hydroxytamoxifen/DNA interaction. The association and dissociation rates of both complexes with and from DNA at 15°C were also compared. Whereas the dissociation rates were practically equivalent, the "asso-ciation rates" which include both the activation of the

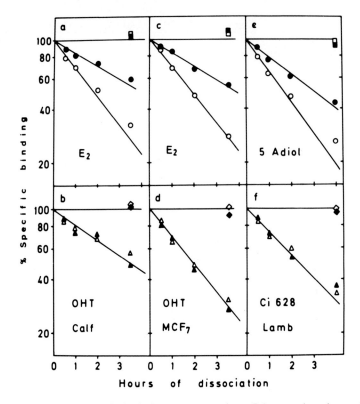

FIG. 2. Effect of Molybdate on the Dissociation Rate of Estrogens and Antiestrogens from the Estrogen Receptor. (a,b). Calf uterine cytosol prepared with (o,△) or without (●,▲) 10 mM MoO_4^{2-} was incubated for 2 h with 5 nM (^3H)estradiol or (^3H) 4-hydroxytamoxifen in the presence or absence of 1 μM unlabeled estradiol. The cytosol estrogen receptor was then heated for 30 min at 25°C and the dissociation rate at 20°C was evaluated as described in Fig. 1. Each value was corrected for non-specific binding. The stability of the complexes was assayed separately (□,■,◇,◆). Results were normalized by taking the pre-dissociation value as 100 %. (c,d). Same experiment with cytosol of the MCF_7 human breast cancer cells. The estrogen receptor was activated at 20°C. (e,f). Dissociation rate at 0°C from lamb uterine cytosol incubated with 20 nM (^3H) androsta-5-ene-3 β,17 β-diol (5 Adiol) or (^3H) CI 628. The estrogen receptor was activated for 30 min at 25°C (from Rochefort and Borgna (15), by permission of editors).

complex and the binding of the activated receptor to DNA, were found to be about three times higher for the estradiol than for the 4-hydroxytamoxifen complex (Fig. 3).

From these studies, it appears that the affinity of the receptor-antiestrogen complex for non-specific DNA is 2 to 3 times lower than that of the estradiol complex. Whether

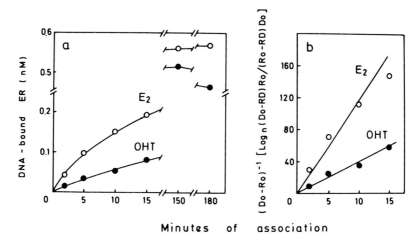

Minutes of association

FIG. 3. Association Rate of Estradiol- and 4-hydroxy-tamoxifen- Estrogen Receptor Complexes with DNA. Calf uterine cytosol incubated at 0°C with 6 nM (^{3}H) estradiol (o) or (^{3}H) 4-hydroxytamoxifen (•) in the presence or absence of 5 µM unlabeled estradiol was treated with charcoal. Aliquots of the supernatants were incubated with aliquots of DNA (150 µg/ml final) adsorbed onto cellulose at 15°C for increasing times. Then, specific binding to DNA was determined as previously described (8). a. Direct representation of the time course of specific binding to DNA. b. Linearization of the binding data, assuming a second order kinetics for the formation of the receptor-DNA complex ; the association rate constant k+ is then directly given by the slope. Ro, R, Do and D are the concentrations of free receptor complex and free DNA expressed as nucleotides, at times 0 and t respectively.

or not this difference is related to the weak agonist activity of antiestrogens is not known since we have not quantified the affinity of the estrogen receptor for specific DNA sequences.

Interaction of the Calf Uterine Complexes with a Monoclonal Antibody

An IgM monoclonal antibody developed by Greene et al (11) against the calf nuclear estrogen receptor, appeared to be an interesting tool for probing the estrogen receptor, since these authors found that the reactivity of the nuclear receptor-estradiol complex for this antibody was greater than that of the corresponding native cytosolic complex. We have used this antibody to compare the activation of the estrogen receptor triggered by estradiol and by 4-hydroxytamoxifen.

Due to the high molecular weight of the IgM class B$_{36}$ monoclonal antibody, B$_{36}$-bound and unbound receptor-

TABLE 2. Relative Affinity of the Different Forms of the Estrogen Receptor for the B_{36} Monoclonal Antibody*

	R_i-E_2	R_i-OHT	R_a-E_2	R_a-OHT
K_A	1	3.0	4.6	11.0

*The relative affinities of the B_{36} antibody for the various forms of the estrogen receptor (activated (Ra) or molybdate-stabilized (Ri) and bound to estradiol (R_a-E_2, R_i-E_2) or to 4-hydroxytamoxifen (R_a-OHT, R_i-OHT)) were derived from the ratio B_{36}-bound receptor/unbound receptor measured in sucrose gradients. Values were standardized by taking the affinity of the B_{36} for the R_i-E_2 complex as 1 (Borgna et al, unpublished results).

estradiol complexes are easily separated in low salt and high salt sucrose gradients (11). Therefore we undertook qualitative and quantitative studies on the receptor/antibody interaction. The 4.5 S (high salt) and 8 S (low salt gradient) molybdate-stabilized or activated receptor-estradiol complexes were shifted by the B_{36} antibody and appeared respectively at ∼13 S and ∼15 S peaks in high salt and low salt sucrose gradients. From the proportion of the receptor-estradiol complexes shifted by the antibody, the reactivity of the activated complex was clearly higher than that of the molybdate-stabilized complex (Borgna et al., unpublished results).

Similar qualitative results were observed with the cytosolic receptor-4-hydroxytamoxifen complexes : they were shifted to the same 13-15 S region of the sucrose gradient ; the reactivity for B_{36} was higher for the activated than for the molybdate-stabilized complex and all the complexes were shifted when using a sufficient concentration of B_{36}. The nuclear complexes extracted from nuclei after in vitro incubation of whole uteri with estradiol or 4-hydroxytamoxifen displayed a similar high reactivity for B_{36}.

Assuming that for a given ionic strength the binding capacity of B_{36} for the receptor is constant (whether the receptor is activated or stabilized by molybdate and bound to estradiol or 4-hydroxytamoxifen), relative K_A values for the interaction of B_{36} with the different forms of the receptor (Table 2) were calculated from the ratio B_{36}-bound receptor/unbound receptor. Regardless of the ligand bound to the receptor, the interaction with B_{36} was higher for the activated receptor than for the molybdate-stabilized receptor. Moreover, the reactivities of the two receptor-antiestrogen complexes were respectively higher than those of the corresponding receptor-estradiol complexes.

Finally, we found that the B_{36} antibody inhibited the DNA binding of the receptor-estradiol and receptor-4-

TABLE 3. Characteristics of the Estrogen
Receptor-Antiestrogens Complex*

---

1. Absence of decreased dissociation rate upon activation.

2. Lower affinity for non-specific DNA sites.

3. Higher affinity for the B_{36} monoclonal antibody.

4. Higher molecular forms in high salt gradient.

5. Interaction with nuclear component(s).

---

*The above differences were observed when the estrogen receptor was bound to antiestrogen instead of estrogen :
    1. in all species studied : human (MCF_7), calf, lamb, rat, mouse (uterus) and chicken (oviduct) using estradiol, estrone, estriol and androsta-5-ene-3 β,17 β-diol as estrogens ; tamoxifen, 4-hydroxytamoxifen and Cl 628 as antiestrogens (15),
    2. with the calf, lamb and rat uterus using estradiol and 4-hydroxytamoxifen (8) or Cl 628 M (rat) (14),
    3. with the calf uterus using estradiol and 4-hydroxytamoxifen (Borgna et al, unpublished results),
    4. with the rat uterus using estradiol and Cl 628 M (14),
    5. with MCF_7 cells using estradiol and Cl 628 M (7).

hydroxytamoxifen complexes. This inhibition was : B_{36} concentration-dependent ; partial ($\leqslant 60$ %) even for concentrations of B_{36} which shifted all the complexes in the sucrose gradient, and slightly more marked for the receptor-estradiol than for the receptor-4-hydroxytamoxifen complex. This observation suggests for the first time that the B_{36}-antigenic and DNA binding sites of the estrogen receptor are related, if not vicinal on the receptor surface. Up to now, no inhibition of receptor-DNA binding by antibodies to steroid receptor had been shown.

CONCLUSION

There is no marked difference between the binding parameters of estradiol and 4-hydroxytamoxifen to the estrogen receptor. Conversely, using three different criteria : the DNA binding, the dissociation rate, and the reactivity for a monoclonal antibody we found quantitative (DNA and B_{36} interactions) and qualitative differences (dissociation rate) between the properties of the two types of complexes as summarized in Table 3 and illustrated in Fig. 4. This strongly suggests that the estrogen receptor activation induced by antiestrogens is different from that induced by estrogens. Therefore the low agonistic activity and the antagonistic activity of non-steroidal antiestrogens could be due to a defective activation of the estrogen receptor by antiestrogens.

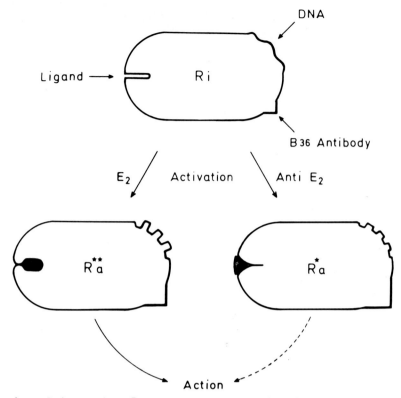

FIG. 4. Schematic Representation of the Calf Estrogen Receptor before and after its Activation by Estradiol or 4-hydroxytamoxifen. The calf uterine estrogen receptor is represented with 3 different binding domains for the ligand, the DNA, and the B_{36} monoclonal antibody. Upon activation of the estrogen receptor, the stabilization of the receptor-ligand complex at the hormone binding site occurs only with estradiol ; the affinity for DNA is more marked for the estrogen complex than for the antiestrogen complex ; conversely, the B_{36} antibody binding domain is more exposed when the receptor is bound to the antiestrogen than when it is bound to the estrogen.

The search for new antiestrogens having purely antagonist activity in humans, and the attempt to improve the efficacy and selectivity in therapy might be guided by an initial screening of the in vitro ability of the antiestrogens to bind and activate the estrogen receptor. The best potential drugs would need to have, a priori, a high affinity for the estrogen receptor, but very weak or zero efficacy in activating the estrogen receptor.

The modification of the biochemical properties of the estrogen receptor when it binds non-steroidal anti-estrogens instead of estrogens strengthens the hypothesis that the antiestrogenic activity of these compounds is mediated by the estrogen receptor. At present, the modified biochemical properties of the estrogen receptor interacting with non-steroidal antiestrogens do not yet enable us to understand the mechanism of action of anti-estrogens at the molecular level.

Work is in progress in an attempt to specify how the different activated receptor complexes interact in chromatin, and modulate transcription at specific regulatory sites.

ACKNOWLEDGMENTS

This study was supported by the "Institut National de la Santé et de la Recherche Médicale", the "Centre National de la Recherche Scientifique", and the "Fondation pour la Recherche Médicale Française". We would like to thank Drs G.L. Greene and E.V. Jensen for their generous gift of B_{36} monoclonal antibody ; Mrs S. Ladrech for her excellent technical assistance and Miss E. Barrié for her skilful preparation of the manuscript. We are grateful to ICI Laboratories for their gifts of tamoxifen and hydroxytamoxifen.

REFERENCES

1. Borgna, J.L., and Rochefort, H. (1980): Mol. Cell. Endocrinol., 20:71-86.
2. Borgna, J.L., and Rochefort, H. (1981): J. Biol. Chem., 256:859-868.
3. Bouton, M.M., and Raynaud, J.P. (1979): Endocrinol., 105:509-515.
4. Capony, F., and Rochefort, H. (1978): Mol. Cell. Endocrinol., 11:181-198.
5. Clark, J.H., Anderson, J.N., and Peck, E.J., Jr (1973): Steroids, 22:707-718.
6. Coezy, E., Borgna, J.L., and Rochefort, H. (1982): Cancer Res., 42:317-323.
7. Eckert, R.L., and Katzenellenbogen, B.S. (1982): J. Biol. Chem., 257:8840-8846.
8. Evans, E., Baskevitch, P.P., and Rochefort, H. (1982): Eur. J. Biochem., 128:185-191.
9. Fromson, J.M., Pearson, S., and Brahma, S. (1973): Xenobiotica, 3:693-709 and 710-714.
10. Furr, B.J., Patterson, J.S., Richardson, D.N., Slater, S.R., and Wakeling, A.E. (1979): In: Pharmacological and Biochemical Properties of Drugs Substances, Vol 2: Tamoxifen, edited by M.E. Goldberg, pp. 355-399. American Pharmaceutical Association, Washington.
11. Greene, G.L., Fitch, F.W., and Jensen, E.V. (1980): Proc. Natl. Acad. Sci. U.S., 77:157-161.
12. Horwitz, K.B., Koseki, Y., and McGuire, W.L. (1978): Endocrinol., 103:1742-1751.
13. Jensen, E.V., Suzuki, T., Numata, M., Smith, S., and DeSombre, E.R. (1969): Steroids, 13:417-427.
14. Katzenellenbogen, B.S., Pavlik, E.J., Robertson, D.W., and Katzenellenbogen, J.A. (1981): J. Biol. Chem., 256:2908-2915.

15. Rochefort, H., and Borgna, J.L. (1981): Nature, 292: 257-259.
16. Rochefort, H., Borgna, J.L., and Evans, E. (1983): J. Steroid Biochem., 19:69-74.
17. Rochefort, H., Garcia, M., and Borgna, J.L. (1979): Biochem. Biophys. Res. Commun., 88:351-357.
18. Rochefort, H., Lignon, F., and Capony, F. (1972): Biochem. Biophys. Res. Commun., 47:662-670.
19. Shyamala, G., and Leonard, L. (1980): J. Biol. Chem., 255:6028-6031.
20. Weichman, B.M., and Notides, A.C. (1977): J. Biol. Chem., 252:8856-8862.
21. Westley, B.R., and Rochefort, H. (1980): Cell, 20: 353-362.
22. Yamamoto, K.R., and Alberts, B. (1972): Proc. Natl. Acad. Sci. U.S., 69:2105-2109.

Progress in Cancer Research and Therapy,
Vol. 31, edited by F. Bresciani, et al.
Raven Press, New York © 1984.

Estrogen Receptor Hormone Binding Activity Is Regulated by Phosphorylation-Dephosphorylation of the Receptor

Ferdinando Auricchio, Antimo Migliaccio, Gabriella Castoria, Secondo Lastoria, and Andrea Rotondi

Istituto di Patologia Generale, I Facoltà di Medicina e Chirurgia, 80138 Naples, Italy

A few reversible covalent modifications regulate the acti vities of many proteins (see Table 1 for the reversible protein modifications)

TABLE 1. REVERSIBLE COVALENT MODIFICATIONS OF PROTEINS INCLUDE:

PHOSPHORYLATION	— DEPHOSPHORYLATION
ACETYLATION	— DEACETYLATION
ADENYLATION	— DEADENYLATION
URYDILATION	— DEURYDILATION
METHYLATION	— DEMETHYLATION

Phosphorylation-dephosphorylation of proteins is controlled by protein kinase and phosphoprotein phosphatase. Some hormone receptors, peptide as well as steroid receptors, are phosphoproteins (see Table 2).

TABLE 2. PHOSPHORYLATED HORMONE RECEPTORS

Epidermal growth factor (EGF) receptor *Cohen S. et al. (7)*
Insulin receptor *Kasuga M. et al. (11)*
17β-estradiol receptor *Migliaccio A. et al. (12)*
Progesterone receptor *Weigel N.L. et al. (18); Dougherty J.J. et al.(8)*
Glucocorticoid receptor *Housley P.R. and Pratt W.B. (10)*

This chapter describes the process of phosphorylation-dephosphorylation of the 17β-estradiol receptor discovered by researchers in our laboratory.

We have recently observed that the addition of nuclei or nuclear extracts from mouse uterus to homologous cytosol rapidly inactivates the cytosol specific estradiol binding activity. Removal of nuclei and the addition of ATP to cytosol rapidly and completely restores the loss of hormone binding (Fig. 1).

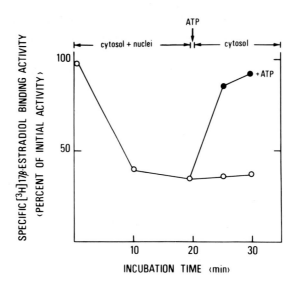

FIG. 1. *Inactivation-reactivation of hormone binding activity of estrogen receptor. Mouse uterine cytosol was labelled in TED (50 mM Tris, 1 mM EDTA, 2 mM dithiothreitol) buffer, pH 7.4, with 12 nM* [³H] *17β-estradiol in the absence and in the presence of an excess of cold 17β-estradiol and incubated at 25° C in the presence of an equivalent amount of uterus nuclei for 20 min (open circles). After centrifugation at 2° C to remove nuclei the sample was supplemented with 10 mM Na_2MoO_4 and divided into two portions. 5 mM $MgCl_2$ and 10 mM ATP (arrow) were added to one portion (black symbols), and $MgCl_2$ without ATP was added to the other (open circles). Temperature was shifted to 15° C and incubation was continued for an additional 10 min. Specific* [³H] *17β-estradiol binding activity was measured at the indicated times. The initial activity was about 1200 fmoles of* [³H] *17β-estradiol binding sites/ml (4)*

We have purified from calf uterus nuclei the enzyme responsible for the inactivation of the receptor hormone binding (2), and from calf uterus cytosol the enzyme responsible for the activation of this binding (4). The first enzyme is a receptor-phosphatase; the second is a receptor-kinase.

Table 3 summarizes the properties of the receptor-phospha tase. This nuclear enzyme is found in mouse uterus and mammary gland, but not in quadriceps muscle, and only trace amounts have been found in liver (1).

TABLE 3. PROPERTIES OF THE PHOSPHATASE THAT INACTIVATES THE 17β-ESTRADIOL BINDING OF THE RECEPTOR

1. Localized in nuclei of estrogen target tissues

2. Purified from calf uterus

3. Stimulated by dithiothreitol

4. Inhibited by zinc, molybdate, fluoride, phosphate, pyrophosphate, and p-nitrophenyl phosphate

5. It inactivates in vitro the hormone binding of crude and pure cytosol and nuclear receptor

6. Km for estrogen-free receptor: 1.5×10^{-9} mol/l

7. Km for estrogen-bound receptor: 0.8×10^{-9} mol/l

8. It apparently inactivates in vivo the hormone binding of the receptor translocated by hormone into nuclei

9. It does not inactivate in vitro the hormone binding of the receptor complexed with antiestrogens

10. It dephosphorylates the 17β-estradiol receptor

It has been extracted from nuclei by sonication in hypotonic buffer and then further purified by CM-cellulose chromatography (2). The lability of the enzyme hinders a more extensive purification. The enzyme is stimulated three-fold by 10 mM dithiothreitol, whereas it is completely inhibited by several phosphatase inhibitors (0.5 mM zinc, 5 mM molybdate, 20 mM fluoride, 1 mM phosphate, 1 mM pyrophosphate) and by 1 mM p-nitrophenyl phosphate, a substrate of several phosphatases. In vitro, the phosphatase inactivates both crude and highly purified calf uterus 17β-estradiol receptor, with a very high affinity for the hormone-bound as well as for the hormone-free receptor. This extraordinary affinity supports the hypothesis that the receptor, which is present in very low concentrations in estradiol target tissues, is the physiological substrate of this enzyme. Evidence from

our laboratory, which will be described later, strongly suggests that in vivo the nuclear phosphatase inactivates the
receptor translocated into nuclei in complex with 17β-estra-
diol. The enzyme does not inactivate cytosol or nuclear receptor complexed with non steroidal antiestrogens such as
tamoxifen and nafoxidine (3). There is a striking remarkable
analogy between these results and the finding that the recep
tor translocated in nuclei by the same antiestrogens is slowly inactivated in intact cells (9). This analogy also suggests that the phosphatase is responsible for the inactivation of the receptor complexed with hormone in the nuclear
compartment of intact cells. Finally, as will be shown in
the next section but only, the phosphatase removes phosphate
from the receptor.

Properties of the receptor kinase

Table 4 summarizes some of the properties of this enzyme
which has been purified by ammonium sulphate precipitation,
heparin-sepharose and DEAE-cellulose chromatographies from
calf uterus cytosol (4).

TABLE 4. PROPERTIES OF THE KINASE THAT ACTIVATES THE
17β-ESTRADIOL BINDING OF THE RECEPTOR

1. Localized in cytosol

2. Purified from calf uterus

3. It sediments at 6 S

4. It reactivates the hormone binding of the
   receptor preinactivated by the nuclear phosphatase

5. Km for the inactivated receptor: 0.3×10^{-9} mol/l

6. Stimulated by Ca^{2+}-calmodulin

7. It phosphorylates the estradiol receptor

The kinase shows an extraordinary affinity for the inactive
(not hormone binding) sites of the receptor. It belongs to
the group of Ca^{2+}-calmodulin-stimulated kinases and it is
not sensitive to cyclic nucleotides, as will be described
in a following section.
   The kinase directly phosphorylates the 17β-estradiol receptor, the phosphorylation being a prerequisite for the hor
mone binding activity of the receptor (see the next section).

Evidence that the kinase phosphorylates the estradiol receptor and that phosphatase dephosphorylates it.
   Calf uterus cytosol receptor, extensively purified by heparin-sepharose and estradiol-agarose chromatographies (15),
was incubated with purified calf uterus nuclear phosphatase
(2). Hormone binding decreased during this incubation. Ad-

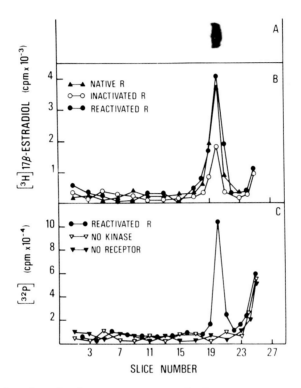

FIG. 2. *Phosphorylation of 17β-estradiol receptor by the kinase*
activating the hormone binding: polyacrylamide gel electrophore-
sis under non denaturing conditions. Purified calf uterus re-
ceptor preparation (native receptor) was incubated with the pho-
sphatase (inactivated receptor), then with the kinase in the
presence of 10 mM MgCl$_2$, 10 mM Na$_2$MoO$_4$, 1.050 mM CaCl$_2$, 2.7 μM
calmodulin/ml and 0.15 mM [γ-^{32}P] ATP (reactivated receptor).
Aliquots of the incubation mixture were submitted to gel electro-
phoresis. Panel A shows the silver staining of a gel lane load-
ed with the native receptor, and panel B the migration pattern
of [^{3}H] 17β-estradiol bound to native (▲), inactivated (O) and
reactivated (●) receptor. Panel C shows the migration pattern
of [^{32}P] of the sample containing the reactivated receptor (●).
Parallel samples incubated without kinase (▽) or without recep-
tor (▼) were run. For further details see Migliaccio et al.(12).

dition of purified calf uterus kinase (4), and $[\gamma\text{-}^{32}P]$ ATP
to the mixture completely restored hormone binding. The reactivated receptor was analyzed by gel electrophoresis in
non denaturing conditions and in SDS and by sucrose gradient centrifugation after incubation with monoclonal antibodies against the receptor (12).

The purified $[^3H]17\beta$-estradiol-receptor complex, after
migration through polyacrylamide gel in non denaturing conditions, shows a single protein band coincident with the peak of $[^3H]17\beta$-estradiol bound to the receptor (panels A and
B of Fig. 2). This peak is reduced by incubation of the receptor with the phosphatase and increased by subsequent incubation with the kinase (panel B). Furthermore, the peak
coincides with a single peak of $[^{32}P]$ obtained with receptor
incubated with the kinase and $[\gamma\text{-}^{32}P]$ ATP (panels B and C).
No $[^{32}P]$ peak is detected when either the receptor or the kinase is omitted from the incubation mixture (panel C). These
findings strongly suggest that the kinase phosphorylates the
receptor and that this phosphorylation requires the kinase.

To ascertain that $[^{32}P]$ has been covalently bound to the
protein, the receptor incubated with the kinase and $[\gamma\text{-}^{32}P]$
ATP was submitted also to SDS-gel electrophoresis (12). Again
a peak of $[^{32}P]$ was observed. It migrates at a molecular weight of about 69,000, which corresponds to the molecular weight of purified 17β-estradiol receptor (13,16).

IgG$_{2A}$ monoclonal antibodies against calf uterus estrogen
receptor are produced by the JS 34/32 clone of hybridoma cells obtained by fusion of myeloma cells with spleen cells
from mice immunized with receptor (14). The receptor reactivated by the kinase using $[\gamma\text{-}^{32}P]$ ATP was divided into two
aliquots; one was incubated with a large excess of antibodies against the receptor (JS 34/32), and the other with a
similar excess of antibodies produced by hybridoma cells derived from the fusion of the myeloma cells with spleen cells
from not immunized mice (control antibodies). Only the receptor incubated with JS 34/32 antibodies interacts with protein A (not shown), which means that the receptor after the
in vitro dephosphorylation-phosphorylation still recognizes
the JS 34/32 antibodies (12). Both aliquots of receptor were
submitted to centrifugation through "high salt" sucrose gradient. $[^3H]17\beta$-estradiol bound to the receptor incubated with
control antibodies sediments in the 4 S region together with
a $[^{32}P]$ peak (Fig. 3). Receptor incubated with JS 34/32 antibodies produces a complex at a molar ratio of 1:1, which sediments in the region of 7.5 S (14). The $[^3H]17\beta$-estradiol peak
of the receptor incubated with JS 34/32 antibodies cosedi-

ments with the $\left[^{32}P\right]$ peak in the 7.5 S region, thereby providing conclusive evidence that the protein phosphorylated during the incubation of receptor with the kinase is indeed the receptor itself.

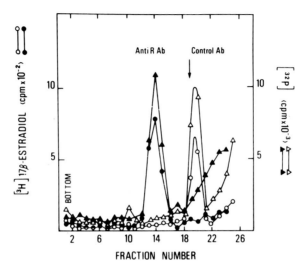

FIG. 3. *Phosphorylation of 17β-estradiol receptor by kinase activating the hormone binding: Sucrose gradient centrifugation of receptor-antibody complexes.* Purified calf uterus receptor was inactivated, then reactivated in the presence of $\left[\gamma-^{32}P\right]$ ATP as described in the legend to Fig. 2. Samples of the reactivated receptor were incubated in the presence of 0.4 M KCl with an excess of control immunoglobulins (open symbols) or of JS 34/32 antibodies (closed symbols), then centrifuged through 10-35% sucrose gradients containing 0.4 M KCl. The arrow indicates the position of the reference protein (bovine serum albumin). Symbols: ○—○, ●—●, $\left[^3H\right]$; △—△, ▲—▲, $\left[^{32}P\right]$. For further details see Migliaccio et al. (12).

Fig. 4 shows the SDS-gel electrophoresis of the receptor phosphorylated with $\left[\gamma-^{32}P\right]$ ATP by the kinase then incubated with and without the phosphatase. This enzyme removes most of the $\left[^{32}P\right]$ incorporated by the receptor during incubation with the kinase. Therefore the nuclear phosphatase inactivating the hormone binding of the estrogen receptor is undoubtly a receptor-phosphatase.

Ca^{2+}-calmodulin stimulates the receptor-kinase activation of estradiol binding of receptor. The activation of hormone binding of purified calf uterus receptor (15) by the purified cytosol kinase was monitored during incubation under different conditions (Fig. 5). Hormone binding is activated in the absence of Ca^{2+} and exogenous calmodulin. Added

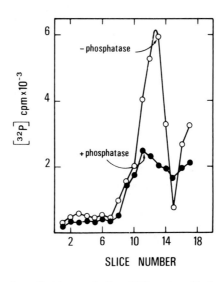

FIG. 4. *Dephosphorylation of the 17β-estradiol receptor by the phosphatase inactivating the hormone binding: SDS-polyacrylamide gel electrophoresis. Purified calf uterus receptor was phosphorylated with [^{32}P] essentially as described in the legend to Fig. 2. Two aliquots of phosphorylated receptor were incubated in the absence and in the presence of purified phosphatase. The samples were dialyzed and then submitted to SDS-gel electrophoresis. The gel lanes were sliced and counted for [^{32}P] radioactivity. Open symbols: receptor incubated without phosphatase; closed symbols: receptor incubated in the presence of phosphatase (6).*

separately Ca^{2+} and calmodulin have no stimulatory effect on this activation, whereas in association they significantly stimulate receptor activation. 25 μM trifluoperazine, which inhibits calmodulin-sensitive enzymes, prevents the stimulation of kinase by the association of Ca^{2+} and calmodulin (Fig. 5). Hence, Ca^{2+} stimulates the receptor-kinase through calmodulin. Cyclic nucleotides have no effect on the purified kinase (not shown).

Evidence that in vivo estradiol receptor translocated into the nuclei is dephosphorylated and released into the cytoplasm. Little is known regarding the mechanism whereby
most of the estradiol receptor translocated in complex with
hormone into the nuclei in intact cells rapidly disappears
(9). We have seen from the foregoing sections that the receptor is a phosphoprotein and that in vitro its phosphorylation-dephosphorylation regulates its hormone binding activity. In addition, our findings suggest that in vivo after
the receptor has translocated into the nuclei the nuclear
phosphatase causes it to lose its hormone binding. The in-

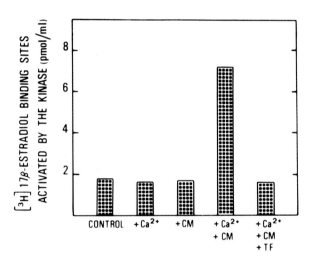

FIG. 5. *Stimulation of kinase activation of hormone binding
of 17β-estradiol receptor by Ca^{2+}-calmodulin.*
    *Purified calf uterus receptor was partially inactivated'
by incubation with the phosphatase, and then used as substrate of the kinase. The binding activation of the receptor by
the kinase was measured after 10 min of incubation at 15° C
in TGD-buffer (50 mM Tris-HCl, pH 7.4, containing 0.2 mM EGTA
and 2 mM dithiothreitol) supplemented with 10 mM $MgCl_2$, 10 mM
Na_2MoO_4, kinase and 0.15 mM ATP. Concentrations of compounds
in the mixture were: 0.8 mM $CaCl_2$, 1.8 μM calmodulin (CM),
25 μM trifluoperazine (TF) (6).*

active and dephosphorylated receptor could be subsequently
released from the nuclei into the cytosol. Should this be
the case, it is reasonable to suppose that nuclear translocation of receptor is followed by the appearance in the cytosol of receptor that does not bind hormone and that can

be reactivated by the cytosol kinase. It also follows that
the amount of receptor so reactivated corresponds to the a-
mount of receptor missing from the cells.

To test this hypothesis, 5 days-ovariectomized mice were
injected with 2 µg estradiol and killed at different times
after injection. Hormone binding activity of receptor was as
sayed in the nuclear fraction by NaSCN exchange method (17)
and in crude cytosol before (cytosol binding activity) and
after 10 min incubation with ATP (5). The increase in hormone binding due to incubation with ATP has been called ATP-
activated cytosol binding activity. Fig. 6 shows the results
averaged from 3 different experiments. In control mice (0 ti
me), most of the hormone binding of the receptor occurs in
the cytosol. No increase of this binding is observed after

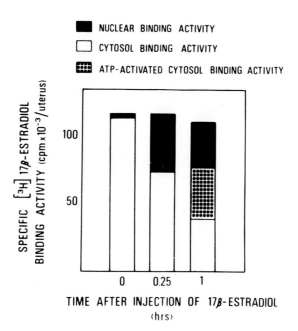

FIG. 6. *Time course of subcellular distribution of 17β-
estradiol receptor and of the appearance of cytosol ATP-
activated receptor from mouse uterus after a single injection of 17β-estradiol.*

incubation of cytosol with ATP. 15 min after hormone injection a significant portion of receptor is translocated into
the nuclei from the cytoplasm. Again incubation of cytosol
with ATP does not modify hormone binding. 1 hour after estra
diol injection the so-called "nuclear processing of receptor"
(9) is observed: nuclear and cytosol hormone binding are

decreased. However this decrease is only apparent since incubation of cytosol with ATP induces an increase of specific
17β-estradiol binding to levels similar to those in control
mice. This result strongly supports our hypothesis that after its nuclear translocation the receptor is inactivated
by the phosphatase, then released into the cytoplasm.

To visualize the kinase-induced activation of hormone
binding of the cytosolic receptor that follows hormone treatment, uterus cytosols from not injected and 1 hr injected
mice were incubated with [³H]17β-estradiol and submitted to
sucrose gradient under "low salt" conditions. In treated mice, most of the cytosol receptor disappears, while in untreated animals it sediments in two peaks (Fig. 7). Incubation with ATP of 1 hr injected mouse uterus cytosol restores the receptor hormone binding.

Receptor can be separated from kinase by heparin-sepharose chromatography of uterus cytosol (4). Cytosol from non
injected and 1 hr 17β-estradiol injected mice has been submitted to this procedure and after separation, receptors
and kinases were mixed to obtain different combinations.
Kinase from untreated or treated mice does not significantly stimulate hormone binding of receptor from not injected
mice, whereas kinase from both treated and untreated animals stimulates binding of receptor from injected mice (5).
This result shows that hormone treatment modifies receptor
rather than kinase and supports our hypothesis that the receptor no longer found in the nuclei, is released into the
cytoplasm in an inactive, dephosphorylated form.

Several conclusions emerge from our results:
1. A phosphatase that dephosphorylates the estradiol receptor and inactivates its hormone binding activity is present
in the nuclei of mouse and calf estrogen target tissues.
2. A kinase that phosphorylates the receptor and activates
its hormone binding activity is present in the cytosol of
mouse and calf uterus. This kinase is stimulated by Ca^{2+}-
calmodulin.
3. Nuclear translocation of receptor in uterus of mice
injected with 17β-estradiol is followed by the appearance
of dephosphorylated receptor in the cytosol, thereby suggesting that the phosphatase is responsible for the disappearance of receptor translocated to nuclei in vivo, and
that the receptor,once dephosphorylated, is released from
the nuclei into the cytosol.
4. Receptor complexed with non steroidal antiestrogens such
as nafoxidine and tamoxifen is not inactivated by the phosphatase; this implies that the long half-life of nuclear

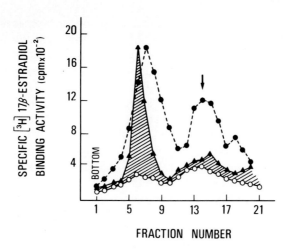

FIG.7. Sedimentation patterns through sucrose gradient of spe-cific [³H]17β-estradiol-binding activity of uterine cytosol from untreated mice and from mice injected with 17β-estradiol.

Two groups of 5 adult ovariectomized mice were used. One group was killed untreated, the other was killed 1 hr after injection with 2 μg 17β-estradiol. Uteri were homogenized and cytosols supplemented with 12 nM [³H]17β-estradiol of high and low specific activity and incubated at 0° C for about 30 min. 10 mM Na₂MoO₄ and 10 mM MgCl₂ were then added and the cytosol was incubated at 15° C for 10 min with and without 10 mM ATP. Samples were left over night at 0° C, then treated with char-coal and 0.3 ml aliquots were layered on the top of 10-35% (w/v) sucrose gradients. Centrifugation was performed at 55,000 rpm for 2 hrs at 2° C. The arrow indicates the peak of the re-ference protein, bovine plasma albumin. Symbols: Binding ac-tivity of uterine cytosol incubated without ATP from untreated mice (●—●) and binding activity of uterine cytosol incubated in the absence (○—○) or in presence of ATP (▲—▲) from hor-mone treated mice. The shaded area represents the ATP-activated cytosol binding activity (5).

receptor-antiestrogen complexes <u>in vivo</u> is the consequence of refractoriness of this complex to the phosphatase activi-ty.

In an attempt to integrate our findings with the general-ly accepted model of mechanism of action of estrogens we pro-pose the following hypothesis: the cytosol receptor must be phosphorylated by the receptor-kinase before it can bind

17β-estradiol. In the presence of 17β-estradiol,the receptor-
hormone complex migrates into nuclei where the phosphatase
inactivates the hormone binding of the receptor; this inacti
vation is prevented when the receptor is translocated into
nuclei in complex with non steroidal antihormones. The pho-
sphatase-inactivated receptor is released into the cytoplasm
where it might be either recycled by the kinase, or irreversibly lost, for instance, by proteolysis. Our hypothetical
model is illustrated in Fig. 8.

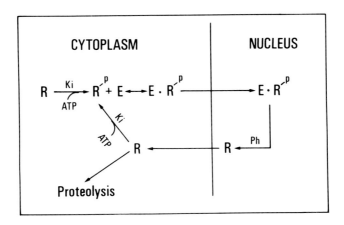

FIG. 8 *Hypothetical model of mechanism of action of estradiol*
Abbreviations: E = estradiol; R = dephosphorylated receptor;
K_i = *receptor-kinase; Ph = receptor-phosphatase; R-P = pho-*
sphorylated receptor

This research was supported by grant no. 82.00220.96
from "Progetto Finalizzato Controllo della Crescita Neo-
plastica".

REFERENCES

1. Auricchio, F. and Migliaccio, A. (1980):FEBS Letters,
   117: 224-226.
2. Auricchio, F., Migliaccio, A. and Rotondi, A. (1981):
   Biochem. J., 194: 569-574.

3. Auricchio, F., Migliaccio, A. and Castoria, G. (1981):
   Biochem. J., 198: 699-702.
4. Auricchio, F., Migliaccio, A., Castoria, G., Lastoria,S.
   and Schiavone, E. (1981): Biochem. Biophys. Res. Comm.,
   101: 1171-1178.
5. Auricchio, F. Migliaccio, A., Castoria, G., Lastoria,S.
   and Rotondi, A. (1982): Biochem. Biophys. Res. Comm.,
   106: 149-157.
6. Auricchio, F., Migliaccio, A., Castoria, G., Rotondi,A.
   and Lastoria, S. (1984): J. Steroid Biochem. in press.
7. Cohen, S., Clinkers, M. and Ushiro, H. (1981): Cold
   Spring Harb. Conference on cell Proliferation. 8:801-808
8. Dougherty, J.J., Puri, R.K. and Toft, D.I. (1982): J.
   Biol. Chem., 257: 14226-14230.
9. Horwitz, K.B. and Mc Guire, W.L. (1978): J. Biol. Chem.
   253: 8185-8191.
10. Housley, P.R. and Pratt, W.B. (1983): J. Biol. Chem.
    258: 4630-4638.
11. Kasuga, M., Karlsson, F.A. and Kahn, C.R. (1982):
    Science, 215: 185-187.
12. Migliaccio, A., Lastoria, S., Moncharmont, B., Rotondi,
    A. and Auricchio, F. (1982): Biochem. Biophys. Res.
    Comm., 109: 1002-1010.
13. Molinari, A.M., Medici, N., Moncharmont, B. and Puca,
    G.A. (1977): Proc. Natl. Acad. Sci. U.S.A., 74: 4886-
    4890.
14. Moncharmont, B., Su, J.L. and Parikh, I. (1982):
    Biochemistry, 21: 6916-6921.
15. Puca, G.A., Medici, N., Molinari, A.M., Moncharmont, B.,
    Nola, E. and Sica, V. (1980): J. Steroid Biochem., 12:
    105-113.
16. Sica, V. and Bresciani, F. (1979): Biochemistry, 18:
    2369-2378.
17. Sica, V., Puca, G.A., Molinari, A.M., Buonaguro, F.M.
    and Bresciani, F. (1980): Biochemistry, 19: 83-88.
18. Weigel, N.L., Task, J.S., Means, A.R., Schraeder, W.T.
    and O' Malley, B.W. (1981): Biochem. Biophys. Res. Comm.
    102: 513-519.

Progress in Cancer Research and Therapy,
Vol. 31, edited by F. Bresciani, et al.
Raven Press, New York © 1984.

Physicochemical Characterization of Estrogen Receptors from a Rabbit Endometrial Carcinoma Model

*Nahid A. Shahabi, *T. William Hutchens, *James L. Wittliff,
**Stephen D. Halmo, **Mary Ellen Kirk, and **Jeffrey A. Nisker

*Department of Biochemistry and James Graham Brown Cancer Center, University of
Louisville, Louisville, Kentucky 40292; and **Department of Obstetrics and
Gynecology, University of Western Ontario, London, Canada*

Steroid hormone receptors are elusive proteins which have been investigated both in regard to their biological significance as well as their physicochemical properties. However, the native state of the estrogen receptor remains uncharacterized largely. There is evidence that steroid hormone receptors exist in multiple forms (6,7,14) which we term isoforms because each component binds the same steroid hormone with high affinity and specificity. Our laboratory has been a proponent of the view that these multiple forms appear to be related to biological function (14,15). This statement is based primarily upon clinical response data from patients with breast cancer (13-15). The fact remains that some of these women (~40%) whose breast tumors contain estrogen receptors are unresponsive to endocrine manipulation suggesting that there may be differences in the intracellular cascade for estrogen action (1,8).

As part of a long term study of the structure/function relationships of the isoforms of estrogen receptors, we initiated studies of their size, shape and surface charge heterogeneity in a variety of hormone target organs, both normal and neoplastic (2,12-16). The present study is directed toward a comparison of these properties of estrogen receptors in an aging rabbit model for endometrial carcinoma. Properties related to receptor size and shape were evaluated simultaneously by sucrose density gradient centrifugation, Sephacryl S-300 chromatography and high performance size exclusion chromatography. In addition their surface charge heterogeneity was determined by high performance chromatofocusing (6). These data suggest that this model tumor exhibits molecular heterogeneity of estrogen receptors and that certain of these isoforms are interrelated. To ascertain if this receptor heterogeneity is related to the neoplastic state of the uterus, a parallel investigation was conducted with normal tissue (Shahabi, Hutchens and Wittliff, in preparation).

METHODS AND MATERIALS

Reagents and Chemicals

The ligand used for this study, $[16\alpha-^{125}I]$iodoestradiol-17ß was obtained from New England Nuclear. Unlabeled diethylstilbestrol (DES), Norite A, Dextran T-70, sodium molybdate and dithiothreitol (DTT) were purchased from Sigma Chemical Co. K_2HPO_4, KH_2PO_4, KCl, disodium ethylene diaminetetraacetic acid (EDTA) and glycerol were obtained from Fisher Scientific Co. Polybuffers 96 and 74, and Sephacryl S-300 gel were purchased from Pharmacia Fine Chemicals. The purified unlabeled proteins used as markers were obtained from Sigma.

Animals and Tissues

Aged (36-42 mo) New Zealand white rabbits were first examined for the presence of endometrial lesions which appeared spontaneously between this age and 55-60 mo (4). Uterine endometria were removed surgically, deep frozen in liquid nitrogen and stored at -86°C.

Preparation of Cytosol

Tissues were minced on ice and homogenized using a Brinkman Polytron (two-10 sec bursts) in 2 vol PEDG buffer (10 mM K_2HPO_4/KH_2PO_4, 1.5 mM EDTA, 1 mM DTT, 10% (v/v) glycerol, pH 7.4 at 4°C) with or without 10 mM sodium molybdate. Homogenates were centrifuged at 40,000 rpm in a Beckman Ti 70.1 rotor for 45 min to sediment particulate material. All procedures were carried out at 0-4°C.

Cytosols were incubated with 2-3 nM [^{125}I]iodoestradiol-17ß for 6-24 hr at 0-4°C (14) in the presence or absence of 200 to 250-fold molar excess of unlabeled competitor (DES). The reactions were terminated by their addition to pellets derived from an equal volume of 1% Dextran-coated charcoal suspension (1% Norite A, 0.5% Dextran). After 10 min incubation, labeled cytosol was centrifuged at 3,000 rpm for 10 min to sediment the charcoal.

Sucrose Density Gradient Centrifugation

Linear gradients of 5-20% (w/v) sucrose were prepared in PEDG buffer with or without 10 mM sodium molybdate, either in the presence or absence of 400 mM KCl, pH 7.4 at 0-4°C. Cytosols (200 µl) prepared in PEDG buffer with or without molybdate were applied to sucrose gradients and centrifuged in a SW60 Ti rotor at 60,000 rpm for 16 hr at 0-4°C ($\omega^2 t$ = 2.25 x 10^{12}).

High Performance Size Exclusion Chromatography (HPSEC)

All chromatography was performed in a cold room at 0-4°C. Estrogen-labeled cytosol (100-200 µl) was applied to Spherogel TSK-3000 SW size exclusion columns (7.5 x 700 mm including a 100 mm guard column) with a Beckman Model 322 HPLC system (11,14). The elution buffer was $P_{50}EDG$ (50 mM KH_2PO_4/K_2HPO_4 containing 1.5 mM EDTA, 1 mM DTT, 10% (v/v) glycerol, pH 7.4 at 4°C) either with or without 10 mM sodium molybdate and/or 400 mM KCl. All buffers were filtered utilizing a 0.45 µM filter (Millipore Corp.). Elution was carried out at a flow rate of 0.5 ml/min.

High Performance Chromatofocusing (HPCF)

SynChropak AX-500 (4.1 mm-ID x 250 mm) anion exchange columns (SynChrom, Inc.) with the Altex Model 210 sample injection valve (Beckman Instruments) were used (14). The column initially was equilibrated with 25 mM Tris-HCl buffer containing 1 mM DTT, 20% glycerol (v/v) pH 8.3 at 0-4°C. Sodium molybdate (10 mM) was included in the column equilibration buffer for certain experiments of molybdate-stabilized receptor components (6).

Two separate polyampholyte buffers were used for elution. The primary eluting buffer was a 30/70 mixture of polybuffers 96 and 74 diluted 1:15 with 20% glycerol and adjusted to pH 5.0 at 0-4°C. The secondary eluting buffer was polybuffer 74 diluted 1:10 with 20% glycerol and adjusted to pH 3.0 at 0-4°C. When cytosol was prepared in the buffer containing molybdate, column

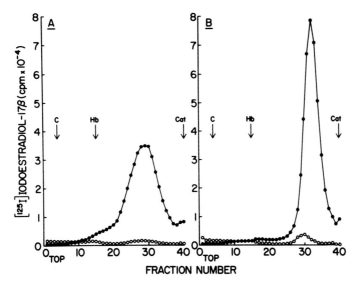

FIG. 1. Separation of Estrogen Receptors Using Sucrose Density Gradient Centrifugation. Cytosol was prepared either without (A) or with 10 mM sodium molybdate (B) and labeled with 2-3 nM [^{125}I]iodoestradiol-17ß in the absence (●) or presence (o) of a 200-fold excess of DES as described in Methods. Estrogen receptors were separated in low salt-containing gradients which had been prepared either without (A) or with molybdate (B). Arrows indicate the positions of the marker proteins; cytochrome C (C), hemoglobin (Hb) and catalase (Cat).

equilibration and primary eluent also contained 10 mM sodium molybdate while the secondary elution polybuffer had no molybdate. For all experiments, 1 ml fractions were collected at 1 ml/min. Columns were regenerated to their starting pH (8.3) with fresh equilibration buffer.

Sephacryl S-300 Chromatography

Sephacryl S-300 gel filtration columns (1.5 cm-ID x 85 cm) were packed according to the manufacturer's protocol (Pharmacia). $P_{50}EDG$ buffer with or without 10 mM sodium molybdate was used for receptor elution. Fractions (1 ml) were collected at 11.3 cm/hr. Blue-Dextran 2000 was used to determine the void volume while a variety of purified proteins served as markers (10).

RESULTS AND DISCUSSION

To ascertain the physicochemical relationship between the different estrogen receptor isoforms, a number of separation methods were utilized. The results presented here represent simultaneous analyses of estrogen receptors by sucrose density gradient centrifugation, size exclusion chromatography using both Sephacryl S-300 and HPSEC with TSK-3000 SW columns, as well as by high performance chromatofocusing.

Sucrose Density Gradient Centrifugation

Although this procedure has limitations regarding its accuracy of assessing receptor size and shape, it has the advantage of evaluating hydrodynamic properties in a gentle and reproducible fashion. Figures 1A and 1B are

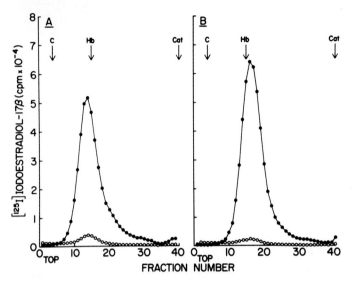

FIG. 2. Separation of Estrogen Receptors Using Sucrose Density Gradient Centrifugation. Cytosol was prepared either without (A) or with 10 mM sodium molybdate (B) and labeled with 2-3 nM [125I]iodoestradiol-17ß in the absence (●) or presence (o) of a 200-fold excess of DES as described in Methods. Estrogen receptors were separated in gradients containing 400 nM KCl which had been prepared either without (A) or with molybdate (B). Arrows indicate the positions of the marker proteins; cytochrome C (C), hemoglobin (Hb) and catalase (Cat).

representative sucrose gradient profiles of cytosolic estrogen receptors of rabbit endometrial carcinoma prepared and sedimented in the presence and absence of 10 mM sodium molybdate at low ionic strength. In each case, only a single form of receptor was readily apparent, always in the 8-9S region. However, if 10 mM sodium molybdate was added to both homogenizing buffer and sucrose solution, the peak activity was sharper (Fig. 1B). All of the profiles indicated very low non-specific binding. In the presence of 400 mM KCl, either in the presence or absence of molybdate, the 8-9S component in the cytosol appeared as 4-5S forms (Fig. 2A,B). The findings are consistent with the results of a number of investigators using a variety of receptors (3,5,9).

Separation of Estrogen Receptors by HPSEC

A representative profile of cytosol proteins separated by HPSEC using a TSK-3000 SW column is shown in Fig. 3. These receptors were extracted in PEDG buffer in the absence and presence of 10 mM molybdate as described in Methods. Under these conditions and in low ionic strength, the specific estrogen binding capacity was distributed primarily as a high molecular weight species (71-76Å) eluting just after the void volume of the column. This component may be analogous to the 8-9S form observed with sucrose gradient centrifugation where again a single species was exhibited. Non-specific binding was virtually absent whether or not molybdate was included.

When the same cytosols were eluted with high ionic strength buffers, a single high molecular weight form (71-61Å) was observed in the presence of molybdate (Fig. 4B). However in the absence of molybdate, two forms of estrogen receptors, a high molecular weight entity (66Å) and a species with Stokes radius of 36Å were identified (Fig. 4A). The non-specific binding in both cases was very low as observed in the other experiments.

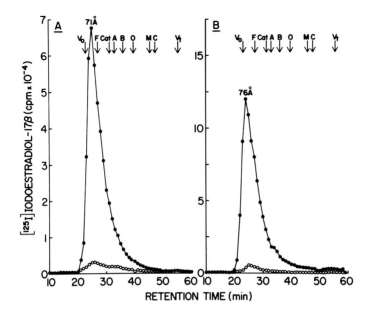

FIG. 3.   Separation of Estrogen Receptors by High Performance Size Exclusion Chromatography.   Cytosols were prepared in PEDG buffer either without (A) or with (B) 10 mM sodium molybdate and incubated with [^{125}I]iodoestradiol-17ß in the absence (●) or presence (○) of a 200-fold excess of DES.   Estrogen receptors were eluted in P$_{50}$EDG buffer without KCl either in the absence (A) or presence (B) of 10 mM sodium molybdate.   Arrows indicate the position of protein markers: ferritin (F), catalase (Cat), human serum albumin (A), bovine serum albumin (B), ovalbumin (O), myoglobin (M), cytochrome C (C); V$_o$ represents the void volume and V$_t$ represents the total volume of the column.

As we have observed earlier with estrogen receptors from lactating mammary gland of the rat and from human breast cancer (11,14), the predominant form exhibits a Stoke's radius of approximately 70Å using HPSEC.   However in the absence of sodium molybdate in high ionic strength buffers, most of the estrogen-receptors in cytosol of endometrial carcinoma separated as a component having a Stoke's radius of 36Å.   The larger species was present also but in smaller amounts.

Separation of Estrogen Receptors using Sephacryl S-300 Chromatography

Using Sephacryl S-300 as a means of separation, three distinct species of estrogen binding proteins were identified in cytosol of the rabbit endometrial carcinoma (Fig. 5).   This profile consists of two high molecular weight isoforms, one appearing immediately after the void volume with Stoke's radius of >85Å and the other with a Stoke's radius of 65Å.   The third isoform which separated from the others as a sharp peak having Stoke's radius of 30Å (Fig. 5A).   Interestingly, when cytosol was extracted with buffer containing 10 mM molybdate, only a single species was exhibited which had a Stoke's radius of 65Å (Fig. 5B).
This type of separation is representative of the isoforms detected in cytosol from rabbit endometrial cancer.

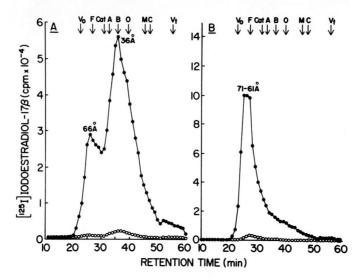

FIG 4.   Separation of Estrogen Receptors by High Performance Size Exclusion Chromatography.   Cytosols were prepared in PEDG buffer either without (A) or with (B) 10 mM sodium molybdate and incubated with [^{125}I]iodoestradiol-17ß in the absence (•) or presence (o) of a 200-fold excess of DES.   Estrogen receptors were eluted in P_{50}EDG buffer with 400 mM KCl either in the absence (A) or presence (B) of 10 mM sodium molybdate.   Arrows indicate the position of protein markers: ferritin (F), catalase (Cat), human serum albumin (A), bovine serum albumin (B), ovalbumin (0), myoglobin (M), cytochrome C (C), V_0 represents the void volume and V_t represents the total volume of the column.

These experiments clearly suggest that sodium molybdate preserves the integrity of a single form (65Å) of the estrogen receptor which may be closely related to the native state.   Similar observations have been reported by other workers (10).   The origin of the high molecular weight species with a Stoke's radius of >85Å is of particular interest to our laboratory.   Currently we are determining if this isoform represents a precursor of the estrogen receptor or simply an aggregate of lower molecular weight forms.

Separation of Estrogen Receptors by HPCF

Recently we have described a new method of rapidly assessing isoforms of estrogen receptors based upon surface charge heterogeneity which give recoveries of >90% (6).   The profile shown in Fig. 6 was generated by chromatofocusing on a AX-500 column using the polybuffers described in Methods. In the absence of sodium molybdate, three distinct species of estrogen binding proteins were eluted at pH 6.8, 6.4 and 5.6.   In contrast when cytosol was prepared with buffer containing 10 mM sodium molybdate, the peaks of activity were focused at pH 4 and 3 as shown in Fig. 7.   When portions of this same cytosol were incubated with the excess of unlabeled competitor (DES) to determine the level of non-specific binding, small amounts of activity were seen at pH 5.5 in the absence of molybdate and at pH 6.2 in the presence of molybdate.

The acidic receptor species in cytosol from rabbit endometrial carcinoma observed in the pH 3-4 region appear similar to those we detected in human uterine cytosol (6).   As seen in our earlier study, the inclusion of sodium

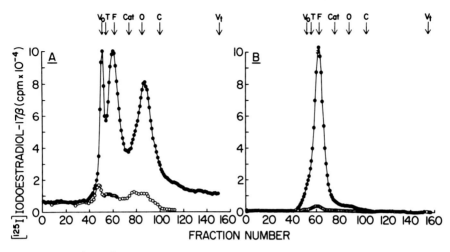

FIG. 5. Separation of Estrogen Receptor Isoforms by Sephacryl S-300. Cytosols were prepared either without (A) or with 10 mM sodium molybdate (B) and labeled with [^{125}I]iodoestradiol-17ß in the absence (●) or presence (o) of a 200-fold excess of DES. After termination of the reaction, a 500 μl aliquot of each was applied to the Sephacryl columns and eluted with P$_{50}$EDG buffer either containing (B) or in the absence (A) of sodium molybdate at a flow rate of 11.3 cm/hr. Arrows indicate the positions of the marker proteins: thyroglobin (T), ferritin (F), catalase (C), ovalbumin (0), cytochrome C (C); V$_O$ represents the void volume and V$_t$ represents the total volume of the column.

molybdate, a commonly used receptor-stabilizing agent, was compatible with HPCF unlike conventional isoelectricfocusing. Whether these isoforms represent intermediates in the processing of larger species of estrogen receptors or dissociation of subunits is the focus of current studies.

SUMMARY

We have examined the size, shape and surface charge properties of estrogen receptors in cytosol prepared from endometrial carcinoma of aging rabbits (Table 1). Sucrose density gradient centrifugation revealed a single form of estrogen receptors with a sedimentation coefficient of 8-9S. Similarly, high performance size exclusion chromatography using a TSK-3000SW column showed the presence of only a single large species (Stokes radius 60-70Å). Only with 0.4 M KCl were smaller 4-5S (30Å) species observed during these analyses. However, under low salt conditions, gel filtration chromatography using Sephacryl S-300 indicated the presence of 3 distinct species with apparent Stokes radii of >85Å, 60-65Å and 28-30Å. Similarly, by high performance chromatofocusing using AX-500 anion exchange columns, 3 species of estrogen receptors were seen with elution pH values of 6.8, 6.4 and 5.4. Interestingly, with 10 mM sodium molybdate, neither the sedimentation coefficient nor the HPSEC profiles were altered while those from Sephacryl S-300 showed the presence of only the 60-70Å species. Sodium molybdate also altered the chromatofocusing profile. As with estrogen receptors from human uterus (6), in the presence of molybdate only 2 relatively acidic species of estrogen receptor were apparent eluting between pH 3 and 4. Currently we are comparing these results with those obtained with normal rabbit endometrial tissues to ascertain the interrelationships of the various forms of estrogen receptors.

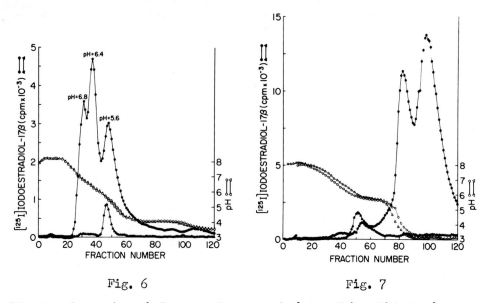

Fig. 6   Fig. 7

FIG. 6.   Separation of Estrogen Receptor Isoforms Using High Performance Chromatofocusing. Cytosol was prepared as described in Methods in the absence of sodium molybdate and labeled with [^{125}I]iodoestradiol-17ß in the absence (•) or presence (o) of a 200-fold excess of DES.   After application to an AX-500 column, elution was accomplished at a flow rate of 1 ml/min using a 30/70 mixture of polybuffers 96/74 diluted 1:15 with 20% glycerol and adjusted to pH 3.5.

FIG. 7.   Separation of Estrogen Receptor Isoforms Using High Performance Chromatofocusing. Cytosol was prepared as described in Methods in the presence of 10 mM sodium molybdate and labeled with [^{125}I]iodoestradiol-17ß in the absence (•) or presence (o) of a 200-fold excess of DES.   After application to an AX-500 column, elution was accomplished at a flow rate of 1 ml/min, first using a 30/70 mixture of polybuffers 96/74 diluted 1:15 with 20% glycerol, and adjusted to pH 5.0.   The second elution was accomplished with polybuffer 74 diluted 1:10 with 20% glycerol and adjusted to pH 3.

Table 1. Summary of properties of estrogen receptor isoforms in the presence and absence of sodium molybdate using different methods of separation.

METHODS	ESTROGEN RECEPTOR ISOFORMS	
	WITHOUT MOLYBDATE	WITH MOLYBDATE
Sucrose Density Gradient Centrifugation	8-9S (4-5S)	8-9S (4-5S)
HPSEC (TSK-3000 SW)	71Å (66 Å & 36 Å)	76Å (71-61Å)
Sephacryl S-300	>85Å & 65Å & 30Å	65Å
HPCF (AX-500)	pH 6.8 & 6.4 & 5.6	pH 4.0 & 3.0

( ) indicate presence of 400 mM KCl.

ACKNOWLEDGEMENTS

The assistance of Mr. Mark Bush is acknowledged. The authors express sincere appreciation to Ms. Debbie Keidel for the preparation of the typescript. This research was supported in part by the Marie Overbey Memorial Grant from the American Cancer Society and by Phi Beta Psi Sorority. N.A.S. is a Research Associate in Cancer Research of the Graduate School.

REFERENCES

1. Anonymous. (1980): Steroid Receptors in Breast Cancer. Cancer, Suppl.46.
2. Daxenbichler, G., Grill, H.J., Wiesinger, H., Wittliff, J.L., and Dapunt, O. (1977): In: Multiple Molecular Forms of Steroid Hormone Receptors, edited by M. K. Agarwal, pp. 163-180. North-Holland Biomedical Press, Elsevier, Amsterdam.
3. Grody, W. W., Compton, J. G., Schrader, W. T., and O'Malley, B. W. (1980): J. Steroid Biochem., 12:115-120.
4. Greene, H.S.N. (1941): J. Exp. Med. 73:273-281.
5. Hutchens, T. W., Markland, F. C., and Hawkins, E. F. (1981): Biochem. Biophys. Res. Commun., 103:60-67.
6. Hutchens, T. W., Wiehle, R. D., Shahabi, N. A., and Wittliff, J. L. (1983): J. Chromatogr., 266:115-128.
7. Kute, T. E., Heidemann, P., and Wittliff, J. L. (1978): Cancer Res., 38:4307-4313.
8. McGuire, W. L., Carbone, P. P. and Vollmer, E. P., eds. (1975): Estrogen Receptors in Human Breast Cancer, Raven Press, New York.
9. Niu, E.M., Neal, R. M., Pierce, V. K., and Sherman, M. R. (1981): J. Steroid Biochem., 15:1-10.
10. Sherman, M. R., Tuazon, FE B., and Miller, L. K. (1980): Endocrinology, 106:1715-1727.
11. Wiehle, R. D., Hofmann, G. E., Fuchs, A., and Wittliff, J. L. (submitted).
12. Wittliff, J. L. (1979): Molec. Aspects Med. 2:395-437.
13. Wittliff, J. L. (1980): Cancer, 46:2953-2960.
14. Wittliff, J. L., Feldhoff, P. W., Fuchs, A., and Wiehle, R. D. (1981): In: Physiopathology of Endocrine Diseases and Mechanisms of Hormone Action, edited by R. S. Soto, A. DeNicola, and J. Blaquier, pp. 375-396. Alan Liss, Inc., New York.
15. Wittliff, J. L., Lewko, W. M., Park, D. C., Kute, T. E., Baker, D. T., Jr., and Kane, L. N. (1978): In: Hormones, Receptors, and Breast Cancer, edited by W. L. McGuire, pp. 325-359. Raven Press, New York.
16. Wittliff, J. L. and Tseng, M. T. (1981): In: Physiopathology of Endocrine Diseases and Mechanisms of Hormone Action, edited by R. Soto, A. F. DeNicola and J. A. Blaquier, pp. 339-373, Alan R. Liss, Inc., New York.

Progress in Cancer Research and Therapy,
Vol. 31, edited by F. Bresciani, et al.
Raven Press, New York © 1984.

Turnover of 3S Androgen Receptors Bound to the Nuclear Matrix of Prostatic Nuclei

P.S. Rennie, N. Bruchovsky, H. Cheng, and J.A. Foekens

Department of Cancer Endocrinology, Cancer Control Agency of British Columbia, Vancouver, B.C., V5Z 3J3 Canada

The nuclear matrix, a spherical, proteinaceous framework structure which is largely devoid of phospholipid and chromatin (2,3), has been implicated as a specific nuclear attachment site for DNA synthesis (11,14) and gene transcription (7,10). Barrack and Coffey (1) reported that nuclear matrices isolated from rat ventral prostate retain over 50% of the total androgen binding sites associated with prostatic nuclei. Subsequently, it was found that these binding sites are due to the presence of 3s androgen receptors tightly bound to the nuclear matrix (9). Since prostatic nuclei contain concentrations of dihydrotestosterone (DHT) several-fold higher than the concentration of androgen receptors (6) and since the functional significance of the nuclear matrix pool of androgen receptors is unknown we performed a series of in vivo experiments to compare the rate of translocation of androgen receptors and the uptake of total androgens into the nuclear matrix and the nuclease/salt extractable chromatin from prostatic nuclei. The results suggest that the androgen receptors associated with the nuclear matrix may regulate the nuclear abundance of non-receptor bound DHT.

ISOLATION OF NUCLEAR MATRICES

Nuclear matrices were isolated from purified nuclei from rat ventral prostates exactly as described by Barrack and Coffey (1). Briefly, the preparation of nuclear matrices involved removal of the nuclear membrane with triton detergent and solubilization of the bulk chromatin with combined DNase I digestion and extraction with 2M NaCl. All buffers used contained 1 mM of the protease inhibitor, PMSF. The isolated nuclear matrices appeared as individual or clumps of intact, spherical structures and retained over 40% of the nuclear protein, 5% of the nuclear DNA and approximately 20% of the nuclear A_{260} units (9). After a pulse injection

(60 min, 150 µCi) of [1,2-^{3}H] testosterone to rats castrated 24 h previously, 50-60% of the total nuclear radioactivity was recovered in association with the nuclear matrices.

ISOLATION OF ANDROGEN RECEPTORS FROM NUCLEAR MATRICES

Following removal of PMSF, brief digestion with the protease, trypsin (0.1 mg/ml, 20°C, 30 min), and centrifugation (20,000 x g for 10 min), approximately 80% of the radioactive androgens retained by the nuclear matrices were recovered in the supernatant fractions. Sucrose density gradient analysis of the supernatant revealed a 3s androgen receptor indistinguishable from the androgen receptor complexes in the nuclease/salt extractable chromatin (9). A similar sedimentation profile was obtained when trypsin digests of prostatic nuclear matrices from non-castrate rats were incubated in vitro at 4°C for 16 h with 1-100 nM of ^{3}H-DHT alone or with a 1000-fold excess of unlabelled DHT (isotope-exchange assay) and applied to sucrose density gradients. Furthermore, the androgen receptors from the nuclear matrices and the bulk chromatin were depleted by over 90% within 24 h after castration. The androgen receptors also possessed similarities with respect to steroid specificities, dissociation constants and concentrations (8,000 to 13,000 androgen receptors per nucleus in each fraction) (9).

NUCLEAR CONCENTRATION OF DHT

A comparison of the total nuclear concentration of androgen receptors (chromatin plus matrix) and the total nuclear concentration of DHT as measured by RIA (6) is shown in Table 1.

TABLE 1.   Nuclear concentration of DHT and androgen receptors in rat prostate

Source of prostates	Concentration (molecules/nucleus)	
	dihydrotestosterone	androgen receptors
Non-castrates	96600 ± 7800 (5)	20500 ± 3750 (4)
Castrates (24 h)	8000 ± 2700 (4)	1500 ± 300 (4)

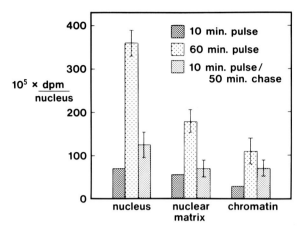

Fig. 1.   The nuclear uptake of ^{3}H-androgens following
administration of ^{3}H-testosterone to 24-h castrate rats.

    In nuclei from the prostates of non-castrate rats only
about 20% of the endogenous nuclear androgen is bound to
androgen receptors. In the prostatic nuclei from castrate
rats there is over a 90% reduction in the concentrations of
both DHT and androgen receptors although the relative ratio
of the two parameters is maintained. This parallelism
together with similarities with regard to steroid specificity, response to anti-androgens (4), and dose relationships (6) suggests that the large nuclear concentration of
non-receptor bound DHT is achieved through a receptor related mechanism. To determine whether the androgen receptors
in the nuclear matrix or in the nuclease/salt extractable
chromatin are involved in this process we compared the
uptake and turnover of radioactive androgens into the matrix
and chromatin following in vivo pulse injections with [3]H-
testosterone (1 µg) and chase injections with unlabelled DHT
(250 µg).

NUCLEAR UPTAKE OF ^{3}H-ANDROGENS

    The results in Fig. 1 show the comparative uptake of
[3]H-androgens into whole nuclei, nuclear matrices and chromatin after a 10 min and 60 min pulse of ^{3}H-testosterone to
24-h castrate rats. Under these conditions the appearance
of radioactivity in each fraction is due to translocation of
androgen receptors (4). After both 10 min and 60 min the
uptake of ^{3}H-androgens into the nuclear matrix occurs at a
slightly faster rate than into the chromatin. This is in
agreement with the observation by Davies et al. (5) that the
nuclease resistant androgen-binding sites in prostatic
nuclei are preferentially replenished relative to the
nuclease sensitive sites in 24-h castrates treated with
androgens.
    In the chase experiments, the 10 min pulse injection
(1 µg) was followed by an injection of unlabelled DHT (250

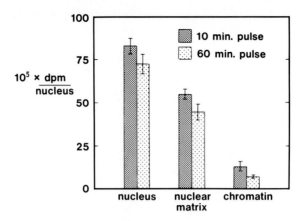

Fig. 2.   The nuclear uptake of ^{3}H-androgens following administration of ^{3}H-testosterone to non-castrated rats.

µg) and then after a further 50 min the radioactivity in each fraction was determined (8).   In the nuclear matrix further accumulation of ^{3}H-androgens beyond the 10 min pulse level was halted; whereas in the chromatin fraction, ^{3}H-androgens continued to increase to a level intermediate between the 10 min and 60 min pulse results.   This indicates that relative to the chromatin the translocation of ^{3}H-androgen-receptor complexes into the nuclear matrix is more readily affected and more sensitive to the dilution of radioactivity caused by the chase dose of DHT.

The results in Fig. 2 show the uptake of ^{3}H-androgens into prostatic nuclei and nuclear fractions following a 10 min and 60 min pulse injection of ^{3}H-testosterone to non-castrated rats.   Since there is very little androgen receptor available for translocation in the prostatic cytosol (12,13), it is likely that most of the ^{3}H-androgen recovered in the nuclear fraction enters through a process not requiring receptor translocation.   The amount of radioactivity re-covered in the whole nuclei after a 10 min pulse is the same as that observed in experiments with the 24-h castrates (Fig. 1) whereas the comparable 60 min pulse levels are considerably lower.   At both time points the concentration of ^{3}H-androgens in the nuclear matrix is several-fold higher than in the chromatin fraction.   This finding implies that under steady state conditions androgens entering the prostatic nucleus accumulate initially in the nuclear matrix.

CONCLUSIONS

Our present results indicate: first, that the 8,000 to 13,000 androgen-binding sites (per nucleus) associated with prostatic nuclear matrices are due to a 3s androgen receptor which can be released by trypsin digestion and which has the same binding characteristics as the 10,000 androgen receptors that are extracted from chromatin with nuclease/salt procedures; second, that in 24-h castrate rats treated with androgens, the replenishment of androgen receptors in the nuclear matrix occurs at a slightly faster rate than in the chromatin; and third, that owing to the preferential accumulation of ^{3}H-androgens in the nuclear matrix under steady state conditions with reduced receptor translocation, it is likely that the large nuclear abundance of endogenous DHT is achieved through a mechanism involving the androgen receptors in the nuclear matrix.

ACKNOWLEDGMENTS

These studies were supported by a grant from the National Cancer Institute of Canada. We thank Cynthia Wells for typing this paper.

REFERENCES

1. Barrack, E.R., and Coffey, D.S. (1980): J. Biol. Chem., 255:7265-7275.

2. Berezney, R. (1980): J. Cell Biol., 85:641-650.

3. Berezney, R., and Coffey, D.S. (1974): Biochem. Biophys. Res. Commun., 60:1410-1417.

4. Callaway, T.W., Bruchovsky, N., Rennie, P.S. and Comeau, T. (1982): The Prostate, 3:599-610.

5. Davies, P., Thomas, P., and Giles, M.G. (1982): The Prostate, 3:439-457.

6. De Larminat, M.-A., Rennie, P.S., and Bruchovsky, N. (1981): Biochem. J., 200:465-474.

7. Faiferman, I., and Pogo, A.O. (1975): Biochemistry, 14:3808-3816.

8. Rennie, P., and Bruchovsky, N. (1973): J. Biol. Chem., 248:3288-3297.

9. Rennie, P.S., Bruchovsky, N., Cheng, H. (1983): J. Biol. Chem., 258:7623-7630.

10. Robinson, S.I., Small, D., Idzerda, R., McKnight, G.S., and Vogelstein, B. (1983): Nucl. Acids Res., 11:5113-5130.

11. Smith, H.C., and Berezney, R. (1982): Biochemistry, 21:6751-6761.

12. Van Doorn, E., and Bruchovsky, N. (1978): Biochem. J., 174:9-16.

13. Van Doorn, E., Craven, S., and Bruchovsky, N. (1976): Biochem. J., 160:11-21.

14. Vogelstein, B., Pardoll, D.M., and Coffey, D.S. (1980): Cell, 22:79-85.

Progress in Cancer Research and Therapy,
Vol. 31, edited by F. Bresciani, et al.
Raven Press, New York © 1984.

Organization and Expression of Prostatic Steroid Binding Protein Genes

Malcolm Parker, Martin Page, and Helen Hurst

Imperial Cancer Research Fund, Lincoln's Inn Fields, London WC2A 3PX, United Kingdom

Prostatic steroid binding protein is the predominant protein secreted into rat prostatic fluid (5). The protein is an oligomer containing C1, C2 and C3 polypeptides (7) whose expression is stimulated by testosterone via effects on transcription rate and RNA turnover (18, 15). In common with other classes of steroid hormone (4, 8) androgens bind to receptors in target cells to form a steroid receptor complex which is translocated into the cell nucleus. To investigate the regulatory role played by testosterone we have cloned the genes for C1, C2 and C3 and characterized their organization (19, 20).

Recent work with other hormone-responsive genes, such as mouse mammary tumour virus whose expression is stimulated by glucocorticoids, suggests that the steroid receptor complex interacts directly with specific DNA sequences adjacent to the viral promoter (23). Evidence that such hormone binding sites operate in vivo comes from gene transfer experiments (10, 12, 13). The role of individual regions of DNA in gene expression can be assessed after introducing mutations into the cloned DNA by analysing the consequences of the mutations after gene transfer.

Our approach to study androgen action has been to introduce the rat C3 genes into a tumour cell line from mouse mammary gland (S115 cells). This cell line was selected because its growth is stimulated by testosterone (26) showing that S115 cells have functional androgen receptors. Selection of transformed cells containing the gene was achieved by using SV2-gpt vectors (14) which contain the gene for the bacterial enzyme xanthine-guanine phosphoribosyl-transferase (gpt). There is no equivalent mammalian enzyme so that wild type cells will not grow in HAT[1] medium containing mycophenolic acid and xanthine because the de novo and salvage pathways for purine biosynthesis are inhibited. However, transformed cells which are expressing the gpt gene will grow providing the medium is supplemented with xanthine. The C3 genes have been introduced into S115 cells either intact or as chimaeric genes. The chimaeric gene consists of putative C3 promoters, and the marker gene interferon (IF), whose expression depends on the C3 promoter. Interferon is secreted from mammalian cells and can be measured in culture medium using a cytopathic effect assay because it

---

[1]Abbreviations: HAT is 250 μg/ml hypoxanthine, 2 μg/ml aminopterin and 10 μg/ml thymidine

confers resistance on cells to viral infection. Thus it is possible to
analyse the effect of different C3 promoters on interferon production
and thereby investigate promoter and regulatory DNA function.

MATERIALS AND METHODS

Reagents

   The following materials were gifts:- reverse transcriptase
(J.Beard, Life Sciences Inc., U.S.A.); mycophenolic acid (V. Mason,
Lilly Research Centre, U.K.); pSV2-gpt (P. Berg, Stanford University,
U.S.A.); mouse S115 cells (R. King, I.C.R.F., London); cyproterone
acetate (Schering AG, Berlin); human β-interferon cDNA (W. Fiers,
State University of Ghent, Belgium); polyoma MboI DNA fragment which
contains poly(A) addition sites (M. Fried, I.C.R.F., London).

Isolation and Characterization of Genomic DNA Clones

   Genomic DNA clones were isolated from Sprague Dawley rat DNA which
had been cloned in bacteriophage λ (19, 20). The clones are designated
as follows: λ11A contains the C1 gene; λ21B contains the C2 gene; λ6
contains the C3(1) gene and λ11B contains the C3(2) gene. The
organization of the four genes was determined by restriction enzyme
mapping. The DNA sequence of the genes for C3 was obtained by subcloning restriction enzyme fragments into the bacteriophage M13
followed by dideoxy sequencing (11).

Construction of Vectors

   The intact C3(1) and C3(2) genes were inserted into SV2-gpt (14) by
digesting λ6 and λ11B with Eco RI and Bam HI respectively and ligating
the genes into the unique Eco RI and Bam HI sites in SV2-gpt as
previously described (16). After transformation of E. coli HB101,
plasmid DNA was isolated using lysozyme and SDS treatment in alkaline
conditions (1).
   The chimaeric gene was constructed by ligating a MboI polyoma DNA
fragment which contains early and late poly(A) addition sites (24) to
human β-interferon cDNA (3). This DNA was then ligated in both
orientations to λ6 DNA from nucleotide -800 to +20 in the C3(1) gene.
The chimaeric gene was then inserted between the Bam HI and Eco RI
sites in SV2-gpt. Full details of the constructions will be published
elsewhere.

Cell Cultures and Transfection Procedures

   S115 cells were maintained and transfected using the calcium
phosphate coprecipitation method as previously described (16).
Interferon was quantitated using a cytopathic effect bioassay (CPE).
Media, which contained interferon was serially diluted onto 10^4 human
embryo fibroblast cells in 96 well dishes for 6 h at 37°C and then
infected with 10^4 pfu of encephalomyocarditis (EMC) virus. After
approximately 30 h cells were stained with crystal violet.

RNA Analysis

Cytoplasmic RNA was isolated using phenol/chloroform (17), C3

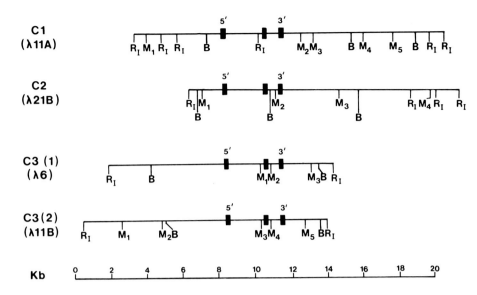

FIG.1.Restriction Enzyme Maps of Prostatic Steroid Binding Protein Genes
The maps were constructed on the basis of restriction enzyme analysis
and R-loop analysis of genomic clones: λ11A for C1, λ21B for C2; λ6 for
C3(1) and λ11B for C3(2). Solid blocks represent exons. The following
restriction enzymes are presented: Bam HI (B), Eco RI (RI) and Msp I (M).

mRNA transcripts were mapped by primer extension using a 70 bp Xba I-
Alu I DNA fragment from the 5' end of pA34 a cDNA clone specific for
C3 mRNA (11).

RESULTS

Gene Organization

The organization of the genes which code for prostatic steroid
binding protein was determined by analysis of genomic DNA clones λ11A
for C1, λ21B for C2, λ6 for C3(1) and λ11B for C3(2). Restriction
enzyme mapping of the recombinant clones indicated that all four genes
were approximately 3.2 Kb and consisted of three exons separated by
two introns (Fig. 1). The genes for C1 and C2 share 76% DNA sequence
homology (19) and the two genes for C3 share 97% DNA sequence homology
(11), suggesting that these two pairs of genes were derived by gene
duplication. The DNA sequence homology between the genes for C1 and
C3 and between the genes for C2 and C3 is less striking being
approximately 35%. However, in view of the similarity in their
organization it is quite conceivable that all four genes have arisen
by a series of gene duplications from a single ancestral gene followed
by divergent evolution (Fig. 2).

Expression of Intact C3 Genes in S115 Cells

Both C3(1) and C3(2) have been introduced into S115 cells using the
SV2-gpt vector shown in Fig. 3.

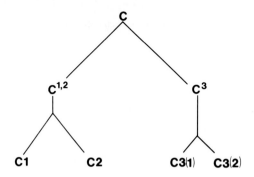

FIG.2.A Putative Evolutionary Tree for Prostatic Steroid Binding Protein
      Genes

     The amount of DNA upstream of the genes ranged from 6,000 bp to 800 bp
for C3(1) and was 4,000 bp for C3(2). Transformed clones were isolated,
checked for the presence of intact C3 genes by Southern blotting and
then analysed for gene expression. Primer extension analysis was used
to map C3 RNA since it both assesses the accuracy of initiation of
transcription and also quantitates the abundance of RNA. C3 RNA from
rat ventral prostate results in major products of 130 nucleotides (T_1)
and a minor product of 170 nucleotides (T_2). Both C3(1) and C3(2) were
accurately transcribed in S115 cells resulting in a major T_1 transcript
and in certain cases a T_2 transcript is just visible (Fig. 4). We
estimate that there are 100–1,000 RNA copies per integrated gene per
cell which represents 0.1–1.0% of the in vivo concentration.

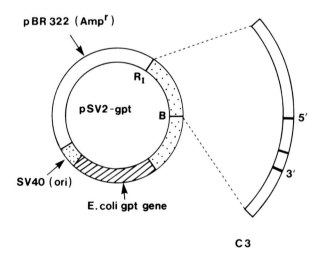

FIG.3.Construction of DNA Vectors which contain the Rat C3 Gene
Genomic clones which contained C3(1) and C3(2) were cloned into pSV2-gpt
(14). The recombinant clones consist of rat C3 exons (solid blocks),
rat C3 introns or flanking DNA (open blocks), plasmid DNA labelled,
pBR322, SV40 DNA (stippled blocks) and E. coli guanine phosphoribosyl
transferase (hatched blocks).

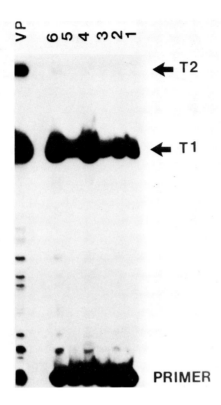

FIG.4.Primer Extension Analysis of C3 RNA expressed in Mouse S115 Cells
Primer extension analysis was carried out with RNA from rat ventral
prostate (VP) and individual mouse S115 clones expressing the C3 gene.
The major extension product of 130-131 nucleotide is labelled T_1 and
the minor extension product of 170 nucleotides is labelled T_2.

The effect of testosterone on C3 gene expression was investigated
by growing the clones in the absence or presence of $10^{-8}M$ testosterone
using 2% foetal calf serum which had been stripped of endogenous
steroids with dextran charcoal treatment (Fig. 5). Individual clones
varied in their response to testosterone irrespective of the amount of
DNA upstream of the C3 gene. About one-third of the clones produced up
to 5-fold more C3 mRNA in the presence of testosterone than in its
absence. Thus in certain clones 800 bp DNA upstream of the C3 gene was
sufficient to confer a small androgenic response. The possibility that
non-responsive clones had lost androgen receptors was ruled out because
their rate of proliferation was still stimulated by testosterone.

Expression of Chimaeric Genes in S115 Cells

We have investigated whether the effect of testosterone on C3 gene
expression was directly on the promoter by analysing the expression of
chimaeric genes. A C3 DNA fragment from the start of transcription to
800 nucleotides upstream was ligated to a marker gene, interferon
(Fig. 5). The putative C3 promoter was inserted in a 5'-3' and 3'-5'
orientation relative to the interferon gene and then ligated into the

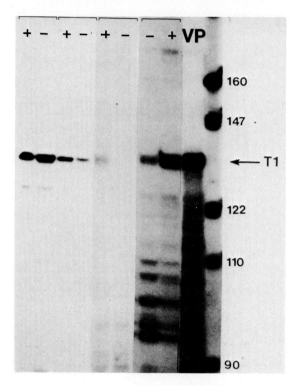

FIG.5.Effect of Testosterone on C3 Gene Expression
Primer extension analysis was carried out with RNA from rat ventral
prostate (VP) and four individual mouse S115 clones which expressed the
C3 gene. The clones were grown in absence (-) or presence (+) of
10^{-8}M testosterone for 3 days prior to the analysis. The major extension
product of 130-131 nucleotides is labelled T_1 and a minor extension
product of 170 nucleotides is just visible. DNA size markers are shown
on the right-hand side.

SV2-gpt vector (14). After transfection into S115 cells, transformed
clones were isolated in HAT medium containing mycophenolic acid plus
xanthine. Six clones contained the promoter in a 5'-3' orientation and
five clones contained the promoter in a 3'-5' orientation. Interferon
gene expression was examined for each clone by testing for interferon
production in the medium using a cytopathic effect bioassay. Human
interferon confers resistance on human embryo fibroblasts to EMC
viral infection and can be quantitated by serial dilution.
    Interferon was produced by $^5/_6$ clones in which the promoter was
inserted in a 5'-3' orientation but not by clones in which the promoter
was inserted in the opposite orientation. This result indicates that
the rat C3 promoter is being used to transcribe interferon mRNA.
Androgen sensitivity was tested as above by growing clones in the
presence or absence of testosterone. None of the clones consistently
produced more than 2-fold more interferon in the presence of testosterone than in its absence as shown in Table 1 and is considered
insignificant.

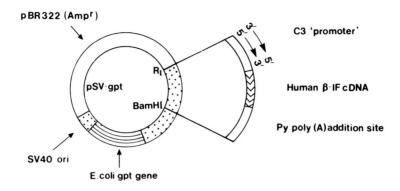

C3 'promoter'

Human β-IF cDNA

Py poly (A) addition site

FIG.6.Construction of DNA Vectors which contain Rat C3 Chimaeric Genes
Chimaeric genes were constructed which consisted of rat C3(1) DNA from
nucleotide -800 to +20 (relative to the 5' end of the gene), human
β-interferon cDNA (IF) and a polyoma poly(A) addition DNA fragment. The
rat DNA was inserted in a 5'-3' and a 3'-5' orientation relative to the
β-interferon cDNA. The chimaeric genes were then cloned between in the
Eco RI and Bam HI sites in pSV2-gpt (14).

DISCUSSION

The introduction of cloned genes into recipient cells and the
analysis of their expression provides an approach for investigating the
role of individual regions of DNA in transcription, RNA processing,
RNA stability and translation. By this means there has been
considerable progress in identifying hormone responsive regions
associated with the gene promoter in the genome of mouse mammary tumour
virus (10, 12, 13) and certain egg white genes (2, 21, 22). This paper
describes our initial attempts to identify testosterone-responsive
regions in the genes which code for C3.

In the rat there are two C3 genes, one of which C3(1), is responsible
for the production of C3 polypeptide and one of which is transcribed
poorly, if at all (11). It has been found that in ventral prostate
the C3(1) gene is demethylated between days 14 and 21 of development
(25) which correlates with the period when prostatic steroid binding
protein can be first detected (6, 9) whereas the C3(2) gene remains

TABLE 1. Effect of Testosterone on IF Production by C3 Chimaeric Gene

Culture conditions	IF titre(medium dilution)	IF/Cell No.(arbitrary units)
4 days +T	32	16.8
4 days -T	24	10.0
4 days -T + CA	32	7.2

Clone 17 was grown in 2% dextran charcoal stripped FCS containing HAT +
MPA selection medium in the presence or absence of testosterone (T) or
cyproterone acetate (CA) as indicated above. Fresh medium was provided
after 3 days and assayed for IF after 4 days using a cytopathic effect
assay.

hypermethylated. In contrast, after transfection into mouse S115 cells, both genes are expressed similarly albeit at a concentration of less than 1% that in ventral prostate. This result indicates that C3(2) is not a pseudogene and that it can be transcribed providing it is unmethylated as was the case in these transfection studies. The obvious question is why the C3(2) gene is not transcribed in vivo especially since the DNA sequence between nucleotide -235 and the first intron of both genes is identical with the exception of 1 nucleotide. We conclude that the promoter for each gene is similar but that DNA signals which are involved in gene activation and perhaps DNA methylation are different in C3(1) and C3(2) and do not reside within the proximal 5' flanking DNA.

We have demonstrated that testosterone stimulated the expression of both C3 genes in certain transformed cell lines when the intact gene was used. However, the hormone does not appear to stimulate trans-cription by interacting with DNA upstream of the gene, at least in these heterologous mouse cells. This result contrasts with that for several glucocorticoid responsive genes such as mouse mammary tumour virus (10, 12, 13) or tryptophan oxygenase (22) but resembles that found for chicken ovalbumin and lysozyme genes. These latter genes respond to hormone in chick oviduct cells but not mammalian cells (2, 21, 22). Therefore it is possible that hormone regulation of certain genes requires tissue specific factors in addition to the steroid receptor complex. To investigate this further, we are analysing the expression of the C3 gene, as a chimaeric gene, in primary cultures of rat ventral prostate.

Acknowledgements. We should like to thank Dr. M. Fried for his advice, Mr. R. White and Mr. M. Needham for their technical assistance and Mrs. M. Barker for typing the manuscript.

REFERENCES

1. Birnboim, H.C., and Doly, J. (1979): Nucleic Acids Res., 7:1513-1523.
2. Dean, D.C., Knoll, B.J., Riser, M.E., and O'Malley, B.W. (1983): Nature 305:551-554.
3. Derynck, R., Content, J., Declercq, E., Volckaert, G., Tavernier, J., Devos, R., and Fiers, W. (1980): Nature 285:542-547.
4. Gorski, J., and Gannon, F. (1976): Ann.Rev.Physiol., 38:425-450.
5. Heyns, W., and DeMoor, P. (1977): Eur.J.Biochem., 78:221-230.
6. Heyns, W., Vandamme, B., and DeMoor, P. (1978): Endocrinology 103: 1090-1095.
7. Heyns, W., Peeters, B., Mous, J., Rombauts, W., and DeMoor, P. (1978): Eur. J. Biochem., 89:181-186.
8. Higgins, S.J., and Gehring, U. (1978): Adv.Cancer Res., 28:313-393.
9. Higgins, S.J., Smith, S.E., and Wilson, J. (1982): Mol.Cell Endocrinol., 27:55-56.
10. Huang, A.L., Ostrowski, M.C., Berard, D., and Hager, G.L. (1981): Cell 27:245-255.
11. Hurst, H., and Parker, M.G. (1983): EMBO J., 2:769-774.
12. Hynes, N.E., van Ooyen, A.J.J., Kennedy, N., Herrlich, P., Ponta, H., and Groner, B. (1983): Proc.natn.Acad.Sci.U.S.A., 80:3637-3641.
13. Lee, F., Mulligan, R., Berg, P., and Ringold, G. (1981): Nature 294: 228-232.
14. Mulligan, R.C., and Berg, P. (1981): Proc.natn.Acad.Sci.U.S.A., 78: 2072-2076.
15. Page, M.J., and Parker, M.G. (1982): Mol. Cell. Endocrinol., 27: 343-355.

16.Page, M.J., and Parker, M.G. (1983): Cell 32:495-502.

17.Parker, M.G., and Mainwaring, W.I.P. (1977): Cell 12:401-407.

18.Parker, M.G., Scrace, G.T., and Mainwaring, W.I.P. (1978): Biochem. J., 170:115-121.

19.Parker, M.G., Needham, M., White, R., Hurst, H., and Page, M. (1982): Nucleic Acids Res. 10:5121-5132.

20.Parker, M.G., White, R., Hurst, H., Needham, M., and Tilly, R. (1983): J.Biol.Chem., 258:12-15.

21.Renkawitz, R., Beng, H., Graf, T., Matthias, P., Grez, M., and Schütz, G. (1982): Cell 31:167-176.

22.Renkawitz, R., Danesch, U., Matthias, P., and Schütz, G. (1983): J. Steroid Biochem. (in press).

23.Scheideret, C., Geisse, J., Westphal, H.M., and Beato, M. (1983): Nature 304:749-752.

24.Soeda, E., Arrand, J.R., Smolar, N., Walsh, J.E., and Griffin, B.E. (1980): Nature (London) 283:445-453.

25.White, R.W., and Parker, M.G. (1983): J.Biol.Chem., 258:8943-8948.

26.Yates, J., and King, R.J.B. (1981): J. Steroid Biochem., 14:819-822.

Progress in Cancer Research and Therapy,
Vol. 31, edited by F. Bresciani, et al.
Raven Press, New York © 1984.

Interaction of Glucocorticoid Hormone Receptors with Defined DNA Sequences of Inducible Genes

C. Scheidereit, P. Krauter, H.M. Westphal, and M. Beato

Institut für Physiologische Chemie, Universität Marburg, D-3550 Marburg, Federal Republic of Germany

The mechanism by which steroid hormones control gene expression has attracted the attention of many biochemists during the past two decades. Similarities to inducers and repressors of gene activity in procaryotes let this system appear as a suitable model for the study of gene regulation in higher organisms. As their low molecular weight analogues in procaryotes steroid hormones do not act directely on the genome of their target cells. Instead they have first to form a complex with specific proteins called receptors, that mediate their effects on mRNA levels.

The molecular mechanisms of the interaction between the hormone-receptor complex and the genome have been intensively studied during the past ten years. In particular the question of whether specific chromosomal proteins, DNA, or both, act as acceptors for the hormone-receptor complex has been the object of considerable debate, but has remained elusive until recently. The availability of purified receptor preparations and of cloned inducible genes has allowed us to obtained conclusive evidence for an involvement of defined nucleotide sequences in the interaction of steroid hormone receptors with their target genomes.

In this contribution we want to summarize what is known on the binding of glucocorticoid receptors to DNA, and to speculate on the mechanisms by which this interaction could influence transcription of the hormone inducible genes.

FILTER BINDING STUDIES

We have previously shown that activated hormone-receptor complexes have a general affinity for all kind of DNA (3, 6). Indeed differential chromatography on calf thymus DNA cellulose has been one of the main steps used for receptor purification in several laboratories. In order to detect an hypothetical preference for specific DNA sequences it is necessary to quantitate and compare the affinity of the hormone-receptor complex for individual DNA fragments. To this end we have used the well established nitrocellulose filter binding assay, that had yielded good results in procaryotic systems (24). This assay is based on the observation that, under certain conditions, only proteins but not nacked DNA will bind to the filters. Therefore, in an incubation of DNA fragments and receptor, only those DNA fragments that bind to the receptor protein will be retained upon filtration. As source of DNA fragments we decided to use cloned inducible genes since in the procaryotic systems regulatory sequences have been located close to the regulated promoters.

For the initial experiments we choose mouse mammary tumor virus (MMTV) DNA because gene transfer experiments had made very likely that this genetic unit carries the sequences required for its hormonal induction (4,11,12,17). After digestion with appropriate restriction enzymes, the DNA fragments were end-labelled with ^{32}P, and incubated with different preparations of partially purified rat liver glucocorticoid receptor (28,30). We found preferential binding of the hormone receptor complex to DNA fragments containing the right half of the long terminal repeat (LTR), as well as to several fragments originating from the env-gene region and from mouse flanking sequences (12). Similar results were obtained by other groups using either the filter binding technique (20,21), or a competition assay based on binding to calf thymus DNA cellulose (22).

Since the LTR region of MMTV is known to contain the main promoter for viral transcription, we focussed our attention on the interaction of the receptor with this region of MMTV. A set of deletion mutants in this region was used for filter binding studies and for a more specific binding assay based on the immunoprecipitation of receptor-DNA complexes with monoclonal antibodies to the receptor (25,29). With these procedures we could define a region of 152 bp, located between position -50 and -202 upstream of the transcription initiation site, that is essential for receptor binding (25). The same region of the LTR was shown to be required for hormonal inducibility in gene transfer experiments (5,13,31). Thus, these results delimited a glucocorticoid regulatory element that is recognized by the hormone receptor.

Since this element is located within proviral DNA it could represent an exceptional situation evolved by the viral genome to cope with the requirements of viral integration and replication. In order to test the general validity of our findings we decided to study a glucocorticoid inducible cellular gene of non-viral origin. We choose the human metallothionein II$_A$ gene (hMT-II), because it was known to be inducible by glucocorticoids in gene transfer experiments and, therefore, could be expected to carry a glucocorticoid regulatory element (16). Appropriate deletion mutants of this gene were used for gene transfer experiments and filter binding studies and helped to delimit a DNA region, between positions -235 and -300, that is required for both receptor binding and hormonal inducibility (15). Thus, the concept of a clucocorticoid regulatory element that is recognized by the hormone-receptor complex, seems to apply for both viral as well as cellular inducible genes.

DNase I PROTECTION EXPERIMENTS

A direct identification of the DNA sequences involved in the interaction with the hormone-receptor complex was attempted in 'foot-print' experiments (25). In this type of experiments specific binding of a protein to DNA results in protection against DNaseI digestion of that DNA region covered by the binding protein (8). The results of 'foot-print' experiments with the LTR region of MMTV are summarized in Figure 1a. Two strong and two weak binding sites for the glucocorticoid receptor were detected between positions -71 and -192, within the glucocorticoid regulatory element (25). The two strong binding sites, between -105 and -122 and between -163 and -192, are of about the same length and exhibit extensive sequence homology. The two weaker binding sites, between -71 and -102, are shorter and contain the hexanucleotide 5'-TGTTCT-3', that is also present in the strong binding sites (Fig. 1a). Similar results have been obtained by K. Yamamoto and his collaborators, who have also analysed glucocorticoid receptor binding sites in MMTV outside of the LTR (personal communication).

In the case of the hMT-II gene, 'foot-print' experiments also served to delimit a region between positions -242 and -267, that is protected against DNaseI digestion in the presence of the receptor (15). In addition, a weak binding of the receptor to a site around position -324 is also seen (Fig. 1b). Examination of the nucleotide sequence in the binding region of hMT-II, shows that the strong binding site exhibits sequence homology to the corresponding sites in the LTR region of MMTV (Fig. 1). The weaker binding site around position -324 of hMT-II contains the hexanucleotide 5'-TGTCCT-3' in the antisense strand. Since the nucleotides upstream of -280 can be deleted without reducing the extend of hormonal induction in gene transfer experiments, we conclude that binding of the receptor to the -324 site of hMT-II is not required for induction (15).

A comparison of the two strong binding sites in the LTR region of MMTV to the strong binding site in hMT-II, shows that 10 out of 17 nucleotides are preserved in all three sites (Fig. 2). Thus, we can formulate a consensus sequence for the glucocorticoid regulatory element that is recognized by the activated hormone-receptor complex (Fig. 2.). This sequence has been chemically synthesized and will be tested for its ability to bind the receptor and to confer hormon sensitivity to an heterologous promoter.

MECHANISM OF BINDING

Since some nucleotide positions within the consensus sequence are not exactly preserved, probably not all nucleotides protected by the receptor against DNaseI digestion are equally relevant for receptor binding. In an attempt to define more precisely the nature of this interaction we have used the assays of methylation protection and methylation interference.

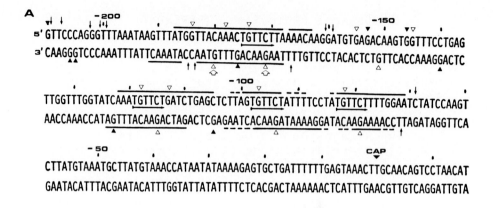

A

```
              -200                                                    -150
5' GTTCCCAGGGTTTAAATAAGTTTATGGTTACAAACTGTTCTTAAAACAAGGATGTGAGACAAGTGGTTTCCTGAG
3' CAAGGGTCCCAAATTTATTCAAATACCAATGTTTGACAAGAATTTTGTTCCTACACTCTGTTCACCAAAGGACTC

                                                   -100
TTGGTTTGGTATCAAATGTTCTGATCTGAGCTCTTAGTGTTCTATTTTCCTATGTTCTTTTGGAATCTATCCAAGT
AACCAAACCATAGTTTACAAGACTAGACTCGAGAATCACAAGATAAAAGGATACAAGAAAACCTTAGATAGGTTCA

      -50                                                   CAP
CTTATGTAAATGCTTATGTAAACCATAATATAAAAGAGTGCTGATTTTTTGAGTAAACTTGCAACAGTCCTAACAT
GAATACATTTACGAATACATTTGGTATTATATTTTCTCACGACTAAAAAACTCATTTGAACGTTGTCAGGATTGTA
```

B

```
                                                        -300
5' CGCGCTAACGGCTCAGGTTCGAGTACAGGACAGGAGGGAGGGGAGCTGTGCACACGGCGGAGGCGCACGGCGTGG
3' GCGCGATTGCCGAGTCCAAGCTCATGTCCTGTCCTCCCTCCCCTCGACACGTGTGCCGCCTCCGCGTGCCGCACC

                  -250
GCACCCAGCACCCGGTACACTGTGTCCTCCCGCTGCACCCAGCCCCTTCAGCCCGAGGCGTCCCCGAGGCGCAAG
CGTGGGTCGTGGGCCATGTGACACAGGAGGGCGACGTGGGTCGGGGAAGTCGGGCTCCGCAGGGGCTCCGCGTTC

   -200                                    -150
TGGGCCGCCTTCAGGGAACTGACCGCCCGCGGCCCGTGTGCAGAGCCGGGTGCGCCCGGCCCAGTGCGCGCGGCC
ACCCGGCGGAAGTCCCTTGACTGGCGGGCGCCGGGCACACGTCTCGGCCCACGCGGGCCGGGTCACGCGCGCCGG

                    -100
GGGTGTTTCCCTTGGAGCCGCAAGTGACTTCTAGCGCGGGGCGTGTGCAGGCACGGCCGGGGCGGGGCTTTTGCA
CCCACAAAGGGAACCTCGGCCGTTCACTGAAGATCGCGCCCCGCACACGTCCGTGCCGGCCCCGCCCCGAAAACGT

   -50                                    CAP
CTCGTCCCGGCTCTTTCTAGCTATAAACACTGCTTCCCGCGCTGCACTCCACCACG
GAGCAGGGCCGAGAAAGATCGATATTTATGACGAAGGGCGCGACGTGAGGTGGTGC
```

Figure 1. <u>Nucleotide sequence around the promoters of the inducible</u>
<u>genes</u>
The nucleotide sequence upstream of the transcription initiation site,
'cap', is shown for a) MMTV-LTR and b) hMT-II. The regions protected
against DNaseI in the presence of the receptor are underlined. Broken
lines denote the uncertainty in establishing the limits of the protected
regions. Sites of enhanced sensitivity to DNaseI in the presence of the
receptor are indicated by arrows. The purine residues undermethylated
in the presence of the receptor are marked by an open triangle, whereas
those which methylation is enhanced by the receptor are indicated by
dark triangles. Numbers refer to positions upstream of the 'cap'site(+1).

Methylation protection

In this assay specific binding of a protein to DNA pro-
tects against methylation by dimethyl sulphate (DMS) only
those purine residues that are in contact with the protein
(19). The methylated residues are identified in sequencing
gels after strand cleavage at the modified positions. Using
this technique we have defined a series of purine residues
within and around the binding sites that are in direct contact with the hormone-receptor complex (Fig. 1 and 2). In all
cases the G:C base pairs within the conserved hexanucleotide
5'-TGTTCT-3' are protected against methylation by DMS in the
presence of the receptor. In general protected G-residues
are separated by 10 ($\frac{+}{-}$) nucleotides and therefore will be
located in one face of the Watson-Crick double helix. Since
the G-residues are selectively methylated at the N7 position
located in the major groove (26), it appears that the receptor contacts the DNA helix from one face through an interaction with residues located in the major groove.

$$5' \qquad\qquad 3'$$

MMTV I	-186	TGGTTACAAACTGTTCT	-170
MMTV II$_A$	-129	TGGTATCAAA·TGTTCT	-113
HMT-II$_A$	-263	CGGT·ACACTGTGTCCT	-248

CONSENSUS: TGGT·ACAAA·TGTTCT
c--- T--CT ---c--

Figure 2. DNA consensus sequence for the binding of the
glucocorticoid receptor

The nucleotide sequence of the two strong binding sites in the LTR
region of MMTV and of the main binding site of hMG-II are aligned to
yield maximal homology. The numbers refer to positions upstream of the
corresponding 'cap' sites. Other symbols are as described in the
legend to Figure 1.

Methylation interference

In this assay partial methylation of the purine residues
is performed prior to the addition of the binding protein.
The influence of methylation at specific sites on protein
binding is analysed by separating protein bound and free DNA
molecules by filtration through nitrocellulose filters,
followed by strand cleavage at the modified positions and
electrophoresis in sequencing gels (26). If methylation at a
particular position interferes with receptor binding, DNA
molecules carrying this modification will be underrepresen-
ted or absent in the population of filter bound DNA fragments. Thus the corresponding band will be weaker or undetectable in sequencing gels from bound DNA molecules, whereas

it will be enhanced in sequencing gels of the free DNA molecules. The results of these experiments essentially confirm
those obtained in methylation protection experiments, and
support the model of receptor binding to the double helix
proposed above.

MECHANISM OF TRANSCRIPTION ACTIVATION

After the demonstration that the hormone-receptor complex
recognizes specific DNA sequences in the neighbourhood of
inducible promoters, the next question concerns the mechanism by which receptor binding leads to enhanced transcription. Gene transfer experiments with chimaeric plasmids have
shown that binding of the receptor to the regulatory element
in the LTR of MMTV activates transcription not only from the
LTR promoter but also from a HSVtk promoter located more
than 400 bp downstream (13). It is also known that the LTR
regulatory element is still active when inserted in the in-
verted orientation more than 800 bp upstream of the HSVtk
promoter (7). These findings are compatible with the idea
that the glucocorticoid regulatory element is transformed into an enhancer upon binding of the hormone-receptor complex.
Enhancer sequences were first discovered in animal viruses
as elements able to stimulate transcription of heterologous
genes, acting in cis over several kilobases irrespective of
their position and orientation (2). Similar tissue specific
elements have been recently described near the immunoglobulin promoter (1,10,23). Unfortunately, little is known about
the mechanism by which enhancer elements stimulate transcription and about DNA sequences required for enhancer activity. In SV40 the 'core' sequence 5'-GTGGtttG-3' is essential for enhancer activity, and this sequence is also found
in other enhancers. Sequences partially homologous to this
'core' element are found in the LTR region of MMTV between
the two strong binding sites for the glucocorticoid receptor
(Fig. 1a, positions -127 to -136 and -141 to -149).

Another interesting feature of the enhancer element of
SV40 is the fact that it contains several Z-DNA segments
(18). It is known that the junctions between B and Z-DNA act
as sites of conformational flexibility of the double helix,
since they are specifically recognized by S1 nuclease (27).
Therefore, these junctions could conceivably serve as entry
sites for RNA polymerase or transcription factors. Interestingly, alternating purine/pyrimidine sequences with the
potential to adopt Z-DNA configuration are present between
the receptor binding sites and the 'cap' site in both the
LTR of MMTV and the hMT-II gene (Fig. 1a, positions -56 to
-47; Fig. 1b, positions -85 to -72 and -304 to -295) it
could be tested in vitro whether binding of the receptor
alters the DNA conformation around these sites.

To elucidate the molecular mechanism of transcriptional
activation it will be ultimately necessary to develop an in
vitro transcription system, in which the receptor function
can be tested under cell-free conditions. Considerable
effort is presently devoted in several laboratories, inclu-

ding our own, to the development of such a cell-free transcription system. Whatever the outcome of these experiments, however, we should not forget that all the receptor binding studies reported till now have been carried out with nacked DNA. Even though the good agreement of these data with the results of gene transfer experiments suggests that a similar binding is taking place in intact cells, binding experiments with chromatin will be needed to study a possible influence of nucleosomal organization on the interaction of receptors with DNA regulatory elements. For this purpose constructions having the regulatory sequences incorporated into an episomal element able to replicate stably in target cells will be of invaluable help. It appears that the glucocorticoid regulatory element of MMTV-LTR is functional under these conditions (G. Hager, personal communication), whereas the regulatory element of the hMT-II gene is not operative in such constructions (14). Further work is needed to clarify these discrepancies.

Specific minichromosomes containing the regulatory elements could be obtained from different cell types and be used for receptor binding studies and cell-free transcription experiments. These studies may help to define the structural features of chromatin that determine accessibility of the hormone regulatory elements. In fact this may be a fundamental aspect of cell differentiation as different cells respond differentially to the same hormone, by expressing a different set of regulated genes, although the regulatory elements of the individual genes are probably the same in different cells. Since the glucocorticoid receptors of different tissues appear to be very similar or identical, other cell specific factors have to determine which set of genes is modulated in a particular cell type. Understanding this aspect of cell differentiation may actually become the main challenge facing those interested in the regulation of gene expression in higher organisms.

Acknowledgements. This work was supported by grants from the Deutsche Forschungsgemeinschaft and from the Fonds der Chemischen Industrie.

REFERENCES

1. Banerji, J., Olson, L., and Schaffner, W. (1983): Cell, 33: 729-740.
2. Banerji, J., Rusconi, S., and Schaffner, W. (1981): Cell, 27: 299-308.
3. Beato, M., Kalimi, M., Konstam, M., and Feigelson, P. (1973/: Biochemistry, 12: 3372-3379.
4. Buetti, E., Diggelmann, H. (1981): Cell, 23: 335-345.
5. Buetti, E., and Diggelmann, H. (1983): EMBO J., 2: 1423-1429.
6. Bugany, H., and Beato, M.(1977): Mol. Cell. Endocr., 7: 49-66.
7. Chandler, V.L., Maler, B.A., and Yamamoto, K.R. (1983): Cell, 33: 489-499.
8. Galas, D.J., and Schmitz, A. (1978): Nucleic Acid Res. 5: 3157-3170.

9. Geisse, S., Scheidereit, C., Westphal, H.M., Hynes, N.E., Groner, B., and Beato, M. (1982): EMBO J., 1: 1613-1619.
10. Gilles, S.D., Morrison, S.L., Oi, V.T.,and Tonegawa, S. (1983): Cell, 33: 717-728.
11. Huang, A.L., Ostrowski, M.C., Berard, D., and Hager, G.L. (1981): Cell, 27: 245-255.
12. Hynes, N.E., Kennedy, N., Rahmsdorf, V., and Groner, B. (1981): Proc. Natl. Acad. Sci. U.S.A., 78: 2038-2042.
13. Hynes, N.E., van Ooyen, A.J.J., Kennedy, N., Herrlich, P., Ponta, H., and Groner, B. (1983): Proc. Natl. Acad. Sci. U.S.A., 80: 3637-3641.
14. Karin, M., Cathala, G., and Nguyen-Huu, M.C. (1983): Proc. Natl. Acad. Sci. U.S.A., 80: 4040-4044.
15. Karin, M., Haslinger, A., Holtgreve, H., Richards, R.I., Krauter, P., Westphal, H.M., and Beato, M. (1983): Nature (submitted).
16. Karin, M., and Richards, R. (1982): Nature, 299: 797-802.
17. Lee, F., Mulligan, R., Berg, P., and Ringold, G. (1981): Nature, 294: 228-232.
18. Nordheim, A., and Rich, A. (1983): Nature, 303: 674-679.
19. Ogata, R.T., and Gilbert, W. (1978): Proc. Natl. Acad. Sci. U.S.A.,75: 5851-5854.
20. Payvar, F., Firestone, G., Ross, S.R., Chandler, V.L., Wrange, Ö., Carlstedt-Duke, J., Gustafsson, J.-A., and Yamamoto, K.R. (1982): J. Cell. Biochem. 19: 241-247.
21. Payvar, F., Wrange, Ö., Carlstedt-Duke, J., Okret, S., Gustafsson, J.-A., and Yamamoto, K.R. (1981): Proc. Natl. Acad. Sci. U.S.A., 78: 6628-6632.
22. Pfahl, M. (1982): Cell, 31: 475-482.
23. Queen, C., and Baltimore, D. (1983): Cell, 33, 741-748.
24. Riggs, A.D., Suzuki, H., and Bourgeois, S. (1970): J. Mol. Biol., 48: 67-83.
25. Scheidereit, C., Geisse, S., Westphal, H.M., and Beato, M. (1983): Nature, 304: 749-752.
26. Sibenlist, U., Simpson, R.B., and Gilbert, W. (1980): Cell, 20: 269-281.
27. Singleton, C.K., Klysik, J., and Wells, R.D. (1983): Proc. Natl. Acad. Sci. U.S.A., 80: 2447-2451.
28. Westphal, H.M., and Beato, M. (1980): Eur. J. Biochem., 106: 395-403.
29. Westphal, H.M., Moldenhauer, G., and Beato, M. (1982): EMBO J., 1: 1467-1471.
30. Wrange, Ö., Carlstedt-Duke, J.C., Gustafsson, J.A. (1979): J. Biol. Chem., 254: 9284-9290.
31. Yamamoto, K.R., Payvar, F., Firestone, G.L., Maler, B.A., Wrange, Ö., Carlstedt-Duke, J., Gustafsson, J.A., and Chandler, V.L. (1983): Cold Spring Harbor Symp. XLVII, 977-984.

Progress in Cancer Research and Therapy,
Vol. 31, edited by F. Bresciani, et al.
Raven Press, New York © 1984.

Changes in the Expression of Differentiated Functions of Dexamethasone-Resistant Hepatoma Cells

A. Venetianer, Zs. Bösze, and K. Kovács

Institute of Genetics, Biological Research Center, Hungarian Academy of Sciences, H-6701 Szeged, Hungary

It is known that glucocorticoid hormones have multiple effects on differentiation, however, the mechanisms responsible for these effects are still poorly understood. In order to get insight into the role of glucocorticoids in differentiation the examination of hormone-responsive cell lines expressing differentiated functions may provide a useful tool. Hepatoma cells express a wide range of liver-specific functions, some of which are under glucocorticoid regulation. Cell lines derived from the Reuber H35 rat hepatoma exhibit numerous functions of hepatocytes of adult liver, including production and secretion of serum albumin, basal and glucocorticoid-induced activities of tyrosine aminotransferase (TAT), the liver specific isozymes of aldolase (ALD-B), alcohol dehydrogenase (ADH-L) (4), as well as activities of gluconeogenic enzymes (3). It has been shown earlier that the growth of well differentiated cells derived from the Reuber H35 rat hepatoma (13,14) is inhibited by glucocorticoids such as dexamethasone (17). We have isolated a series of stable, dexamethasone-resistant variants ("growth resistant") from a hormone-sensitive, well differentiated parent hepatoma cell line (Faza 967; 4,17) and examined whether the dexamethasone-resistance of the cells does influence or not the expression of differentiated functions.

Previously we have found that hormone-sensitive Faza 967 cells maintained in long term culture undergo spontaneous changes (19) that must be taken into account in evaluating the possible effects of hormone resistance on the properties of the cells. In this study we show that the hormone-resistant cells undergo even more dramatic changes in the expression of many liver specific functions. The purpose of this work was to examine whether it is possible to dissociate the expression of various hormone-mediated responses in these hepatoma cells. It had been shown earlier that dexamethasone--resistant Faza 967 cells continue to show TAT inducibility although the specific activity of both basal and induced TAT was significantly decreased (17). Therefore, we have examined the state of both constitutive (ALD-B, ADH and FDPase) and hormone-inducible (TAT, albumin and PEPCK) liver specific functions in various Faza 967-derived cell clones. In particular we have addressed the question whether there is a special decrease in the expression of those liver functions which are normally regulated by glucocorticoid hormones.

METHODS

Cell lines and culture conditions. The glucocorticoid-sensitive and resistant cell lines and the culture conditions have been described (4,17,19,20). Dexamethasone (Dex; 9-α--fluoro-16-α-methyl-prednisolone) was added to the culture medium at a concentration of $2x10^{-6}M$. Dexamethasone-containing medium was replated with steroid free medium 4-6 days before performing the different assays.

The differentiated 8-azaguanine-resistant cell clone Faza 967 was derived from the H4IIEC3 rat hepatoma cell line (4). Dex-resistant Faza 967 cells were obtained by Dr M.C.Weiss (Centre de Genetique Moleculaire du C.N.R.S., Gif-sur-Yvette France) by growing Faza 967 cells in the presence of increasing concentration of dexamethasone (from $1x10^{-7}$ to $2x10^{-6}M$) for 4 months. The pedigree of Dex-resistant clones and subclones is published elsewhere (20). Faza 967 and Dex-resistant Faza 967 cells have been cultivated in our laboratory since September 1978, the age of the cells is calculated from this time. By subcloning the Dex-resistant Faza 967 cells in medium containing $2x10^{-6}M$ Dex we have obtained a clone designated D2 (17). This clone and the Dex-Faza 967 cells were grown for about 8 months in a medium containing $2x10^{-6}M$ Dex. Cells of clone D2 and Dex-resistant Faza 967 cells were then divided and grown either in the presence or in the absence of Dex. D2 cells and Dex-Faza 967 cells grown without Dex are designated "clone 2" and "cell line No. 14", respectively (the latter cells are derivatives of uncloned Dex-resistant Faza 967 cells). This scheme permitted us to analyze the effect of the continuous presence of hormone and to compare the properties of cultures of resistant cells with those of clones derived from them. Subclones of the resistant cells were derived by isolation of colonies following single cell plating and were examined a few months later.

Assays.
- Induction of tyrosine aminotransferase (TAT: E.C. 2.6.1.5) was performed according to Deschatrette and Weiss (4) except that cells were exposed to $1x10^{-6}M$ Dex for 18 h. TAT activity was assayed according to Diamondstone (5). Protein was assayed according to the technique of Lowry et al. (9) using bovine serum albumin as standard.
- For electrophoretic analysis of alcohol dehydrogenase (ADH: E.C.1.1.1) and aldolase (E.C.4.1.2.13) extracts were prepared and electrophoresis was carried out on gelatinized cellulose acetate strips (Chemotron, Milan, Italy) (1,2,11,12).
- The amount of albumin secreted into the medium was determined using the electro-immundiffusion method of Laurell (8). Indirect immunofluorescent staining of albumin producing cells was carried out according to Mevel-Ninio and Weiss(10). Rabbit antisera against rat serum albumin was a generous gift of Dr M.C.Weiss.

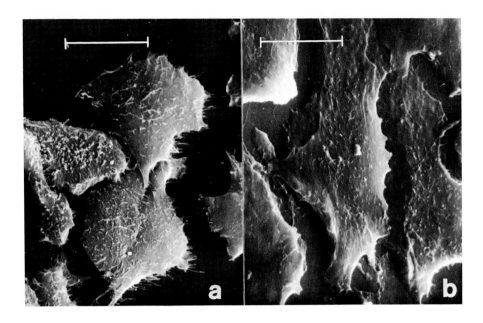

FIG. 1. Scanning electron micrographs of Faza 967 (a) and
clone 2 (b) cells. Bar: 20 μm. Cells were fixed on glass
coverslips in 2.5% glutaraldehyde in 4.2% Na-cacodylate buffer pH 7.3, and post-fixed in 2% OsO₄.

- Binding of dexamethasone to hepatoma cells was determined
as described (16,17). The experimental data were plotted according to Scatchard (15).

RESULTS

In the course of cultivation of dexamethasone-resistant
(Dex-resistant) cells we noticed that the morphology of most
resistant variants changed drastically (18,20) (Fig. 1).
In view of reports on a correlation between morphology and
expression of differentiated functions of the Reuber hepatoma
cells (4) we examined whether the expression of liver-specific functions had been changed in these Dex-resistant cells.
  TAT activity
Figure 2 shows the time course of the changes in basal and
hormone-induced TAT activity of sensitive and Dex-resistant
cells. The reduction in induced TAT activity occurred more
rapidly in the Dex-resistant cells and clones examined than
in Faza 967 cells (20,19). The fact that the TAT activity
decreased drastically in Faza 967 cells, in the resistant
clones and in the uncloned Dex-resistant population, indicates that change of TAT activity is characteristic for all
derivatives of Faza 967 cells, irrespective of their Dex-
sensitive or Dex-resistant state. Obviously, reduction of
TAT activity is an intrinsic property of Faza 967 cell cultures under those conditions we have used, and occurs much
more rapidly in the Dex-resistant cells.
  Albumin production
Synthesis of serum albumin was evaluated using both sen-

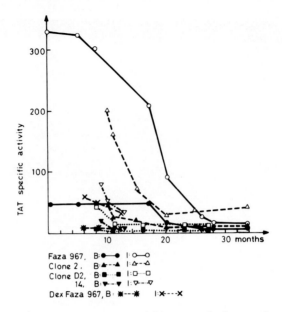

Faza 967, B ●—● I: ○—○
Clone 2, B ▲--▲ I: △---△
Clone D2, B ■--■ I: □····□
    14, B ▼--▼ I: ▽--▽
Dex Faza 967, B ✱--✱   I: ✖---✖

FIG. 2. Changes in the TAT specific activity of parental
and Dex-resistant hepatoma cells. Induction of TAT was performed according to Deschatrette and Weiss (4) except that
cells were exposed to 10^{-6}M dexamethasone for 18 h. Control
(B) and induced (I) cells were treated and harvested in parallel. TAT activity was assayed according to Diamondstone(5).
Results are expressed as mU/mg protein. Values given are the
average of 2-3 experiments. SD is less than 10% of the values
shown (Venetianer A. and Bősze Zs.: Differentiation (1983)
25: 70-78).

sitive immunofluorescence microscopy, for intracellular
albumin, and the electroimmunodiffusion method of Laurell(8).
When maintained in continuous culture, the Dex-sensitive Faza
967 cells showed a dramatic decrease in albumin production
after about 1 year (Fig. 3; 19).
Albumin production by the Dex-resistant cells also decreased
with culture time, showing variations of the time course of
reduction in the diverse resistant variants (Fig. 3). In
contrast to the situation encountered in the case of TAT, the
decline in albumin production was usually slower in the Dex-
-resistant than in the sensitive cells (Figs. 2 and 3).
  Isozyme patterns of hormone-resistant variants
   Aldolase B activity could be detected in the differentiated
Faza 967 cells in the form of A-B heterotetramers during
about 40 months of investigation. In contrast to the hormone-
-sensitive parent cells, the relative amounts of the liver-
-specific B component in the A-B heterotetramers appeared to
be reduced in the Dex-resistant variants (Fig. 4).
Some aldolase B was retained in all variants for at least 20
months of cultivation but finally disappeared. Similarly, the
liver specific isozyme of alcohol-dehydrogenase (ADH-L) disappeared after about 1 year of cultivation in the Dex-resistant variants. The presence of ADH-L could be detected in the

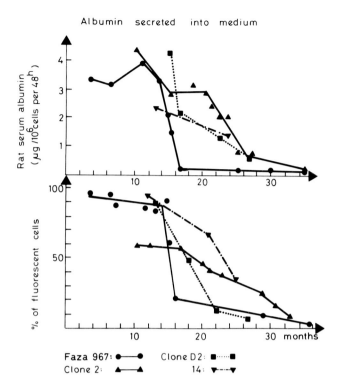

FIG. 3. Changes in the albumin production of parental and Dex-resistant hepatoma cells. Upper graph: The amount of albumin secreted into medium was determined using the electro-immundiffusion method of Laurell (8). The results are the average of at least 3 independent determinations. SD is less than 10% of the values shown. Lower graph: Indirect immuno-fluorescent staining of albumin-producing cells were carried out according to Mevel-Ninio & Weiss (10). The data are based upon the analysis of at least 500 cells in each case. Both brightly and weakly fluorescent cells are considered to be positive (Venetianer A. and Büsze Zs.: Differentiation(1983) 25: 70-78).

extracts of Faza 967 cells for about 30 months of observation (for details see 19,20). These results show that the Dex-resistant variants tend to lose the liver specific isozymes of aldolase and ADH during long-term culturing whereas these proteins are stably expressed in the Dex-sensitive parent Faza 967 cell line.

Glucocorticoid receptors of resistant variants

All of the resistant variants contained specific glucocorticoid receptors quantitated by Scatchard analysis using whole cell uptake methods. The number of receptors per cell and the dissociation constants of the receptors for dexamethasone (K_d) were comparable in the TAT inducible, differentiated (about 10-months old) and in the TAT non-inducible, dedifferentiated (36-48-months old) variants (Table 1) (17).

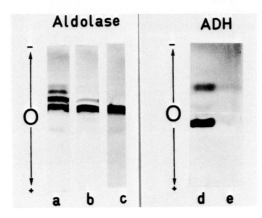

FIG. 4. Isozyme pattern of aldolase (a,b,c) and alcohol dehydrogenase (d,e). Equal amounts of extracts prepared from
the same numbers of cells were applied in all cases. Aldolase:
Cell extracts were prepared from 5.5 months old Faza 967
cells (a), from 14.5 months old D2 clone cells (b) and from
29 months old 2a subclone cells (c). A4 homotetramer migrates
nearest to the origin, it is followed by the A3B1 (a,b), A2B2
and A1B3 heterotetramers (a). Alcohol dehydrogenase: Cell
extracts were prepared from 16 months old Faza 967 cells (d)
and from 37 months old clone 2 cells (e). The cathodally migrating liver-specific isozyme (L-ADH) and the anodally migrating "stomach" ADH are visible on the gel of Faza 967
extracts (d), while only traces of ADH activity can be seen
in clone 2 cell extracts (e) (Venetianer A. and Bõsze Zs.:
Differentiation (1983) 25: 70-78).

TABLE 1. Binding of (^{3}H) Dexamethasone in Sensitive and Resistant Hepatoma Variants

Cell line	Age[1] (in months)	Dex. sensitivity[2]	Dex.binding sites/cell[3] (x 10^4)	K_d[3] (x10^{-8}M)
Faza 967	10	S	6.4	0.9
Dex-Faza 967	10	R	3.5	1.1
Clone D2	10	R	5.4	1.4
Clone D2	36	R	5.4	1.6
Clone 2	10	R	5.7	2.3
Clone 2	48	R	7.5	0.9

[1]Faza 967 and Dex-resistant Faza 967 cells have been cultivated in our laboratory since 1978, the age of the cells is
calculated from this time.
[2]R=resistant, S=sensitive to 2x10^{-6}M dexamethasone (17).
[3]Binding of dexamethasone to hepatoma cells was determined
as described (16,17). Each value represents the average of
3-6 independent experiments. Table taken in part from Venetianer A., Pinter Zs. and Gal A.: Cytogenet. Cell Genet.
(1980) 28: 280-283.

These results show that neither the dexamethasone resistance nor the dedifferentiation of the different Faza 967 clones are due to the absence of glucocorticoid receptors.

DISCUSSION

Our results show that the expression of liver-specific functions can change drastically in dexamethasone-resistant cultures and clones derived from differentiated steroid sensitive Faza 967 cells. The decrease in expression is not specific to those functions whose activity is normally regulated by glucocorticoids. We have reported earlier the dissociation of growth resistance and resistance to TAT induction in different Dex-Faza 967 clones (17). Our present data provide evidence for the existence of growth resistant Faza 967 cells which continue to express all the differentiated functions examined, i.e. the cells were Dex-resistant before they lost the liver-specific functions, i.e. became "dedifferentiated". This means that the dedifferentiation of Faza 967 cells is not a prerequisite for Dex-resistance and that growth sensitivity and the expression of differentiated functions is not controlled in a coordinated way. It does not mean, however, that the steroid resistance has no effect on the state of differentiation of Faza 967 cells. In contrast to the Dex-sensitive Faza 967 cells which, during prolonged cultivation partially also dedifferentiate (19), the expression of all liver-specific functions have been changed in the Dex-resistant clones and in uncloned Dex-resistant cell populations.

The changes in the Dex-resistant cells are not the consequences of long term cultivation as such because these functions do not change in the same way in Faza 967 cells grown for about the same time. In most cases the continuous presence of glucocorticoid is not necessary for the alteration of specific functions. It seems, however, that dexamethasone may induce or stabilize phenotypic changes that can occur spontaneously. Moreover, the sequence of dedifferentiation is not the same in the sensitive and the Dex-resistant cells, suggesting that perhaps mechanisms and programs are involved that are different in hormone sensitive and resistant cells.

One important conclusion of this study is that differentiated Faza 967 Reuber hepatoma cells may become glucocorticoid-resistant which demonstrates that dedifferentiation is not an obligatory prerequisite for the appearance of hormone-mediated growth resistance in these cells. The examination of different human breast cancer cell lines and transplantable rat prostatic adenocarcinoma cell lines also has revealed that differentiated cells can be hormone-sensitive as well insensitive (6,7). Thus, the lack of coordinate regulation of the expression of differentiated functions seems to be rather general, at least in continuous tissue culture of malignant cells. It is interesting, however, that in spite of the independent regulation of glucocorticoid controlled and other differentiated functions, the expression of all liver-specific functions has changed in the resistant hepatoma cells. We do not know the mechanism(s) by which dexamethasone promotes or provokes the changes of differentiated functions of the resistant cells. We have previously shown that the resist-

ance of several Faza 967 clones to the growth inhibitory effect of glucocorticoids is not due to the absence of functional receptors (17). Resistant cells which have been cultivated for over 3 years and have lost the expression of all
differentiated functions still contain specific glucocorticoid receptors comparable in quantity to the well differentiated cells. In the same vein, our results indicate that
the altered phenotype of the resistant cells cannot be explained by the absence of glucocorticoid receptors. Further
analysis of Dex-resistant hepatoma cells may help to elucidate the multiple effects of glucocorticoid hormones and to
decide whether the effects observed are specific for the
cell line examined and whether the dedifferentiated state is
irreversible.

REFERENCES

1 Bertolotti, R. and Weiss, M.C. (1972): J. Cell Physiol.
      79:211-224.
2 Bertolotti, R. and Weiss, M.C. (1972): Biochimie, 54:
      195-201.
3 Bertolotti, R. (1977): Somat. Cell Genet., 3:365-380.
4 Deschatrette, J. and Weiss, M.C. (1974): Biochimie, 56:
      1603-1611.
5 Diamondstone, T.L. (1966): Analyt. Biochem.,16:359-401.
6 Engel, L.W., and Young, N.A. (1978): Cancer Research,
      38:4327-4339.
7 Isaacs, J.T., Heston, W.D.W., Weissman, R.W., and Coffey,
      D.S. (1978): Cancer Research, 38:4353-4359.
8 Laurell, C.B. (1966): Anal. Biochem., 15:45-52.
9 Lowry, O.H., Rosebrough, N.J., Lewis Farr A., and Randall,
      R.J. (1951): J. Biol. Chem., 193:265-275.
10 Mevel-Ninio, N., and Weiss, M.C. (1981): J. Cell Biol.,
      90:339-350.
11 Ohno, S., Stenius, C., Christian, L., Harris, C., and
      Yvey, C. (1970): Biochem. Genet., 4:565-577.
12 Penhoet, E., Rajkumar, T., and Rutter, W.J. (1966):
      Proc. Nat. Acad. Sci. USA, 56:1275-1282.
13 Pitot, H.C., Peraino, C., Morse, P.A., and Potter, V.R.
      (1964): Nat. Cancer. Inst. Monograph., 13:229-242.
14 Reuber, M.D. (1961): J. Nat. Cancer Inst., 26:891-899.
15 Scatchard, G. (1949): Ann. N.Y. Acad. Sci., 51:660-672.
16 Venetianer, A., Bajnoczky, K., Gal, A., and Thompson,
      E.B. (1978): Somat. Cell Genet., 4:513-530.
17 Venetianer,A., Pinter, Zs., and Gal, A. (1980): Cyto-
      genet. Cell Genet., 28:280-283.
18 Venetianer, A., Gal, A., and Büsze, Zs. (1981): Acta
      Biologica ASH, 32:175-187.
19 Venetianer, A. and Büsze, Zs. (1983): Somat. Cell
      Genet., 9:85-93.
20 Venetianer, A. and Büsze, Zs. (1983): Differentiation,
      25:70-78.

Progress in Cancer Research and Therapy,
Vol. 31, edited by F. Bresciani, et al.
Raven Press, New York © 1984.

Corticosteroid-Induced Remodeling of the Lipid Content of Membranes

D.H. Nelson, Darrell K. Murray, and Thomas M. Kelly

Department of Internal Medicine, Division of Endocrinology and Metabolism, University of Utah, School of Medicine, Salt Lake City, Utah 84132

One of the outstanding features of corticosteroid action is their ability to affect multiple biologic functions in almost every tissue in the body. There is considerable data illustrating effects of corticosteroids upon membrane receptors, transport through membranes, and membrane bound enzymes, all of which suggest a major effect of these hormones upon membranes (5). The classical mechanism of steroid action upon new protein synthesis, without an intermediate mediator, would necessitate effects upon numerous enzymes to specifically influence each of the cellular functions modified by corticosteroids. A search was begun a number of years ago by two of us (D. H. N. and D. K. M.), therefore, to find a mechanism by which corticosteroid action upon one or a few enzymes might produce the known permissive and protective actions of these hormones. It became apparent in the course of this investigation that many of the functions of the corticosteroids are related to modification of reactions occurring in membranes, and particularly in the plasma membrane of cells. Many of these enzymatic or other biologic functions can be modified by an alteration in the lipid environment in which the reaction takes place. Studies were initiated, therefore, to determine whether corticosteroids altered the lipid nature of cell membranes (2).

These studies, as outlined below, have demonstrated an effect of corticosteroids to markedly, and specifically, alter the phospholipid composition of cellular membranes and particularly the plasma membrane, of a number of cell types. Phospholipid changes are associated with alterations of biologic effects such as glucose transport in fat cells or fibroblasts, or superoxide anion production by leukocytes. These findings are consistent with the theory that many effects of the corticosteroids are mediated through alterations in the lipid composition of cellular membranes.

BACKGROUND

Corticosteroid effects upon rat epididymal fat cell membranes.
Initial studies of corticosteroid action upon membrane lipids were carried out in isolated rat epididymal fat cells (2). Ghosts were prepared from epididymal fat cells from adrenalectomized rats incubated with or without 8×10^{-8} molar dexamethasone for three hours. Incuba-

tion with dexamethasone produced a 61% increase in membrane sphingo-myelin without producing any significant change in other phospholipids, cholesterol, or the fatty acid components of the phospholipids. There was a very significant effect (P <0.025) upon the sphingomyelin content of the ghosts of these cells without causing any significant alteration in other membrane lipids. (Table I).

TABLE I. Effect of dexamethasone on the phospholipid content of epid-idymal fat cell ghosts obtained from adrenalectomized rats (micrograms of phosphorus per mg protein)

Phospholipids	Control	Dexamethasone	P
Sphingomyelin	0.835 ± 0.133	1.344 ± 0.122	<0.025
Phosphatidylethanolamine	2.082 ± 0.102	2.137 ± 0.094	>0.2
Phosphatidylcholine	5.173 ± 0.184	5.362 ± 0.163	>0.2
Phosphatidylserine and phosphatidylinositol	0.458 ± 0.081	0.478 ± 0.076	>0.5
Total phospholipids	8.545 ± 0.442	9.288 ± 0.365	>0.05
Total phospholipids - sphingomyelin subtracted	7.709 ± 0.323	7.968 ± 0.292	>0.2

Phosphorus and protein were measured in ghosts from fat cells which had been incubated for 3 hours with or without 8×10^{-8}M dexamethasone. Each value represents the mean ± SE from 12 experiments, expressed as micrograms of phosphorus per mg protein. Total phospholipid content was calculated as the sum of the above individually measured phospholipids. (Reproduced with permission frm Ref. 2)

These initial studies with fat cell ghosts were carried out **in vitro**. Additional studies were then undertaken to determine whether corticosteroids may have more long term **in vivo** effects upon membrane lipid composition. Sprague-Dawley rats of approximately 250 g were adrenalectomized for three days during which time they were maintained on normal saline but given no steroid therapy. At the end of this time, rat epididymal fat cell ghosts were isolated as carried out in the previous experiments and the lipid content of the isolated membranes determined (4). There was a 33% decrease in the sphingomyelin content of the isolated ghosts in the adrenalectomized animals and a 59% de-crease in the cholesterol content of the adrenalectomized animals as compared with the intact animals (Table II). These data demonstrate an effect of adrenalectomy, the removal of normal secretion of corticoster-oids, to markedly influence the lipid content of the cellular membranes in vivo.

TABLE II. Effect of three day adrenalectomy upon the sphingomyelin and cholesterol content of ghosts from rat epididymal fat cells (Mean ± SE).

	Sphingomyelin (µg P/mg protein)	Cholesterol (µg/mg protein)
Intact	1.03 ± 0.12	151 ± 17.2
Adrenex	0.69 ± 0.06	62 ± 6.0
P value	<0.05	<0.005

Studies, not shown, demonstrated an apparent correlation between the action of the corticosteroids to alter the membrane lipid content and their ability to inhibit glucose transport. Corticosteroids are well known to inhibit the insulin effect to stimulate glucose transport. In those studies insulin induced membrane lipid changes were blocked by corticosteroid effects (3). Whether the effect is upon insulin receptor action or glucose transport itself is, at this time, not determined. Changes in the lipid environment in which both of these functions take place may be important in influencing either or both activities.

Corticosteroid effects upon lipid composition of 3T3-L1 cell membranes.

In order to more clearly demonstrate whether the corticosteroid effect upon membrane lipids affected other cell types and to begin to understand the mechanism by which these changes are brought about, 3T3-L1 cells were incubated with 0.1μ molar dexamethasone for four hours and a plasma membrane enriched fraction from these cells isolated. As had been seen in the rat epididymal fat cells, this resulted in a marked increase, 50% (P <0.05), in the sphingomyelin of the plasma membrane enriched fraction (7). No change was seen in the other major lipid constituents of the membrane. The phospholipid change in sphingomyelin and lack of change in phosphatidylcholine are demonstrated in Table III. As the lipid values are reported in terms of milligrams protein, careful measurements of cellular protein were carried out and no change was seen during the short period of incubation. There was not a significant change in phosphatidylcholine after this short incubation with corticosteroid.

TABLE III. Choline-containing phospholipids isolated from whole cells and a plasma membrane-enriched fraction from 3T3-L1 fibroblasts after a 4-hour incubation with or without 0.1 μM dexamethasone.

Lipid	Treatment	Whole cells, μg P/mg of protein	Plasma Membrane fraction μg P/mg of protein
Sphingomyelin	Control	1.34 ± 0.26	7.34 ± 0.91*
	Dexamethasone	1.48 ± 0.25	11.02 ± 1.63*
Phosphatidyl-choline	Control	2.54 ± 0.42	10.69 ± 2.7
	Dexamethasone	2.23 ± 0.23	11.49 ± 2.4

Values are means ± SEM; n = 12. *P<0.05. (Reproduced with permission from Ref. 7).

When sphingomyelin synthesis from phosphatidylcholine by the phosphatidylcholine:ceramide cholinephosphotransferase pathway was determined, it was found that dexamethasone had a marked effect upon this enzymatic activity. After exposure to the steroid for a period of four hours, an 83 % increase in the transferase was seen (FIG. 1). This dexamethasone stimulated increase in sphingomyelin formation was blocked by the addition of cyclohexamide (2μg/ml) with the dexamethasone. When the activity of the enzyme CDP-choline:ceramide cholinephosphotransferase was determined, there was much less incorporation of cytidine diphophoso-[methyl-^{14}C] choline than there had been of phosphatidyl (methyl-^{14}C) choline into sphingomyelin by the plasma membrane enriched fraction. There was no stimulation of the CDP-choline pathway when dexamethasone

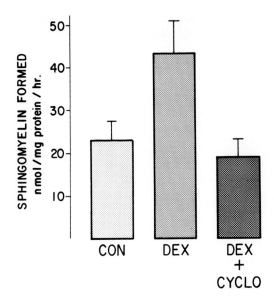

FIG. 1. Formation of sphingomyelin from phosphatidylcholine by a plasma membrane-enriched fraction from 3T3-L1 cells treated with dexamethasone (Dex) or dex with cycloheximide (Cyclo). Dex, 0.1 μM dex added; Dex and Cyclo, 0.1 μM dex and cyclo at 2 μg/ml added. Values are means ± SEM; n = 7. Control vs. Dex, P <0.025; Dex vs. Dex and Cyclo, P <0.05. Results obtained after incubation with cyclo alone were not significantly different from control in five experiments. (Reproduced with permission from Ref. 7).

was added. These data demonstrate that a significant mechanism by which corticosteroids alter the phospholipid content of the plasma membrane is by stimulation of a specific transferase in the plasma membrane of the cells.

Unpublished studies have also demonstrated that as the corticosteroids alter the phospholipids of the plasma membrane, they reduce the uptake of glucose by the cells and partially inhibit insulin stimulated glucose uptake by the cells. Thus, in agreement with the findings in the rat epididymal fat cells, corticosteroid-induced changes in the phospholipid membrane can be related to the biologic action of corticosteroids to inhibit insulin induced glucose transport.

Corticosteroid effects upon human leukocyte lipids.

Preliminary studies showed some change in phospholipids of leukocytes incubated with dexamethasone, which appeared to relate to the ability of the corticosteroid to inhibit superoxide anion production by the cells. These studies were not totally satisfactory, however, as a mixed leukocyte population was employed for the experiments. In more recent studies, a preparation of specifically isolated, viable, polymorphonuclear leukocytes was obtained from normal fasted male and female subjects and incubated for two hours with 3×10^{-9} to 8×10^{-5} M dexamethasone (8). There was a statistically significant increase in the concentration of sphingomyelin in the cells incubated with dexamethasone (Table IV). Smaller changes occured when the concentration was in-

TABLE IV. Effect of incubation for 2 hours with dexamethasone $(8 \times 10^{-8} M)$ and/or cycloheximide (2µg/ml) on the sphingomyelin content of human PMN (mean ± SE)

	n	Sphingomyelin (µg phosphorus/ mg protein)	Significance vs. control
Control	10	0.356 ± 0.067	
Dexamethasone	10	0.437 ± 0.075	<0.05
Cycloheximide	5	0.332 ± 0.151	NS
Cycloheximide + dexamethasone	5	0.338 ± 0.154	NS

creased or decreased from this level (FIG. 2). The addition of cyclohexamide blocked this steroid-induced increase in sphingomyelin in the human polymorphonuclear leukocyte preparation as it had in the 3T3-L1 cells.

Concurrent with the increase in sphingomyelin an increase in "sphingomyelinase" was also demonstrated. As the technique used for the

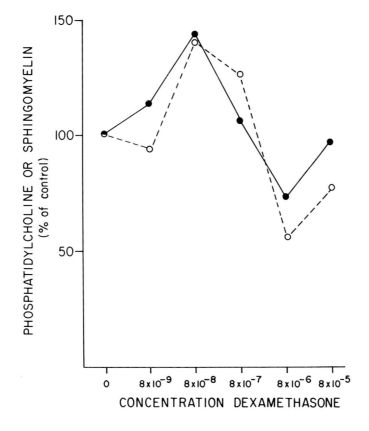

FIG. 2. Effect of increasing concentrations of dexamethasone incubated with human PMN for 2 hours, ●—●, Phosphatidylcholine; O--O, sphingomyelin. Each point represents the mean of three determinations. (Reproduced with permission from Ref. 8).

estimation of "sphingomyelinase" would be consistent with the reverse reaction of the phosphatidylcholine:ceramide cholinephosphotransferase which was demonstrated to be increased in the 3T3-L1 cells after treatment with dexamethasone, it seems likely that this same activity was responsible for the changes seen.

The correlation of corticosteroid induced changes in phospholipids and the known action of lipid changes to alter activity of the oxidase responsible for superoxide anion formation by the leukocytes, again suggests an important relationship between the action of the corticosteroids to alter membrane lipids and their biologic activity. As the result of these findings, studies have been undertaken in humans to determine if individuals exposed to increased levels of corticosteroids have phospholipid changes in circulating polymorphonuclear leukocytes.

METHODS

Approximately 50 ml of blood was obtained at 8 a.m. from fasted subjects and added to an equal volume of dextran/ACD solution and allowed to stand for 60 minutes. The supernatant was added to two volumes of 0.87% ammonium chloride solution and centrifuged at 155 g for ten minutes at 4°C. The pellet was washed x 2 with 10 ml Dulbecco's buffer, centrifuged, and taken into solution in 2 ml buffer. Polymorphonuclear cells were separated by layering on Ficoll-Hypaque. Approximately 10^7 cells in suspension were added to glass Petri dishes which were incubated for 30 minutes at 37°. Nonadhering cells were washed free with buffer while the viable cells continued to adhere. Viability was determined by Trypan blue exclusion which demonstrated 94% viable cells. Cells were scraped from the dish, and sonicated for ten seconds on ice x 2. The sonicated cell preparation was centrifuged for 20 minutes at 27,000 g to obtain a crude membrane preparation. Lipids were extracted from this membrane preparation with methanol:choloroform (2:1), and phospholipids were determined by either thin layer chromatography and phosphorus measurement, or flame ionization detection in an Iatroscan following chromatography on chromarods.

Blood samples were obtained from three types of patients. The first group were patients with Cushing's syndrome, as determined by standard techniques, all of whom have required therapy since the studies were performed. The second group were patients receiving therapy with prednisone in the amount of 20-60 mg/day for a period of two days to many months. Thirdly, normal subjects have been studied who were given ten mg prednisone b.i.d. for six days with determination of polymorphonuclear leukocyte lipids before and after administration of the corticoid.

Results of the studies carried out on patients with Cushing's syndrome are illustrated in Table V. It can be seen that there was a highly significant change in the phosphatidylcholine to sphingomyelin ratio of these patients who were secreting increased quantities of cortisol from their adrenal glands. The values are clearly different from those obtained from studies carried out on polymorphonuclear leukocytes isolated from normal subjects with a P <0.005. It is of interest that the changes are more clearly in phosphatidylcholine in these studies, as compared with incubations for a few hours in which the most significant change was found in the sphingomyelin.

TABLE V.   Phospholipids of PMN membranes of patients with Cushing's syndrome and of control subjects

Patient	μg PC/mg Protein μg Sph/mg Protein	Sphingomyelin	Phosphatidylcholine
VC	4.4	10.5	46.3
SB	4.0	17.8	71.1
MS	4.0	15.0	59.8
DK	7.0	8.1	56.8
Cushing's(M ± SEM)	4.8 ± 0.6	12.8 ± 1.9	58.5 ± 4.4
Controls(n=8)	2.3 ± 0.3	17.8 ± 2.0	44.1 ± 10
P value	<0.005	-	-

Studies were then performed to determine relative amounts of lipids in polymorphonuclear leukocytes from the patients receiving prednisone. As can be seen in Table VI, age matched control subjects had a mean ratio of phosphatidylcholine to sphingomyelin of 2.6 ± 0.3.   All patients on prednisone had a mean value of 4.3 ± 0.2. Comparison of the mean amounts of the two phospholipids in the membranes from PMNS from control subjects and those from patients receiving prednisone demonstrate a relative increase in phosphatidylcholine and decrease in sphingomyelin to account for these changes.

Figure 3 illustrates the effect of administration of prednisone, 10 mg b.i.d. for six days to a normal subject.   Phosphatidylcholine, although not significantly changed after two days administration, was markedly increased after six days with resulting increase in the phosphatidylcholine to sphingomyelin ratio.   There was a simultaneous

TABLE VI.   Comparison of the phospholipid content of polymorphonuclear leukocyte membranes from patients receiving prednisone and from control subjects.

	Phosphatidylcholine(Pc)	Sphingomyelin(Sph) (μg lipid/mg protein)	Pc/Sph
Patients receiving prednisone			
1	65.7	16.2	4.0
2	40.0	10.0	3.8
3	76.0	15.5	4.7
4	68.2	13.2	4.8
5	58.9	13.7	4.2
6	75.5	18.2	4.1
Mean ± SEM	64.1 ± 5.5	14.5 ± 1.2	4.3 ± 0.2*
Control subjects (n=6)			
Mean ± SEM	52.3 ± 12.7	19.7 ± 2.3	2.6 ± 0.3*

*P <0.001, as compared with the control group value by unpaired student's t-test.

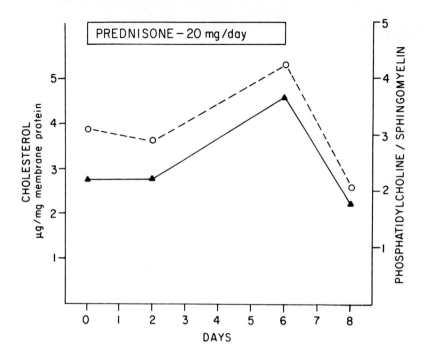

FIG. 3.   Effect of prednisone, 10 mg b.i.d. for six days given to a
normal subject, upon the cholesterol content and phosphatidylcholine to
sphingomyelin ratio of a crude membrane fraction of human polymorphonuclear leukocytes. Cholesterol ▲——▲. Phosphatidylcholine/sphingo-
myelin O----O.

increase in the cholesterol content of these cells, but sphingomyelin
was essentially unchanged.   No change in the choline containing
phospholipids was detected in lymphocytes obtained from these patients
as compared with a control group of subjects (PC/Sph ratio 3.2 in control subjects, and 3.1 in patients receiving prednisone).

DISCUSSION

The studies presented clearly demonstrate an action of corticosteroids to modify the relative concentrations of phospholipids, and cholesterol in cellular membranes. In relatively short term incubations of
a few hours, dexamethasone produced a marked increase in the sphingomyelin content of epididymal rat fat cell ghosts, human polymorphonuclear leukocytes, and a plasma membrane enriched fraction obtained
from 3T3-L1 cells. In the latter cells it has been demonstrated that
this increase is mediated by a considerable increase in the activity of
phosphatidylcholine:ceramide cholinephosphotansferase. This pathway of
sphingomyelin synthesis appears to be the major mechanism for synthesis
of sphingomyelin and alteration of its content in the plasma membrane.
In short term incubations there appeared to be an increase in phosphatidylcholine in the leukocyte preparation, but this was not found to be
statistically significant.

In vivo experiments comparing lipids of ghosts of rat epidiymal fat cells from adrenalectomized animals with normal controls, revealed a marked decrease in the sphingomyelin content of the membranes from the adrenalectomized animals. Of further interest in these studies was a decrease in cellular cholesterol which paralleled the fall in fat cell ghost sphingomyelin following adrenalectomy. It is well known that there is a tendency for cholesterol and sphingomyelin to associate in membranes, and this affinity may have accounted for the simultaneous changes in cholesterol. Alternatively, however, recent studies have demonstrated an effect of sphingomyelin to increase the synthesis of cholesterol in cultured human skin fibroblasts, and thus, cholesterol changes may also have occurred due to effects on synthesis within the cell (1).

When corticosteroids were administered to normal subjects in fairly large doses (10 mg b.i.d. for six days) significant changes in membrane lipids were again found. In the longer experiments there was an increase in phosphatidylcholine with a significant increase in the phosphatidylcholine to sphingomyelin ratio. The finding of similar changes in phosphatidylcholine to sphingomyelin ratio in the membranes of polymorphonuclear leukocytes obtained from patients with Cushing's syndrome and those receiving prednisone, suggests that this is a general effect of high corticosteroid dosage. Such large changes in the lipids of the plasma membrane appear likely to have marked effects upon membrane related processes. One study carried out in this laboratory has shown an effect of corticosteroid treatment associated with such lipid changes to inhibit receptor mediated changes in other membrane lipids (3).

CONCLUSIONS

The studies reported here demonstrate an effect of Cushing's syndrome, and chronic or subacute administration of prednisone to produce changes in the phospholipids and cholesterol of human polymorphonuclear leukocytes. There is an increase in phosphatidylcholine in a crude membrane preparation of the cells with a resultant increase in the phosphatidylcholine to sphingomyelin ratio. Associated with these changes is an increase or decrease in cholesterol which appears to parallel the exposure to corticosteroid. Previously reported effects of the corticosterids were to increase sphingomyelin synthesis and content of cellular membranes. Corticosteroid effects are, therefore, upon both of the choline containing phospholipids of a variety of cells. An acute increase in sphingomyelin occurs after exposure to corticosteroid. This is followed by an increase in phosphatidylcholine and cholesterol. Many studies have shown alterations in tumor lipids associated with malignancy. It appears likely that corticosteroid induced alterations in the lipid membranes of these cells may relate to effects of corticosteroids to inhibit growth, alter responsivity to a variety of stimuli, and exert many of their beneficial therapeutic effects (5,6).

REFERENCES

1. Kudchodkar, B.J., Albers, J.J., Bierman, E.L.(1983), Atherosclerosis, 46:353-367.
2. Murray, D.K., Ruhmann-Wennhold, A., and Nelson, D. H. (1979), Endocrinology, Vol. 105, No. 3, pp. 774-777.

3. Murray, D.K., and Nelson, D.H.(1981), Endocrinology, Vol. 108, No. 5, pp. 2014-2016.
4. Murray, D.K., Ruhmann-Wennhold, and Nelson, D.H.(1982), Endocrinology, Vol. 111, No. 2, pp. 452-455.
5. Nelson, D.H.(1980), Endocrine Reviews Vol.1, No. 2, pp. 180-199,
6. Nelson, D.H., Murray, D.K., Ruhmann-Wennhold, A.(1980), Adv. Physiol. Sci. Vol. 13, Endocrinology, Neuroendocrinology, Neuropeptides, E. Stark, G.B. Makara, Zs. Acs, E. Endroczi (eds), pp. 77-81.
7. Nelson, D.H., and Murray D.K.(1982), Proc. Natl. Acad. Sci. USA, Vol. 79, pp. 6690-6692.
8. Nelson, D.H., Murray, D.K., and Brady, R.O.(1982), Journal of Clinical Endocrinology and Metabolism, Vol. 54, No. 2, pp. 292-295.

Progress in Cancer Research and Therapy,
Vol. 31, edited by F. Bresciani, et al.
Raven Press, New York © 1984.

Effects of High-Dose Medroxyprogesterone Acetate on Plasma Membrane Lipid Mobility

*H. Bojar, *M. Stuschke, and **W. Staib

*Onkologische Chemie, **Physiologische Chemie II, Universität Düsseldorf,
D-4000 Düsseldorf, Federal Republic of Germany

Biological membranes crucially participate in nearly all cellular functions under normal conditions as well as in malignancy. In a current membrane model (7) proteins are supposed to be embedded into a heterogeneous lipid matrix forming lipid clusters (5) or lateral phase separations (7,10). The mobility of membrane proteins is influenced by lipid-protein interactions, lateral protein-protein associations, exclusion from specific lipid domains, restraint by peripheral membrane components at the inner or outer membrane surface and interactions with the membrane-associated cytoskeleton (7).Thus, the lipids of the plasma membrane may in part regulate the activities of membrane-associated enzymes, the availibilty of membrane-bound receptors to their ligands, the interaction of receptors with each other, the antigenicity of cells as well as their susceptibility to lysis.

Malignantly transformed cells exhibit an altered 'social behavior', in which the cell surface membrane is also believed to play a crucial role. An association of changes in lipid lateral diffusion rates with malignant cell transformation has been recently reported (9).

In this report we present evidence for changes in membrane lipid lateral mobility upon treatment of isolated cells with high-dose medroxyprogesterone acetate (MPA). The fundamental reasons for the study are

(i) The apparent need for high doses of MPA for effective treatment of hormone-dependent human neoplasias, which has brought up the idea that, in addition to the wellknown receptor-mediated mechanism of action of the progestational compound, receptor-nonmediated mechanisms of action (direct cytotoxic effects) of MPA might occur at the extraordinarily high concentrations of the ligand;

(ii) Reportedly effective high-dose MPA therapy of certain human malignancies, as for example renal cell carcinoma, which do not contain significant quantities of progestin receptors.

The action of MPA was investigated on the plasma membrane of isolated intact hepatocytes. The rationale for using hepatocytes as experimental model for the study is as follows.

(i) The cells do not contain significant amounts of progestin receptors, thereby offering the advantage that participation of the progestin

receptor in mediating biological response can be excluded.
(ii) Assumed direct interactions of steroids with cell membranes are most
likely to occur in normal as well as malignant cells.

MATERIALS AND METHODS

Medroxyprogesterone acetate (MPA) was kindly supplied by Dr. P. Lanius,
Farmitalia Carlo Erba GmbH, Freiburg, FRG.
1-acyl-2-(N-(4-nitrobenzo-2-oxa-1,3-diazolyl)aminocaproyl)phosphatidyl-
choline (NBD-PC)was purchased from Avanti Polar Lipids (Birmingham,
Alabama). 5-(hexadecanoylamino)fluorescein ($F-C_{16}$) was from
Molecular Probes (Junction City, Oregon).
Livers from male Wistar rats, 250 g average body weight, fed ad libitum
were used in the study. Hepatocytes were enzymatically isolated as
described earlier (3).
Intact hepatocytes suspended in 1 ml Dulbecco's modified Eagle's medium
(MEM-D) (10 mg cell wet weight / ml of medium) containing 0.3 % bovine
serum albumin (BSA) were incubated with MPA for 6C min under gentle
periodic agitation at room temperature. After centrifugation the
preincubated cells were resuspended in 1 ml of BSA-free MEM-D, mixed with
the fluorescent lipid probe dispersions (either $F-C_{16}$ or NBD-PC at a
final concentration of 5 ug/ml, containing 0.5 % ethanol) and labeled for
10 min at $4^{o}C$. During labelling MPA was also present at
concentrations as indicated in the Tables. The cells were then collected
by centrifugation and washed four times with MEM-D containing 0.3 % BSA.
The hepatocytes were stored at $0^{o}C$ under gentle periodic agitation
for no longer than 30 min, thereby preventing the dye from cytoplasmic
uptake and labeling of internal structural elements. Immediately before
photobleaching the labeled cells were allowed to adjust to room
temperature for two minutes.
Our instrument for measuring fluorescence recovery after photobleaching
(FRAP) is similar to that described by Koppel et al. (4). It is based on
a modified fluorescence microscope (Leitz) and an argon ion laser (CR 6,
Coherent). In principal, a small area of the upper plasma membrane of a
fluorescently labeled hepatocyte is irradiated with a focused laser beam
at a low intensity. The fluorescence signal of the irradiated spot (IS)
is picked up by a photocounting system (Ortec, 5 C 1) equipped with a
thermoelectrically cooled ($-40^{o}C$) photomultiplier (RCA, type C 31043)
 and registered using a DC amplifier recorder. By a short increase of the
laser light intensity (10,000 fold) an irreversible photolysis of the
fluorescent lipid probes in the IS is induced. After attenuation of the
laser light power to the initial low intensity an asymptotically
increasing fluorescence signal from the IS is observed indicating a
diffusion of fluorophores from the surrounding unirradiated area of the
plasma membrane into the bleached IS. The half-time ($t_{1/2}$) of the
fluorescence recovery, related to the diffusion coefficient D by

(1) $$D = \gamma_{D} \, w^2 / 4t_{1/2},$$

was obtained by a three point fit on smoothed data (2).
(γ_{D} is a parameter which, for a Gaussian intensity profile of the
laser beam, is related to the degree of photobleaching; $t_{1/2}$ is the
 time for which the fractional fluorescence recovery

$$f = (F_{(t)} - F_{(0)}) / (F_{(\infty)} - F_{(0)}) = 0.5,$$

($F_{(-)}$, $F_{(0)}$, $F_{(\infty)}$: measured IS-fluorescence before, immediately after, and long time after photobleaching); w: $1 / e^2$ radius of the Gaussian laser beam profile in the sample plane).
The mobile fraction (R) of the fluorescent lipid probes was derived from equation
(2) $$R = (F_{(\infty)} - F_{(0)}) / (F_{(-)} - F_{(0)}).$$

For excitation of the fluorescent lipid probes the 488 nm line of the argon laser in TEM 00 mode was used. Light intensity (bleaching light power in the object plane: 0.5 - 4 mW) and puls length (100 - 300 ms) of the laser for photolysis, attenuation factor (10,000 - 40,000) for the laser power in the period before and after photolysis, and sampling time (0.1-1s) of the photocounting system were adjusted to obtain the same amount of bleaching ($(F_{(-)} - F_{(0)}) / F_{(-)} = 60$ %) and a similar photon statistic for each fluorescent probe. The fluorescence intensity distribution in the IS was analyzed by an optical multichannel analyzer (OMA II, E G & G). To determine the $1 / e^2$ radius of the IS a Gaussian curve was fitted to the measured intensity profile by the computer. For each cell preparation and each dye a reference radius was determined from measurements on 10 cells (w = 2.7+/-0.1 μm). To account for the effect of nonplanarity of the hepatocyte plasma membrane caused by microvilli the diffusion coefficients were corrected according to D' = 2 D (1). FRAP measurements were restricted to cells of 24 +/- 1 μm. Of those only cells exhibiting good peripheral staining were exepted for measurement.Statistics. Analysis of variance was performed according to the method of unweighted means (8). A mixed model was used (rat effect: random, treatment effect: fixed). Data were tested for normality and for homogeneity of variance in the different subgroups.

RESULTS

The fluorescent lipid analogues NBD-PC and F-C$_{16}$ predominantly labeled the plasma membranes of the hepatocytes giving an intense homogeneous ring stain. For both lipid probes the recovery was about 80%. We could demonstrate that 10^{-6} as well as 10^{-5} mol/l MPA significantly retarded the diffusion coefficients of both fluorescently labeled lipid analogues.

TABLE 1. Effect of high-dose MPA (10^{-5}mol/1) on NBD-PC diffusion

Cell preparation	*No. of cells	Control D'x10^9 (cm^2/s)	MPA D'x10^9 (cm^2/s)	ΔD' (%)
C	12	1.9+/-0.2	1.4+/-0.1	-25+/-9
D	8	1.8+/-0.3	1.5+/-0.3	-14+/-21
E	10	1.9+/-0.2	1.5+/-0.2	-22+/-13
F	9	2.1+/-0.3	1.6+/-0.3	-28+/-18
Total	39	1.9+/-0.1	1.5+/-0.1	-22+/-8

ANOVA F test for treatment effect: $F_{(1,3)} = 36.1$; $p < 0.01$

*No. of cells in each of the groups

As can be seen in the series of experiments summarized in Table 1, the diffusion coefficient D' of the membrane incorporated fluorochrome NBD-PC amounted to about 1.9×10^{-9} cm^2/s in the control groups. When the cells were incubated with 10^{-5} mol/l MPA for 60 min at room temperature prior to labeling with the fluorochrome, the diffusion coefficients decreased to a mean value of 1.5×10^{-9} mol/l. In the experimental series of Table 1 as well as those of Table 2 and 3, neither an effect depending on the cell preparation nor an interaction effect depending on both the cell preparation and the treatment (cell preparation x treatment) could be found. The treatment effect, a 22 % decrease of the diffusion coefficients as compared those of the controls, proved to be significant at the level of $p < 0.01$. The mobile fraction of NBD-PC was unaffected by MPA.

As can be seen in Table 2, in a further series of experiments, also using NBD-PC as fluorescent lipid probe, MPA at 10^{-6} mol/l could be demonstrated to retard lateral diffusion of the fluorochrome to an extent similar to that of MPA at the higher dose (22 % inhibition, $p < 0.05$). Again, there was no effect of MPA on the fraction of fluorophore free to diffuse.

TABLE 2.   Effect of high-dose MPA (10^{-6} mol/l) on NBD-PC diffusion

Cell preparation	No. of cells	Control D'x10^9 (cm^2/s)	MPA D'x10^9 (cm^2/s)	ΔD' (%)
D	8	1.8+/-0.3	1.5+/-0.3	-18+/-21
G	10	1.9+/-0.2	1.5+/-0.2	-18+/-14
H	12	1.9+/-0.2	1.3+/-0.2	-30+/-13
Total	30	1.9+/-0.2	1.4+/-0.2	-22+/-10

ANOVA F test for treatment effect: $F_{(1,2)}$ = 21.7; $p < 0.05$

As is summarized in Table 3, with the lipid analogue F-C$_{16}$ as fluorescent probe for the lipid layer of the plasma membrane higher basal diffusion constants were observed as compared to NBD-PC . MPA at 10^{-5} mol/l resulted in a significant ($p < 0.05$) decrease of the diffusion coefficients to 70 % of those of the controls. The mobile fraction of F-C$_{16}$ was found to be not sensitive to MPA treatment.

TABLE 3.   Effect of MPA (10^{-5} mol/l) on F-C$_{16}$ diffusion

Cell preparation	No. of cells	Control D'x10^9 (cm^2/s)	MPA D'x10^9 (cm^2/s)	ΔD' (%)
A	11	3.9+/-0.4	2.8+/-0.4	-27+/-13
B	10	3.8+/-0.3	2.5+/-0.2	-32+/-7
Total	21	3.9+/-0.3	2.7+/-0.2	-30+/-7

ANOVA F test for treatment effect: $F_{(1,1)}$ = 319; $p < 0.05$

DISCUSSION

Our results support the hypothesis that one of the action mechanisms of high-dose MPA involves modulation of the lipid mobility of the plasma membrane. Recently, Searls and Edidin (9), also by applying FRAP technique, could demonstrate that fluorescently labeled lipid probes diffused more rapidly in plasma membranes of teratocarcinoma-derived cell lines as compared to embryo-derived cell lines. When the embryonal carcinoma lines were induced to differentiate, diffusion constants were reduced to levels similar to those of normal endodermal cell lines. This changes were paralled by differences in the content of the essential membrane steroid cholesterol. Membrane free cholesterol levels were inversely related to the observed changes in the diffusion constants. Considering the MPA-induced decrease of the lateral diffusion coefficients observed in our study, the steroidal compound MPA might be able to induce 'pseudonormality' of membrane dynamics in malignant cells.

Steroid-induced changes in plasma membrane fluidity and conformation have been proposed by several authors. By incorporation of cholesteryl hemisuccinate into the cell membranes a marked increase in specific immunogenicity of tumor cells could be achieved (11). Cholesteryl hemisuccinate is a strong lipid rigifier and is assumed to mediate the exposure of latent tumor associated antigens to the immunsystem. In general, it has been hypothesized by Shinitzky (11) that changes in lipid fluidity can expose or mask antigenic determinants in the plasma membrane. It remains to be elucidated, wether or not MPA by a similar mechanism might be able to increase tumor immunogenicity.
Massa et al.(6), when analysing the effect of hormones on the activity of membrane-bound acetylcholinesterase and Na^+/K^+-ATPase, concluded that cortisol effected the enzymes by an enhancement of membrane fluidity. Interestingly, the above authors also quoted their own preliminary data on the effect of progesterone on acetylcholinesterase. In contrast to cortisol, progesterone at 10^{-7} mol/l decreased membrane fluidity.
In conclusion, we believe that for obvious, discussed reasons the MPA-induced decrease in the lateral mobility of membrane lipids may play a role in the antitumor activity of MPA.

REFERENCES

1. Aizenbud, B.M., Gershon, N.D. (1982): Biophys. J., 38: 287-293
2. Axelrod, D., Koppel, D.E., Schlessinger, J., Elson, E., Webb, W.W. (1976): Biophys. J., 16: 1055-1069
3. Bojar, H., Balzer, K., Reiners, K., Basler, M., Reipen, W., Staib, W. (1975): J. Clin. Chem. Clin. Biochem., 13: 25-30
4. Koppel, D.E., Axelrod, D., Schlessinger, J., Elson, E.L:, Webb, W.W. (1976): Biophys. J., 16: 1315-1329
5. Lee, A.G., Bridsall, N.J., Metcalfe, J.C., Toon, P.A., Warren, G.B. (1974): Biochemistry,13: 3699-3705
6. Massa, E.M., Morero, R.D., Bloj, B., Farias, R.N. (1975): Biochem. Biophys. Res. Commun., 66: 115-122
7. Nicolson, G.L. (1976): Biochim. Biophys. Acta, 457: 57-108
8. Searle, S.R. (1971): Linear models. Wiley, New York
9. Searls, D.B., Edidin, M. (1981): Cell, 24: 511-517
10. Shimshick, E.J., McConnell, H.M.(1973): Biochemistry, 12: 2351-2359
11. Shinitzky, M., Skornick, Y. (1982): In: Membranes in tumour growth. edited by T. Galeotti et al. , pp. 61-68. Elsevier Biomedical Press Amsterdam, New York, Oxford

Progress in Cancer Research and Therapy,
Vol. 31, edited by F. Bresciani, et al.
Raven Press, New York © 1984.

Prostatic Epithelial Morphogenesis, Growth, and Secretory Cytodifferentiation Are Elicited Via Trophic Influences from Mesenchyme

G.R. Cunha

Department of Anatomy, University of California, San Francisco, California 94143

In vivo studies have demonstrated that injection of testosterone into castrated males stimulates prostatic epithelial DNA synthesis and proliferation (1,7,11,51). Since it is not possible to determine from animal studies whether androgens stimulate prostatic epithelial growth via direct, androgen-receptor-mediated mechanisms within the epithelial cells themselves, organ and cell cultures have been used as a means of providing a more simplified system to study androgenic effects upon the prostate. Prostatic explants maintained in organ culture retain the histotypic architectural association of epithelium and stroma which may facilitate or may be required for eliciting androgen-induced epithelial proliferation (2,23). Prostatic epithelial hyperplasia, defined histologically as an increase in epithelial cells/acinus, has been elicited by addition of androgens to prostatic organ cultures (5,31,32). Utilizing epithelial labelling index or biochemical incorporation of precursors into DNA as a means of investigating growth in organ culture, many investigators have demonstrated a direct effect of testosterone on prostatic growth (26,27,38,40). By contrast, prostatic epithelial cells grown in monolayer culture are neither dependent upon nor sensitive to testosterone or its metabolites for proliferation (6,8,9,22,25,34,35,39,42,44,48,50,52). Thus, although androgens may stimulate prostatic growth in organ culture by direct (presumably androgen receptor mediated) mechanisms, it is unclear whether androgen stimulation of prostatic epithelial proliferation can be elicited directly in these cells or whether other prostatic cells play a role in this process. The presence of androgen receptors (29,30,46,49) within both epithelial and stromal cells of the prostate clearly raises the possibility that androgen-induced prostatic epithelial growth may be mediated either directly via intra-epithelial androgen receptors or indirectly via trophic influences from androgen stimulated stromal cells. The fortuitous correlation of intra-epithelial androgen receptors with androgen-induced epithelial growth (increased ^{3}H-thymidine labelling) cannot be construed as indicating that prostatic epithelial growth is mediated via these intra-epithelial androgen receptors. This reasonable (but probably incorrect) conclusion completely disregards the distinct possibility that androgen-receptor-positive stromal cells may play a role as essential mediators or regulators of prostatic epithelial growth. Resolution of the questions posed above is not possible through biochemical analysis of prostatic homogenates which destroy the morphological integrity of the prostate. However, regulation of prostatic epithelial growth is amenable to cell biological analysis of tissue recombinants composed of epithelium and mesenchyme derived from Tfm and wild-type mice. The insensitivity to androgens of Tfm mice (or humans) is due to

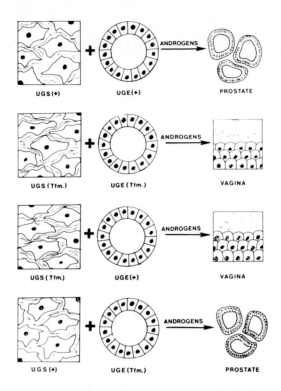

Fig. 1. Recombination experiments between urogenital sinus epithelium and mesenchyme from Tfm and wild-type mouse embryos. Prostatic morphogenesis occurs only when wild-type mesenchyme is utilized irrespective of the source of the epithelium (wild-type or Tfm). Conversely, vaginal differentiation occurs when either wild-type or Tfm epithelium is grown in association with Tfm mesenchyme. From Cunha et al (17).

abnormalities in androgen receptor activity which may be undetectable, present in reduced levels (in comparison to normal controls), or may be thermally unstable (3,4,21,53,54). Moreover, it can be argued that residual androgen-binding activity in Tfm individuals is not indicative of true androgen receptor activity since this residual activity is not coupled to biologic response of androgens, e.g. development of male internal and external genitalia. Thus, because of this insensitivity to androgens, the urogenital sinus of Tfm mice never develops prostatic tissue (36,41).

Despite the insensitivity of Tfm tissues to androgens, urogenital sinus epithelial cells of Tfm fetuses can be induced to form prostatic tissue (Fig. 1) when associated with urogenital sinus mesenchyme (UGM) derived from androgen-receptor-positive wild-type fetuses, provided the tissue recombinants are grown in intact male hosts (16,17,33). Prostatic epithelial development can also be induced in adult Tfm bladder epithelial cells by wild-type UGM (15,17). By contrast, when Tfm mesenchyme is utilized, prostatic development is never observed whether the epithelium is derived from wild-type or Tfm mice (Fig. 1). These observations are in complete agreement with the earlier reports of Tfm/wild-type tissue recombinations performed on the developing mammary gland (20,28). All studies of this type demonstrate that the mesenchyme is the actual target and mediator of androgenic effects upon the epithelium, a concept proposed earlier from studies on developing male accessory sexual glands (12-14).

Prostatic development elicited in Tfm epithelium, whether derived from urogenital sinus (UGE) or bladder epithelium (BLE) (15-17) involves three fundamental processes all of which are androgen dependent: glandular arborization (epithelial morphogenesis); epithelial growth; and secretory cytodifferentiation. All of these processes are androgen-dependent (since they only occur in tissue recombinants grown in intact and not castrated male hosts 19), and all are expressed in androgen-insensitive Tfm epithelium which remains deficient in nuclear androgen-binding sites (47). By contrast, the associated wild-type stromal cells of these Tfm/wild-type tissue recombinants exhibit nuclear androgen binding sites. These wild-type stromal cells are thought to provide the basis for androgenic sensitivity in these tissue recombinants.

To directly assess the androgenic dependency of epithelial morphogenesis and growth in tissue recombinants composed of wild-type urogenital sinus mesenchyme and Tfm bladder epithelium (UGM + Tfm BLE), tissue recombinants were grown in either intact or castrated male hosts for 7 days. Two hours before sacrifice the hosts were injected with ^{3}H-thymidine (1uCi/g body weight). In UGM + Tfm BLE recombinants grown in castrated male hosts, prostatic morphogenesis did not occur, and the epithelium was maintained as bladder epithelium. As expected labelling index within the Tfm BLE was extremely low. By contrast, in intact male hosts prostatic morphogenesis proceeded and epithelial labelling index was dramatically elevated in UGM + Tfm BLE recombinants (Fig. 2).

Differentiation of a simple columnar secretory epithelium occurs in tissue recombinants prepared with wild-type UGM and either Tfm UGE or BLE. In both cases a stratified transitional epithelium gives rise to a highly differentiated secretory epithelium. Epithelial height and secretory cytodifferentiation are androgen-dependent since castration of hosts bearing UGM + Tfm BLE recombinants leads to epithelial atrophy, a condition that can be reversed by administration of testosterone. Restoration of a tall secretory epithelium by testosterone can be inhibited by co-administration of an excess of cyproterone acetate (15).

These observations demonstrate that wild-type urogenital sinus mesenchyme is the actual target and mediator of androgenic effects upon the epithelium. Moreover, androgen-receptor-deficient Tfm epithelial cells express androgen-induced morphogenesis, growth, and secretory cytodifferentiation when grown in association with wild-type UGM. Since each of these processes is androgen-dependent and presumably mediated via androgen receptors, we conclude that androgenic effects expressed in Tfm epithelial cells must be mediated via trophic factors produced by the wild-type mesenchymal cells. Significantly, autoradiographic analysis of the developing prostate and mammary gland demonstrates the presence of androgen receptors in mesenchymal cells of these organ rudiments of wild-type embryos (18,24,45,46). Furthermore, in UGM + Tfm BLE recombinants the stromal cells derived from wild-type UGM are androgen-receptor positive while the Tfm glandular epithelial cells are devoid of nuclear androgen-binding sites (19,47).

Another approach in evaluating the mechanism of androgenic action within the prostate is to assess and compare androgenic action in mature UGM +Tfm BLE recombinants versus that in fully differentiated wild-type prostate. These two types of prostatic specimens exhibit one fundamental difference. In wild-type prostate both epithelial and stromal cells possess androgen receptors, whereas in UGM + Tfm BLE recombinants, only the wild-type stromal cells exhibit this activity (19,47,49). Androgen-deprivation causes prostatic epithelial atrophy which is reversed by administration of androgen (43).

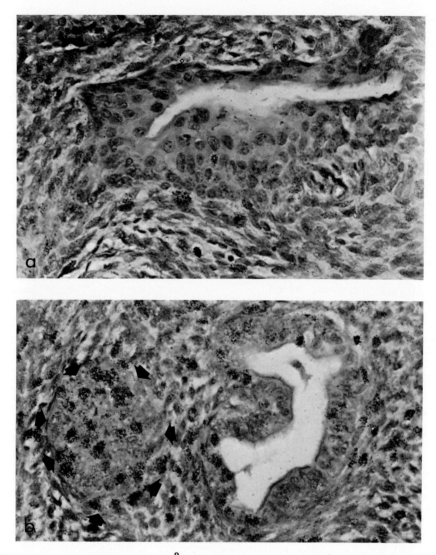

Fig. 2.   Autoradiographs of ^{3}H thymidine incorporation in recombinants composed of wild-type UGM + Tfm BLE.   (a) Recombinants grown in castrated male hosts do not undergo prostatic morphogenesis. Instead the epithelium remains unchanged and labelling is essentially nil. (b) UGM + Tfm BLE recombinant grown in an intact male host. Note the solid (arrows) and canalized prostatic ducts, which demonstrate that prostatic morphogenesis and cytodifferentiation is occurring in the Tfm epithelium. Labelling of the Tfm epithelium with ^{3}H-Thymidine is substantial. 400X. From Cunha et al (19).

Epithelial cytodifferentiation in UGM + Tfm BLE recombinants undergoes identical changes, being tall and well differentiated in intact or testosterone-treated castrated hosts and atrophic in castrated hosts or in castrated hosts injected with testosterone plus cyproterone acetate (15).

Prostatic DNA synthesis is induced when androgens are injected into

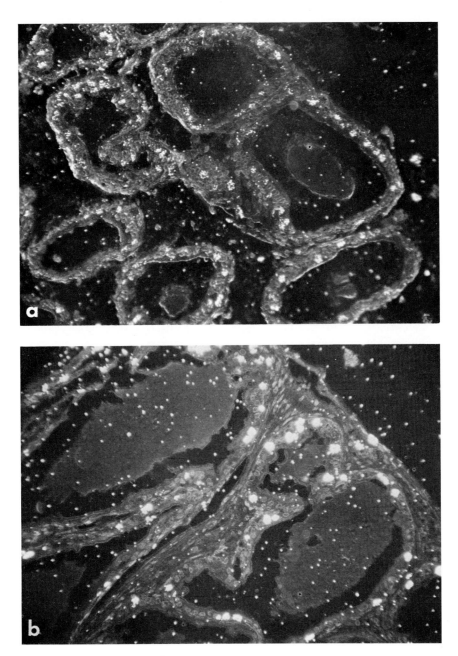

Fig. 3. Autoradiograms of ^{3}H-thymidine in (a) wild-type prostate and (b) wild-type UGM + Tfm BLE recombinants. Recombinants were grown for 1 month in intact male hosts, which were then castrated. Two weeks post-castration, the hosts were injected daily with testosterone propionate (TP). Seventy hours after initiation of TP treatment the host mice were injected with ^{3}H-thymidine (1uCi/g body weight) and sacrificed 2 hours later. Paraffin sections were prepared and processed autoradiographically. (a) is the wild-type prostate of the host bearing the grafted UGM + Tfm BLE recombinant (b). Note that nuclear labelling is similar in both specimens (400X).

previously castrated wild-type rodents (10).   Comparison of incorporation of ^{3}H-thymidine in wild-type prostate, UGM + Tfm BLE recombinants and in urinary bladder demonstrates that testosterone propionate injected daily stimulates DNA synthesis in both wild-type prostate and UGM + Tfm BLE recombinants; the peak of DNA synthesis occurs on day 3 of androgen stimulation. By contrast, DNA synthesis in the urinary bladder is unresponsive.   Preliminary results of parallel autoradiographic studies demonstrate comparable ^{3}H-thymidine labelling in epithelial cells of the wild-type prostate and UGM + Tfm BLE recombinants, which indicates that much of the DNA synthetic activity measured biochemically is in fact due to thymidine incorporation into the Tfm epithelial cells (Fig. 3).

Another effect of androgens is stimulation of protein synthesis in the prostate (37). Therefore, protein synthetic activity was assessed in the urinary bladder, wild-type prostate, and UGM + Tfm BLE tissue recombinants by 2-dimensional gel electrophoresis. Results of this study indicate that organs such as the prostate and urinary bladder express distinctive patterns of protein synthetic activity. Moreover, UGM + Tfm BLE recombinants exhibit a pattern of protein synthetic activity which is very similar to that of the prostate. However, despite this similarity it must be recognized that the UGM + Tfm BLE recombinants exhibit some subtle differences in proteins synthesized relative to wild-type prostate.

Hormonal response is usually correlated with the expression of hormone receptor activity within the responding cells. In the prostate, biochemical and autoradiographic evidence demonstrates that prostatic epithelial cells possess nuclear androgen receptors (29,30,49).   Furthermore, animal studies have demonstrated that proliferative activity of prostatic epithelium is stimulated by androgens.   This has lead many to assume that the growth response of prostatic epithelium to androgens is elicited directly via androgen receptor activity within prostatic epithelial cells. Arguing against this conclusion is the observation that prostatic epithelial cells grown in monolayer culture proliferate whether androgens are present or absent (6,9,42,44,48,50). Moreover, Franks et al (23) have demonstrated that apposition of epithelial and stromal tissues is required for prostatic epithelial DNA synthesis. This concept receives considerable support from analyses of androgenic response in tissue recombinants composed of wild-type UGM + Tfm BLE. Tfm epithelium (UGE or BLE) is unequivocally insensitive to androgens and lacks androgen receptors as judged autoradiographically (19,47).   Despite this, glandular arborization, epithelial DNA synthesis, and secretory cytodifferentiation are elicited by androgens in Tfm epithelial cells of UGM + Tfm BLE recombinants grown in male hosts. The fundamental difference between wild-type prostate and UGM + Tfm BLE recombinants is the presence of androgen receptors in wild-type prostatic epithelium and their absence in UGM +Tfm BLE recombinants. In both cases the stromal cells of these specimens possess androgen receptors.

The fact that a variety of androgen-induced epithelial effects can be elicited in androgen-receptor deficient Tfm epithelial cells in UGM + Tfm BLE recombinants indicates that expression of these effects does not require androgen-receptor mechanisms within the responding   epithelial cells themselves.   To the contrary, these results suggest that many androgenic effects expressed within prostatic epithelium are elicited via trophic influences emanating from mesenchymal or stromal cells whose biosynthetic activity is regulated, in part, by androgens. From this body of evidence it is apparent that attention must now be focused upon the stromal component of the developing and mature prostate.   It is evident that elucidation of the mechanism of androgenic effects upon the prostate will have to resolve function of stromal cells at the molecular level in relation to regulation of epithelial growth and development.   (Supported by NIH grants AM 25266, CA27418, and AMCA 16570).

References

1. Allen, J.M. (1958): Exptl. Cell Res., 10:523-532.
2. Aumuller, G. (1983): Prostate, 4:195-214.
3. Attardi B., and Ohno, S. (1974): Cell, 2:205-212.
4. Bardin, C.W., and Bullock, L.P. (1974): J. Inves. Dermatol., 63:75-84.
5. Baulieu, E.E., Lasnitzki, I., and Robel, P. (1968): Nature, 219: 1155-1156.
6. Brehmer, B., Marquardt, H., and Madsen, P.O. (1972): J. Urol., 108:890-96.
7. Bruchovsky, N., Lesser, B., and Van doorn, E. (1975): Vitamins and Hormones, 33:61-101.
8. Burleigh, B.D., Reich, E., and Strickland, S. (1980): Endocrinology, 19:183-196.
9. Chevalier, S., Bleau, G., Roberts, K.D., and Chapdelaine, A. (1981): Endocrinology, 24:195-208
10. Chung, L.W.R and Coffey, D.S. (1971): Biochem. Biophys. Acta., 247:584-596.
11. Coffey, D.S. (1974): In: Male Accessory Sex Organs: Structure and Function in Mammals, edited by D. Brandes, pp. 307-328. Academic Press, New York.
12. Cunha, G.R. (1972a): Anat. Rec., 172:179-196.
13. Cunha, G.R. (1972b): Anat. Rec., 172:529-542.
14. Cunha, G.R. (1972c): Anat. Rec., 173:205-212.
15. Cunha, G.R and Chung, L.W.K. (1981): J. Steroid Biochem., 14:1317-1321.
16. Cunha G.R, and Lung, B. (1978): J. Exptl. Zool., 205:181-194.
17. Cunha G.R., Chung, L.W.K, Shannon, J.M., and Reese, B.A. (1980): Biol. of Reprod., 22:19-42.
18. Cunha G.R, Shannon, J.M., Neubauer, B.L., Sawyer, L.M., Fujii, H., Taguchi, O., and Chung L.W.K (1981): Human Genetics, 56:68-77.
19. Cunha G.R., Chung L.W.K., Shannon J.M., Taguchi O., and Fujii, H. (1983): Recent Prog. Hormone Res., 39:559-598.
20. Drews, U., and Drews, U. (1977): Cell, 10:401-404.
21. Fox, T.O., and Wieland, S.J. (1981): Endocrinology, 109:790-797.
22. Fraley, E.E., Ecker, S., and Vincent, M.M. (1970): Science, 170:540-542.
23. Franks, L.M., Riddle, P.N., Carbonell, A.W., and Gey, G.O. (1970): J. Pathol., 100:113-119.
24. Heuberger, B., Fitzka, I., Wasner, G., and Kratochwil, K. (1982): Proc. Natl. Acad. Sci., 79:2957-2961.
25. Hudson, R.W. (1981): Physiol. and Pharmacol., 59:949-956.
26. Johansson, R. (1975): Acta. Endoc., 80:761-774.
27. Johansson, R., and Niemi, M. (1975): Acta. Endoc., 78:766-780.
28. Kratochwil, K., Schwartz, P. (1976): Proc. Natl. Acad. Sci. USA, 73:4041-4044.
29. Krieg, M., Klotzl, G., Kaufman, J., and Voigt, K.D. (1981): Acta. Endocrinol. 96:422-432.
30. Lahtonen, R., Bolton, N.J., Kontturi, M., and Vihko, R. (1983): Prostate, 4:129-139.
31. Lasnitzki, I. (1974)): In: Male Accessory Sex Organs: Structure and Function in Mammals, edited by D. Brandes, pp 348-382. Academic Press, New York.
32. Lasnitzki, I., Whitaker, R.H., Withycombe, J.F.R. (1975): Br. J. Cancer, 32:168-178.
33. Lasnitzki I., and Mizuno, T. (1980): J. Endoc., 85:423-428.
34. Lechner, J.F., Naayan, K.S., Ohnuki, Y., Babcock, M.S., Jones, L.W., and Kaighn, M.E. (1978): J. Nat'l. Cancer Inst., 60:797-801.
35. Lewis, R.W., Kaack, B., Roth, J.K., and Fussell, E.N. (1981): Invest. Urol., 18:251-257.

36. Lyon M.F., Cattanach, B.M., and Charlton, H.M. (1981): In: Mechanisms of Sex Determination in Animals and Man, edited by C.R. Austin and R.G. Edwards, pp. 329–386. Academic Press, New York.

37. Mainwaring, W.I.P. (1977): The Mechanism of Action of Androgens, Springer-Verlag, New York.

38. McRae, C.U., Ghamadian, K., Fatherby, K., and Chrisholm, G.D. (1973): Br. J. Urol., 45:156.

39. Merchant, D.J. (1979): In: Prostatic Cancer, edited by G.P. Murphy, pp. 75–88. PSG Publishing Co., Littleton, Mass.

40. Mistry, D., Buchanan, L., Dattani, G., Weaver, P., and Riches, A. (1982): Prostate 3:291–299.

41. Ohno, S. (1979): Major Sex Determining Genes. Springer-Verlag, New York.

42. Okada, K., Laudenbach, I., and Schoeder, F.H. (1976): J. Urology, 115:164–167.

43. Price, D., and Williams-Ashman, H.G. (1961): In: Sex and Internal Secretions 3rd Ed., edited by W.C. Young, pp. 366–448. Williams and Wilkins, Baltimore.

44. Shain, S.A., Boesel, R.W., Kalter, S.S., and Heberling, R.L. (1982): In: Hormones and Cancer, edited by Wendell W. Leavitt, pp. 337–351. Plenum Pub. Corp., New York.

45. Shannon, J.M., Cunha, G.R., and Vanderslice, K.D. (1981): Anat. Rec., 199:232A.

46. Shannon, J.M., Cunha, G.R. (1983a): Prostate 4:367–373.

47. Shannon, J.M., Cunha G.R. (1983b): Biol. of Reprod., (In Press).

48. Stone, K.R., Stone, M.P., and Paulson, D.F. (1976): Invest. Urol., 14:79–82.

49. Stumpf, W.E., Sar, M. (1976): Autoradiographic localization of estrogen, androgen, progestin, and glucocorticosteroid in "target tissues" and "non-target tissues." In: Receptors and Mechanism of action of steroid hormones, J.R. Pasqualini ed. pp 41–84. Marcel Dekker Inc., New York.

50. Syms, A.S., Haysen, M.E., Buttersby, S., and Griffiths, K. (1982): J. Urology, 127:561–567.

51. Tuohimaa, P., and Niemi M. (1974): In: Male Accessory Sex Organs: Structure and Function in Mammals, edited by D. Brandes, pp. 329–343. Academic Press, New York.

52. Webber, M.M. (1974): J. Urol., 112:798–801.

53. Wieland, S.J., and Fox, T.O. (1979): Cell, 17:781–787.

54. Wilson, J.D., Griffin, Leshin, M., and George, F.W. (1981): Human Genetics, 58:78–84.

Progress in Cancer Research and Therapy,
Vol. 31, edited by F. Bresciani, et al.
Raven Press, New York © 1984.

Growth Arrest of Mammary Tumors by Proline Analogs

William R. Kidwell, Susan Taylor, Mozenna Bano, and Flora Grantham

Laboratory of Pathophysiology, Cell Cycle Regulation Section, National Cancer Institute, Bethesda, Maryland 20205

Proline analogs such as cis-hydroxyproline, 4-thio-proline and L-azetidine carboxylate have been found to be good inhibitors of the growth of rat mammary tumors in vivo. An analysis of this phenomenon has indicated that the sensitivity to these analogs is a function of the degree of differentiation of the tumors and in particular is correlated with the ability of the tumor to make basement membranous material. The studies have indicated that the production of the basement membrane is important for the growth of such tumors because these proline analogs selectively inhibit collagen synthesis and block basement membrane assembly before cell death occurs. Basement membrane production by the tumors appears to be regulated in an autocrine fashion. Tumors that produce this material also make a growth factor that is very potent in stimulating production of the three major components of the basement membrane; collagen, laminin and glycosaminoglycan. Tumors that do not make a basement membrane do not make the growth factor. They are also resistant to the effects of the proline analogs in vivo. The results obtained with the experimental animal model systems are probably applicable to the human breast cancer situation. In the present report we (a) review the observations that indicate a necessity for basement membrane production for certain types of mammary tumor growth (b) demonstrate the specificity and utility of proline analogs in blocking production of this matrix material and (c) examine the mechanisms whereby basement membrane synthesis is controlled in tumors that make this substance.

PROLINE ANALOG EFFECTS ON TUMOR GROWTH

A range of types of mammary tumors has been evaluated for sensitivity to cis-hydroxyproline. Both primary and transplantable rat mammary tumors have been found to be very responsive (3). Highly differentiated tumors such as N'-methylnitrosourea-induced tumor, the 7,12-dimethylbenz (α)anthracine-induced tumor and the transplantable MTW9 tumor are responsive. Poorly differentiated tumors that have been analyzed include the DMBA-1, the T-NMU and the MTW9a, all of which are maintained by serial transplantation. None of these are sensitive to the analogs. Examples of the most extremes of histological types are depicted in fig. 1 a,b. In fig. 1a, is depicted the primary NMU-induced tumor

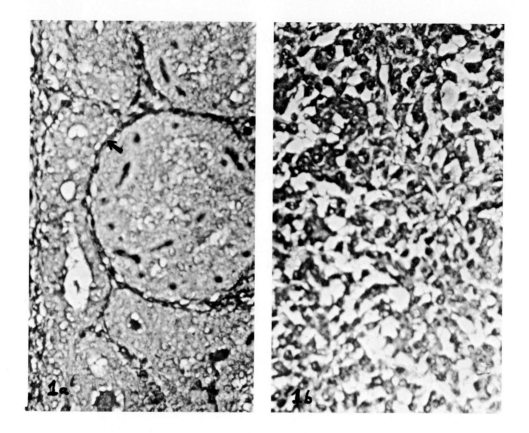

Fig. 1. Examples of well differentiated and poorly differentiated rat
mammary tumors. Well differentiated, primary NMU-induced (1a) and the
poorly differentiated transplantable NMU tumor, fig. 1b. Tumors stained
with PAMS, periodic acid Schiff-silver. The basement membrane is illustrated by the arrow in fig. 1a. Note the lack of staining for this
material in the poorly differentiated tumor.

and in 1b is the transplantable NMU tumor. The tumor sections have
been stained for basal lamina and this material is readily demonstrated
in the primary tumor but is absent in the transplantable one. Consistent with the presence of basement membranous material is the fact that
the primary NMU-induced tumors synthesize type IV collagen, a collagen
species that is uniquely localized in basement membranes. In contrast,
the transplantable NMU tumor derived from the primary by serial transplantation (Miorana, A., NIH) synthesizes stromal collagen and little or
no type IV collagen (fig. 2 a,b).

Structures and Biological Activities of Proline Analogs

The structures of the proline analogs we have evaluated extensively
are depicted in fig. 3. Like proline, they are imino acids and all have

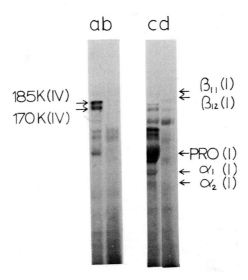

Fig. 2. Identification of the type of collagen made by the well differentiated and the poorly differentiated rat mammary tumors. Primary cultures of the two types of epithelium were prepared and incubated with ^{14}C-proline to label proteins. The collagens were extracted and electrophoresed according to methods described by Timpl, et al. (6). Autoradiography was performed to identify the newly synthesized collagen. 2a,b; collagen samples from the well differentiated tumor. 2c,d; collagen samples from the poorly differentiated tumor. In lanes b and d are the samples that were digested with collagenase before electrophoresis. In a and c are the corresponding samples without collagenase digestion. Arrows indicate the electrophoretic mobility of type IV collagen species (left margin) and the type I collagen species (right margin). As is evident, the well differentiated tumor produces only type IV collagen, the collagen of basement membranes, while the poorly differentiated tumor produces predominantly type I collagen in the precursor form, Pro (I). The same results have been obtained when comparing the primary and the transplantable DMBA tumors. I.e., the production of type IV collagen is seen only with the differentiated tumor and the Pro (I) collagen with the poorly differentiated tumor. Reproduced from reference 3.

been shown to be taken up into cells and incorporated into proteins in place of and in competition with proline. Their effect on collagen in particular is due to the fact that this protein is on average about 8 times richer in proline than are the total cellular proteins. Prockop's group (2) has shown that the incorporation of the proline analog into collagen has the effect of destabilizing the collagen triple helix making the protein more susceptible to intracellular degradation.

Effects of Proline Analogs on Collagen Synthesis in Tumor Cell Cultures

All of the proline analogs listed in fig. 3 are good inhibitors of collagen synthesis by primary cultures of rat mammary tumor cells as

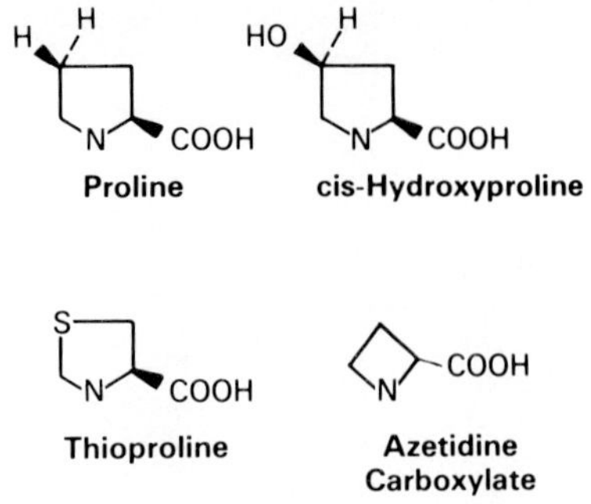

Fig. 3. Structure of some biologically active proline analogs.

shown in Table 1. Primary NMU or DMBA-induced mammary tumor epithelium
was incubated with the analogs at a concentration of 25 µg/ml medium
(Serum-free IMEM containing insulin, hydrocortisone, epidermal growth
factor, transferrin and fetuin as described by Salomon (5). The incorporation of ^{3}H lysine into collagenase sensitive protein was differentially reduced by 4 to 27 fold after 3 days of culture as shown in
Table 1.

Table 1.   Selective effects of proline analogs
on collagen synthesis

Proline Analog*	% Inhibition of Collagen Synthesis % Inhibition of Total Protein Synthesis
CHP	4
TP	14
LACA	27

*The abbreviations are: CHP, cis-hydroxyproline, TP, Thioproline and
LACA, L-azetidine carboxylate.

Proline Analog Effects on Tumor Growth

Based on the ability of cis-hydroxyproline to block the growth of
the normal rat mammary epithelium (7) it was postulated that mammary
tumors might also be responsive to the proline analog. Accordingly,
rats bearing tumors induced with either NMU or DMBA were administered
cis-hydroxyproline either orally in drinking water or by s.c. injection. The total dose given was 100 mg/kg twice daily by the injection
route or the same amount in the volume of water that the average
animal would consume/day. Tumor growth was assessed on the basis of
change in tumor volume with time. The results obtained with the analog
given by the s.c. route are presented in fig. 4a. As seen there was an
immediate cessation of growth after analog administration was begun.
The drug caused no deleterious effects on the host animals at this concentration as determined from body weight measurements and histological

examination of cartilage, bone, liver, muscle and intestinal tissue. Electron microscopy revealed areas in which the basal lamina was missing and the tumor epithelium was apposed to stromal collagen. There was also areas in which folded lamina existed and others where basal cells were filled with material that appeared to be unsecreted lamina. Essentially the same results were obtained when the analog was given by the oral route.

The cis-hydroxyproline effects differed when tested on animals bearing the poorly differentiated mammary tumor, the transplantable NMU tumor as seen in fig. 4b. The proline analog given at the same concentration by the s.c. route was completely inactive. Since there was the possibility that the difference in responsiveness was a property of the transplantability of a tumor, a comparison was made of the effects of cis-hydroxyproline on differentiated and undifferentiated tumors that were transplantable. The conclusion reached from these studies was that the sensitivity to cis-hydroxyproline related to the degree of differentiation or the tumors.

The two other proline analogs, TP and LACA, have also been evaluated for their effects on mammary tumor growth. The results obtained are essentially the same as those presented in fig. 4a. With primary NMU or DMBA induced tumors there is a growth arrest seen at 100 mg thioproline/kg body weight. This analog actually causes tumor regression to about 1/2 of the tumor volume at the time of initiation of analog treatment after two weeks treatment. The LACA was also an efficient blocker of tumor growth. Consistent with its greater potency in blocking collagen synthesis in tumor cell cultures, the analog was also active in vivo at concentrations 1/2 to 1/3 that required for tumor growth arrest by cis-hydroxyproline. A near complete growth arrest was seen at a dose of 50 mg LACA/kg when administered s.c.

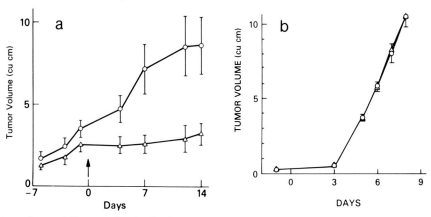

Fig. 4a. Effect of cis-hydroxyproline on the growth of primary NMU-induced mammary tumors. Tumor growth was followed for about 1 week prior to initiating treatment by s.c. injection. Arrow indicates the time injections begun. Triangles are the treatment group and the circles are the saline controls. Values age given with the standard deviations. After 14 days, the groups differ in tumor volume by a factor of about 2.5. The difference is statistically significant (p value of <0.03). Reproduced from reference 3.

Fig. 4b. Lack of effect of cis-hydroxyproline on the growth of transplantable NMU-induced tumors in vivo. The protocol is essentially as outlined for fig. 4a. Reproduced from reference 1.

REGULATION OF BASEMENT MEMBRANE PRODUCTION BY MAMMARY TUMORS

The results obtained to date are all suggestive of a requirement of mammary adenocarcinomas for the production of a basement membrane for tumor growth. The ability of the proline analogs, cis-hydroxyproline, thioproline and L-azetidine carboxylate in blocking the growth of this type of tumor but having no effect on tumors which do not make this type of matrix material is consistent with this postulate. However, other information recently obtained also strongly suggests this possibility. We have found, (1) that basement membrane producing tumors of the rat mammary gland make a growth factor that is very potent in differentially enhancing the production of a basement membrane. This factor is a protein of 68,000 molecular weight and pI of 5.9, in the case of rat tumors. In cultures of normal rat or mouse mammary cells it stimulates type IV collagen, laminin and glycosaminoglycan production by 2 to 10 fold more than it stimulates total cell protein synthesis. Most interestingly, this growth factor does not affect the tumor cells from which the factor is derived. This indicates that the factor acts in an autoregulatory fashion and is produced in optimal amounts by such tumor cells.

Table 2. Collagen synthesis stimulating activity
production by various mammary tumors

Tumor extract[a]	Differentiation[b]	CSSF[c]	68 K Protein[d]
Primary NMU	High	380	1.0
Transp. NMU	Low	40	0.1
Primary DMBA	Moderate	210	0.4
Transp. DMBA	Low	10	0.0
Transp. MTW9	Moderate	150	0.3
Transp. MTW9a	Low	0	N.T.

[a]Tumor extracts were prepared by acid-ethanol extraction and ether precipitation as described by Roberts (4). The biological activity is recoverable as a soluble protein from the ether precipitate.
[b]The degree of differentiation was estimated from random sections of 5-6 tumors that had been stained with PAMS.
[c]CSSF is a measure of the collagen synthesis stimulating activity present in the tumor extract. It is estimated by determining the amount of labeled amino acid incorporated into collagen, normalized against total amino acid incorporation, and converted to a percentage. Thus, cells incubated with primary NMU extract made collagen 380% more abundantly than they did when incubated with the MTW9a extract.
[d]The amount of the 68 K protein in the tumor extract was quantitated by SDS-gel electrophoresis of the pI 5.9 fraction of the various tumor extracts. The biological activity in the extract was previously shown to reside in this protein. Details of the purification and bioassays are given in reference 1. The amount of stainable protein on the gels is expressed relative to that of primary NMU tumor extracts.

The production of collagen synthesis stimulating factor is also related to the degree of differentiation of the rat mammary tumors as indicated in table 2. The most differentiated tumors contain the most extractable activity while the least differentiated contain the least activity.

We would like to present two other recent observations and formulate a model outlining our concept of how production of the basement membrane is regulated and the significance of this process. First, we have found that normal mammary cells which produce less than optimal amounts of the collagen synthesis stimulating factor respond to the exogenous addition of the factor. However, their response is dependent on the substratum on which the cells are plated. For example, the cells produce about 6 times as much type IV collagen in response to the factor when the cells are cultured on type I collagen surfaces (stromal collagen) as they do when plated on type IV collagen, the collagen on which the normal mammary epithelium rests in vivo. A second observation which is pertinent is that proline auxotrophy is seen by both normal and tumor epithelium (from primary, well differentiated tumors) when the cells are grown on the stromal collagen substrata but not when the cells are grown on type IV collagen or plastic substrata.

Taken together with the other observations presented these results lead to the conclusion that the well differentiated tumors resemble normal mammary epithelium in that they recognize the basement membrane as the natural surface on which they should reside. (This is logical since the cells from either source are responsible for the synthesis of the basement membrane.) Not only do the tumor and normal cells recognize the appropriate substratum, but they also recognize a "foreign" substratum such as stromal collagen. Their response to such a foreign substratum is an increased sensititivity to hormones and growth factors such as the collagen synthesis stimulating activity, and an increased requirement for nutrients such as proline. In the event that hormones, growth factors or proline, etc. are not optimal for the production of new basement membrane during the growth into stroma, both the normal and tumor cells stop dividing. Teleologically this behavior makes good sense for it provides a mechanism for maintaining the epithelium as an organized, continuous structure. Differences between the well differentiated and poorly differentiated tumors may be, then, a difference in the ability of the cells therein to recognize stroma as a "foreign" substratum and hence a difference in proline auxotrophy. In other words, the well differentiated tumor epithelium and the normal mammary epithelium are more responsive to the proline analogs than the epithelium from poorly differentiated tumors because the former have a greater requirement for proline than the latter.

REFERENCES

1. Bano, M., Zwiebel, J., Salomon, D. and Kidwell, W. R. (1983): J. Biol. Chem., 258:2729-2735.
2. Bruckner, P., Eikenberry, E., and Prockop, D. (1981): Eur. J. Biochem., 118:607-613.
3. Lewko, W. M., Liotta, L. A., Wicha, M. S., Vonderhaar, B. K. and Kidwell, W. R. (1981): Cancer Res., 41:2855-2862.
4. Roberts, A. B., Lamb, L. C., Newton, D. L., Sporn, M. B., Delarco, J. E., and Todaro, G. J. (1980): Proc. Nat'l. Acad. Sci. U.S.A., 77:3494-3498.
5. Salomon, D. S., Liotta, L. A. and Kidwell, W. R. (1981): Proc. Nat'l. Acad. Sci. U.S.A., 78:382-386.
6. Timpl, R., Martin, G. R., Bruckner, P., Wick, G. and Wiedemann, H. (1978): Eur. J. Biochem., 84:43-49.
7. Wicha, M. S., Liotta, L. A., Vonderhaar, B. K. and Kidwell, W. R. (1980): Dev. Biol., 80:253-266.

Progress in Cancer Research and Therapy,
Vol. 31, edited by F. Bresciani, et al.
Raven Press, New York © 1984.

Establishment of Estrogen-Responsive Clonal Cell Lines in Tissue Culture from an Estrogen-Dependent, Prolactin-Secreting Rat Pituitary Tumor

*Martin Posner, † Anthony L. Rosner, **James Pellegrini, and ‡ Nelson A. Burstein

*Departments of *Physics and **Biology, University of Massachusetts/Boston, 02125; †Department of Pathology, Harvard Medical School and Beth Israel Hospital, 02215; and ‡Department of Pathology, St. Elizabeth's Hospital, Boston, Massachusetts 02135*

The physiologic effects of estrogen on target tumor cells in long term culture have been studied in detail by a number of investigators. Such tumor cell lines are derived from tumors of estrogen target tissues, e.g. mammary and mamotropic pituitary cells, possess characteristic estrogen receptor proteins, and require estrogen for in vivo growth in suitable syngenic host animals (21,24,25,29).

A number of recent studies on cell lines established from estrogen dependent tumor lines in inbred strains of rodents have failed to detect any direct effects of estrogen on cell growth (12,22,26,29,). Such negative results have led some investigators to postulate indirect modes of action of estrogen dependent tumors (11,22,23,27,28). In contrast, the work of Lippman, et.al. (1,4,15,17) on the MCF-7 and other human mammry tumor cell lines in culture indicated that direct stimulatory effects of estrogen on cell growth in vitro could be obtained utilizing estrogen deficienct culture medium and/or by the use of anti-estrogen drugs as Tamoxifen. Other investigators have failed to confirm these results on the MCF-7 cells (3,20). Recently, Amara and Dannies (2) have obtained estrogen stimulation of cell growth in culture for the GH_4C_1 cell line utilizing castrated horse serum.

The effects of estrogen on prolactin secretion are also contradictory. Short term studies on normal pituitary cells in culture show a stimulation by estrogen of prolactin secretion by a mechanism involving the induction of prolactin specific m-RNA synthesis (13,14,16,31,32). However, studies in culture on the cell line GH_3 and sub-lines have been inconsistent, with some studies indicating a position effect of estrogen on prolactin secretion (2,9,10) but others demonstrating no effect of estrogen (6).

The present studies were undertaken to try to resolve these descrepancies by establishing new tumor cell lines in culture from an estrogen dependent tumor line whose in vivo dependence on estrogen for growth was well documented. The Furth, mammotropic pituitary tumor line, MtT/W13, was chosen for this purpose because it is an estrogen induced tumor that

has been propagated exclusively in female, estrogen primed Wistar-Furth
rats (reference 7, and 8, and unpublished information from the EGG-Mason
Research Institute, Worcester, Massachusetts, USA).

Since endogenous estrogen in the serum component of the culture medium
was a possible cause of the contradictions in the other experiments cited,
a systematic attempt was made in these studies to eliminate such effects
by the use of estrogen deficient serum. Castrated calf serum, i.e.,
steer serum (SS), turned out to be the most effective serum utilized for
this purpose. It was determined by 17β-estradiol (E_2) radioimmunoassay
(RIA) that the E_2 concentration of steer serum was less than $3x10^{-11}$ M as
compared to $(1-2)x10^{-9}$ M for fetal calf serum (FCS). In the prolactin
secretion experiments the anti-estrogen drug Tamoxifen was also utilized
to suppress the possible stimulatory effects of endogenous estrogen in
the serum component of the culture medium.

MATERIALS AND METHODS
Establishment of Permanent Cell Lines in Culture

Transplants of the Furth Mammotropic pituitary tumor line, MtT/W13,
were obtained from the Mason Foundation tumor bank in Worcester, Massachusetts, USA, implanted in Wistar-Furth female host rats which were injected with 5 mg of estradiol valerate every three weeks.

Primary cultures of tumor cells were made by lancing and mincing
tumor transplants in Hanks Balanced Saline Solution (HBSS) and resus-
pending the cells in Dulbecco's Modified Eagle Medium (DMEM) plus fifteen
percent fetal calf serum (FCS). The cells were plated at approximately
10^6 cells per 100 mm culture dish in culture medium supplemented with
17β-estradiol (E_2) at 10^{-8} M.

After one to two weeks in culture and several medium changes, the surviving cells were harvested using trypsin, resuspended in fresh culture
medium, and reinjected subcutaneously into estrogen primed, Wistar-Furth
female host rats (5 mg of estradiol valerate IM every three weeks).
Tumors developed in two to three months and were again cultured as described above. Serial passage in culture and transplantation in vivo
in estrogen primed host animals was repeated several times, until single
cell plating techniques were successful in isolating several clonal cell
lines.

Single cell suspensions were obtained by treatment of stock cultures
with trypsin (0.25%) plus EDTA (0.2 mg/ml) at 37 °C for five to ten minutes. The cells were resuspended in DMEM plus nutrient mixture F-12
(1:1) supplemented with FCS (15%) and E_2 at 10^{-8} M. Single cell platings
were made into Falcon multi-well microtest plates (E3034), and clones
were selected from colonies growing up in wells originally containing a
single cell. One of the original clones was recloned several times to
obtain a number of sub-clones.

Growth Experiments.

Cultures to be used for seeding growth experiments were first grown
up in DMEM plus FCS and then pre-incubated for several days in estrogen
deficient culture medium with daily medium changes and saline rinses.
The estrogen deficient medium generally used was DMEM plus five percent
castrated calf serum, i.e., steer serum (SS).

Single cell suspensions were prepared after preincubation using trypsin plus EDTA as described above and replicate culture dishes were plated
with approximately 3,000 cells per dish (35 or 60 mm culture dishes) in
DMEM-F12 (1:1) culture medium with SS (5%). Finally, E_2 and Tamoxifen

at varying concentrations were added to replicate culture dishes (in duplicate or triplicate).

Experiments were incubated in an air-CO_2 incubator at 37 °C with all replicate plates in an experiment placed directly on an incubator shelf. Medium changes were made every four to five days and experiments were generally incubated from two to four weeks time, until the faster growing cultures reached saturation cell densities at approximately $(1-2)x10^6$ cells per 35 mm culture dish.

In growth curve experiments replicate culture dishes from each subset were harvested sequentially at time intervals approximately equal to cell doubling times. In dose response experiments all culture dishes were harvested at the end of the experiment.

The cells from harvested culture dishes were dispersed into single cell suspensions using trypsin-EDTA, rinsed once with serum containing medium and then twice with Hanks Balanced Saline Solution (HBSS). They were resuspended in HBSS, appropriately diluted, and counted on a Biophysics Systems Cytograf (Model 6300A). Representative cell suspensions were also counted with a hemocytometer to verify the accuracy of the cytograf counts. The cell counts from replicate culture dishes were averaged and the Standard Error of the Mean calculated.

Hormone Secretion Experiments.
Studies on the stimulation of prolactin secretion by estrogen were carried out for short term periods of a few days in DMEM-F12 medium (1:1) plus SS, as well as for longer periods of time in culture medium supplemented with FCS (10-15%) plus Tamoxifen at $(1-2)x10^{-6}$ M. In the latter case the growth rate was identical in all culture dishes irrespective of exogenous estrogen added to the culture medium and all plates contained approximately equal numbers of cells at all times during the experiment.

At the end of a hormone secretion experiment both the cells and culture medium were harvested from each culture dish for cell counts (as previously described) and prolactin concentration in the culture medium determined by a double antibody, rat prolactin RIA (NIH-NIAMD rat prolactin RIA kit). This RIA was sensitive to rat prolactin levels in the culture medium down to 1 ng/ml and the assay had a reproducibility of 5 to 10 percent for duplicate samples. Prolactin concentrations in the culture medium were expressed on a per cell basis.

Estrogen Receptor Assays.
Cells were grown up in 100 mm dishes in DMEM plus FCS (10%). After the cultures reached saturation cell densities (5-7 million cells/dish) they were pre-incubated in estrogen deficient medium, i.e., DMEM plus SS (5%), for four days with daily medium changes and saline rinses. At the end of the pre-incubation period the cell cultures were rinsed once with Ca/Mg free HBSS, pooled, and pelleted using a clinical centrifuge. They were then resuspended in HBSS and spun down a final time. Approximately 0.3 ml of Ca/Mg free HBSS was added to the pellet which was then broken up by mechanical pipetting and transferred to a cellulose acetate freezing vial (Vangard International NUNC serum tube, #1076-02). The vials were then stored in a liquid nitrogen cryostat until the receptor assay could be performed.

The concentration and affinity of specific estrogen receptor binding sites in the cells were determined by measuring the binding of tritiated

FIG. 1:
E_2-CELL PROLIFERATION DOSE
RESPONSE IN DMEM-F12 MEDIUM PLUS
SS (5-10%). REPLICATE CULTURE
DISHES PLATED WITH 12-13 THOUSAND
CELLS AND GROWN UP FOR 12-14 DAYS
WITH EACH E_2 CONCENTRATION IN
DUPLICATE.
A. WITHOUT TAMOXIFEN (UPPER).
B. WITH TAMOXIFEN AT 10^{-6} M
     (LOWER).

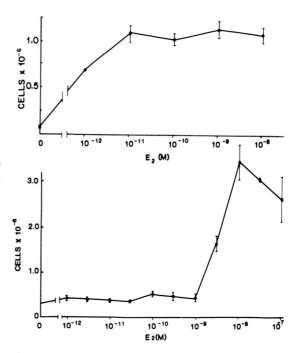

E_2 to cytoplasmic extracts of the cells at 4 °C with and without 100
fold excess of Diethylstilbesterol (DES). Bound E_2-receptor complexes
were separated from estradiol using a hydroxylapatite filtration method
(19). Protein determinations on cell extracts were also performed using
the microburet method.

EXPERIMENTAL RESULTS

Initial single cell platings yielded three permanent cell lines.
One of these three was recloned yielding a particular clone of
exceptional homogeneous morphology and epitheliod appearance. Karyo-
typic analysis of this clone indicated a near diploid karyotype. All
subsequent studies were carried out on this clone and sub-clones isolated from it.

GROWTH EXPERIMENTS

Figure 1 shows E_2-cell proliferation dose response experiments on the
original clone with and without Tamoxifen. Figure 2 shows similar data
from experiments on two sub-clones (3F3, 4E10). Both experiments were
carried out in culture medium supplemented with steer serum (SS).
The data in Figures 1 and 2 clearly demonstrate that the cell lines
are sensitive for cell growth down to sub-physiologic concentrations of
E_2 of 10^{-11} or less, in agreement with results on other estrogen responsive cell lines (2,15,17). The shift in dose response curve in the
presence of Tamoxifen (FIG. 1B) clearly indicates that this anti-estrogen drug acts as a competitive inhibitor of E_2 with a relative binding
affinity for the E_2 receptor of approximately 0.3-1 percent that of E_2,
in agreement with the results of other investigators (5,18).
Finally, the lack of any detectible growth in the control dishes with-

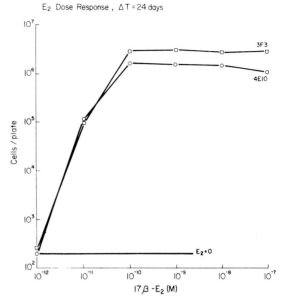

FIG. 2:
E_2-CELL PROLIFERATION DOSE
RESPONSE IN DME-F12 MEDIUM PLUS
SS (5%). REPLICATE CULTURE DISHES
WERE PLATED AT 3000 CELLS PER DISH
AND GROWN UP UNTIL E_2 TREATED CUL-
TURES REACHED SATURATION DENSITIES
(24 DAYS).

out E_2 in the experiments on the sub-clones (FIG. 2) indicates that few,
if any, cells are capable of proligeration without E_2, i.e., that these
sub-clones are virtually hormone dependent.

The extreme sensitivity of the cells to small quantities of estrogen
in the culture medium can also be inferred from the cell growth experiment in FIG. 3. The addition of even a very small quantity of estrogen
rich FCS ($1-3\times10^{-9}$ M E_2) to the estrogen deficient culture medium
(10^{-12} M E_2) apparently adds sufficient estrogen to stimulate cell
growth without directly adding E_2, thus eliminating any observable effect
on the cell of exogenous E_2.

Kinetic data on the E_2 stimulation of cell growth of sub-clone 1E7 are
shown in Figures 4 and 5. Figure 4 shows growth curves taken for over a

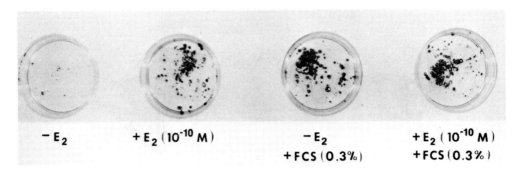

FIG. 3: PHOTOGRAPH OF STAINED CULTURES FROM E_2 CELL GROWTH EXPERIMENT
ON SUB-CLONE 4E10. REPLICATE CULTURE DISHES PLATED AT 3000 CELLS PER
DISH IN DMEM-F12 PLUS SS (5%). CULTURES HARVESTED AT 28 DAYS, RINSED
THREE TIMES WITH HBSS, FIXED WITH METHANOL-ACETIC ACID (3:1) AND
STAINED WITH HEMATOXYLIN-EOSIN.

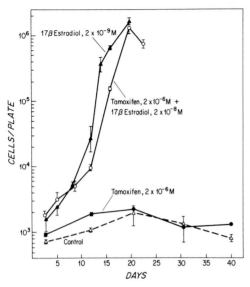

FIG. 4: GROWTH CURVES OF SUB-CLONE
1E7 WITH AND WITHOUT E_2 IN THE
PRESENCE AND ABSENCE OF TAMOXIFEN
IN DMEM-F12 MEDIUM (1:1) PLUS SS
(5%).

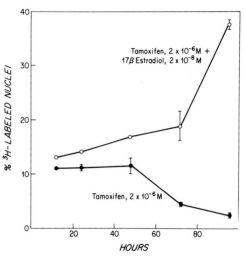

FIG. 5: ^{3}H-THYMIDINE UPTAKE EXPERI-
MENT ON CLONE 1E7 IN DME-F12 MED-
IUM PLUS SS (5%) and TAMOXIFEN AT
2×10^{-6} M. ON HARVESTING, CULTURE
DISHES RINSED TWICE WITH HBSS AND
FIXED WITH ETHANOL (95%) AND OVER-
LAYED WITH NUCLEAR TRACK PHOTO-
GRAPHIC EMULSION FOR ONE WEEK.
AFTER DEVELOPING, THE PLATES WERE
STAINED WITH GIEMSA AND THE LABEL-
ING INDEX OF CELL NUCLEI IN EACH
CULTURE DISH WAS DETERMINED FROM
MICROSCOPICALLY SCORING AT LEAST
ONE HUNDRED CELLS PER DISH.

month in DME-F12 medium (1:1) plus SS (5%). Lack of observable growth in
the cultures without E_2 over this long time span indicates that this sub-
clone is virtually estrogen dependent. Figure 5 shows the results of an
autoradiographic experiment on E_2 stimulation of tritiated Thymidine (^{3}H-
Thy) uptake into cell nuclei on DME-F12 (1:1) medium plus SS (5%) and
Tamoxifen at 2×10^{-6} on the same clone, 1E7. These results indicate
that E_2 is capable of directly stimulating DNA synthesis by a factor of
almost 10 under these culture conditions (with Tamoxifen) over a period
of several days. Qualitatively similar results have been obtained on E_2
stimulated ^{3}H-Thy nuclear uptake without using Tamoxifen, but the factor
of enhancement is smaller (factor of 2-3 over a period of several days).

PROLACTIN SECRETION EXPERIMENTS

Figures 6 and 7 show experiments on prolactin secretion carried out in
DMEM plus FCS (10-15%). In both cases replicate culture dishes were plated with 10 to 20 thousand cells and grown up to saturation densities
with the concentrations of Tamoxifen and E_2 indicated (in triplicate).
In all cases there were no significant differences in growth rate of
final cell numbers, but in any case, all listed prolactin values are

FIG. 6:
PROLACTIN SECRETION-TAMOXI-
FEN DOSE RESPONSE WITH AND WITHOUT
E_2.   REPLICATE 60 MM CULTURE DISH-
ES WERE PLATED AT SEVERAL THOU-
SAND CELLS PER DISH AND GROWN UP
TO SATURATION DENSITIES IN THE
INDICATED CONCENTRATIONS OF E_2
AND TAMOXIFEN FOR TWENTY DAYS (IN
TRIPLICATE).   THE PROLACTIN
VALUES INDICATED ARE FOR THE
FINAL 48 HOUR INCUBATION.

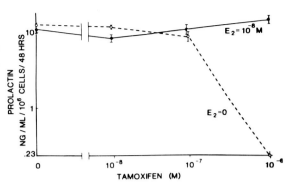

normalized to total cells per plate.   These prolactin values represent
the concentrations in the culture medium after a final 48 hour incubation.

Figure 6 shows a prolactin secretion-Tamoxifen dose response experi-
with and without E_2 at 10^{-8} M.   These results show that Tamoxifen can
exert a strongly inhibitory effect on prolactin secretion under these
culture conditions (15% FCS) at concentrations above 10^{-7} M.   This inhibition can be completely overcome with an E_2 concentration (10^{-8} M)   approximately one-hundreth the Tamoxifen concentration.

Figure 7 shows a prolactin secretion-E_2 dose response under similar
culture conditions (10% FCS) and protocol.   In this experiment all
plates were grown up in 10^{-6} M Tamoxifen.   These results show that E_2
can stimulate prolactin secretion by up to a factor of at least forty
under these culture conditions with maximal stimulation in the range of
10^{-8} M E_2.

The data in Figure 7 (and indirectly, Figure 6) show that estrogen
stimulation of prolactin secretion can be obtained under culture conditions such that there is no significant stimulation of cell growth (10-
15% FCS plus 10^{-6} M Tamoxifen).   Hence, the E_2 stimulation of prolactin
secretion in these pituitary tumor cell lines is direct and independent
of E_2 effects on cell growth.

Figure 8 shows a prolactin secretion-E_2 dose response curve taken in
DMEM-F12 (1:1) medium plus SS (5%) and Tamoxifen (10^{-6} M).   The cell cultures were grown up in DMEM plus FCS and then preincubated in DMEM-F12

FIG. 7:
PROLACTIN SECRETION-E_2 DOSE
RESPONSE EXPERIMENT IN DMEM PLUS
FCS (10%) and TAMOXIFEN (10^{-6} M).
EXPERIMENTAL PROTOCOL THE SAME AS
DESCRIBED IN FIGURE 6.

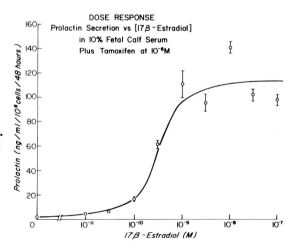

FIG. 8:

PROLACTIN SECRETION-E_2 DOSE
RESPONSE CURVE IN DMEM-F12 (1:1)
PLUS SS (5%) ON 4E10 CELLS. REPLI-
CATE CULTURE DISHES WERE PLATED
IN DMEM PLUS FCS (10%) AND GROWN
UP TO SATURATION DENSITIES
FOLLOWED BY THREE DAYS OF PRE-
INCUBATION IN DMEM-F12 PLUS SS
(5%) WITH DAILY MEDIUM CHANGES
AND SALINE RINSES (HBSS). THE
CULTURES WERE THEN INCUBATED IN
DMEM-F12 PLUS SS (5%) FOR THREE
DAYS WITH E_2 AND TAMOXIFEN AS IN-
DICATED (IN DUPLICATE) WITH ONE
MEDIUM CHANGE. THE PROLACTIN
VALUES INDICATED ARE FOR THE FINAL
48 HOUR INCUBATION.

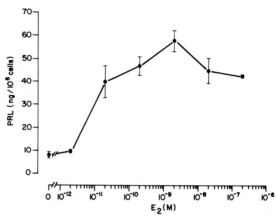

SS and Tamoxifen as indicated for several days. Under these conditions
a factor of E_2 stimulation of prolactin secretion of five or six could be
obtained with optimal E_2 concentrations again occuring in the range of
10^{-8} M. All prolactin values were normalized to the total number of
cells on each plate.

Estrogen Receptor Studies
Figure 9 shows a Scatchard plot of data from an estrogen receptor

FIG. 9:

SCATCHARD PLOT OF ^{3}H-E_2
BINDING TO CYTOSOL PREPARATIONS
FROM CELLS PREINCUBATED FOR FOUR
DAYS IN DMEM PLUS SS (5%) WITH
DAILY MEDIUM CHANGES AND SALINE
RINSES (HBSS). THE PROTOCOL FOR
PROCESSING AND RECEPTOR ASSAY IS
DESCRIBED IN THE MATERIALS AND
METHODS SECTION.

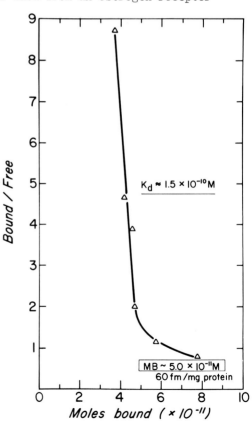

assay on cytosol extracts from cultures of an estrogen responsive sub-clone prepared and assayed as described. The results are typical of the clones tested for concentrations of cytoplasmic estrogen receptor binding sites and their E_2 affinity. All seem to have high affinity binding sites in the range of 10-50 fentamoles per milligram of cell protein with a K_d of about 10^{-10} M for the equilibrium constant of E_2-receptor binding. From the break in the Scatchard plot it appears that lower affinity binding sites may also be present.

DISCUSSION AND SUMMARY

A number of clonal cell lines and sub-lines have been established in culture from an estrogen induced, estrogen dependent, prolactin secreting rat pituitary tumor line (MtT/W13) which possess cytoplasmic estrogen of binding affinity and concentration characteristic of estrogen target cells.

In addition, Tamoxifen can suppress the effects of E_2 on cell pro-liferation and prolactin secretion at relative concentrations of 100 to 1. Assuming a competitive binding mode of anti-estrogen action, the results indicate a relative binding affinity of 100 to 1 or more for E_2 and Tamox-ifen to the estrogen receptor, in agreement with other investigations (5,18).

These results are in agreement with the work of Lippman, et.al. (4, 15,17), on human breast tumor cell lines and the recent work of Amara and Dannies (2) on a rat pituitary tumor cell line. Our results differ from investigations in which no stimulatory effects of estrogen on cell growth were obtained (12,20,21,26,29). The reasons for this descrepancy may be due to the sensitivity of the cells to very low concentrations of estrogen and the prolonged retention of estrogen by target cells in culture (30).

ACKNOWLEDGEMENTS

The authors wish to thank Richard Hudson, Donna Margolis and Richard Viscarello for technical assistance, and Dr. Richard B. Cohen, Department of Pathology, Harvard Medical School (HMS) and Beth Israel Hospital (BIH) for his advice and guidance. In addition, we would like to thank Dr. Joanna Pallotta, Director, RIA Lab, HMS and BIH, for technical assistance and Dr. Arthur E. Bogden, Director, EGG-Mason Research Institute, for donation of the tumor transplants. This research was supported by an American Cancer Society Grant, BC-250.

REFERENCES

(1) Allegra, J.C., and Lippman, M.E. (1980): *Eur. J. Cancer Clin. Oncol.,* 16:1007-1015.

(2) Amara, J.F., and Dannies, P.S. (1983): *Endocrinology,* 112:1151-1156.

(3) Barnes, D., and Sato, G.H. (1979): *Nature,* 281:388-389.

(4) Bronzart, D.A., Monaco, M.E., Pincus, L., Aitken, S., and Lippman, M.E. (1981): *Cancer Res.,* 41:604-610.

(5) Coezy, E., Borgna, J.L., and Rochefort, H. (1982): *Cancer Res.,* 42:317-323.

(6) Dannies, P.S., Yen, P.M. and Tashjian, Jr., A.H. (1977): *Endocrinology,* 101:1151-1156.

(7) Furth, J., Clifton, E.L. and Buffet, R.F. (1956): *Cancer Res.,* 16: 608-616.

(8) Furth, J., and Clifton, E.L. (1966): In: *The Pituitary Gland,* edited by G.W. Harris and B.T. Donovan, pp. 460-497, Butterworth London.

(9) Haug, E., and Gautvik, K.M. (1976): *Endocrinology,* 99:1482-1489.

(10) Haug, E. (1979): *Endocrinology,* 104:429-437.

(11) Ikeda, T., Liu, Q.F., Danielpour, D., Officer , J.B., Iilo, M., Leland, F.E., and Sirbasku, D.A. (1982): *In Vitro,* 18:961-969.

(12) Lee, Davis, I.J., Soto, A.M., and Sonnenschein, C. (1981): *Endocrinology,* 108:990-995.

(13) Lieberman, M.E., Maurer, R.A., Gorski, J. (1978): *Proc. Natl. Acad. Sci.,* 75:5946-5959.

(14) Lieberman, M.E., Maurer, R.A., Claude, P., and Gorski, J. (1982): *Mol. Cell Endocrinol.,* 25:277-294.

(15) Lippman, M.E., Bolan, G., Huff, K., (1976): *Cancer Res.,* 36:4595-4601.

(16) Maurer, R.A. (1982): *Endocrinology,*110:1515-1520.

(17) Monaco, M.E., and Lippman, M.E.: In: *Endocrine Control in Neoplasia,* Edited by R.K. Sharma and W.E. Criss, pp. 209-230, Raven Press, New York.

(18) Nicholson, R.I., Syne, J.S., Daniel, C.P., Griffiths, K. (1979): *Eur. J. Cancer Clin. Oncol.,* 15:317-329.

(19) Rosner, A.L. Teman, G.H., Bray, C.L., Burstein, N.A. (1980): *Eur. J. Cancer Clin Oncol.,* 16:1495-1502.

(20) Shafie, S.M. (1980): *Science,* 201:701-702.

(21) Sirbasku, D.A. (1978): *Cancer Res.,* 38:1154-1165.

(22) Sirbasku, D.A. (1978): *Proc. Natl. Acad. Sci.,* 75:3786-3690.

(23) Sirbasku, D.A. and Benson, R.H. (1979): In: *Hormones and Cell Culture,* Edited by G.H. Sato and R. Ross, Cold Spring Harbor Conferences on Cell Proliferation, Volume 6, pp.477-497, Cold Spring Harbor, New York.

(24) Sonnenschein, C., Posner, M., Saiduddin, S., Krasnay, M. (1973): *Exp. Cell Res.,* 78:41-46.

(25) Sonnenschein, C., Posner, M., Sahr, K. Farookhi, R., Brunelle, R. (1974): *Exp. Cell Res.,* 84:399-411.

(26) Sonnenschein, C., and Soto, A.M. (1979): *J. Natl. Cancer Inst.,* 63:835-841.

(27) Sonnenschein, C., and Soto, A.M. (1980): *J. Natl. Cancer Inst.,* 64:211-215.

(28) Sonnenschein, C., and Soto, A.M. (1980): In: *Estrogens in the Environment,* Edited by J.A. McLachlan, pp.169-190, Elsiever/ North Holland, Inc., New York.

(29) Sorrentino, J.M., Kirkland, W.L., and Sirbasku, D.A. (1976): *J. Natl. Cancer Inst.,* 1149-1154.

(30) Stroble, J.S., and Lippmen, M.E. (1979): *Cancer Res.* 39:3319-3327.

(31) Vician, L., Shupnik, M.A., and Gorski, J. (1979): *Endocrinology,* 104:736-743.

(32) West, B., and Dannies, P.S. (1980): *Endocrinology,* 106:1108-1113.

Progress in Cancer Research and Therapy,
Vol. 31, edited by F. Bresciani, et al.
Raven Press, New York © 1984.

Estrogen-Regulated 52 K Protein and Control of Cell Proliferation in Human Breast Cancer Cells

Françoise Vignon, Françoise Capony, Dany Chalbos,
Marcel Garcia, Frédéric Veith, Bruce Westley,
and Henri Rochefort

*Unité d'Endocrinologie Cellulaire et Moléculaire, U 148 INSERM,
34100 Montpellier, France*

The response of some breast cancers to various endocrine therapies (ablative, additive or substitutive) has for some time suggested that estrogens stimulate the proliferation of such tumors. However, clinical trials or in vivo experiments in animals (mostly rodents) have not allowed a specification of the mechanism by which estrogens might regulate breast cell growth. The need for in vitro systems has led to the establishment of various human breast cancer cell lines in continuous cultures such as MCF7 (34), ZR75-1 (13), and T47D (19), all derived from breast cancer metastases, and containing receptors for 4 classes of steroid hormones (estrogens, androgens, progestins and glucocorticoids) (16). In such systems, estrogens were shown both to regulate the expression of multiple specific proteins (15)(44)(12) and to modulate more general pleiotypic effects such as cell proliferation (14)(7). While the estrogen-specific effects have been widely reproduced, the effect on cell proliferation initially described by M. Lippman's group (23) has remained controversial and has prompted various models of estrogen regulation of cell growth.

We will successively :

1. show the in vitro effect of estradiol on the proliferation of breast cancer cells and discuss several models.

2. describe the effect of estrogens on the production of specific proteins with a particular emphasis on a 52 K glycoprotein released by the cells.

3. discuss the possible relationship between such estrogen-inducible proteins and cell proliferation.

IN VITRO EFFECT OF ESTRADIOL ON CELL PROLIFERATION

The evidence for a direct in vitro effect of estradiol on cell growth is controversial, since some laboratories

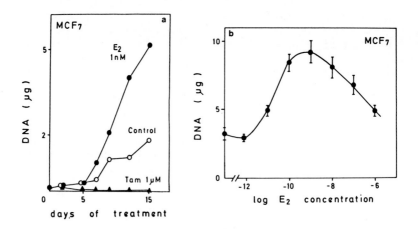

FIGURE 1

Hormonal control of cell proliferation in MCF7 cells
a. time-course effect of E_2 and tamoxifen
b. E_2 dose-response curve

MCF7 cells were cultured for 5 days in steroid-stripped serum (FCS/DCC) to ensure efficient withdrawal from endogenous steroids. They were then plated in F12/DEM containing 3 % FCS/DCC in the absence of insulin and later treated with E_2 (1 nM) or tamoxifen (1 µM) (1-a) or with increasing concentrations of E_2 (1 pM to 1 µM) (1-b) in the presence of 1 % FCS/DCC. DNA content was evaluated by the DABA fluorescence assay (20) on triplicate dishes and mean ± 1 SD represented as a function of time (1-a) or concentration (1-b).

have failed to show such an effect (15)(31)(33), in contradiction with the initial observations described in MCF7 (23) and ZR75-1 (2) cell lines. The discrepancy thus observed between in vivo and in vitro systems has prompted the hypothesis that estrogens might act indirectly on mammary cells via the liberation of estrogen-inducible growth factors (estromedins) from various target organs such as the uterus, the kidney, and the pituitary (32). We have reexamined the hormonal control of the proliferation of various cell lines in controlled culture conditions, particularly with regard to cell withdrawal from endogenous estrogens (39). Providing that the fetal calf serum, routinely used to grow these cells, was efficiently stripped of estrogens, a stimulatory effect of estradiol was confirmed in MCF7 cells and demonstrated in T47D by several types of evaluation (DNA assay, cell counts and thymidine incorporation) (7). Hormonal effect was restricted to the estrogen receptor positive cell lines (T47D clone 11 - MCF7) and displayed a biphasic-dose response curve (7) (Fig. 1a-b). Estradiol produced a 2 to 10 fold stimulation which became statistically different

from the control after 16 hours of treatment when evaluating DNA synthesis and after 5-6 days when measuring cell
number or total DNA. This effect was restricted to
estrogens, and physiological concentrations of other
steroid hormones (androgens, progestins, glucocorticoids)
did not stimulate cell growth.

Other laboratories (9)(10)(22)(28)(42) have also
recently reported that estrogens can stimulate the growth
of breast cancer cells in culture and it is likely that
the failure to demonstrate such an effect was due to
different experimental conditions or to the use of cells
which had lost their estrogen responsiveness for growth.

Therefore, the in vitro mitogenic effect of estradiol
is now substantially supported by the experimental data
gathered in different responsive cell lines, thus
indicating that estradiol is able to act directly on the
epithelial mammary cells. However, the precise mechanism
by which estrogens directly promote breast tumor growth
remains unclear and might be the result of several
interaction modes of the hormone as suggested in Figure 2.
Estrogen itself might directly stimulate cell division in
a one-step pathway (c) but its precise level of action on
the cell cycle kinetics remains to be determined.
Estrogens could favor the mitogenic effect of an unidentified serum factor, thus exerting a direct permissive
effect (d). This possibility will probably soon be
confirmed or ruled out with the use of chemically defined
media. Finally, estrogens could regulate cell proliferation through an autocrine control, by favoring the
induction or release of specific growth factors which
behave as true mitogens for the mammary cells (e). The
autocrine regulatory growth control was first proposed by
Todaro (36) on the basis of the observation that malignant
cells require lower concentrations of exogenous growth
factors than normal cells for optimal growth and that the
transformed cells had less accessible EGF receptors than
their normal counterparts. The evidence for numerous transforming growth factors (35) which stimulate cell division
of normal fibroblasts, interact with the membrane
receptors for EGF and promote anchorage independent agar
growth now substantially support this system. We will
later present evidence in favor of the autocrine mechanism
to explain the in vitro effect of E_2 on the growth of
human breast cancer cells in culture.

The in vivo situation might be even more complex since
several estrogen target organs could simultaneously
respond to a hormonal message, and the interactions among
various cell types have to be considered. Therefore one
cannot exclude the possibility that in vivo estrogen-
inducible factors such as estromedines (32) exert an
endocrine regulation on mammary cell growth, in addition
to the direct control of estrogen (Fig. 2a). Finally,
estrogens could promote the in vivo growth and dissemination of mammary cancer cells with the help of proteases
(such as plasminogen activator (4) or collagenase) or yet
unknown inhibiting factors, at the expense of surrounding

FIGURE 2
Regulation of cell
growth by estrogens:
Possible mechanisms

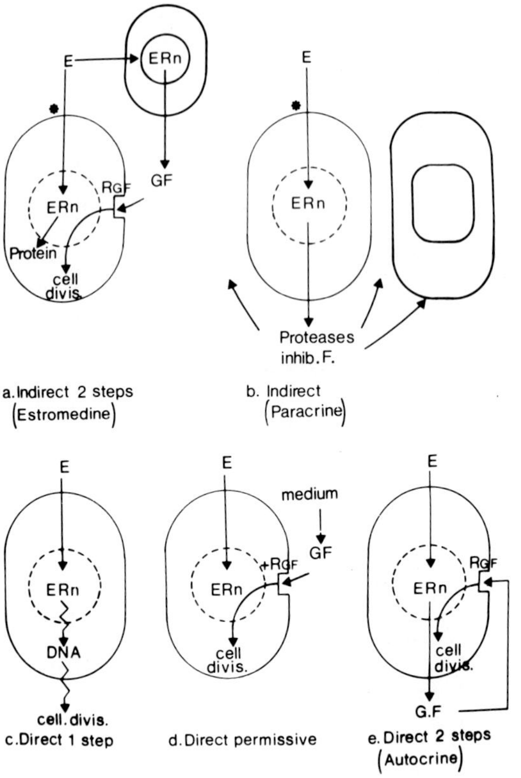

a. "Endocrine" regula-
tion : in various
target organs (kidney,
pituitary, uterus..)
(small cell) estrogens
stimulate the release
of estromedines (GF)
which are the true mito-
gens for the mammary
cell (*).

b. "Paracrine" regula-
tion : estrogens could
increase the synthesis
of proteases or inhibi-
ting factors in mammary
cells (*) thus favoring
the spread and dissemi-
nation of the responsi-
ve cancer cells to the
detriment of the
surrounding stromal
cells.

c. Direct one-step re-
gulation : estrogens
stimulate DNA synthesis
and consequently cell
division by various

a.Indirect 2 steps
(Estromedine)

b. Indirect
(Paracrine)

c.Direct 1 step

d.Direct permissive

e. Direct 2 steps
(Autocrine)

possible interactions on the mammary cell cycle (increase
in the recruiting of cycling cells, decrease in cell loss,
decrease in the duration of the cell cycle (G_1-S)).

d. Direct permissive effect : estradiol itself has no
stimulatory effect on cell division but rather acts as a
permissive agent for an unidentified serum growth factor.

e. Direct two-step "autocrine" regulation : estrogens
specifically trigger the release of growth factors by
mammary cells, which autostimulate their proliferation.

stromal and adipose tissues, through a paracrine mechanism
(Fig. 2b).

ESTROGEN-REGULATED PROTEINS

In addition to the progesterone receptor (15), several
specific estrogen-regulated intracellular proteins have
now been identified by double-labelling experiments (^{3}H,
^{14}C), such as the 24 K cytosolic protein (12), or by
single labelling (^{35}S) of the cells, such as the 4

cytosolic proteins (24) with 46, 52, 54 and 60 K molecular weights. We found several estradiol-stimulated proteins by using ^{35}S-methionine labelling of proteins which could be resolved by two-dimensional gel analysis. Some of these cellular proteins could have potential interests. However, they can only be assayed in tumor samples collected during surgery. We have therefore preferred to search for estrogen induced proteins which might be secreted by the cells, in an attempt to find potential circulating marker(s) of hormone-dependent breast cancers.

Using protein labelling by ^{35}S-methionine followed by SDS polyacrylamide gel electrophoresis and fluorography, we have analysed the proteins released into the culture medium by several breast cancer cell lines which are either hormone responsive (MCF7, ZR75-1 and T47D) or hormone unresponsive (BT20, HBL100 - clone 8 of T47D). We found that estrogens stimulated the general production of proteins which were released into the medium (44)(45). One in particular, representing 20 to 40 % of these secretory labelled proteins, had a molecular weight of 52,000 daltons [*1] in denaturating conditions. The increased production of this protein was specifically triggered by physiological concentrations of estrogens. Antiestrogens, such as Tamoxifen, which are potent antiproliferative agents in the hormone-responsive cell lines did not affect the 52 K production and specifically inhibited the E_2 induced production (Fig. 3) in a dose-dependent manner.

Progesterone and dexamethasone were inactive. But any steroid able to fully activate the RE after binding was also able to induce this protein, which therefore provides a very useful in vitro test to assess the estrogenic activity of ligands (29). For instance, the 52 K protein was also induced by the estrogen 3-sulfate but not the 17-sulfate in MCF7 cells (39). Androgens were also able to stimulate this protein but only when their concentrations or affinities for RE were sufficient to occupy the RE sites (30). Thus, pharmacological concentrations of DHT (0.5 µM) and physiological concentrations (1) of adrenal androgens such as 5-androstenediol and DHEA are able to induce the 52 K protein in vitro. These results indicate that steroids structurally defined as androgens can also be biologically active estrogens and that the plasma concentration of adrenal androgens, particularly in post-menopausal or ovariectomized women, may play a role in stimulating the growth of hormone-dependent cancer.

Other hormones (prolactin (11)(43), insulin (26)(3)) or growth factors (charcoal-treated fetal calf serum and EGF) (27)(17) which were shown to increase the human mammary cell proliferation, were inactive in stimulating the production of the 52 K protein (Fig. 4), thus showing that this protein is not triggered by all mitogens but is

---

*1. The molecular weight was first found to be 46,000 daltons when using 15 % polyacrylamide gels. It appears to be closer to 52,000 daltons in 10 % polyacrylamide gels and using the NEN protein markers.

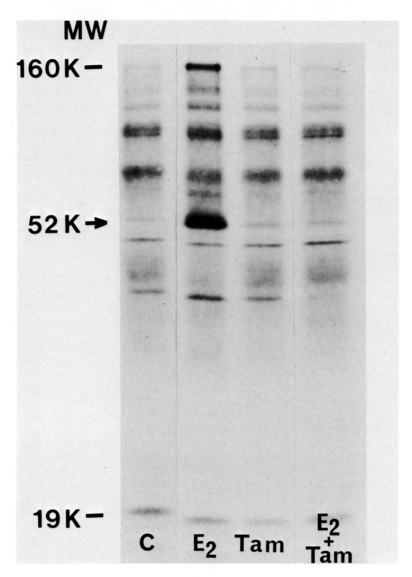

FIGURE 3

The 52 K E$_2$-regulated protein released by MCF7 cells

MCF7 cells were grown in DEM containing 10 % FCS/DCC (4 days of withdrawal). They were then plated in 96 µ well-dishes and either treated with 1 nM E$_2$, 1 µM tamoxifen, E$_2$ + tamoxifen (1 nM + 1 µM) or with the solvent alone (control). After 2 days of treatment, the cells were labelled for 6 hours with ^{35}S-methionine. The labelled proteins of the medium were analyzed by SDS-polyacrylamide gel (15 %) electrophoresis and processed for fluorography (45) (from (44) with permission).

strictly estrogen-specific. A similar stimulation of the production of the 52 K protein was recently demonstrated in serum-free conditions, thus confirming that the 52 K protein does not require the presence of unidentified serum factors but is a direct response to estrogens (Vignon, unpublished). Some physico-chemical properties of this protein have now been defined and have made it possible to raise polyclonal rabbit antibodies against 52 K (5). The 52 K protein is a glycoprotein, as shown by its labelling with ^{3}H fucose and mannose, its selective retention on Concanavalin A Sepharose, and its sensitivity to neuraminidase and tunicamycine. A regulation at the transcriptional level is likely, as suggested by the effects of actinomycin D and α-amanitin (Garcia et al., in preparation). The identity of the 52 K protein, whose concentration in culture medium is low (10-20 ng/ml) is presently unknown. We can however assume that it is not a major milk protein such as human casein or α-lactalbumin, which have different molecular weights and have not yet been proved to be present or estrogen inducible in MCF7 cells.

The relation of the 52 K protein with other estrogen-regulated proteins (24 K protein, plasminogen activators) or with virus-related proteins (gp52) which are present in MCF7 cells has been questioned by immunological and biochemical approaches, and is unlikely (O. Massot et al. ; D. Chalbos, unpublished experiments). The functions of such a secreted factor associated with the known effects of estradiol in human breast cancer could be multiple, such as a transforming and/or a growth activity. By analogy with the autocrine model described in transformed cells by Todaro (35) and on the basis of the parallel controls of 52 K induction and cell growth by E_2, we have further investigated the mitogenic properties of the estrogen-inducible proteins.

52 K PROTEIN AND CONTROL OF CELL PROLIFERATION

Several indirect results support the hypothesis that the regulation of the proteins released into the medium is correlated to, if not responsible for, the regulation of cell growth by estrogens and antiestrogens.

Estrogens sequentially stimulate both responses

In the RE positive cell lines (MCF7 - ZR75-1 - T47D Clone 11) the same physiological concentrations of estrogens _in vitro_ stimulate both the production of the 52 K (or 60 K) protein and cell proliferation. In the BT20 breast cancer cell line (21) which is unresponsive to estrogen for growth, a constitutive level of 52 K protein was demonstrated by antigenic reactivity with poly-

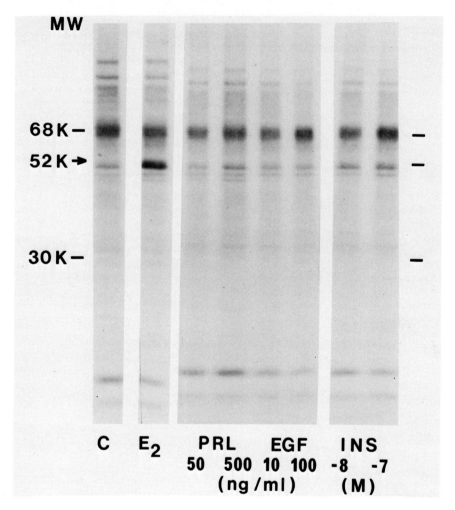

FIGURE 4
Effect of several peptides with potential
mitogenic activities

MCF7 cells were grown in DEM containing 10 % FCS/DCC
for 2 days then switched to 3 % FCS/DCC for 2 additional
days. They were then plated in 96 μ well-dishes at a
density of 30,000 cells/well in DEM with 3 % FCS/DCC
without insulin. After 2 days, they were treated with E_2
(1 nM), prolactin (ovine - NIH) (50-500 ng/ml), EGF
(mouse - Collaborative Research) (10-100 ng/ml), insulin
(bovine - Collaborative Research) (10-100 nM) or remained
in the same medium (control). After 2 days of treatment
(with a medium change every day) the cells were labelled
with ^{35}S-methionine (5 μCi/well). The media were analyzed
by SDS-polyacrylamide gel (12 %) electrophoresis and
processed for fluorography as described (45).

clonal antibodies (F. Capony, in preparation). However, its concentration remained unaffected by estrogen treatment. Similarly in two other unresponsive cell lines (T47D Clone 8 or HBL 100 normal mammary milk cells) there was a strict parallel in the absence of response to estrogens for both the 52 K protein and cell proliferation. These results show that the estrogen regulation of the 52 K protein production is always associated with a parallel regulation of cell growth. The effect of E_2 on protein production occurred after 12 hours and was optimal after 2 days of treatment, which clearly anticipates the stimulation of cell growth (5-6 days). Such a timing is therefore in agreement with a possible role of these proteins in the E_2 growth regulation.

The concentration of 52 K protein, evaluated by silver staining of the non-radioactive culture medium, is low (10-20 ng/ml) and in the range of concentrations of the known peptide growth factors. Finally, the effect of E_2 is amplified when the culture media are changed less often during the cell growth test, suggesting that the medium could be conditioned by an accumulation of estrogen-inducible growth factors released by the cells.

Several Antiestrogens (Progestins and Triphenylethylene Derivatives) Inhibit both Responses at the same Concentrations

In MCF7 cells, tamoxifen is totally inactive in inducing the 52 K protein but prevents E_2 action in a molar ratio of 10^3. Monohydroxy tamoxifen, a metabolite of tamoxifen which binds RE with a high affinity, is 100 times more potent than tamoxifen itself for blocking the cell growth (8) and the induction of the secreted 52 K protein by E_2 (45).

On the other hand, in tamoxifen-resistant clones of MCF7, such as the R27 cell line established by Nawata et al. (25), or RTx6 established by Jozan et al. (18), tamoxifen no longer inhibits cell growth. In these 2 resistant clones, we have shown that both tamoxifen and hydroxytamoxifen markedly stimulate the biosynthesis of the 52 K protein and thus behave as a full estrogen agonist for this particular response (F. Vignon et al., submitted).

Progestins such as R5020 are able to inhibit sequentially, and at the same concentrations, the production of estrogen-induced released proteins and estrogen-stimulated cell proliferation (40)(6).

The timing of 52 K protein induction and the regulation of the 52 K protein production by estrogens and anti-estrogens implies a possible role of the 52 K protein in the hormonal control of cell growth. In order to address this question more directly, we prepared serum-free conditioned media enriched in estrogen-inducible proteins to evaluate their mitogenic activity directly.

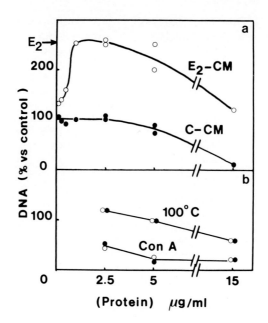

FIGURE 5
Growth stimulatory effects of conditioned media

a. Aliquots of conditioned media from control (C-CM) (●) or E_2 treated (E_2-CM) (o) MCF7 cells were added at increasing protein concentrations to recipient MCF7 cells cultured in the presence of 1 % FCS/DCC and without insulin. DNA was measured after 10 days of culture on triplicate wells. Results are expressed as percentages of control cells not treated by conditioned media. The effect of estradiol (⟶) is shown for comparison.

b. The same experiment was performed with C-CM (●) and E_2-CM (o) either preheated at 100° for 3 mn or passed over a Con A Sepharose column (from (41) by permission).

Mitogenic Effects of Estrogen-Regulated Proteins from Serum-Free Conditioned Media

We prepared two series of serum-free conditioned media from control (C-CM) or E_2-treated cells (E_2-CM). The 52 K protein induction was monitored in each experiment by ^{35}S-methionine labelling and by silver staining of poly-acrylamide gel electrophoresis. We showed that E_2-CM stimulates the growth of MCF7 cells (equivalent to E_2 stimulation) while C-CM is either ineffective or even inhibitory at high protein concentrations (41) (Fig. 5a). Protease digestions (pronase, trypsine) or heat treatment (100°C – 3 mn) suppressed, the mitogenic activity. The passage through a Concanavalin A Sepharose, which retained the glycoproteins including the 52 K protein, similarly led to a complete loss of the mitogenic effect (Fig. 5b).

TABLE 1

Effect of conditioned media on the growth of MCF7 cells

Expt	DNA (% of control)			52 K induction
	E_2	C-CM	E_2-CM	E_2-CM/C-CM
1	248	102	207	3.25
2	211	114	140	2.75
3	180	107	143	3.17
4	226	77	230	2.25
mean	216	100	180	2.85
± 1 SD	±28	±16	±45	±0.46

Student's E_2/E_2-CM   = 1.2   NS
  t test E_2-CM/C-CM = 1.8   p<0.01

C-CM and E_2-CM conditioned media were prepared with the optimal conditions described in (41) (6 hrs of conditioning in experiments 1, 2 and 3 and 17 hrs in experiment 4).
a. The effect of C-CM and E_2-CM conditioned media, containing 5 μg protein per ml, on the growth of recipient MCF7 cells was evaluated in the conditions described under Fig. 5. The effect of estradiol alone was tested in parallel for comparison.
b. The percentages of 52 K protein in C-CM and E_2-CM were evaluated after labelling with ^{35}S methionine and scanning of the fluorographs of the labelled media analyzed by polyacrylamide gel electrophoresis. The degree of induction of 52 K protein represents the ratio of the percentages obtained in the presence of estradiol versus those measured in its absence (E_2-CM vs C-CM). In experiments 1 and 4, silver staining of the polyacrylamide gels confirmed the evidence of a preferential accumulation of the 52 K protein in E_2-CM versus C-CM.
(From (41) with permission).

The E_2-conditioned medium also induced the appearance of numerous microvilli on the cell surface (41) thus reproducing the results previously obtained with E_2 alone under the same conditions (38). Identical results were obtained when the mitogenic activity was evaluated by DNA growth assay in long-term experiments or by a thymidine incorporation test on short-term experiments (F. Vignon, unpublished) with a mean stimulatory effect of twice the control, which is equivalent to the effect of E_2 alone (Table 1) (41).
These results suggest that glycoproteins present in the medium might act as growth factors, mediating, as second

extracellular messengers, the mitogenic effect of estrogen on mammary cells. The 52 K protein is a good candidate for being such a growth factor since it is the major estrogen-regulated protein of the medium. However, we have shown both by fluorography of the labeled medium and by silver staining of the non-radioactive media that other minor proteins are also estrogen-regulated. The availability of several specific monoclonal antibodies recently developed against the 52 K protein (Garcia et al., in preparation) should now allow us to prove whether or not the 52 K protein is the growth factor responsible for the stimulatory activity of media conditioned in the presence of estrogens.

CONCLUSIONS

Estrogen-responsive breast cancer cell lines (MCF7, ZR75-1, T47D) provide excellent in vitro experimental systems for studying both the regulation of the expression of specific markers and the modulation of cell growth. Several estrogen-inducible proteins have been detected in these cell lines, among which a 52 K glycoprotein which is released by the cells and could therefore be a breast cancer circulating marker. Its induction, which was initially established in various cell lines has been confirmed in primary cultures of breast cancer metastases thus supporting its potential clinical interest (37).
The evidence for an in vitro stimulatory effect on cell growth will permit a study of the mechanism by which estrogen stimulates the growth of epithelial breast cancer cells. Our experimental data support the idea of an autocrine control through the 52 K protein or other estrogen-induced factors. Such factors could be produced constitutively in hormone independent cancer (BT20) or be under hormonal control in responsive cancer (MCF7, ZR75-1, T47D). However, we do not exclude the occurrence of additional indirect regulatory mechanisms to explain the in vivo effect of E_2 on cell proliferation.
The availability of several specific monoclonal antibodies against the 52 K protein will help us to determine whether the 52 K protein or other estrogen-regulated proteins or peptides are mitogens and to further assess the clinical relevance of this estrogen-regulated protein.

ACKNOWLEDGMENTS

This study was supported by the "Institut National de la Santé et de la Recherche Médicale", the NCI-INSERM cooperation on "Hormones and Cancer", the "Fondation pour la Recherche Médicale Française" and the "Fédération Nationale des Centres de Lutte contre le Cancer". We would like to thank Mrs D. Derocq, Mr C. Rougeot and Mrs C. Prébois for their excellent technical assistance and Miss E. Barrié for her skilful preparation of the manuscript. We are grateful to Drs. M. Lippman, I. Keydar, F. Bayard, the Mason Research Institute, and the Michigan Cancer Foundation for their gifts of mammary cell lines.

REFERENCES

1. Adams, J., Garcia, M., and Rochefort, H. (1981): Cancer Res., 41:4720-4726.
2. Allegra, J.C., and Lippman, M.E. (1980): Eur. J. Cancer, 16:1007-1015.
3. Butler, W.B., Kelsey, W.H., and Goran, N. (1981): Cancer Res., 41:82-88.
4. Butler, W.B., Kirkland, W.L., and Jorgensen, T.L. (1979): Biochem. Biophys. Res. Commun., 90:1328-1334
5. Capony, F., Garcia, M., Veith, F., and Rochefort, H. (1982): Biochem. Biophys. Res. Commun., 108:8-15.
6. Chalbos, D., and Rochefort, H. J. Biol. Chem., in press.
7. Chalbos, D., Vignon, F., Keydar, I., and Rochefort, H. (1982): J. Clin. Endocrin. Met., 55:276-283.
8. Coezy, E., Borgna, J.L., and Rochefort, H. (1982): Cancer Res., 42:317-323.
9. Coosen, R., De Jong, W.J., and Schwarz, F. (1982): Mol. Cell. Biochem., 42:155-160.
10. Darbre, P., Yates, J., Curtis, S., and King, R.J.B. (1983): Cancer Res., 43:349-354.
11. Dilley, W.G., and Kister, S.J. (1975): J. Natl. Cancer Inst., 55:35-36.
12. Edwards, D.P., Adams, D.J., Savage, N., and Mc Guire, W.L. (1980): Biochem. Biophys. Res. Commun., 93:804-812.
13. Engel, L.W., Young, N.A., Tralka, T.S., Lippman, M.E., O'Brien, S.J., and Joyce, M.J. (1978): Cancer Res., 38:3352-3364.
14. Hershko, A., Mamont, P., Shields, R., and Tomkins, G.M. (1971): Nature New Biology, 232:206-211.
15. Horwitz, K.B., Koseki, Y., and Mc Guire, W.L. (1978): Endocrinology, 103:1742-1751.
16. Horwitz, K.B., Zava, D.T., Thilagar, A.K., Jensen, E.M., and Mc Guire, W.L. (1978): Cancer Res., 38: 2434-2437.
17. Imai, Y., Leung, C.K.H., Friesen, H.G., and Shiu, R.P.C. (1982): Cancer Res., 42:4394-4398.
18. Jozan, S;, Elalamy, H., and Bayard, P. (1981): C. R. Acad. Sci., 297:767-770.
19. Keydar, I., Chen, L., Karby, S., Weiss, F.R., Delarea, J., Radu, M., Chaitcik, S., and Brenner, H.J. (1979): Eur. J. Cancer, 15:659-670.
20. Kissane, J.M., and Robins, E. (1958): J. Biol. Chem. 233:184-193.
21. Lasfargues, E.Y., and Ozzello, L. (1958): J. Natl. Cancer Inst., 21:1131-1147.
22. Leung, B.S., Quresai, S., and Leung, J.S. (1982): Cancer Res., 42:5060-5066.

23. Lippman, M.E., Bolan, G., and Huff, K. (1976): Cancer Res., 36:4595-4601.
24. Mairesse, N., Deuleeschonver, N., Leclercq, G., and Galand, P. (1980): Biochem. Biophys. Res. Commun., 97:1251-1257.
25. Nawata, H., Bronzert, D., and Lippman, M.E. (1981): J. Biol. Chem., 256:5016-5021.
26. Osborne, C.K., Bolan, G., Monaco, M.M., and Lippman, M.E. (1976): Proc. Nat. Acad. Sci., 73:4536-4540.
27. Osborne, C.K., Hamilton, B., Titus, G., and Livingston, R.B. (1980): Cancer Res., 40:2361-2366.
28. Page, M.J., Field, J.K., Everett, N.P., and Green, C.D. (1983): Cancer Res., 43:1244-1250.
29. Rochefort, H., Coezy, E., Joly, E., Westley, B., and Vignon, F. (1980): In: Progress in Cancer Research and Therapy. Hormones and Cancer, edited by S. Iacobelli, R. King, H. Lindner, and M. Lippman, Vol. 14, pp. 21-29. Raven Press, New York.
30. Rochefort, H., Garcia, M., Vignon, F., and Westley, B. (1980): In: Steroid Induced Uterine Proteins, edited by M. Beato, pp. 171-182. Elsevier/North-Holland Biomedical Press, Amsterdam, New York, Oxford.
31. Shafie, S.M. (1980): Science, 209:701-702.
32. Sirbasku, D.A. (1978): Proc. Natl. Acad. Sci. (USA), 75:3786-3790.
33. Sonnenschein, C., and Soto, A.M. (1980): J. Natl. Cancer Inst., 64:211-215.
34. Soule, H.D., Vazquez, J., Long, A., Albert, S., and Brennan, M.A. (1973): J. Natl. Cancer Inst., 51: 1409-1413.
35. Sporn, M.B., and Todaro, G.J. (1980): New England J. Med., 303:878-880.
36. Todaro, G.J., De Larco, J.E., and Cohen, S. (1976): Nature, 264:26-31.
37. Veith, F.O., Capony, P., Garcia, M., Chantelard, J., Pujol, H., Veith, F., Zajdela, A., and Rochefort, H. (1983): Cancer Res., 43:1861-1868.
38. Vic, P., Vignon, F., Derocq, D., and Rochefort, H. (1982): Cancer Res., 42:667-673.
39. Vignon, F., Terqui, M., Westley, B., Derocq, D. and Rochefort, H. (1980): Endocrinology, 106:1079-1086.
40. Vignon, F., Bardon, S., Chalbos, D., and Rochefort, H. (1983): J. Clin. Endocrin. Met., 56:1124-1130.
41. Vignon, F., Derocq, D., Chambon, M., and Rochefort, H. (1983): C. R. Acad. Sci., 296:151-156.
42. Weichselbaum, R.R., Hellman, S., Piro, A.J., Nove, J.J., and Little, J.B. (1978): Cancer Res., 38: 2339-2342.
43. Welsch, C.W., Dombroske, S.E., Mc Manus, M.J., and Calaf, G. (1979): B. J. Cancer, 40:866-871.
44. Westley, B., and Rochefort, H. (1979): Biochem. Biophys. Res. Commun., 90:410-416.
45. Westley, B., and Rochefort, H. (1980): Cell, 20:353-362

Progress in Cancer Research and Therapy,
Vol. 31, edited by F. Bresciani, et al.
Raven Press, New York © 1984.

Altered Estrogen and Anti-Estrogen Responsiveness in Clonal Variants of Human Breast Cancer Cells

C.D. Berg, H. Nawata, D.A. Bronzert, and M.E. Lippman

Medicine Branch, National Cancer Institute, National Institutes of Health, Bethesda, Maryland 20205

Breast cancers are among the few human malignancies responsive to endocrine manipulation. This responsiveness was recognized clinically long before the demonstration of cytoplasmic estrogen receptors. It had been hoped that the ability to assay estrogen receptors in mammary tumors would lead to the identification of a subset of patients whose tumors would all be responsive to hormonal therapy. Unfortunately, only 60% of breast cancer patients have tumors which are positive for estrogen receptors and of that 60%, nearly half are unresponsive to endocrine manipulations (23). Therefore, the factors that affect the presence of receptors and their function if present are crucial to understanding the growth modulating effect of steroids on breast cancer. Fortunately, some breast cancer cell lines have been shown to have hormonal responsiveness mimicking the clinical situation. The study of such lines and clonally selected variants with altered hormonal sensitivity should help to shed light on the mechanism(s) of such clinical resistance to hormonal therapy.

For several years our laboratory has been interested in the study of hormone responsiveness and resistance in breast cancer clinically and in tissue culture. We decided to study the problem using the MCF-7 cell line and have pursued this goal in part through the development of hormone resistant cell line variants. The MCF-7 breast cancer cell line was initially isolated from a pleural effusion in a woman with metastatic breast cancer and was subsequently found to contain estrogen receptor (22,3). We have previously shown that this cell line responds to a wide variety of hormonal manipulations under controlled conditions (14-17). In the absence of insulin, a marked growth response to estradiol (E_2) can be demonstrated, with maximal stimulation occurring at an estradiol concentration of 10^{-9}M. Since maximal growth can occur without estradiol, it is necessary to document other evidence of estrogenic activity in the cell line. Responses to estrogen which have been measured include increased nucleoside incorporation and induction of thymidine kinase. Progesterone receptor(PgR) can also be induced (11). This is of particular clinical importance, as tumors which contain both estrogen receptor (ER) and progesterone receptor (PgR) are most sensitive to hormonal manipulation (19).

Several specific proteins have been shown to be under estrogenic control, including thymidine kinase (2), lactic dehydrogenase (LDH) isoenzymes (4), a secreted protein with a molecular weight, 52,000 daltons, of unknown function(28), plasminogen activator(5), and a 24,000 and a 36,000 dalton pair of cytoplasmic proteins induced by estradiol after initial nafoxidine block(7).

Effects of anti-estrogens on MCF-7 cells have also been evaluated. Tamoxifen, a triphenylethylene derivative, has both antagonistic and agonistic effects. It inhibits cell growth (14) an effect which can be blocked by high concentrations of estradiol. Tamoxifen increases the progesterone receptor concentration(11), while the concentration of the 52,000 dalton secreted protein which is increased by estradiol remains unaffected (28). Tamoxifen is thought to act through the estrogen receptor because its effects are blocked by simultaneous incubation with estradiol. In addition, radiolabeled ligand studies suggest equivalence in the number of sites for estrogen and anti-estrogen binding in the MCF-7 cells and there is no inhibition by this anti-estrogen in cells without ER. However, there is other evidence that saturable anti-estrogen binding sites (AEBS) distinct from the estrogen receptor exist. These sites are cytosolic, high affinity and specific for anti-estrogens. Sex steroids are unable to compete with anti-estrogens for binding to these sites. Recently, an endogenous ligand for this AEBS has also been discovered(6).

Therefore, we thought that by selecting for tamoxifen resistance in MCF-7 cells we could better study mechanisms of steroid hormone action in response to estrogens and anti-estrogens (18,20,21). The technique we employed, modified from Sibley and Tomkins(30), was to select for clones resistant to high concentrations of tamoxifen. MCF-7 cells were grown in monolayer culture for two weeks, treated with tamoxifen at 10^{-6}M for 24 hours and then cloned in soft agar in the continued presence of tamoxifen at 10^{-6}M for six to eight weeks. The cloning efficiency of MCF-7 cells in tamoxifen was approximately 10^{-4} compared to 10^{-1} for wild-type cells grown in the absence of tamoxifen. The surviving clones were isolated with a sterile Pasteur pipette and grown up in 24-well dishes, progressing to larger flasks with IMEM(improved minimal essential medium) and 5% fetal calf serum. The vast majority of the colonies remained tamoxifen sensitive when growth curves were done. Two clones, R3 and R27, demonstrated tamoxifen resistance and were selected for further study.

R3 and R27 demonstrated karyotypes identical to the original wild-type MCF-7 cell line, containing the specific marker chromosomes of the MCF-7 cell(18). In addition, they showed alloyzme phenotypes identical to the wild-type cells(performed by Dr. Stephen J. O'Brien, NCI).

Our next step was to characterize the differences in hormonal responsiveness between the cloned variants and the MCF-7 cell line. The first clone to be studied was R3 (21). Under growth conditions employed to evince estradiol effect, the R3 cells have a doubling time of 2.4 days as compared to the MCF-7 cells which doubled slightly more quickly (every 2 days). The response to hormonal stimulation differed. As can be seen in Figure #1 (Growth Curve R3), the effect of estradiol on cell growth was apparently much smaller in R3 than MCF-7 cells. The growth constant increased from 0.26 ± 0.06 days^{-1} to 0.33 ± 0.05 days^{-1} in MCF-7 but increased only from 0.14 ± 0.01 days^{-1} to 0.18 ± 0.02 days^{-1} in R3 with 10^{-8}M estradiol treatment. This was a significant difference ($p<0.001$). The addition of 10^{-6}M tamoxifen to cells in culture results in growth inhibition of both MCF-7 and R3, but R3 was more resistant to tamoxifen than MCF-7. The growth constants for MCF-7 and R3 in 10^{-6}M tamoxifen were 0.18 ± 0.07 days^{-1} and 0.09 ± 0.02 days^{-1}, respectively, which were significantly different ($p<0.02$).

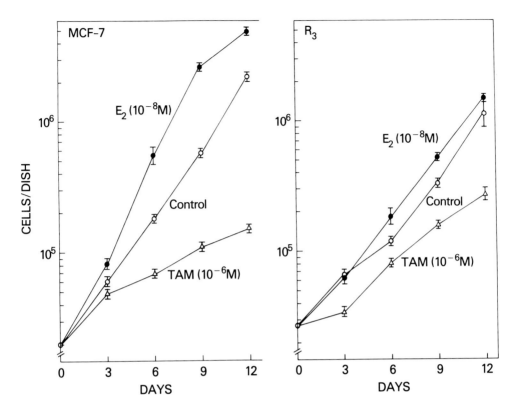

Figure 1. Effect of Hormones on Cell Proliferation of MCF-7 and the R3 Variant.
Hormones were added at 0 time. O controls, ●, 10^{-8} M E_2, Δ, 10^{-6} M TAM. Triplicate dishes of cells were harvested every 3 days and counted in a Coulter counter.

Estradiol at a concentration of 10^{-8}M stimulated thymidine incorporation by 50% over control in MCF-7 cells(10,11). Thymidine incorporation in MCF-7 cells was inhibited by 60% at 5 x 10^{-6}M tamoxifen. In the R3 clone, estradiol did not increase thymidine incorporation while a concentration of 10^{-6}M tamoxifen decreased thymidine incorporation by only 5%.

Four days of estradiol treatment of MCF-7 cells resulted in an eight to ten-fold increase in progesterone receptor as measured by sucrose gradient centrifugation. When R3 cells were subjected to the same treatment, no induction of progesterone receptor was observed. Therefore, at least two major estrogen responses, thymidine incorporation and progesterone receptor induction, were not intact in the R3 cell line.

Cytosolic estrogen receptor was determined by dextran-coated charcoal assay and nuclear estrogen receptor was determined by hydroxylapatite assay. Saturation curves and Scatchard analyses were then done. Nuclear receptor has a slightly higher apparent binding affinity for estradiol than cytoplasmic receptor in both MCF-7 and R3. The K_d of the cytosol (MCF-7 -- 1.18 + 0.3 x 10^{-10}M and R3 1.59 + 0.28 x 10^{-10}M) and nuclei (MCF-7 2.6 + 0.19 x 10^{-10}M and R3 2.61 + 0.25 x 10^{-10}M) were similar.

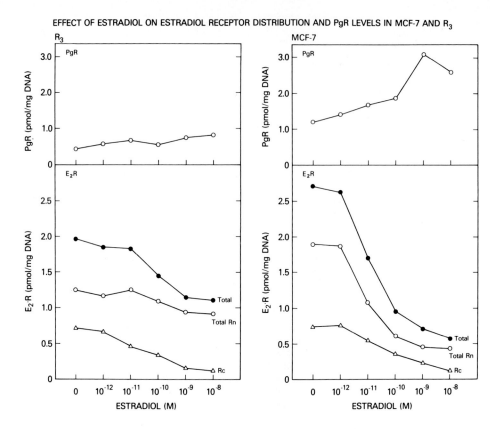

Figure   2.   Effect of E_2 on PgR Levels and ER Distribution.
               Two T-150 flasks/point were treated 4 days with increasing
               E_2 concentrations (0.001 to 10nM) added to IMEM containing
               stripped calf serum and insulin. Control flasks received
               the same medium with E_2. Unoccupied cytoplasmic receptors.
               (Δ, Rc 4°C incubation), total nuclear receptor (0, Rn 37°C
               incubation) and total cell receptors (Rc + Rn) were then
               determined.

Concentrations of receptors were measured, R3 contains at least as much
binding activity in both cytoplasmic and nuclear components as MCF-7.
Binding of radiolabeled ligand occurred with apparently normal affinity,
however the ability of this receptor complex to function in subsequent
steps was still undetermined.
   High affinity binding of estradiol by R3 did not exclude the possibility that the R3 receptor had an altered affinity for anti-estrogens.
We therefore performed competition experiments with estradiol and tamox-
fen against tritiated estradiol. These competition experiments demonstrated no differences between MCF-7 and R3. As has been described in
MCF-7 cells, and now shown in R3, tamoxifen had an approximately 100-fold
lower affinity for the receptor than estradiol. Similar results were
obtained with nafoxidine and clomiphene.
   Sucrose gradients and Sephadex G-100 column chromatography of cytoplasmic estrogen receptor demonstrated no significant differences between

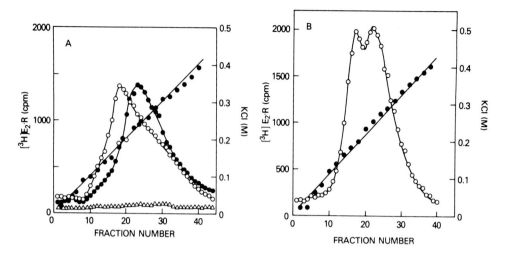

Figure 3. DNA Cellulose Column Chromatogrpahy.
Activated [^{3}H]E$_2$ receptor complexes were applied to a DNA
cellulose column. After the columns were rinsed to remove
unbound [^{3}H]E$_2$, bound receptor in the column was eluted
with a KCl gradient (●). △ , MCF-7 or R3 with [^{3}H]E$_2$ and
100-fold excess unlabled E$_2$. Figure A-MCF-7 with [^{3}H]E$_2$
(O) and R3 with [^{3}H]E$_2$ (◐) and Figure B- shows MCF-7 and
R3 incubated with 0.1 M KCl before they were mixed. The
same pattern was obtained by incubation with 0.1 M KCl
after they were mixed.

MCF-7 and R3 receptor. Sedimentation coefficients (S value) for cytoplasmic receptor, in the absence of 0.4M KCl were 8.7S in MCF-7 and 9.2S
in R3. Molecular weight estimations by Sephadex G-100 gel filtration
were also identical(51,000 daltons). Since molybdate and protease inhibitors were not included in these experiments this probably represented
the characterization of a receptor fragment rather than the whole
receptor.

We measured over the course of five hours the concentrations of
cytosolic and nuclear estrogen-receptor complexes. In both cell lines,
initially we saw a decrease in cytosolic receptor and an increase in
nuclear receptor consistent with translocation. Therefore, translocation
was not the site of the defect.

At five hours, 60% of the total amount of original receptor-complex in
MCF-7 cells translocated into the nucleus by estradiol was no longer detectable by salt extraction followed by hydroxylapatite exchange assay
(referred to as processing). In R3 cells less than 20% of the receptor
complex eluded detection at five hours. As can be seen in Figure 2,
we found that the processing defect in R3 cells occurred at the estradiol
concentration PgR production was expected. This suggested a role for
"processing" in steroid hormone action (Figure #2).

Cytosol from MCF-7 and R3 were mixed, DNA-cellulose column chromatography of each of the two receptor complexes remained unaltered with two
distinct peaks seen (Figure #3). This result was consistent with R3
containing an altered receptor. If a cytosolic factor were responsible
for the alteration in behavior of the R3 receptor one would have expected

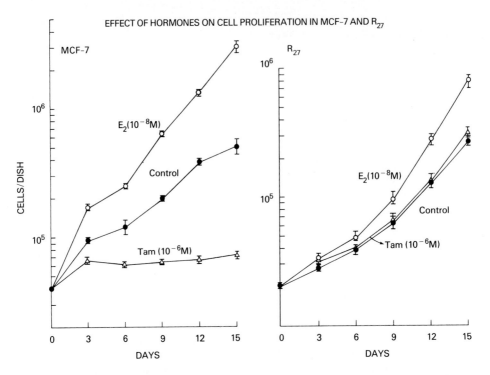

Figure 4.   Effect of Hormones on Cell Proliferation in MCF-7 and R27.
            Hormones were added at 0 time. Triplicate dishes of cells
            were harvested every 3 days and counted in a Coulter counter.
            Results are means + S.D.   ●, control;   O, estradiol (E₂),
            Δ, 10⁻⁶M tamoxifen.

an alteration in binding of the MCF-7 receptor. Somatic cell hybridization studies between R3 and MCF-7 which would unequivocally demonstrate
the distinctness of the two receptors have not yet been done.
    We have concluded from these studies that R3 was an MCF-7 variant
cell line which failed to demonstrate a growth response to estradiol or
substantial inhibition by anti-estrogens. The receptor had normal
affinity for estrogen and anti-estrogen. Sucrose density gradient
analysis and Sephadex chromatography were identical for R3 and MCF-7.
The receptor from R3, however, bound more tightly than normal to DNA-
cellulose and after 5 hours was processed minimally as compared with
that from MCF-7.
    Another cell line, R27 was also cloned from the wild-type MCF-7
cells in soft agar in the presence of 10⁻⁶M tamoxifen. An evaluation
of several characteristics of this cell line was undertaken analogous
to the investigation of R3. We initially studied the growth characteristics of the R27 cell line in response to hormonal stimulation.
Estradiol at a concentration of 10⁻⁸M stimulated cell division, but to a
much lesser extent than in MCF-7 cells. But more interestingly, growth
curves failed to demonstrate any inhibition by tamoxifen (Figure #4).
Thus R27 had become altered so that the inhibitory response to antiestrogens had been eliminated, while some estrogenic growth stimulation
persisted. Thymidine incorporation studies were consistent, in R27 cells

estradiol minimally stimulated incorporation while tamoxifen did not change it from baseline.

Scatchard analysis and saturation curves demonstrated similar dissociation constants and quantities of nuclear and cytoplasmic receptors. Sucrose density gradients and Sephadex chromatography demonstrated similar sedimentation coefficients and molecular weight estimates for the estrogen receptor in R27 and MCF-7. Therefore by physical criteria there was nothing to separate the R27 from the MCF-7 receptor.

The affinity of the receptor for estradiol was also identical in MCF-7 and R27. The affinity of both receptors for tamoxifen was identical and was 100-fold less than that for estradiol as was expected.

In R27 cells although translocation of the cytoplasmic receptor complex to the nucleus is apparently normal, "processing" did not appear to occur and the level of detectable nuclear receptor remained constant over time. Preliminary data suggest that nuclear processing of antiestrogen-estrogen receptor complexes in R27 may be diminished as compared to antiestrogen-estrogen receptor complexes in wild-type cells.

We measured DNA-cellulose binding after a variety of activation steps including addition of salt and nucleotides and found that it was decreased in R27 cells compared to MCF-7 cells. This binding alteration and the defect in processing mentioned earlier suggest that the site of the defect may be at the interaction of receptor with nuclear components.

In collaboration with Professor Henri Rochefort, we studied induction of a 52,000 dalton secreted glycoprotein in R27 clonal variants(27). In MCF-7 wild-type cells and R27 this protein was secreted in response to estradiol. The response was similar to that seen in their studies of MCF-7 cells. However, in MCF-7 cells, tamoxifen and OH-tamoxifen (a tamoxifen metabolite with high affinity for estrogen receptor) inhibited 52K protein production. In contrast, R27 cells increased their synthesis of this protein when treated with tamoxifen. The response to OH-tamoxifen was biphasic; at 10^{-8}M OH-tamoxifen there was an increase in 52K production, at higher concentrations, secretion was inhibited. Similarly, progesterone receptor synthesis was also stimulated by tamoxifen and OH-tamoxifen in R27 whereas we never saw induction of PgR by anti-estrogens in wild-type MCF-7 cells (Table #1). Thus R27 had not only escaped antiestrogen inhibition but had actually acquired trophic responses to these compounds. The site of this interesting defect is not known.

Another technique we employed to develop variant MCF-7 cell lines with altered hormonal responsiveness was one in which MCF-7 cells were exposed to $16\alpha^{125}$Iodoestradiol. Cells were exposed at a concentration of 2×10^{-9}M for one hour, centrifuged, viably frozen for two months, recovered, the process was repeated and then the cells were cloned. Cloning efficiency was 0.0004% of control. It was thought that the iodinated estradiol-estrogen receptor complex would bind to chromatin at sites at which estrogen had an effect on transcription and that the irradiation might induce variants with an altered estrogen responsiveness. Alternatively, we had hoped that another way such cells might escape lethal irradiation was by loss of hormone binding activity.

The 55 clonal cell lines that resulted were studied for their responsiveness to hormonal stimulation. Fifty-four of these lines were apparently normal, demonstrating estrogen receptor, progesterone receptor and normal growth characteristics under hormonal stimulation. One of these 55 lines however, I13, was quite unusual and has been further characterized (manuscript in preparation). The I13 cells upon exposure to estradiol would grow normally for four to six days (i.e. like the wild-type MCF-7 cells). However, then the cell number plateaued, the cells began

TABLE 1. Summary of Effects of Estradiol and Antiestrogens on Induction of Progesterone Receptor in Wild Type MCF-7 Cells and Clone R27

	MCF-7				R27			
Exp. No.	Control	OH-Tam (20nM)	TAM (20nM)	E_2 (10nM)	Control	OH-Tam (20nM)	TAM (20nM)	E_2 (10nM)
	111.1*	19.8	204	1574.7	42.8	37.4	149.6	427.3
	287	124	168	1377	96.9	575	413	640
	549	214	427	1786	130	400	440	392
	590	624	659	2087	332	1284	1298	1849
	476	ND	576	1743	202	218	181	1178
Avg. % Change		-48.5	+6.8	+488		+196	+218	+519
p value†		.07	NS	.02		.04	.04	.02

* all values are femtomoles/mg protein
† signed rank test

Progesterone receptor concentration was determined by dextran-coated charcoal assay. Cells were grown in Dulbecco's Modified Eagle's medium plus 5% charcoal treated calf serum for two weeks. Antiestrogens, estradiol or vehicle were added 48 hours prior to harvest.

to become round morphologically, detach from the plate and die(Figure 5). This phenomenon was seen with estradiol concentrations as low as 10^{-10}M. The response of the I13 cell line to tamoxifen was like that of the wild-type MCF-7 cells. Cell growth was inhibited.

Next, we looked for the site of alteration(s) in the hormone pathway. Tritiated thymidine incorporation was reduced in I13 compared to MCF-7 cells in response to estradiol and tamoxifen. Progesterone receptor induction occurred in I13 in response to estradiol, but only to one-third the amount seen in MCF-7 cells. By binding assays with sucrose density gradients, the characteristics of estrogen receptors in this cell line appeared identical to the wild-type MCF-7 cells. These lines of evidence indicated that the I13 cell line retained responsiveness to hormones, but that this response was altered in comparison with MCF-7 cells.

We theorized that the I13 cell line might be unusual in that it could secrete autocrine factors which would be inhibitory to neighboring cell growth. Secreted factors of this nature might well be found in the media. To test this hypothesis, we harvested media from I13 cells. This media was then added back to other I13 cells under experimental conditions at a time (that of rescue from thymidine block) when maximal growth was expected, and consequently the cells might be most sensitive to inhibition. No inhibitory effects were noted. Furthermore, conditioned media from I13 cells were as stimulatory for wild-type MCF-7 cells as conditioned media from MCF-7 cells. Consequently, a secreted inhibitory factor would be highly unlikely. Therefore, we believed the growth inhibition occurred intracellularly in each cell as a result of hormonal effects. I13 may therefore be a model for studying in vivo killing by pharmacologic concentrations of estradiol.

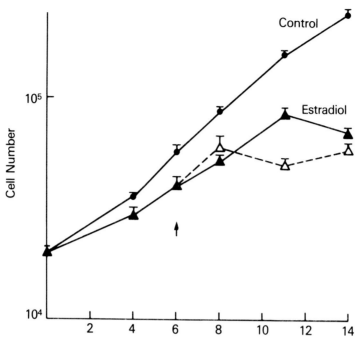

Figure 5. Effect of Hormones on Cell Proliferation in MCF-7 and I13. Hormones were added day 6 (↑). Triplicate dishes of cells were harvested every 3 days and counted in a Coulter counter. Results are means + S.D. ●, control; ▲, estradiol (10^{-8} M), △, tamoxifen, 10^{-6} M.

CONCLUSIONS

Our laboratory has developed three variant clonal cell lines from the MCF-7 parental breast cancer cell line. These clonal lines, R3, R27 and I13, arose with a greater frequency than expected from mutational events; however, even if they are manifestations of epigenetic resistance, the study of their characteristics should shed light on the mechanisms of hormone action and escape from endocrine manipulations in vivo. All of these lines showed altered responsiveness to tamoxifen and estradiol. In addition, their defects did not seem to involve the part of the receptor that binds the steroid hormones. The defects in at least two lines, R3 and R27, were more associated with abnormal receptor complex interactions with DNA and abnormal processing.

We hope that through analysis of these defective cell lines there will evolve an understanding of the cellular and molecular mechanisms involved in the action of steroid hormones. Furthermore, we hope that this study will shed light on the development of resistance in human tumors so as to enhance the probability for successful endocrine therapy of breast cancer.

REFERENCES

1. Aitken, S.C. and Lippman, M.E. (1982): Cancer Res., 42:1727-1735.
2. Bronzert, D.A., Monaco, M.E., Pinkus, L., Aitken, S. and Lippman, M.E. (1981): Cancer Res., 41:604-610.

3. Brooks, S.C., Locke, E.R., and Soule, H.D. (1973): J. Biol. Chem., 248:6251-6253.
4. Burke, R.E., Harris, S.C. and McGuire, W.L. (1978): Cancer Res., 38:2773-2776.
5. Butler, W.B., Kirkland, W.L. and Jorgensen, T.I. (1979): Biochem. Biophys. Res. Commun., 90:1328-1334.
6. Clark, J.H., Winneker, R.C., Guthrie, S.C. and Markaraverich, B.M. (1983): Endocrinology, 113:1167-1169.
7. Edwards, D.P., Adams, D.J., Squage, N. and McGuire, W.L. (1980): Biochem. Biophys. Res. Commun., 93:804-812.
8. Gulino, A. and Pasqualini, J.P. (1980): Cancer Res., 40:3821-3826.
9. Horwitz, K.B. and McGuire, W.L. (1975): Steroids, 25:497-505.
10. Horwitz, K.B. and McGuire, W.L. (1978): J. Biol. Chem., 253:2223-2228.
11. Horwitz, K.B. and McGuire, W.L. (1978): J. Biol. Chem., 253:8185-8191.
12. Horwitz, K.B. and McGuire, W.L. (1980): J. Biol. Chem., 255:9699-9705.
13. Horwitz, K.B. and Mockus, M.B. and Lessey, B.A. (1982): Cell, 28: 633-642.
14. Lippman, M.E., Bolan, G. and Huff, K.K. (1976): Cancer Treat. Rep., 60:1421-1430.
15. Lippman, M.E., Bolan, G. and Huff, K.K. (1976): Cancer Res., 36:4595-4601.
16. Lippman, M.E., Bolan, G. and Huff, K.K. (1976): Cancer Res., 36:4602-4609.
17. Lippman, M.E., Bolan, G. and Huff, K.K. (1976): Cancer Res., 36:4610-4618.
18. Lippman, M.E. and Nawata, H. (1982): In: The Role of Tamoxifen in Breast Cancer, edited by S. Iacobelli, M.E. Lippman and G. Robustelli Della Cuna, pp 9-16, Raven Press, New York.
19. McGuire, W.L., Carbone, P.P. and Vollmer, E.P. (1974): Estrogen Receptors in Normal and Neoplastic Tissues, Raven Press, New York.
20. Nawata, H., Bronzert, D.A. and Lippman, M.E. (1981): J. Biol. Chem., 256:5016-5021.
21. Nawata, H., Chong, M.T., Bronzert, D.A. and Lippman, M.E. (1981): J. Biol. Chem., 256:6895-6902.
22. Soule, H.D., Vazquez, J., Long, A., Albert, S. and Brennan, M. (1973): J. Natl. Cancer Inst.. 51:1409-1413.
23. Strobl, J.S. and Lippman, M.E. (1979): Cancer Res., 39:3319-3327.
24. Strobl, J.S., Monaco, M.E. and Lippman, M.E. (1980): Endocrinology, 107: 450-460.
25. Sutherland, R.Z., Murphy, L.C., Foo, M.S., Green, M.D., Whybourne, A.M. and Krozowski, Z.S. (1980): Nature, 288:273-275.
26. Ucker, D.S., Ross, S.R. and Yamamoto, K.R. (1981): Cell 27:257-266.
27. Vignon, F., Lippman, M.E., Nawata, H. and Rochefort, H., (1983): J Biol. Chem., (submitted).
28. Westley, B. and Rochefort, H. (1980): Cell 20:353-362.
29. Yamamoto, K.R., Stampfer, M.R. and Tomkins, G.M. (1974): Proc. Nat. Acad. Sci., 71:3901-3905.

*Progress in Cancer Research and Therapy,
Vol. 31,* edited by F. Bresciani, et al.
Raven Press, New York © 1984.

Isolation and Properties of Endocrine and Autocrine Type Mammary Tumor Cell Growth Factors (Estromedins)

*Tatsuhiko Ikeda, **David Danielpour, and **David A. Sirbasku

*Faculty of Nutrition, Kobe-Gakuin University, Igawadani-cho Arise, Nishi-ku, Kobe, Japan 673; and **Department of Biochemistry and Molecular Biology, The University of Texas Medical School, Houston, Texas 77225*

Growth of both normal and malignant mammary, pituitary, kidney and uterine tissue is under estrogen control *in vivo*. Although there has been intensive interest in establishing the molecular basis for this phenomenon, the central unanswered question remains what is the mechanism or mechanisms responsible for steroid regulation of growth? Of the many hypotheses being tested, only a small number will be reviewed here.

Our study of estrogen-responsive growth began with attempts to develop permanent tissue culture cell lines from estrogen responsive tumors of each of the major target tissues. The goal of these studies was to confirm *in vitro*, the well recognized growth phenomenon always demonstrable with estrogens *in vivo*. Our working hypothesis at that time (1972 to 1978) was that estrogens were directly mitogenic, and that isolation of permanent tissue culture cell lines from responsive tumors would allow a detailed study of the estrogen receptor-mediated growth of target tissues *in vitro*. We successfully obtained permanent tissue culture cell lines from estrogen (and androgen) responsive tumors of the uterus (ULMS-A and UCS-A hamster cells) (18), kidney (H-301 hamster cells) (41), mammary (MTW9/PL rat cells) (36) and pituitary (GH3/C14 rat cells) (16,47,48), and were able to show that with the exception of the uterine origin tumor cells these were either estrogen-responsive (36,47) or estrogen-dependent (21) for growth *in vivo*.

Additional characterization of these cell lines showed that the MTW9/PL (17), GH3/C14 (30) and the H-301 cells (D. Danielpour and D.A. Sirbasku, unpublished) have estrogen-specific receptors in the expected concentrations with binding constants for 17β-estradiol that were within the recognized molar concentrations of the respective normal target tissues. With these cell lines in hand, it seemed a relatively simple matter to demonstrate direct effects of estrogens on growth *in vitro*; this proved not to be the case. For our experiments (16-18,30,41), as well as reports by others (3,6,7,9,10,22,31,32,34,35,44-46,51-53), it is apparent that substantial (i.e. greater than 2-fold) estrogen responses are far more complex to demonstrate *in vitro* than initially conceived.

The current state of the matter is that some investigators propose that estrogens are directly mitogenic and present evidence interpreted to support this position (2,5,23-27), while others using similar or identical cell systems, report little if any effect of estrogens on

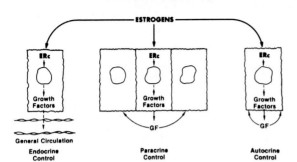

New Concepts in Control of Estrogen-Responsive Tissue Growth

FIG. 1. *Possible roles of estrogen-inducible growth factors in target tissue growth. The definitions of endocrine, autocrine and paracrine control have been presented elsewhere (42).*

growth (3,4,7,11,15,35). Even those who earlier reported large direct mitogenic effects (23,27) now report minimal responses to physiological concentrations of steroid (1,33,49). Yet another group has suggested that cells attached to an appropriate synthetic or natural basal lamina may become estrogen responsive (8), although to date, the evidence available in this area is far from conclusive. The discrepancies in the available data led to our proposal in 1978 (37) of an alternative mechanism by which estrogens may regulate target cell growth. More detailed summaries have been presented elsewhere (17,40,42) of our reasons for not accepting the hypothesis that estrogens are directly mitogenic, and for proposing the possible role of polypeptide mediator growth factors.

Our working hypothesis to be discussed here, is that estrogens promote growth of normal target tissue cells and hormone-responsive tumors via two new levels of regulation. These are summarized in Fig. 1. We propose that one of these levels of regulation may be that estrogens induce production of endocrine or circulating type growth factors which have their primary action in distant target tissues (a classical endocrine mechanism). These types of growth factors would be mediators of estrogen mitogenicity, and hence, we have tentatively designated them estromedins. For mammary cells we have identified uterus, kidney and pituitary as potential sources of endocrine estromedins. Clearly, a great body of information links pituitary origin hormones and/or growth factors to mammary growth. The possibility that uterus and kidney are involved also is a new proposal (37).

A second type of control (Fig. 1) may be that estrogens act locally on the target tissue cells to induce biosynthesis and/or secretion of estromedin growth factors whose primary site of action is either adjacent cells (paracrine mode of action) or directly back on the tumor cell or origin (autocrine mode of action). Such growth factors would not necessarily appear in significant concentrations in plasma, but may be consumed within the target tissue.

In this report we will describe the purification and properties of three possible endocrine estromedins from sheep uterus, mature ewe kidney and whole sheep pituitaries. These purified mitogens are of molecular weights ranging between 3,900 and 4,200 daltons, and are biologically active with MTW9/PL rat mammary tumor cells at concentrations of 10^{-10} to 10^{-9} M in completely serum-free medium. The purifications of the uterine, kidney and pituitary derived mitogens will be described next, as will the characterization of an estrogen-inducible autocrine

TABLE 1

Purification of Sheep Uterine Mammary Tumor Cell Growth Factor (UDGF)

Steps	Specific Activity (G_{50}, ng/ml)	Total Protein (mg)
Lyophilized Uterine Powder	450,000 (a)	(500g) (b)
0.1M Acetic Acid Extraction	1300	20,600
93°C Treatment	370	4800
SP-Sephadex Chromatography	82	970
Sephadex G-50	21	212
CM-Sephadex C-25	8	40 to 50

(a) Specific Activity of pH 7.2 PBS Extract

(b) Total Dry Weight of Powder Used to Initiate Isolation

type growth factor (estromedin) from MTW9/PL cells in culture. Also, preliminary work will be presented showing that the human estrogen-re sponsive MCF-7 and T-47D mammary tumor cells also possess potent auto-crine growth factor activities.

Purification and Properties of Endocrine Estromedins

Uterine derived growth factor (UDGF)

The purification of UDGF from lyophilized powders of early pregnant sheep uteri is presented in detail elsewhere (14); only a summary of those results will be described here. The purification of UDGF was mon-itored by following the stimulation of incorporation of tritium labeled thymidine into DNA of MTW9/PL rat mammary cells in culture as described before (13,14). Using only purified UDGF, the activity was monitored by a cell number increase assay (13,14). Unless otherwise noted, all puri-fications were performed at 4°C.

Beginning with lyophilized powder of early (i.e. < 49 days) pregnant sheep uteri, this material was extracted for 24 hours in 0.1 M acetic acid. After this period the residue was removed by centrifugation and the active supernatant heated at 93°C for 5 min. The large inactive precipitate was removed by centrifugation and Sulphopropyl Sephadex C-25 (equilibrated in 0.1 M acetic acid) was added to the supernatant. This mixture was stirred overnight, the inactive supernatant poured off, and the ion exchange Sephadex washed with 0.1 M acetic acid, 0.001 M acetic acid and then eluted (in a glass column) with 0.3 M ammonium acetate, pH 7.2. The active eluant was pooled, lyophilized, redissolved in a small volume of 0.1 M acetic acid and chromatographed on Sephadex G-50 equilibrated in the same acid. The activity eluted in the < 5,000 dal-ton volume. This was pooled, lyophilized, redissolved in 10 mM sodium phosphate, pH 6.0 and chromatographed on CM-Sephadex C-25 equilibrated in the same buffer. The UDGF was eluted with a linear sodium chloride gradient, and the final active fraction desalted by Sephadex G-25 chro-matography in 0.1 M acetic acid.

A summary of the purification is presented in Table 1. From 500 g of powder 40 to 50 mg of UDGF was obtained in an overall yield of 33%. Cal-culated from Table 1, UDGF represented 0.02% of the dry weight of the uterine powder. From assays shown in Table 1, the specific activity of each step of the purification yielded decreasing G_{50} values (the amount of protein required to one-half replace the MTW9/PL cell growth response

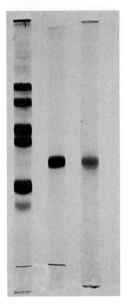

FIG. 2. *The 8 M urea, 0.1% SDS PAGE and Coomassie Blue staining analysis of the CM-Sephadex Step 5 purified UDGF preparation. The molecular weight markers used are shown in the left lane (horse heart myoglobin and the sequenced fragments of the myoglobin, M_r = 16,947, 14,404, 8,159, 6,214 and 2,512, respectively). The middle lane shows the migration position of a single band found after application of 75 µg of UDGF, and in the right lane, application of 10 µg of the same UDGF.*

to 10% fetal calf serum) to a final amount of 8 ng/ml. Estimation of the degree of homogeneity of the final preparation eluted from CM-Sephadex was made by 8 M urea, 0.1% SDS 12.5% polyacrylamide gel electrophoresis (PAGE) as shown in Fig. 2. One Coomassie Blue stained band was observed.

Experiments were conducted which showed that the stained band corresponded to the only area of elution of UDGF from unstained gels run in parallel (14). The state of homogeneity was further characterized by non-SDS PAGE at different acrylamide concentrations at pH 8.5 and pH 4.5, hydrophobic chromatography on octylsepharose, HPLC analysis on a C8 reverse phase column, HPLC TSK-125 molecular sieve analysis, and by isoelectric focusing (14). In all of these studies > 90% homogeneity was found. The isoelectric point of UDGF has been determined as pI = 7.3 ± 0.4. The molecular weight of UDGF was estimated at 4,200 daltons by 8 M urea, 0.1% SDS, 12.5% PAGE (Fig. 3). The data obtained thus far indicate that UDGF is an acid and heat stable, low molecular weight peptide with half-maximal biological activity (G_{50}) at 1.90×10^{-9} M with MTW9/PL rat mammary tumor cells growing under completely serum-free conditions. Throughout the isolation process, the mitogenic activity of UDGF was monitored by following the effect of the factor upon labeled precursor incorporation into MTW9/PL cell DNA. However, to define UDGF as a true growth factor, it was necessary to demonstrate its ability to promote growth as measured by logarithmic increase in cell number. As shown in Fig. 4, UDGF promotes the continuous growth of MTW9/PL cells in serum-free medium supplemented with a non-growth promoting concentration (i.e. 16 µg/ml) of neutral buffer extract of uterine powder. We have reviewed elsewhere (14) the preparation and significance of this requirement for supplementation of the serum-free medium with neutral uterine extract. From the data presented in Fig. 4, we conclude that by the criteria of promoting logarithmic cell growth, a potent mammary tumor cell growth factor has been isolated. In additional experiments described previously (14), it has been shown that UDGF activity is not

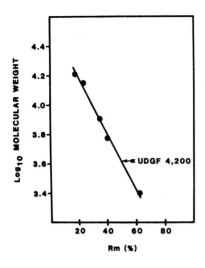

FIG. 3. *Estimation of UDGF molecular weight by 8 M urea, 0.1% SDS PAGE. From the data presented in Fig. 2, and using the relative mobilities of the myoglobin markers, the molecular weight of UDGF was calculated.*

replaceable by any of the other known purified growth factors such as EGF, FGF, SmC (IGF-I), MSA (mixture of IGF-I and IGF-II), PDGF or insulin.

The cell type specificity of UDGF has been characterized partially (14). UDGF is a potent mitogen for the estrogen-dependent H-301 hamster kidney tumor cells (G_{50} = 42 ng/ml), estrogen-induced uterine UCS-A cells (176 ng/ml) and estrogen-responsive GH3/C14 rat pituitary tumor cells (1,400 ng/ml). However, UDGF whose concentration was 50 µg/ml, was not mitogenic for rat fibroblasts. In data not presented here (T. Ikeda *et al.*, manuscript in preparation), we have shown that purified

FIG. 4. *Demonstration of UDGF as a promoter of cell growth as measured by logarithmic cell number increase. The methods used were those described in the cell population doubling assay (14). Cell growth was measured daily in DME only (open triangles); DME supplemented with 100 ng UDGF/3.0 ml medium (closed squares); DME supplemented with only 50 µg of neutral uterine extract per 3.0 ml medium (open squares); DME supplemented with 50 µg of neutral uterine extract and 100 ng/3.0 ml of medium (closed circles). On days 2 and 4 (shown*

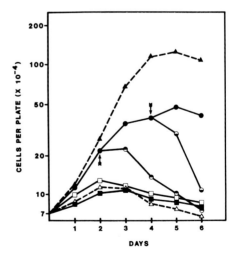

by arrows) additional UDGF (100 ng/plate) was added to those cultures which had already received 50 µg/plate of neutral uterine extract. These cultures continued to grow (closed circles). When UDGF was not added on either day 2 or day 4, the cell numbers per plate decreased as shown by the half-closed circles. Closed triangles represent growth in response to 10% fetal calf serum.

TABLE 2

Purification of Sheep Pituitary Mammary Tumor Cell Growth Factor (PitDGF)

Steps	Specific Activity (G_{50}, ng/ml)	Total Protein (mg)
Lyophilized Pituitary Powder	22,000 (a)	(10g) (b)
0.1M Acetic Acid Extraction	702	439
93°C Treatment	176	136
SP-Sephadex Chromatography	61	40
Sephadex G-50	29	8 to 10

(a) Specific Activity of pH 7.2 PBS Extraction
(b) Total Dry Weight of Powder Used to Initiate Isolation

UDGF is mitogenic for normal rat uterine cells in culture. This is potentially a very important observation. The data available from both purified sheep UDGF (14) and partially purified rat UDGF suggest that these growth factors may serve as autocrine controls of normal and malignant uterine growth, as well as potential endocrine estromedins for mammary tissue. This possible dual role of UDGF is now under active investigation.

Pituitary derived growth factor (PitDGF)

The purification of PitDGF was initiated with 10 g amounts of lyophilized powder of mixtures of male and female whole sheep pituitary glands (Table 2). A more detailed description of these results has been presented elsewhere (12). PitDGF specific activity was monitored by the radioassay method described before (13,14). The method of purification of PitDGF was identical to the first four steps of UDGF (14) with the single exception that individual steps were conducted on 1/50 scale. In the final step of purification (Sephadex G-50 eluted with 0.1 M acetic acid), a single peak of protein corresponded to the elution volume of the PitDGF activity (Fig. 5). Analysis of the components of this peak by 8 M urea, 0.1% SDS, 12.5% PAGE followed by Coomassie Blue staining showed one major protein peak (Fig. 5). The molecular weight of PitDGF was estimated at 3,900 ± 200 daltons (Fig. 6). From 10 g of powder, a total of 8 to 10 mg of PitDGF can be obtained in 50% overall yield. Calculated from Table 3, PitDGF is 0.16% of the dry weight of sheep pituitary powder. PitDGF showed G_{50} = 29 ng/ml (7.4 x 10^{-9} M) with MTW9/PL cells (Fig. 7) when assayed under completely serum-free culture condi-

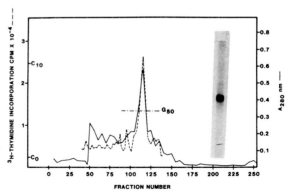

FIG. 5. *Elution of PitDGF activity from Sephadex G-50 equilibrated and eluted with 0.1 M acetic acid. PitDGF activity and protein elution (A 280 nm) are shown. Insert shows the 8 M urea, 0.1% SDS PAGE and Coomassie Blue stain localization of the 50 µg of protein from the pooled Sephadex G-50 peak.*

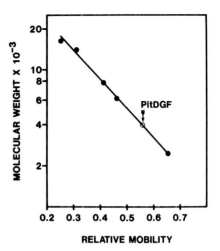

FIG. 6. *Estimation of PitDGF molecular weight by 8 M urea, 0.1% SDS PAGE. Molecular weight estimation was done as described in Fig. 3.*

tions and in the absence of all other known growth factors, nutrients and hormones required for mammary cell growth (3,4,23). Additional data presented in Fig. 7 and in another report (14), show that PitDGF activity cannot be replaced by other known hormones or growth factors.

Since we had shown previously (13) that MTW9/PL cells grew more rapidly *in vivo* in response to the growth hormone (GH) (MW = 22,000 daltons) and prolactin (PRL) (MW = 24,000 daltons) secretions from GH3/C14 cells (13), it is of particular significance that PitDGF is a potent mitogen, while these other well established hormones are not. In view of the controversy surrounding the role of PRL as a mammary cell mitogen (28,29), the identification of a new low molecular weight pituitary factor suggests the possibility that the PitDGF could represent a new pituitary hormone that is an active mitogen for mammary tissue. Further confirmation of this possibility was obtained when PitDGF, PRL and GH were compared for mitogenic effects on human MCF-7 and T-47D mammary tumor cells in culture. Growth of both of these cell lines in athymic nude mice has been shown to be pituitary hormone and/or pituitary factor

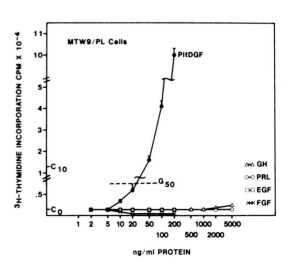

FIG. 7. *Effect of PitDGF, bovine-GH (growth hormone), bovine-PRL (prolactin), mouse EGF and bovine pituitary FGF on MTW9/PL cell growth. Assays were conducted as described in (13,14). Purified EGF and FGF were obtained from Collaborative Research Corp., Lexington, MA.*

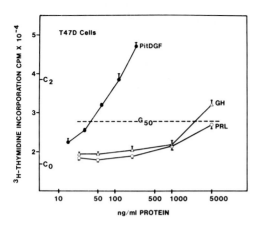

FIG. 8. *Effect of PitDGF, bovine-GH (growth hormone) and bovine-PRL (prolactin) on T-47D cell growth. Assays were conducted as described elsewhere (12). The assay methods for T-47D cells were significantly different from those used for MTW9/PL cells.*

responsive (20,50). The T-47D cells respond to PitDGF (G_{50} = 46 ng/ml, 1.2 x 10^{-8} M), while under similar serum-free assay conditions, concentrations of 3,000 (1.3 x 10^{-7} M) to 5,000 (2.1 x 10^{-7} M) ng/ml of GH and PRL, respectively, were required for G_{50} level responses (Fig. 8). Similar experiments conducted with the MCF-7 cell line (12) showed responsiveness to PitDGF (G_{50} = 75 ng/ml, 1.9 x 10^{-8} M), but no response over serum-free controls to GH or PRL at concentrations of up to 5,000 ng/ml. Thus, sheep PitDGF appears to be a mitogenic agent active in serum-free culture at 10^{-9} to 10^{-8} M concentrations for rat and human mammary tumor cells. Studies are now in progress to determine what other nutrients, attachment factors or hormones will facilitate the action of purified PitDGF on mammary cells. Addition of these may alter significantly the G_{50} of purified PitDGF. Parallel assays of PitDGF with human foreskin fibroblasts and rat ear fibroblasts show little or no mitogenic activity (12).

Further characterization of the degree of homogeneity of PitDGF are in progress, as are experiments designed to better define the *in vivo* significance of this new mammary cell mitogen.

Kidney derived growth factor (KDGF)
Purification of KDGF was initiated with the first two steps used with UDGF (14). Thereafter, the methods were modified significantly from those used with UDGF. These modifications were made because KDGF is an acidic (negatively charged) peptide at neutral pH, while UDGF (pI = 7.3) is slightly basic. Again, the purification of KDGF was monitored by the radioassay method described before (13,14). Beginning with lyophilized powder of mature ewe kidney, extraction was done with 0.1 M acetic acid for 24 hours. The inactive residue was removed by centrifugation and the supernatant treated at 95°C for 5 min. The large inactive precipitate was removed by centrifugation and the supernatant applied directly to a Bio-Rad AG50W x 8 column. This column was washed successively with 0.1 M acetic acid and then 0.001 M acetic acid and eluted with 10 mM ammonium hydroxide. The fractions containing KDGF were pooled, lyophilized and redissolved in 10 mM sodium acetate pH 5.8. Then the redissolved KDGF was applied to a DEAE-Sepharose CL-6B column equilibrated in the same buffer. The activity was eluted with a linear sodium chloride gradient to a second DEAE-Sephadex CL-6B column equilibrated at pH 6.2 in 10 mM sodium acetate; the activity was eluted with a sodium chloride gradient from 0 to 0.3 M. The final step of the purification was chro-

TABLE 3

Purification of Sheep Kidney Mammary Tumor Cell Growth Factor (KDGF)

Steps	Specific Activity $(G_{50}, ng/ml)$	Total Protein (mg)
Lyophilized Kidney Powder	345,000 (a)	(500g) (b)
0.1M Acetic Acid Extraction	2700	31,600
95°C Treatment	310	3,145
BIO-RAD AG50W-X8	58	285
DEAE-Sepharose CL-6B pH 5.8	41	79
DEAE-Sepharose CL-6B pH 6.2	29	24
Sephadex G-50	19	11

(a) Specific Activity of pH 7.2 PBS Extract

(b) Total Dry Weight of Powder Used to Initiate Isolation

matography on Sephadex G-50 in 0.1 M acetic acid. A summary of the results of the purification is presented in Table 3.

From 500 g of kidney powder, 8 to 14 mg of KDGF was isolated in an
overall yield of 5%; KDGF represents a calculated 0.04% of the dry
weight of the sheep kidney powder. The purified KDGF showed G_{50} = 19
ng/ml (4.5×10^{-9} M) with MTW9/PL cells in serum-free medium without any
other supplements. The lower yield of KDGF compared to UDGF represents
the problem of removing the considerably greater number of copurifying
proteins and peptides extracted from the kidney powder by 0.1 M acetic
acid. Characterization of the state of homogeneity was performed by 8 M
urea, 0.1% SDS, 12.5% PAGE (Fig. 9). Further evaluations of homogeneity are in progress. Estimation of the apparent molecular weight of
KDGF was made at 4,200 ± 400 daltons by the same methods described for
UDGF using 8 M urea, 0.1% SDS, 12.5% PAGE. On the basis of molecular
weight alone, UDGF and KDGF appear closely related. However, estimation
of pI of KDGF gave values of 4.2 to 4.7 (T. Ikeda and D.A. Sirbasku,

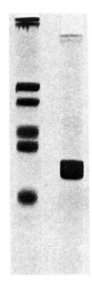

FIG. 9. *The 8 M urea, 0.1% SDS PAGE and
Coomassie Blue staining analysis of the
purified KDGF preparation from the Sephadex G-50 column step. The migration
position of the known molecular weight
markers of myoglobin and myoglobin
fragments are shown (see legend Fig. 2).
The migration of a 50 µg sample of KDGF
is shown as a single Coomassie Blue
stained band.*

unpublished) which clearly distinguishes the kidney factor from UDGF (pI = 7.3).

Studies are now in progress to define the cell specificity range of KDGF, and to determine whether KDGF and UDGF are capable of synergistically stimulating mammary cell growth in culture.

Estrogen-Inducible Autocrine Growth Factors in MTW9/PL Cells and Autostimulatory Factors Extracted from MCF-7 and T-47D Human Mammary Tumor Cells

One of the interesting observations made during our work with UDGF was that this mitogen promoted growth of normal and malignant uterine origin cells (14). Since both an increased uterine growth and an estrogen or pregnancy induction of elevated tissue levels of UDGF were correlated in rats (37) and sheep (14), and an acid extractable, heat stable UDGF was identified in estrogen induced accumulations of rat uterine luminal fluid under uterine growth promoting conditions (19,42,43), the possibility existed that UDGF may have a role in the uterus as an estrogen-regulated autocrine growth factor.

If we assumed this to be the case, then it became equally possible that regulation of growth of other estrogen target tissues was occurring locally. This would mean that estrogen-inducible autocrine growth factors should be identifiable in estrogen-responsive tumors growing *in vivo*, and if these were truly biosynthetic products of responsive cells, identification should be possible *in vitro*. Our first efforts, reported elsewhere (13,17,38,42), were to identify autocrine growth factors for rat MTW9/PL cells in extracts of estrogen-responsive MTW9/PL tumors growing in female rats. Those studies demonstrated potent mitogenic activities which appeared to be estrogen-related. MTW9/PL tumors which remained static or which regressed in ovariectomized females had 2-fold lower specific activity of the autostimulatory factor than tumors which continued to grow in response to normal levels of estrogens in intact females.

The methods of approach used in these earlier studies were to prepare extracts of washed (to remove residual blood) MTW9/PL tumors in neutral (pH 7.2) phosphate buffered saline, followed by preparation of high speed centrifugation supernatants (100,000 x g), and finally, assay of the growth factor activity with MTW9/PL cells in serum-free culture either by the cell population doubling assay or by the radioassay described before (13,14). More recently, the autostimulatory activity of the MTW9/PL tumors has been partially purified (D. Danielpour and D.A. Sirbasku, unpublished results) by a procedure beginning with 0.1 to 0.3 M acetic acid extraction and heating at 95°C for 5 min. Molecular weight estimations of the tumor associated activity (MTDGF) showed that extraction into 0.1 M acetic acid yielded > 90% of the activity at a MW of approximately 5,000 daltons; comparable extractions with neutral pH buffers gave activities ranging in MW between 50,000 and 80,000 daltons. We assume that the higher apparent MW for MTDGF in neutral buffer represents the association of the growth factor with high molecular weight proteins of the extract. The sum of the data obtained at that time suggested that the tumor associated activity did not originate from residual serum or extracellular fluids in the tumor, although it remained to be established conclusively that the autostimulatory factor was a biosynthetic product of MTW9/PL cells.

In a series of experiments designed to resolve this problem (D. Dan-

FIG. 10. *Growth responses of MTW9/PL rat mammary and MCF-7 human mammary tumor cells to 0.1 M acetic acid extracts of these same cell types. Both cell lines were grown under serum-free conditions for 4 days (with daily medium changes), then harvested and acetic acid extracts prepared. The upper panel shows the responses of extracts of MTW9/PL cells to extracts of MTW9/PL and MCF-7 cells; the bottom panel shows the responses of MCF-7 to similar extracts of MCF-7 and MTW9/PL cells. The MTW9/PL assays were conducted as described before (13,14), while the MCF-7 cell assays were conducted as described in another report (12).*

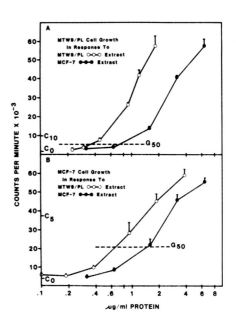

ielpour and D.A. Sirbasku, unpublished), we have shown that the auto-stimulatory factor of MTW9/PL cells was identifiable in acetic acid extracts of those cells growing in serum-free medium (after at least four daily serum-free medium changes); cycloheximide treatment caused complete loss of the activity from MTW9/PL cell extracts within three days. The activity also was found in the serum-free conditioned medium of MTW9/PL cells, although at greatly reduced concentrations compared to the cell extracts. We have obtained data showing that the MTW9/PL MTDGF is rapidly consumed by the cells in culture, resulting in a low available concentration in the serum-free conditioned medium. These data were extremely important when considering whether to purify MTDGF from cell extracts or conditioned medium.

Data presented in Fig. 10 demonstrated the specific activity (G_{50}) of rat MTW9/PL cell derived factor when assayed directly on the same estrogen-responsive MTW9/PL cells (top panel), and when assayed on the estrogen-responsive human MCF-7 cells (bottom panel). Similarly, acetic acid extracts of MCF-7 cells growing in serum-free medium showed mitogenic activity toward rat MTW9/PL cells (Fig. 10, top panel) and activity toward human MCF-7 cells (Fig. 10, bottom panel). Thus, an acetic acid and heat stable MTDGF was identified in acid extracts of rat and human breast cancer cells. Since the rat and human cell extracts each promoted growth of the breast cancer cells from the other species, the activities appeared to have a broad biological range.

We have conducted the essential test of establishing the estrogen-inducibility of these activities using both MTW9/PL rat and MCF-7 human cells in culture. The results with the MTW9/PL activity are presented in Fig. 11. In culture under serum-free conditions, concentrations of 10^{-9} to 10^{-8} M estradiol induced a 2-fold increase in MTDGF specific activity in MTW9/PL cells. Higher estrogen concentrations (i.e. 10^{-7} M) did not induce above the no estrogen controls, while lower levels (i.e. 10^{-11} to 10^{-10} M) were equally ineffective. Induction occurred within the concentration range compatible with the $K_d = 1.9 \times 10^{-9}$ M of the es-

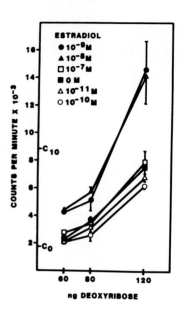

FIG. 11. *Estrogen-induction of MTW9/PL autostimulatory activity in culture. The MTW9/PL cells were grown under serum-free conditions for 4 days with only estradiol supplemented at the designated concentrations. Cell extracts were prepared as before by acetic acid treatment, and assays were based on deoxyribose, rather than protein, to correct for differences in cell number. Assays were conducted as described before (13,14).*

tradiol receptor of MTW9/PL cells (17). Similar experiments with MCF-7 cells showed induction of MTDGF between 40% and 60% (D. Danielpour and D.A. Sirbasku, unpublished). Efforts are now underway to further optimize the estrogen induction conditions for the MCF-7 autostimulatory growth factor by application of hormonally defined serum-free culture conditions.

At present, purification of MTDGF from human cells in culture is planned, and methods of approach are now under development. The implications of our results are numerous with regard to estrogen-responsive growth in general, and particularly with regard to the concepts of the roles of estrogens in mammary tumor growth. Isolation of new estrogen regulated autocrine factors from hormone-responsive breast cancer cells would open broad new avenues to diagnosis and treatment of these neoplasms.

Summary of Our Working Hypothesis

The following is a brief summary of the possible roles of growth factors in estrogen-induced growth of normal and neoplastic target tissues:

1. Estrogen-dependent (responsive) growth is, at least in part, regulated by growth factors.

2. Three levels of estrogen-inducible growth factor regulation are involved.

   A. Estrogen may induce endocrine (circulating) type growth factors. For example, mammary cell growth factors could be synthesized and secreted by uterus, kidney and pituitary, while pituitary cell estromedins may be produced by uterus, kidney and hypothalamus.

B. Also, estrogen may induce locally acting autostimulatory growth factors by direct action on target cells. Such factors would be mitogenic in the microenvironment of the producing cells.

C. Estrogens may induce growth factors whose primary action is local (e.g. uterine derived growth factor promotes growth of uterine cells), but which may reach the general circulation and coordinately regulate another estrogen-responsive tissue (i.e. mammary gland) as an endocrine factor.

The possible consequences of these mechanisms may be summarized as follows:

1. Both endocrine and autocrine growth factors are required for optimal estrogen-responsive growth *in vivo*. Endocrine types of estromedins may be more important in normal tissue growth control or early highly dependent tumors, whereas, autocrine estromedins may play a greater role in later stages of hormone-responsive growth leading to complete autonomy.

2. Locally produced autostimulatory activity is under regulation of the estrogen receptor. Hence, a high correlation between receptor positive tumors and estrogen responsiveness would be expected; this is clearly what is observed by most investigators, including our laboratory.

3. Tumors may escape estrogen-dependence by increases in unregulated production of autostimulatory growth factors. This would result in gradual conversion of estrogen-dependent cells to fully autonomous cells in a gradient-like process, which is completely consistent with the observed pattern of conversion from tumor dependence to autonomy. Thus, autonomy is not the loss of steroid hormone or polypeptide hormone receptors as suggested by many workers, but is the gradual gaining of the ability to produce autostimulatory factors without estrogen regulation. As a consequence, hormone autonomous tumors could be estrogen-receptor positive or negative and still exhibit autonomous growth. This is, in fact, what we as well as many other groups have observed. Clearly, autonomous tumors possess apparently normal numbers of estrogen receptors (D. Danielpour and D.A. Sirbasku, unpublished). The ability to produce growth factors in an unregulated manner would be expected to provide selective advantage to autonomous cells over dependent cells, and thus, account for the gradual process of conversion to autonomy seen with most hormone dependent tumors.

ACKNOWLEDGMENTS

The authors wish to thank Ms. Judy Roscoe for her expert technical assistance and preparation of the photographs, Ms. Wilda Ward for typing this manuscript and Mr. Mark Kunkel for editing. Also, we thank Mr. Tadao Sawada for assistance in the PitDGF purification. DD is supported by a Predoctoral Fellowship in Cancer Research from the Rosalie B. Hite Foundation, Houston, Texas, and DAS is a recipient of an American Cancer

Society Faculty Research Award, FRA-212. This work was supported by an American Cancer Society grant, BC-255 and by a National Cancer Institute grant, CA26617.

REFERENCES

1. Aitken, S.C. and Lippman, M.E. (1982): *Cancer Res.*, 42:1727-1737.
2. Allegra, J.C. and Lippman, M.E. (1978): *Cancer Res.*, 38:3823-3829.
3. Barnes, D. and Sato, G.H. (1979): *Nature (London)*, 231:388-389.
4. Barnes, D. and Sato, G.H. In: *Cell Biology of Breast Cancer*, edited by C. McGrath, M.J. Brennan and M.A. Rich, pp. 277-287. Academic Press, Inc., New York (1980).
5. Chalbos, D., Vignon, F., and Rochefort, H. (1982): In: *Cold Spring Harbor Conferences on Cell Proliferation, Vol. 9, Cell Growth in Hormonally Defined Media*, edited by G.H. Sato, A.B. Pardee and D.A. Sirbasku, pp. 845-848. Cold Spring Harbor Laboratory, Cold Spring Harbor, New York.
6. Dao, T.L., Sinha, D.K., Nemoto, T., and Patel, J. (1982): *Cancer Res.*, 42:359-362.
7. Edwards, D.P., Murphy, S.R., and McGuire, W.L. (1980): *Cancer Res.*, 40:1722-1726.
8. Gospodarowicz, D., Greenburg, G., and Birdwell, C.R. (1978): *Cancer Res.*, 38:4155-4171.
9. Hallowes, R.L., Rudland, P.S., Hawkins, A.R., Lewis, D.J., Bennett, D., Durbin, H. (1977): *Cancer Res.*, 37:2494-2504.
10. Henson, J.C., Pasteels, J.L., Legros, N., Henson-Steinnon, J., and Leclerq, C. (1975): *Cancer Res.*, 35:2039-2048.
11. Horowitz, K.B., and McGuire, W.L. (1978): *J. Biol. Chem.*, 253:8185-8191.
12. Ikeda, T., Danielpour, D., and Sirbasku, D.A. (1983): *In preparation*.
13. Ikeda, T., Liu, Q.-F., Danielpour, D., Officer, J.B., Iio, M., Leland, F.E., and Sirbasku, D.A. (1982): *In Vitro*, 18:961-979.
14. Ikeda, T., and Sirbasku, D.A. (1983): *J. Biol. Chem.*, (in press).
15. Jozan, S., Moure, C., Gillois, M., and Bayard, F. (1979): *J. Steroid Biochem.*, 10:341-342.
16. Kirkland, W.L., Sorrentino, J.M., and Sirbasku, D.A. (1976): *J. Natl. Cancer Inst.*, 56:1159-1164.
17. Leland, F.E., Danielpour, D., and Sirbasku, D.A. (1982): In: *Cold Spring Harbor Conferences on Cell Proliferation, Vol. 9, Growth of Cells in Hormonally Defined Media*, edited by G.H. Sato, A.B. Pardee and D.A. Sirbasku, pp. 741-750. Cold Spring Harbor Laboratory, Cold Spring Harbor, New York.
18. Leland, F.E., Iio, M., and Sirbasku, D.A. (1981): In: *Functionally Differentiated Cell Lines*, edited by G.H. Sato, pp. 1-46. Allen Liss, Inc., New York.
19. Leland, F.E., Kohn, D.F., and Sirbasku, D.A. (1983): *Biol. Reprod.*, 28:1243-1266.
20. Leung, C.K.H. and Shiu, R.P. (1981): *Cancer Res.*, 41:546-551.
21. Liehr, J.G., DaGue, B.B., Ballatore, A.M., and Sirbasku, D.A. (1982): In: *Cold Spring Harbor Conferences on Cell Proliferation Vol. 9, Growth of Cells in Hormonally Defined Media*, edited by G.H. Sato, A.B. Pardee and D.A. Sirbasku, pp. 445-458. Cold Spring Harbor Laboratory, Cold Spring Harbor, New York.

22. Lin, C.Y., Loring, J.M., and Villee, C.A. (1982): *Cancer Res.*, 42: 1015-1019.
23. Lippman, M.E., Allegra, J.C., and Strobl, J.S. (1979): In: *Cold Spring Harbor Conferences on Cell Proliferation, Vol. 6, Hormones and Cell Culture*, edited by G.H. Sato and R. Ross, pp. 545-558. Cold Spring Harbor Laboratory, Cold Spring Harbor, New York.
24. Lippman, M.E. and Bolan, G. (1975): *Nature (London)*, 256:592-593.
25. Lippman, M.E., Bolan, G., and Huff, K. (1976): *Cancer Res.*, 36: 4595-4601.
26. Lippman, M.E., Bolan, G., Monaco, M.E., Pinkus, L., and Engel, I. (1976): *J. Steroid Biochem.*, 7:1045-1051.
27. Lippman, M.E., Strobl, J., and Allegra, J.C. (1980): In: *Cell Biology of Breast Cancer*, edited by C. McGrath, M. Brennan and M. Rich, pp. 265-275. Academic Press, Inc., New York.
28. Mittra, I. (1980): *Biochem. Biophys. Res. Commun.*, 95:1750-1759.
29. Mittra, I. (1980): *Biochem. Biophys. Res. Commun.*, 95:1760-1767.
30. Moo, J.B., Stancel, G.M., Heindel, J.J., and Sirbasku, D.A. (1982): In: *Cold Spring Harbor Conferences on Cell Proliferation, Vol. 9, Growth of Cells in Hormonally Defined Media*, edited by G.H Sato, A.B. Pardee and D.A. Sirbasku, pp. 429-444. Cold Spring Harbor Laboratory, Cold Spring Harbor, New York.
31. Pasteels, J.L., Henson, J.C., Henson-Steinnon, J., and Legros, N. (1976): *Cancer Res.*, 36:2162-2170.
32. Pietros, R.J. and Szego, C.M. (1975): *Endocrinology*, 96:946-954.
33. Scholl, S.M., Huff, K.K., and Lippman, M.E. (1983): *Endocrinology*, 113:611-617.
34. Seaver, S.S., van der Bosch, J., Sato, G.H., and Baird, S.M. (1982): In: *Cold Spring Harbor Conferences on Cell Proliferation, Vol. 9, Cell Growth in Hormonally Defined Media*, edited by G.H. Sato, A.B. Pardee and D.A. Sirbasku, pp. 1171-1186. Cold Spring Harbor Laboratory, Cold Spring Harbor, New York.
35. Shafie, S.M. (1980): *Science*, 209:701-702.
36. Sirbasku, D.A. (1978): *Cancer Res.*, 38:1154-1165.
37. Sirbasku, D.A. (1978): *Proc. Natl. Acad. Sci. USA*, 75:3786-3790.
38. Sirbasku, D.A. (1981): *Banbury Rep.*, 8:425-443.
39. Sirbasku, D.A., and Benson, R.H. (1979): In: *Cold Spring Harbor Conferences on Cell Proliferation, Vol. 6, Hormones and Cell Culture*, edited by G.H. Sato and R. Ross, pp. 477-497. Cold Spring Harbor Laboratory, Cold Spring Harbor, New York.
40. Sirbasku, D.A. and Benson, R.H. (1980): In: *Cell Biology of Breast Cancer*, edited by C. McGrath, M.J. Brennan and M.A. Rich, pp. 289-314. Academic Press, Inc., New York.
41. Sirbasku, D.A. and Kirkland, W.L. (1976): *Endocrinology*, 98:1260-1272.
42. Sirbasku, D.A. and Leland, F.E. (1982): In: *Biochemical Actions of Hormones, Vol. 9*, edited by G. Litwack, pp. 115-140. Academic Press, Inc., New York
43. Sirbasku, D.A. and Leland, F.E. (1982): In: *Hormonal Regulation of Mammary Tumors, Vol. 2, Peptide and Other Hormones*, edited by B.S. Leung, pp. 88-122. Eden Press, Montreal, Canada.
44. Sonnenschein, C. and Soto, A.M. (1980): *J. Natl. Cancer Inst.*, 64: 211-215.
45. Sonnenschein, C., Ucci, A.A., and Soto, A.M. (1980): *J. Natl. Cancer Inst.*, 64:1141-1145.

46. Sonnenschein, C., Ucci, A.A., and Soto, A.M. (1980): *J. Natl. Cancer Inst.*, 64:1147-1151.

47. Sorrentino, J.M., Kirkland, W.L., and Sirbasku, D.A. (1976): *J. Natl. Cancer Inst.*, 56:1149-1154.

48. Sorrentino, J.M., Kirkland, W.L., and Sirbasku, D.A. (1976): *J. Natl. Cancer Inst.*, 56:1155-1158.

49. Strobl, J. and Lippman, M.E. (1978): In: *Hormones, Receptors and Breast Cancer,* edited by W.L. McGuire, pp. 85-95. Raven Press, New York.

50. Welsch, C.W., Swim, E.L., McManus, M.J., White, A.C., and McGrath, C.M. (1981): *Cancer Lett.*, 14:309-316.

51. Yang, J., Guzman, R., Richards, J., Imagawa, W., McCormick, K., and Nandi, S. (1980): *Endocrinology*, 107:35-41.

52. Yang, J., Richards, J., Bowman, P., Guzman, R., Enami, J., McCormick, K., Hamamoto, S., Pitelka, D.R., and Nandi, S. (1979): *Proc. Natl. Acad. Sci. USA*, 77:2088-2092.

53. Yang, J., Richards, J., Guzman, R., Imagawa, W., and Nandi, S. (1980): *Proc. Natl. Acad. Sci. USA*, 77:2088-2092.

Progress in Cancer Research and Therapy,
Vol. 31, edited by F. Bresciani, et al.
Raven Press, New York © 1984.

Effects of Antiestrogens and Estrogens on Proliferation of Human Breast Cancer Cells: *In Vitro* and *In Vivo* Models

C. Kent Osborne

*Department of Medicine/Oncology, University of Texas Health Science Center
at San Antonio, San Antonio, Texas 78284*

The mechanisms by which estrogens and antiestrogens regulate human breast cancer growth have not been totally defined. The bulk of evidence to date suggests that these hormones regulate tumor growth by a direct effect on human breast cancer cells which contain estrogen receptors. Estrogens and antiestrogens have been shown to influence several biochemical pathways leading to the synthesis of macromolecules or important enzymes, but the net effect of these biochemical events on actual cell proliferation is not totally clear. Our laboratory has initiated studies of the effects of estrogens and antiestrogens on breast cancer cell proliferation using human breast cancer cells growing in vitro in tissue culture as well as human breast cancer cells growing in vivo in athymic nude mice. Our studies suggest that the major effect of these hormones is to regulate the transit of breast cancer cells through the cell cycle.

METHODS

In vitro studies.

MCF-7 human breast cancer cells were used for these studies. The cell culture techniques used for the propagation of these cells have been described in detail (3). For cell kinetic experiments, cells were grown in monolayer for 24 hrs in culture medium supplemented with 1.0 nM insulin and 5% bovine serum. Medium was then replaced with medium supplemented with 5% charcoal-stripped serum. After 24 hrs, hormones or vehicle control were added directly to the cultures. The tritiated thymidine labeling index or flow cytometry of mithramycin-stained cells were used to assess the effects of hormonal manipulation on cell cycle distributions (2). G_1 cells were further classified as early or late G_1 by the morphology of prematurely condensed chromosomes as previously described (1, 2).

In vivo studies.

Four to six week old female intact or ovariectomized BALB/c nu+/nu+ athymic mice were used. MCF-7 cells (5×10^6 cells/0.2 ml medium) were injected s.c. in the axillary region. Estrogen supplementation was performed by the placment of s.c. pellets of 17β estradiol (0.25-0.5 mg) purchased from Innovative Research. The antiestrogens tamoxifen or LY156758 were given by s.c. injections of the drug in peanut oil. Tumor volume was calculated from the formula $\frac{width^2 \times length}{2}$.

Tumor mitotic index was measured by fixing tumors in formalin, and processing paraffin-embedded sections for histological assessment and staining with hematoxylin-eosin. The number of mitoses per 2000 cells was determined.

RESULTS

In vitro studies.

The addition of tamoxifen (1 μM) to MCF-7 cells growing in medium with 5% stripped bovine serum resulted in a slowing of cell proliferation compared to controls. By day 4 twice as many cells were present in control dishes compared to those treated with tamoxifen, and by day 6 there was a 3-fold difference. During this time cell number actually increased 2-fold in tamoxifen-treated dishes and at no time was there a reduction in cell number. Growth simply plateaued. This suggested that tamoxifen was exhibiting a cytostatic rather than cytocidal effect.

To determine the effect of tamoxifen on the fraction of cells in S phase, the thymidine labelling index (TLI) was used. As shown in Table 1, tamoxifen caused a time dependent reduction in the S fraction. By 72 hrs, less than 5% of tamoxifen treated cells were in S phase. The TLI in control cells also decreased as the cells neared confluence.

TABLE 1. Effect of tamoxifen on the TLI.

	TLI%	
Time (hrs)	Control	Tamoxifen
0	37	37
24	30	25
48	28	12
72	21	5

We next examined the effect of tamoxifen on the fraction of cells in G_1 and S phase using flow cytometry. A dose dependent reduction in the S phase population and an increase in G_1 cells was observed (Table 2).

TABLE 2: Effect of tamoxifen concentration.

Tam	% G_1	% S
0	72	21
0.1 nM	71	16
10 nM	79	13
1 μM	92	7

Concentrations higher than 1.0 μM were not tested since this concentration approaches the level observed in patients receiving the drug. Identical effects were observed with other antiestrogens including nafoxidine and LY156758.

These data suggest that antiestrogens inhibit cell proliferation by causing cells to accumulate in G_1 phase. Since some growth inhibitors block progression of cells at the G_1-S interface, whereas others block cells earlier in G_1, we next asked where in G_1 phase does the tamoxifen block occur. Using the morphology of prematurely condensed chromosomes, cells can be classified as occurring

early or late in G_1 based upon the criteria of Hittleman and Rao (1). The majority (65%) of tamoxifen-treated cells were found to be in early G_1. In contrast,
62% of control cells were in late G_1. Thus, antiestrogens induce a transition
delay in the early to mid G_1 phase of the cell cycle.

An important question is whether or not tamoxifen-inhibited G_1 cells are
permanently blocked and are destined to die. To answer this question in vitro,
MCF-7 cells were incubated in control or tamoxifen-containing media for 96 hrs.
At that time, 17β estradiol (10 nM) was added directly to the culture plates. As
shown in Table 3, estrogen caused a time dependent increase in the fraction of
cells leaving G_1 and entering S phase. Control cells grown in stripped serum only
for 96 hrs, began to leave G_1 and enter S phase by 12 hrs. By 24 hrs, 43% of
these cells were in S phase. Tamoxifen-treated cells were also "revived" with
estrogen, although the lag time was longer as might have been predicted from
the data showing that the majority of these cells were in early G_1 at the time of
estrogen addition. By 24 hrs, 56% of these cells were in S phase. Thus, the
tamoxifen block is not permanent as it can be reversed by adding a 100-fold
lower concentration of estradiol. This block can also be partially reversed by
simply changing to tamoxifen-free medium.

TABLE 3. Effect of estrogen rescue

Time after estrogen	Control (%)		Tamoxifen treated (%)	
	G_1	S	G_1	S
0 hrs	72	22	85	6
6	65	22	80	7
12	48	40	80	7
24	40	43	40	56

In vivo studies.
We next examined the in vivo effects of estrogen and antiestrogen on MCF-7
tumor development and growth in athymic nude mice. Similar to other reports (4,
5), tumor development after s.c. inoculation was estrogen dependent. Small
nodules persisted at the inoculation site in ovariectomized mice, but sustained
tumor growth did not occur. More than 90% of mice supplemented with an 0.25
mg estrogen pellet developed progressively growing tumors. After 28 days, the
average tumor size in estrogen supplemented mice was 9.2 mm. MCF-7 cells
remained viable for prolonged periods even in ovariectomized mice. Estrogen
supplementation of these mice more than 30 days after cell inoculation resulted
in tumor growth.

An interesting pattern of tumor growth was observed in ovariectomized mice
treated with the antiestrogens tamoxifen or LY156758 (Table 4). Initially,
tumors grew in all mice treated with antiestrogen and by day 12, tumors were
twice as large as those present in ovariectomized mice but half the volume of
those in estrogen supplemented mice. Thereafter, tumor growth stopped in
antiestrogen treated mice. This initial stimulation of tumor growth by the
antiestrogen may reflect initial estrogen-agonist activity which is then followed
by the antiestrogen effect. A clinical correlate may be the "tumor flare"
phenomenon occasionally observed with tamoxifen therapy in patients. Again,
the cells in tamoxifen-treated mice remained viable, since placement of an
estrogen pellet on day 30 restored tumor growth in these mice (not shown).

TABLE 4. Effect of antiestrogen on tumor development.[a]

Group	Tumor Volume (mm^3)	
	Day 12	Day 25
+ Estrogen	250	600
+ Tamoxifen	125	105
+ LY156758	130	120
Ovariectomy	70	43

[a]Ovariectomized mice without or with hormone treatments were inoculated with MCF-7 cells on Day 1. Tumor volume was measured on Days 12 and 25. Estrogen, .25 mg pellet; tamoxifen 25 μg/day s.c. in oil; LY156758 25 μg/day s.c. in oil.

In the next series of experiments we examined the effect of estrogen and antiestrogen on growth of already established tumors. On day 0 estrogen supplemented ovariectomized mice were inoculated with MCF-7 cells. On day 7, when tumors were growing rapidly, mice were divided into 5 groups (Table 5).

TABLE 5. Effect of hormones on growth of established tumors

Group	Tumor Volume (mm^3)	
	Day 12	Day 33
+ Estrogen	242	881
+ Estrogen + Tamoxifen	267	625
- Estrogen[a]	220	205
- Estrogen[a] + Tamoxifen	195	208
- Estrogen[a] + LY156758	200	204

[a]Estrogen pellet removed.

Tumors continued to grow in estrogen supplemented mice. Tamoxifen partially antagonized the estrogen effect. Tumor growth ceased, but tumor regression did not occur in estrogen deprived mice without or with antiestrogens. Regression of tumors failed to occur even when mice were treated for as long as 60 days (not shown). Tumor cells remained viable histologically despite prolonged antiestrogen treatment although the mitotic index was markedly reduced. Fifty mitoses per 2000 cells were observed in tumors from estrogen supplemented mice compared to only 8 mitoses per 2000 cells in tumors from estrogen-deprived tamoxifen-treated mice.

DISCUSSION

These studies demonstrate that a major effect of estrogens and antiestrogens is to regulate the progression of cells through the cell cycle. Similar to the work of Sutherland (6), we find that antiestrogen treatment of cells in vitro results in their accumulation in G_1 phase. Furthermore, the majority of cells are in early G_1 suggesting that tamoxifen causes a block or transition delay in early to mid G_1. The effect of tamoxifen is not permanent or lethal, at least at concentrations less than or equal to 1.0 μM and with a duration of exposure of several days. The block can be partially reversed by simply changing cultures to tamoxifen free medium, and it can be fully reversed by adding a 100-fold lower concentration of 17β estradiol. This tamoxifen block followed by estrogen "rescue" results in a marked synchronization of cells in S phase. The ability to synchronize breast cancer cells by this hormonal manipulation might be used to therapeutic advantage in the clinic by combining hormonal therapy with appropriately timed cytotoxic chemotherapy.

In vitro studies are limited by several factors, including the restriction to short-duration experiments. Thus, we have also used human breast cancer cells growing as tumors in nude mice to study the proliferative effects of estrogens and antiestrogens. Confirming previous results (4, 5), growth of MCF-7 tumors in nude mice is estrogen dependent. Inoculation of tumor cells into estrogen-deprived mice does not result in tumor development, but cells remain viable for prolonged periods. Replacement of estrogen results, then, in sustained tumor growth.

Treatment of mice carrying established MCF-7 tumors with estrogen withdrawal and/or antiestrogen therapy results in a cessation of tumor growth but not in actual tumor regression. Again, cells remain viable for weeks in such mice, and tumor growth can be restored by replenishment with estrogen. Not surprisingly the mitotic index in these plateau-phase tumors is significantly lower than in estrogen-treated mice with rapidly growing tumors. These cummulative data further support the hypothesis that estrogen deprivation or antiestrogen therapy inhibit breast cancer growth by reversibly blocking cell proliferation rather than by a direct cytocidal effect. Actual regression of tumor in patients treated by antiestrogen therapy may require immune mediated events which are deficient in the nude mouse.

REFERENCES

1. Hittleman, W. N. and Rao, P. N. (1978): J. Cell Physiol., 95:333-342.

2. Osborne, C. K., Boldt, D. H., Clark, G. M., and Trent, J. M. (1983): Cancer Res., 43:3583-3585.

3. Osborne, C. K., Monaco, M. E., Lippman, M. E., and Kahn, C. R. (1978): Cancer Res., 38:94-102.

4. Seibert, K., Shafie, S. M., Triche, T. J., Whang-Peng, J. J., O'Brien, S. J., Taney, J. H., Huff, K. K., and Lippman, M. E. (1983): Cancer Res., 43:2223-2239.

5. Shafie, S. M. and Grantham, F. H. (1981): J. Natl. Cancer Inst., 67:51-56.

6. Sutherland, R. L., Green, M. D., Hall, R. E., Reddel, R. R., and Taylor, I. W. (1983): Eur. J. Cancer Clin. Oncol., 19:615-621.

Progress in Cancer Research and Therapy,
Vol. 31, edited by F. Bresciani, et al.
Raven Press, New York © 1984.

Effects of Antioestrogens on Human Breast Cancer Cells *In Vitro.* Interactions with High Affinity Intracellular Binding Sites and Effects on Cell Proliferation Kinetics

Robert L. Sutherland, Leigh C. Murphy, Rosemary E. Hall, Roger R. Reddel, Colin K.W. Watts, and Ian W. Taylor

Ludwig Institute for Cancer Research (Sydney Branch), University of Sydney, New South Wales 2006, Australia

Many hormones, growth factors and drugs exert their effects on target cells through interactions with high affinity, saturable, cell surface or intracellular binding sites. The nonsteroidal antioestrogens, a group of synthetic compounds with oestrogen antagonist and antitumour activity (38,40), are no exception and have been shown to interact with two distinct high affinity binding sites in many tissues. Recent research in this laboratory has centred on understanding the mechanisms by which the antioestrogenic, anticancer agent, tamoxifen, inhibits the proliferation of human cancer cells. In particular we have studied the interaction of this and other structurally related compounds with two intracellular high affinity binding sites, oestrogen receptor (ER) and antioestrogen binding site (AEBS), in MCF 7 human mammary carcinoma cells and investigated their effects on the proliferation kinetics of this cell line. In this chapter some of the data contributing to our present understanding of the effects of antioestrogens on human breast cancer cell proliferation in vitro are presented.

INTERACTIONS WITH HIGH AFFINITY INTRACELLULAR BINDING SITES

Oestrogen Receptors

The MCF 7 cell line was derived from a pleural effusion from a woman with metastatic breast cancer (35) and was subsequently shown to contain specific receptors for oestrogens (3) and other steroid hormones (14). Synthetic nonsteroidal antioestrogens were shown to be competitive inhibitors of the binding of oestradiol to the oestrogen receptor (3,21) and potent inhibitors of the growth of this cell line in vitro (19,20). These important observations led to the widespread use of MCF 7 cells for studies on the molecular modes of action of nonsteroidal antioestrogens (1,4,6,7,8,15,16,29,34). Many of these studies illustrated that the effects of antioestrogens could be reversed by the simultaneous or subsequent administration of oestradiol providing strong evidence that these drugs exert most of their effects through interactions with the oestrogen receptor molecule (1,4,8,15,19,20). There are, however, some effects of antioestrogens that appear not to be completely reversed by oestradiol (2,22,32,41,42) and are therefore difficult to explain in terms of oestrogen receptor-mediated events.

During the course of studying those structural features of the antioestrogen molecule that influence their affinity for the AEBS we discovered that, although both ER and AEBS bound antioestrogens with relatively high affinity, the structural specificity of the two sites was markedly different (24,26,43,48). For example, while aromatic hydroxylation of tamoxifen to form 4-hydroxytamoxifen (4OHT) enhanced affinity for ER at least 30 fold it significantly reduced affinity for AEBS (Fig.1, Table 1). By contrast structural modifications in the basic aminoether side chain of tamoxifen often had relatively minor effects on binding to ER but markedly reduced e.g. N-desmethyltamoxifen (DMT), or abolished e.g. ICI 145680, affinity for AEBS (Table 1).

It therefore appeared likely that detailed studies of the specificity of these two high affinity binding sites in MCF 7 cells might reveal compounds that had similar affinity for one site and significantly different affinity for the other and that such compounds could provide valuable research tools for evaluating the contribution of each binding site to the overall effect of the drug. Such an approach was adopted with some success in the present studies and the results are presented later (Figs 10,11).

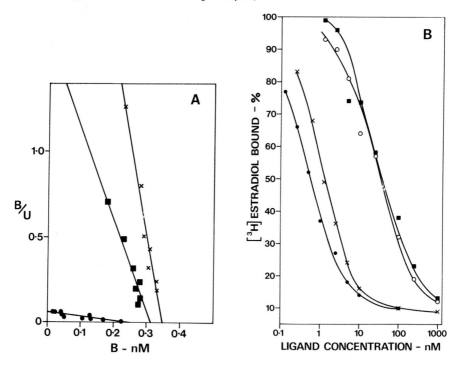

FIG.1. Binding data for the interactions of tamoxifen metabolites with MCF 7 cytoplasmic ER. A. Scatchard plots of binding data for the direct interactions of [^{3}H]oestradiol (**✕**), trans-4-[^{3}H]hydroxytamoxifen (**■**) and [^{3}H]tamoxifen (**●**) with cytosol. B. Competition of oestradiol (**●**) 4OHT (**✕**), DMT (**■**) and tamoxifen (O) for the binding of [^{3}H]oestradiol to cytoplasmic ER. From Reddel <u>et al</u> (31).

Antioestrogen Binding Sites

   Following the initial documentation in a number of oestrogen target
tissues of a high affinity intracellular binding site with narrow
specificity for antioestrogens of the triphenylethylene series (37,43)
there have been several reports confirming the presence of this site in
MCF 7 cells and describing some of its properties (9,17,23,24,26-28,
48). Initial studies described the presence of the specific antioestrogen binding site (AEBS) in the cytosol of these cells (24,43) but

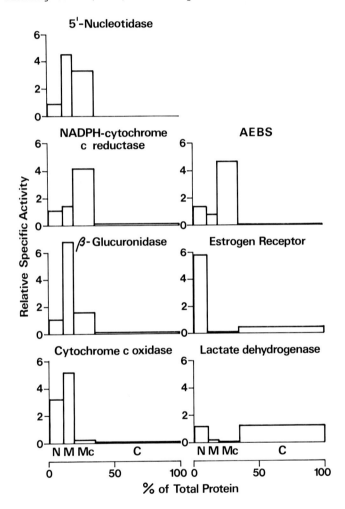

FIG.2. Subcellular localization of AEBS in MCF 7 cells. MCF 7 cell
homogenates were separated into nuclear (N), mitochondrial (M),
microsomal (Mc) and cytosol (C) fractions by differential
centrifugation. The distribution of marker enzymes for plasma membranes
(5'nucleotidase), endoplasmic reticulum (NADPH cytochrome c reductase),
lysosomes (β-glucuronidase), mitochondria (cytochrome c oxidase) and
cytosol (lactate dehydrogenase) and the distribution of AEBS and ER in
each fraction are shown. From Watts et al. (48).

the inability of some research groups to repeat this observation (4,7) prompted a more rigorous subcellular localization study which revealed that AEBS was located predominantly in the microsomal fraction. Fig.2 shows the distribution of AEBS, ER and the enzyme markers for mitochondria (cytochrome c oxidase), lysosomes (β-glucuronidase), plasma membranes (5' nucleotidase), endoplasmic reticulum (NADPH cytochrome c reductase) and cytosol (lactate dehydrogenase) between the cytosol, mitochrondrial, microsomal and nuclear fractions of MCF 7 cells prepared by differential centrifugation.

The AEBS was concentrated in the microsomal fraction and throughout the fractions tended to parallel the distribution of the endoplasmic reticulum marker enzyme. Purified nuclei showed an 80% reduction in specific binding activity of tamoxifen cf. the crude preparation (results not shown), and this suggested that the majority of AEBS found in the crude nuclear fraction was due to the presence of unbroken cells (as evidenced by a significant proportion of the lactate dehydrogenase activity in the nuclear fraction) and/or contaminating organelles. The distribution of ER was very different from that of the AEBS and its predominant nuclear location would be predicted for cells grown in foetal calf serum containing oestrogen.

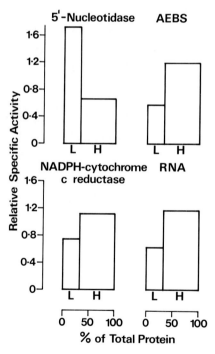

FIG.3. Subfractionation of the MCF 7 microsomal fraction. Microsomes were separated on a discontinuous sucrose gradient containing CsCl into heavy (H) and light (L) fractions. The distribution of marker enzymes for plasma membranes (5'nucleotidase) and endoplasmic reticulum (NADPH cytochrome c reductase) and the distribution of AEBS and RNA are shown. From Watts et al. (48).

   Since the microsomal fraction contained a large proportion of the
5'nucleotidase and the majority of the NADPH cytochrome c reductase
activity, this fraction was separated into light and heavy fractions in
an attempt to further separate these activities. The results of this
subfractionation are presented in Fig.3 where it is seen that the
5'nucleotidase activity was concentrated in the light fraction and
NADPH cytochrome c reductase activity in the heavy fraction. AEBS
concentration again paralleled distribution of the endoplasmic
reticulum marker. In replicates of this experiment the AEBS
concentration always followed the distribution of RNA more closely than
that of NADPH cytochrome c reductase activity. While this is suggestive
of an association of the AEBS with rough endoplasmic reticulum, further
studies are needed to clarify this observation.
   Because the [^{3}H]tamoxifen binding properties of pelleted and
resuspended microsomes were not demonstrably different from those of
the postmitochondrial fraction (microsomal fraction plus cytosol), the
latter preparation was used, for convenience, in subsequent studies.
Data from saturation analysis studies on the interactions between
[^{3}H]tamoxifen and binding sites in the microsomal fraction are shown in
Fig.4A. At concentrations below 3 nM the relationship between B and U
was curvilinear, indicating the presence of saturable, high affinity
sites for tamoxifen. When the data were analysed according to the
Scatchard transformation and correction made for non-specific binding

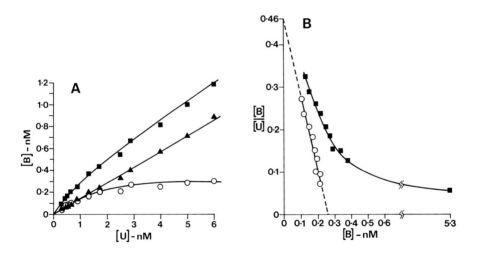

FIG.4. Saturation analysis of the binding of tamoxifen by MCF 7 cell
microsomes. Incubation was for 16 hr at 4°C with increasing
concentrations of [^{3}H]tamoxifen in the absence (total binding) or
presence (non-specific binding) of 1 μM unlabelled tamoxifen.
Charcoal/dextran adsorption (30 min at 4°C) was used to separate bound
(B) and unbound (U) ligand. (A). [B] is plotted against [U]. Specific
binding (O) was determined as the difference between total binding
(■) and non-specific binding (▲). (B). Scatchard plot of the
interaction between [^{3}H]tamoxifen and the AEBS. Data are plotted before
(■) and after (O) correction for non-specific binding. From Watts
et al. (48).

components the relationship between B/U and B was linear, demonstrating the presence of a single class of non-interacting, high affinity saturable binding sites (K_D = 0.97 ± 0.15 nM, C = 4.5 ± 0.7 pmol/mg microsomal protein = 140,000 ± 20,000 microsomal sites/cell).

A number of other properties of the AEBS from MCF 7 cells have been investigated in detail and are presented elsewhere (48). Some of the more interesting properties of this binding site are the temperature independence of the K_D for tamoxifen, its resistance to heat inactivation, the sensitivity of binding to lipase and phospholipase digestion as well as protease treatment (an observation which is compatible with localization in endoplasmic reticulum and a requirement for lipid in maintaining binding integrity), a narrow pH optimum for binding around pH 7.5 and narrow ligand specificity for basic ether derivatives of triphenylethylene. In general the binding data with MCF 7 microsomal AEBS agree well with results obtained with AEBS from other tissues (9-12,17,18,23,36,49).

Together these data confirm the existence of a distinct AEBS which can be distinguished from the classical ER by a number of criteria including: affinity for tamoxifen, cellular concentration, tissue distribution, subcellular localization, kinetics of interaction, pH optimum of binding, resistance to denaturation by elevated temperature, susceptibility to enzyme degradation and ligand specificity.

It is the latter property which we have investigated most thoroughly since detailed studies of the structural requirements for binding have revealed interesting ligands that have facilitated further studies on the function of AEBS in the control of cell proliferation. The results are presented in detail elsewhere (48) and are summarized briefly here.

The majority of the changes in substituents on the triphenylethylene portion of the molecule at positions R_1, R_2 and R_3 (see Table 1) resulted in only minor effects on affinity. However, hydroxylation at R_1 resulted in a 20 - 45% decrease in affinity, presumably because of the disruptive effects of hydrogen-bonding at this position. Substitution of an ethyl group at position R_2 (tamoxifen series) with -Cl (clomiphene series) resulted in a large increase in binding affinity while a $-NO_2$ substitution (CI 628 series) was without effect (48).

A basic side chain at R_4 was necessary for binding to the AEBS. Absence of the side chain e.g. metabolite E, or replacement with a non-basic side chain e.g. ICI 145680, resulted in complete loss of affinity. An increase in chain length from 2 to 3 methylene units (enclomiphene vs 6866) resulted in a decrease in affinity (Table 1). Increasing the size of the substituents on the N atom resulted in a decrease in affinity, but for compounds hydroxylated at R_1 a slight increase in affinity was seen (48). The orientation of the side chain with respect to the triphenylethylene moiety also influenced affinity. Geometric isomers of these compounds had either similar (tamoxifen vs ICI 47649) or reduced affinity (enclomiphene vs zuclomiphene), while replacement of the ether O atom with a N atom diminished affinity by 90% (enclomiphene vs 10222, Table 1). Compounds which had side chains containing tertiary amine groups e.g. (tamoxifen, enclomiphene and CI 628) displayed the highest affinity. Affinity was reduced by greater than 75% if the side chain contained a secondary amine group e.g. DMT, 9599 (Table 1).

TABLE 1. Relative binding affinities (RBA) of some tamoxifen and clomiphene derivatives for ER and AEBS of MCF 7 cells

Compound	R_1	R_2	R_4	RBA AEBS	RBA ER
Tamoxifen	H	C_2H_5	$OCH_2CH_2N(CH_3)_2$	100	1.3 ± 0.3
4 hydroxy-tamoxifen	OH	C_2H_5	$OCH_2CH_2N(CH_3)_2$	80 ± 4	41 ± 3
N-Desmethyl-tamoxifen	H	C_2H_5	$OCH_2CH_2NHCH_3$	19 ± 2	2 ± 1
ICI 145680	H	C_2H_5	$OCH_2CHOHCHOH$ (with CH_3)	0	1.4 ± 0.3
Metabolite E	H	C_2H_5	OH	0	0.8 ± 0.1
Clomiphene	H	Cl	$OCH_2CH_2N(C_2H_5)_2$	142 ± 5	2
6866	H	Cl	$OCH_2CH_2CH_2N(C_2H_5)_2$	44 ± 5	6
9599	H	Cl	$OCH_2CH_2NHC_2H_5$	37 ± 2	0.7
10222	H	Cl	$NHCH_2CH_2N(C_2H_5)_2$	15 ± 1	5

R_3 = H in all cases. Oestradiol has a RBA for ER of 100.

The triphenylethylene moiety also appeared necessary for maximal binding. Thus other di- and tri-cyclic compounds bearing amino alkylether side chains were either unable to bind to the AEBS (e.g. local anaesthetics) or displayed markedly weaker binding affinity than tamoxifen e.g. triphenylethanol derivatives, bibenzyl and stilbene derivatives, the new benzothiophene antioestrogen LY 117018 and analogues of the cytochrome P-450 inhibitor SKF-525A (48).

EFFECT ON MCF 7 CELL PROLIFERATION KINETICS

The effects of tamoxifen on the growth of MCF 7 cells in exponential growth phase are shown in Fig.5A. Tamoxifen treatment resulted in a dose-dependent decrease in cell proliferation rate with doses as low as

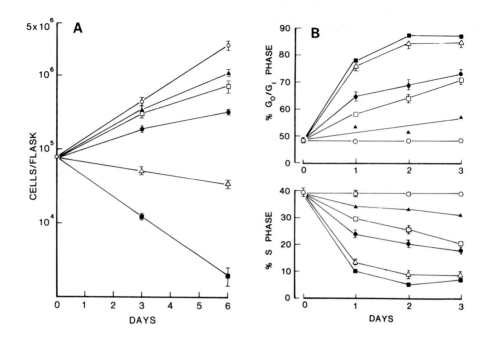

FIG.5. Effect of tamoxifen on (A) the growth and (B) the cell cycle kinetic parameters of MCF 7 cells in exponential growth phase. 5×10^4 cells were plated into 25 cm^2 flasks in 5 ml of medium containing 5% FCS and 24 hr later tamoxifen was added at concentrations of 0 (O), 100 nM (▲), 1 (□), 5 (●), 10 (△) or 12.5 μM (■). Replicate flasks were harvested at the times indicated, viable cell counts were made, and the % G_0/G_1 and % S phase cells calculated from DNA histograms obtained by flow cytometry. From Sutherland <u>et al</u>. (42).

100 nM producing a significant reduction in cell number, c.f. control after 6 days of treatment. At doses of 10 μM and above, cell numbers declined from inocula levels, indicating that at these doses, tamoxifen was probably cytotoxic (Fig.5A). Cell cycle kinetic parameters measured in similar experiments showed that the decreased growth rate was accompanied by a dose-dependent decrease in the proportion of S-phase cells with a concomitant increase in the percentage of G_0/G_1 phase cells (Fig.5B).

To further investigate the cytotoxic effects of tamoxifen, cells were exposed to different doses of tamoxifen for 24 hr, and the surviving fraction was determined. Exposure of exponentially growing cells to doses > 10 μM resulted in a dose-dependent decrease in the surviving fraction with < 20% of cells surviving 24 hr of exposure to 15 μM tamoxifen. At doses of 10 μM and above, the colony size was also reduced significantly by drug treatment, suggesting that 24 hr exposure to high doses of tamoxifen also decreased the subsequent rate of proliferation of surviving cells (42).

In the presence of a 10-fold lower concentration of oestradiol, doses of tamoxifen < 5 μM were without effect on the growth of MCF 7 cells. However, at higher concentrations of tamoxifen, oestradiol could only partially reverse the growth inhibitory effects of tamoxifen and when tamoxifen reached cytotoxic doses the two drugs acted synergistically (Fig.6, 31,41).

When the changes in cell cycle kinetic parameters were measured, it was apparent that, at doses of tamoxifen < 5 µM, simultaneous treatment with oestradiol resulted in cell cycle kinetic parameters that were indistinguishable from those of control. By contrast, the decrease in the percentage of S-phase cells following treatment with higher concentrations was only partially reversed after simultaneous administration of tamoxifen and oestradiol (Fig.6, 30-32,41,42,45). It is therefore concluded that tamoxifen has both oestrogen-reversible and oestrogen-irreversible components to its effects on cell growth and cell cycle kinetic parameters of MCF 7 cells <u>in vitro</u>.

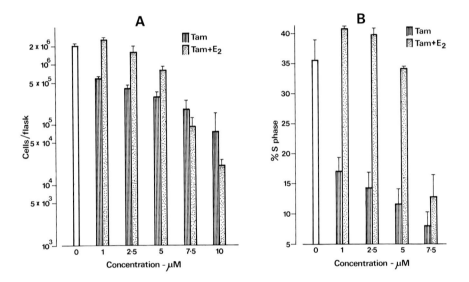

FIG.6. Effect of oestradiol on tamoxifen-induced changes in (A) cell number and (B) % S phase cells. Exponentially growing MCF 7 cells were grown in the presence of tamoxifen, with or without a 10-fold lower concentration of oestradiol. Replicate flasks were harvested after 114 hr of treatment, viable cell counts were made, and the % S phase cells calculated from DNA histograms obtained by flow cytometry. Redrawn from Reddel and Sutherland (30).

In order to test whether cells were irreversibly blocked in G_0/G_1 following tamoxifen treatment or accumulated there due to a tamoxifen-induced increase in the G_1 transit time relative to other phases of the cell cycle, the rate of exit of cells from G_0/G_1 phase was monitored. This was done using the drug ICRF 159 an inhibitor of cytokinesis (13). Therefore, ICRF 159 prevents nuclei from dividing and re-entering the G_0/G_1 peak of the DNA histogram obtained by flow cytometry, enabling measurement of the proportion of cells in G_0/G_1 without contribution from cells re-entering this phase from $G_2 + M$ (46).

A detailed time course of changes in the percentage of G_0/G_1 phase cells following treatment of exponentially growing MCF 7 cells with

ICRF 159 demonstrated that, after a short lag period of about 2 hr, cells began to leave G_0/G_1, with a single exponential rate of decay which was maintained for about 8 hr. By 12 hr, cells were leaving G_0/G_1 again at a rate approximating a single exponential decay, but the $t\frac{1}{2}$ was significantly increased to about 28 hr. These data are interpreted as indicating the presence of 2 populations of MCF 7 cells with markedly different G_1 transit times. We refer to these 2 populations as "rapidly cycling" cells and "slowly cycling" cells. When the rate of efflux of the "rapidly cycling" component was corrected for influence from the "slowly cycling" component, the true half-time of efflux of the "rapidly cycling" cells was shown to be 2.3 hr (42).

The effect of pretreatment with tamoxifen on the rate of efflux of cells from G_0/G_1 phase is presented in Fig.7A. It is apparent from these data that tamoxifen causes a dose-dependent decrease in the proportion of MCF 7 cells leaving G_0/G_1 phase. A significant decrease was apparent at 100 nM, and at 10 µM, tamoxifen had almost completely arrested cell cycle progression. When the $t\frac{1}{2}$ and the size of the "slowly cycling" pool were calculated, it became obvious that tamoxifen decreased the rate of disappearance of cells from this pool and increased the proportion of "slowly cycling" cells (Table 2).

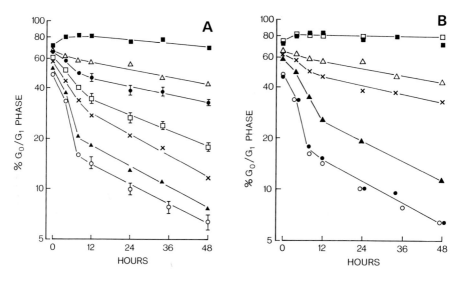

FIG.7. Effect of administration of tamoxifen with or without oestradiol on the rate of efflux of MCF 7 cells from the G_0/G_1 phase of the cell cycle. 2×10^5 cells in exponential growth phase were plated into 25 cm^2 flasks in 5 ml of medium containing 5% FCS and tamoxifen with or without a 10-fold lower concentration of oestradiol. After 42 hr exposure to drug, ICRF 159 was added to a final concentration of 100 µg/ml. Replicate flasks were harvested at the times indicated and the proportion of the cell population remaining in G_0/G_1 phase was calculated from DNA histograms obtained by flow cytometry. (A) control (O), 100 (▲), 500 nM (✖), 1 (□), 5 (●), 7.5 (△) and 10 µM (■) tamoxifen. (B) control (O), 5 µM tamoxifen (✖), 5 µM tamoxifen + 500 nM oestradiol (●), 7.5 µM tamoxifen (△), 7.5 µM tamoxifen + 750 nM oestradiol (▲), 10 µM tamoxifen (■), 10 µM tamoxifen + 1 µM oestradiol (□). From Sutherland et al. (42).

The effect of oestradiol on these parameters was also investigated. Oestradiol alone (100 nM and 1 µM) had no significant effect on the rate of disappearance of MCF 7 cells from the G_0/G_1 phase. When a 10-fold lower concentration of oestradiol was administered together with 5 µM tamoxifen, the rate of disappearance was similar to control (Fig.7B). In contrast, 1 µM oestradiol had no effect on the arrest of cells by 10 µM tamoxifen. Pretreatment of cells with 750 nM oestradiol and 7.5 µM tamoxifen resulted in partial reversal of the effects induced by this dose of tamoxifen alone (Fig.7B).

TABLE 2. Effect of tamoxifen on the proportion of "slowly cycling" cells and their half-time of disappearance from G_0/G_1 phase

Tamoxifen Concentration	n	% "Slowly-cycling" cells	$t^{\frac{1}{2}}$ (hr)	r^2
0	30	18.4	28.9	0.704
100 nM	9	23.8	28.6	0.818
500 nM	8	39.0	26.2	0.937
1 µM	14	41.9	39.0	0.928
5 µM	13	50.5	75.0	0.718
7.5 µM	5	68.0	66.0	0.820
10 µM	4	85.2	171	0.743

n, the number of observations used to calculate the regression equation; r^2, the coefficient of determination. From Sutherland et al. (42).

To further investigate the effects of tamoxifen on cell cycle progression, studies were undertaken with MCF 7 cells that had been synchronized by mitotic selection. One hr after mitotic selection 90 to 95% of the cells were in G_0/G_1 phase as all mitotic cells had divided after harvesting. No significant change in this distribution was seen with time of culture until 7 hr, when cells began to leave G_0/G_1 and progress into S phase (Fig.8A). The G_0/G_1 to S-phase transition occurred over the following 3 hr when the proportion of G_0/G_1 cells fell to 15% and S phase increased to about 80%. By 16 to 20 hr after harvesting, the majority of cells had traversed S phase and, during the following 4 to 6 hr, undergone mitosis, once again returning to G_0/G_1. Estimates of cell cycle time and mean phase durations for G_0/G_1, S and G_2 + M were calculated from the data shown in Fig.8A for untreated cells as 21.3, 9, 9.3, and 3 hr, respectively. In addition, the presence of a more slowly cycling or noncycling subpopulation of MCF 7 cells representing approximately 15% of the cell population could be observed in G_0/G_1 between 10 and 18 hr after mitotic selection (Fig.8A). This result is in close agreement with the size of the "slowly cycling" pool in control asynchronous populations (Table 2).

Tamoxifen treatment of synchronized cells resulted in an increased proportion of cells remaining in G_0/G_1 and a corresponding reduction in the numbers entering S phase. This can be observed clearly when the DNA distributions of cultures treated for 12 and 16 hr with tamoxifen are compared with control (Fig.6B). These data also demonstrate that those cells that entered S phase in tamoxifen treated cultures were able to traverse S phase at a similar rate to untreated cells as judged by the superimposition of the leading edges of the DNA histograms. This observation was supported by the detailed study of the effects of 7.5 μM tamoxifen which showed that, apart from a slight delay at the 8 and 10 hr points, those cells capable of leaving the G_0/G_1 phase progressed through the cell cycle at a rate similar to that for controls. It should be pointed out, however, that the plateauing of G_0/G_1 cells after 24 hr exposure to tamoxifen was found to be unchanged[1] (G_0/G_1 = 84%) when cultures were subsequently analyzed at 46 hr. This suggests that the effects of tamoxifen are cumulative with increasing exposure. Together these data indicate that the major effect of the drug is to reduce the proportion of cells that can exit the G_0/G_1 phase of the cell cycle but with much less effect on the progression of cells through subsequent phases of the cell cycle.

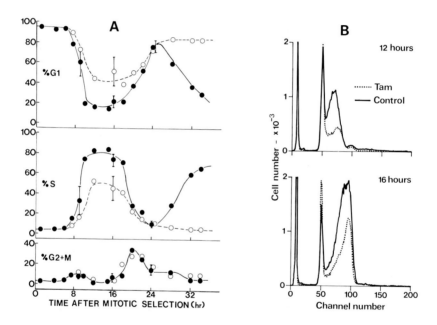

FIG.8. Changes in the cell cycle distribution of MCF 7 cells with time after mitotic selection. (A) time course for non-treated controls (●) and cultures continuously exposed to 7.5 μM tamoxifen (O). (B) DNA histograms of control cultures and cells treated with 5 μM tamoxifen for 12 and 16 hr following mitotic selection. The DNA peak in channel 50 corresponds to G_0/G_1 phase MCF 7 cells. From Taylor et al. (47) and Sutherland et al. (45).

Further experiments in which 2 hr pulses of tamoxifen were administered to synchronous cells during their progression through the cell cycle demonstrated that the major sensitivity to tamoxifen in terms of both inhibition of cell cycle progression and drug cytotoxicity was restricted to a short interval in the middle of G_1 phase. This 2 to 4 hr period of maximum drug sensitivity began approximately 4 hr after mitotic selection, with drug exposures outside this time frame having markedly less effects (Fig.9).

RELATIONSHIP BETWEEN AFFINITY FOR ER AND AEBS AND GROWTH INHIBITION

Since the predominant effect of tamoxifen was to inhibit the progression of cells through G_1 phase by increasing the proportion of cells with prolonged G_1 transit times i.e. "slowly cycling" cells (Fig.7, Table 2) it seemed likely that the proliferation rate of MCF 7

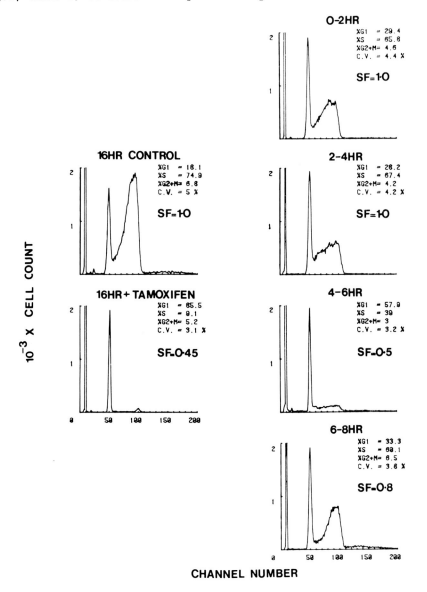

CHANNEL NUMBER

FIG.9. Changes in the cell cycle distribution of MCF 7 cells 16 hr after mitotic selection in the presence or absence of tamoxifen. Cells were exposed to 12.5 μM tamoxifen either continuously or as a 2 hr pulse during the times indicated. The first peak in each histogram corresponds to chicken erythrocytes which act as an internal standard. The DNA peak in channel 50 corresponds to G_0/G_1 MCF 7 cells. C.V. = coefficient of variation of the G_0/G_1 peak and S.F. = surviving fraction obtained from a clonogenic assay. From Taylor et al. (47).

cells in the presence of antioestrogen would be governed by the
proportion of cells that escaped this effect and progressed through the
cell cycle at the normal rate. Thus the proliferation rate would be
expected to correlate with % S phase cells since the duration of S
phase was almost unchanged by drug treatment (Fig.8). In addition one
would predict that in the dose range where the effects of antioestrogen
were reversed by oestradiol, and were thus likely to be mediated via
ER, the potency of a particular analogue in decreasing the proportion
of S phase cells would be related to its affinity for ER. Two
experiments were conducted to test these hypotheses.

In the first experiment exponentially growing cells were treated
with 0.1 - 5 μM tamoxifen and its two metabolites, in the presence or
absence of a 10-fold lower concentration of oestradiol. After 6 days of
treatment the proliferation rate was seen to be highly correlated with
the proportion of S phase cells (Fig.10A) confirming the initial
hypothesis. Furthermore, this and similar experiments (31) demonstrated
that 40HT, the metabolite with enhanced affinity for ER (Fig.1), was at
least 100-fold more potent than tamoxifen and DMT in inhibiting MCF 7
cell growth. In a further experiment, employing a fixed concentration
of six antioestrogens with markedly different affinities for ER, it was
observed that the ability of an antioestrogen to decrease the % S phase
cells was correlated with its affinity for ER (Fig.10B). Together these
data support the concept that oestrogens and antioestrogens compete for

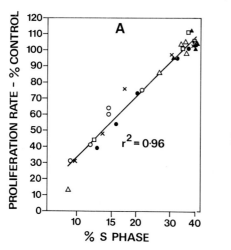
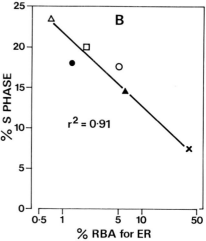

FIG.10. Relationship between (A) MCF 7 cell proliferation rate and the
proportion of cells in S phase of the cell cycle and (B) the relative
binding affinity for ER and percentage of cells in S phase following
treatment with different antioestrogens. Exponentially growing cells
were exposed to antioestrogens in the presence or absence of a 10-fold
lower dose of oestradiol for 6 days. Cell counts were made and the % S
phase cells calculated from DNA histograms obtained by flow cytometry.
(A) 0.01 - 5 μM tamoxifen (●), plus oestradiol (▲); DMT (✗), plus
oestradiol (□); 40HT (○), plus oestradiol (△). (B) 1 μM tamoxifen
(●), clomiphene (□), 6866 (▲), 9599 (△), 10222 (○), or LY
117018 (✗). From Reddel et al. (31).

a common event which regulates the rate of cell proliferation by
controlling the proportion of cells entering S phase and that ER is
intimately involved in this regulatory process since the potency of a
ligand in controlling this event is related to its affinity for ER.

In an attempt to understand the role of AEBS in the control of MCF 7
cell proliferation, studies were performed with tamoxifen analogues
having no detectable affinity for this high affinity binding site. The
analogue studied in most detail was ICI 145680, a triphenylethylene
antioestrogen with a nonbasic side chain and an affinity for ER not
significantly different from that of tamoxifen (Table 1). ICI 145680
was an inhibitor of MCF 7 cell proliferation but was less
potent than tamoxifen over the entire concentration range tested i.e.
0.5 - 20 µM (Fig.11A). The differences between ICI 145680 and tamoxifen
were small but significantly different (p < 0.01) between 0.5 - 2.5 µM
and became greater at concentrations above 5 µM (Fig.11B) where the
oestrogen-irreversible effects of tamoxifen were manifested (Fig.6). At
concentrations of 10 µM and greater, cytotoxicity contributed
significantly to the reduction in cell numbers seen in tamoxifen
treated cultures (42). Although ICI 145680 was able to almost
completely arrest growth at doses of 15 and 20 µM, these doses did not
induce the precipitous decline in cell numbers observed with the same
doses of tamoxifen (41,42). We have tentatively interpreted this result
to indicate that ICI 145680 is a much weaker cytotoxic agent than
tamoxifen.

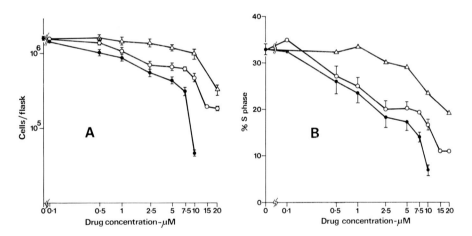

FIG.11. Effect of tamoxifen (●), ICI 145680 (○) and metabolite E
(△) on (A) MCF 7 cell growth and (B) percentage of cells in S phase
of the cell cycle. Exponentially growing cells were innoculated at 5 x
10^4 cells/flask, allowed to reach 10^5 cells/flask then treated with 0.1
- 20 µM drug for 4 days. Cells were harvested, counted and the % S
phase calculated. From Murphy and Sutherland (27).

Growth inhibition induced by ICI 145680 was accompanied by a
decrease in % S phase cells similar to that seen with tamoxifen
(Fig.11B). At doses of 0.5 - 5 µM there was no significant difference
between the effects of the two compounds on % S phase cells. However,
at higher doses tamoxifen was significantly more potent in this regard
(Fig.11B).

Metabolite E, a weakly oestrogenic triphenylethylene derivative with negligible affinity for AEBS, had about half the affinity of tamoxifen and ICI 145680 for ER (Table 1) and was a very weak inhibitor of MCF 7 cell growth (Fig.11A). Cell numbers were slightly reduced at a dose of 10 μM while 20 μM Metabolite E induced a marked reduction in cell growth. These changes were accompanied by a decrease in % S phase cells (Fig.11B).

These data (Fig.11, ref.27) indicate that a triphenylethylene anti-oestrogenic compound with high affinity for the AEBS was a more potent inhibitor of MCF 7 cell growth in vitro than a compound with no affinity for this site but identical affinity for ER. The differences between the two types of compounds became more apparent in the oestrogen-irreversible dose range indicating that the enhanced activity of the compound with high affinity for AEBS was probably mediated by pathways independent of ER. Furthermore ICI 145680 had no cytotoxic activity, as defined by a decrease in cell numbers below innoculation levels, at concentrations where compounds with high affinity for AEBS were extremely cytotoxic (26,31,41,42).

DISCUSSION

The data summarized herein review some of the recent research findings from this laboratory that have enabled development of rational working hypotheses on the mechanisms by which nonsteroidal anti-oestrogens control the growth of human breast cancer cells in vitro.

Our studies have confirmed the presence of a classical ER system in MCF 7 cells and have documented the properties of another high affinity binding site for nonsteroidal antioestrogens in the microsomal fraction of these cells (26-28,48). In addition, detailed studies on structure - affinity relationships for the interaction of antioestrogens with ER and AEBS have identified a number of ligands which have proved to be valuable research tools for probing the role of these binding sites in the control of breast cancer cell proliferation (26-28,31,48).

Three distinct effects of tamoxifen on MCF 7 cell proliferation kinetics have been identified. 1. an oestrogen-reversible inhibition of cell proliferation which is associated with an accumulation of cells in the G_0/G_1 phase of the cell cycle, 2. an oestrogen-irreversible growth inhibitory effect associated with similar cell cycle kinetic changes and 3. a cytotoxic effect (Figs 5,6,7,11, refs 26-28,30,31,41,42).

The first effect may well be the most important from both a physiological and pharmacological point of view since it is likely to be mediated via ER and occurs in the lower dose range which probably approximates the plasma concentrations found in patients on chronic tamoxifen therapy (5). However, the many factors affecting tamoxifen sensitivity in vitro (32) make it difficult to extrapolate to the situation in vivo. In the oestrogen-reversible dose range the decrease in cell numbers following tamoxifen treatment can be attributed almost entirely to a decrease in cell proliferation rate since clonogenic survival assays failed to demonstrate significant cell death at these concentrations (42). Thus the overall effect of the drug was to decrease proliferation rate by increasing the mean cell cycle transit time and this was due to a tamoxifen-induced shift of cells from a "rapidly cycling" pool, with a t½ of efflux from G_1 of 2.3 hr, to a "slowly cycling" pool with a $t\frac{1}{2}$ of efflux from G_1 of > 25 hr (Fig.7, Table 2). Since the length of S phase appeared to be relatively unaffected by tamoxifen treatment (Fig.8) the shift of cells from a pool with a rapid G_1 transit time to one with a 10-fold slower transit time provides the kinetic basis for the accumulation of cells in G_0/G_1 phase following tamoxifen treatment. Further experiments employing synchronized cells and pulses of tamoxifen (Fig.9 and unpublished data) revealed that the effects of tamoxifen on the progession of MCF 7 cells through the cell cycle were confined to a narrow period 2 - 6 hr into the G_1 phase.

As might be expected the oestrogen-reversible effects of tamoxifen and the characteristic cell cycle kinetic changes were confined to ER-positive cell lines (33). This observation in association with the data on potency and affinity for ER (Fig.10), the ability of the response to be "rescued" by subsequent treatment with oestradiol (45) and previously published data on the cell cycle effects of oestrogens (44) provide strong evidence that this effect is controlled by ER mediated pathways within the cell.

The oestrogen-irreversible inhibition of cell proliferation accompanied by a decrease in S phase is very similar to that seen in the oestrogen-reversible dose range and probably shares pathways with that effect. It occurs in a dose-range where significant cytotoxicity is undetectable by clonogenic assay and is accompanied by further accumulation of cells in the G_0/G_1 phase of the cell cycle (42). Furthermore, these cell cycle changes appear to be explained by an oestrogen-irreversible shift of cells from the "rapidly cycling" to "slowly cycling" pool similar to that seen in the oestrogen-reversible dose range (Fig.7B). Interestingly the phenomenon is only apparent in ER-positive cell lines i.e. it has been clearly defined in MCF 7 (30,31,41,42) and T 47D (32,33) cells but was absent in 9 ER-negative cell lines studied under identical conditions (33).

Whilst it is tempting to dismiss this effect as being identical to the first, with the inability to reverse the response with oestrogen resulting from differential rates of metabolism of tamoxifen and oestradiol or some other uncontrolled factor in the experimental design, a number of observations argue against this. For example, varying the oestrogen:tamoxifen concentration ratio over a 1,000-fold range did not change the conclusion (31,32,41) while the potency of a series of analogues in inducing this type of response was unrelated to their affinity for ER (26,27). Compounds with enhanced affinity for AEBS were generally more potent in this dose range (26,27).

The cytotoxic effect occurred at doses of tamoxifen > 7.5 µM and was not reversed by the simultaneous addition of oestradiol. In fact under some circumstances the two drugs had a synergistic effect on cell death (41). At 12.5 µM tamoxifen this cytotoxic effect was confined to a 2 hr period 4 - 6 hr into G_1 phase and was accompanied by accumulation of cells in G_0/G_1 phase (Fig.9, ref.47). A 20 µM dose however, caused only minor perturbations in cell cycle kinetic parameters (41), indicating cell killing throughout the cell cycle. Perhaps the differences between these two results can be explained by a cell cycle phase specific cytotoxic event at lower doses and a truly phase nonspecific cytotoxicity at higher doses. Certainly the cytotoxic event is not a nonspecific response since many steroids and triphenylethylene derivatives lacking a basic aminoether side chain cannot induce this response in the same dose range i.e. 7.5 - 20 µM.

Although we have been able to identify at least three distinct effects of tamoxifen on MCF 7 cells the possibility still exists that they are all mediated through a common mechanism. Indeed the localization of the three effects to a precise locus within G_1 favours such an interpretation. If this were the case one could propose a model whereby a critical factor, pathway or metabolite controlled the rate of progression through G_1 by determining whether cells entered the "rapidly cycling" or "slowly cycling" pool and this event was controlled by antioestrogens through at least two pathways one of which involved ER. The likelihood that interactions with AEBS are also involved in the control of this event is supported to some extent by the data presented in Fig.11 and elsewhere (26,27) but the inability of ER-negative cells containing AEBS to respond to tamoxifen with the same kinetic changes (33) argues against this binding site having a primary role in the control of cell cycle progression. More detailed studies are required to define the antioestrogen-regulated biochemical events controlling cell cycle progression and the functional role of AEBS. Such studies are currently being pursued in this laboratory.

ACKNOWLEDGEMENTS

The authors wish to thank I.C.I. Ltd, Pharmaceuticals Division, Merrell National Laboratories and Lilly Industries Pty Ltd for supply of the drugs, Narelle Hobbis and Pamela Hodson for their excellent technical assistance, Judy Hood for preparation of the manuscript and Professor M.H.N. Tattersall for his continuing interest and critical comments.

REFERENCES

1. Aitken, S.C. and Lippman, M.E. (1982): Cancer Res., 42:1727-1735.
2. Allegra, J.C. and Lippman, M.E. (1978): Cancer Res., 38:3823-3829.
3. Brooks, S.C., Locke, E.R., and Soule, H.D. (1973): J. Biol. Chem., 248:6251-6253.
4. Coezy, E., Borgna, J.-L., and Rochefort, H. (1982): Cancer Res., 42:317-323.
5. Daniel, C.P., Gaskell, S.J., Bishop, H., Campbell, C., and Nicholson, R.J. (1981): Eur. J. Cancer, 17:1183-1189.
6. Eckert, R.L., and Katzenellenbogen, B.S. (1982): Cancer Res., 42:139-144.
7. Eckert, R.L. and Katzenellenbogen, B.S. (1982): J. Biol. Chem., 257:8840-8846.
8. Edwards, D.P., Murthy, S.R., and McGuire, W.L. (1980): Cancer Res., 40:1722-1726.
9. Faye, J.-C., Jozan, S., Redeuilh, G., Baulieu, E.E., and Bayard, F. (1983): Proc. Natl Acad. Sci., 80:3158-3162.
10. Faye, J.C., Lasserre, B., and Bayard, F. (1980): Biochem. Biophys. Res. Commun., 93:1225-1231.
11. Gulino, A. and Pasqualini, J.R. (1980): Cancer Res., 40:3821-3826.

12. Gulino, A. and Pasqualini, J.R. (1982): Cancer Res., 42:1913-1921.
13. Hallowes, R.C., West, D.G., and Hellman, K. (1974): Nature, 247:487-490.
14. Horwitz, K.B., Costlow, M.E., and McGuire, W.L. (1975): Steroids, 26:285-295.
15. Horwitz, K.B., Koseki, Y., and McGuire, W.L. (1978): Endocrinology, 103:1742-1751.
16. Horwitz, K.B. and McGuire, W.L. (1978): J. Biol. Chem., 253:8185-8191.
17. Jozan, S., Elalamy, H., and Bayard, F. (1981): C. R. Acad. Sci. Paris, 292:767-770.
18. Kon, O.L. (1983): J. Biol. Chem., 258:3173-3177.
19. Lippman, M.E. and Bolan, G. (1975): Nature, 256:592-593.
20. Lippman, M.E., Bolan, G., and Huff, J. (1976): Cancer Res., 36:4595-4601.
21. Lippman, M., Bolan, G., Monaco, M., Pinkus, L., and Engel, L. (1976): J. Steroid Biochem., 7:1045-1051.
22. Martin, L. (1981): In: Non-Steroidal Antioestrogens. Molecular Pharmacology and Antitumour Activity, edited by R. L. Sutherland, and V.C. Jordan, pp.143-163. Academic Press, Sydney.
23. Miller, M.A. and Katzenellenbogen, B.S. (1983): Cancer Res., 43: 3094-3100.
24. Murphy, L.C. and Sutherland, R.L. (1981): Biochem. Biophys. Res. Commun., 100:1353-1361.
25. Murphy, L.C. and Sutherland, R.L. (1981): J. Endocr., 91:155-161.
26. Murphy, L.C. and Sutherland, R.L. (1983): J. Clin. Endocr. Metab., 57:373-379.
27. Murphy, L.C. and Sutherland, R.L. (1983): submitted for publication.
28. Murphy, L.C., Watts, C.K.W., and Sutherland, R.L. (1983): In: Rational Basis for Chemotherapy, UCLA Symposia on Molecular and Cellular Biology, Vol.4, edited by B.A. Chabner, pp.195-210. Alan R. Liss, New York.
29. Nawata, H., Bronzert, D., and Lippman, M.E. (1981): J. Biol. Chem., 256:5016-5021.
30. Reddel, R.R. and Sutherland, R.L. (1983): Eur. J. Cancer Clin. Oncol., 19:1179-1181.
31. Reddel, R.R., Murphy, L.C., and Sutherland, R.L. (1983): Cancer Res., 43: in press.
32. Reddel, R.R., Murphy, L.C., and Sutherland, R.L. (1983): submitted for publication .
33. Reddel, R.R., Murphy, L.C., Hall, R.E., and Sutherland, R.L. (1983): submitted for publication.
34. Rochefort, H. and Borgna, J.-L. (1981): Nature, 292:257-259.
35. Soule, H.D., Vazquez, J., Albert, S., and Long, A. (1973): J. Natl Cancer Inst., 51:1409-1413.
36. Sudo, K., Monsma, F.J., and Katzenellenbogen, B.S. (1983): Endocrinology, 112:425-434.
37. Sutherland, R.L. and Foo, M.S. (1979): Biochem. Biophys. Res. Commun., 91:183-191.
38. Sutherland, R.L., and Jordan, V.C., editors (1981): Non-Steroidal Antioestrogens. Molecular Pharmacology and Antitumour Activity. Academic Press, Sydney.

39. Sutherland, R.L. and Murphy, L.C. (1982): Eur. J. Cancer,
        16:1141-1148.
40. Sutherland, R.L. and Murphy, L.C. (1982): Molecular Cellular
        Endocrinology, 25:5-23.
41. Sutherland, R.L., Green, M.D., Hall, R.E., Reddel, R.R., and
        Taylor, I.W. (1983): Eur. J. Cancer Clin. Oncol., 19:615-621.
42. Sutherland, R.L., Hall, R.E., and Taylor, I.W. (1983): Cancer
        Res., 43:3998-4006.
43. Sutherland, R.L., Murphy, L.C., Foo, M.S., Green, M.D., Whybourne,
        A.M., and Krozowski, Z.S. (1980): Nature, 288:273-275.
44. Sutherland, R.L., Reddel, R.R., and Green, M.D. (1983): Eur. J.
        Cancer Clin. Oncol., 19:307-318.
45. Sutherland, R.L., Reddel, R.R., Hall, R.E., Hodson, P.J., and
        Taylor, I.W. (1983): Rational Basis for Chemotherapy, UCLA
        Symposia on Molecular and Cellular Biology, Vol.4., edited by
        B.A. Chabner, pp.195-210. Alan R. Liss, New York.
46. Taylor, I.W. and Bleehen, N.M. (1977): Br. J. Cancer, 35:587-594.
47. Taylor, I.W., Hodson, P.J., Green, M.D., and Sutherland, R.L.
        (1983): Cancer Res., 43:4007-4010.
48. Watts, C.K.W., Murphy, L.C., and Sutherland, R.L. (1983):
        submitted for publication.
49. Winneker, R.C. and Clark, J.H. (1983): Endocrinology,
        112:1910-1915.

Progress in Cancer Research and Therapy,
Vol. 31, edited by F. Bresciani, et al.
Raven Press, New York © 1984.

Cholesterol Biosynthesis in MCF$_7$ Cell Line in Relation to Cell Division: Stimulation by Estradiol and Inhibition by Tamoxifen

C. Tabacik, B. Cypriani, S. Aliau, and A. Crastes de Paulet

INSERM U.58, 34100 Montpellier, France

It is now well established that relationships exist between the processes of cell growth and those of cholesterol biosynthesis ; however, most studies have been focused at the 3-hydroxy-3-methyl glutaryl Co enzyme A (HMG CoA) reductase, the key enzyme of cholesterol biosynthesis (3, 8, 9, 12, 14, 17, 18, 19) : inhibition of HMG CoA reductase is followed by cell growth decrease.

Mevalonic acid, the product of the HMG CoA reductase catalyzed reaction is not committed exclusively to cholesterol biosynthesis, since branching pathways also lead to the synthesis of isopentenyl adenin (6), ubiquinone (5) and dolichol (11). As the commonly used inhibitors are known to interfere with HMG CoA reductase, it is not clear whether the essential metabolite which becomes unavailable and is involved in cell growth is cholesterol or another terpenoid of the branching pathways(16).

- In a previous study with human lymphocytes (21) we observed that the low basal level of cell cholesterol production can be notably increased only when cells are stimulated to divide.

- With cultured fibroblasts (23) we tested a new cholesterol inhibitor,pentadecane-2-one. This compound was shown by Gilbertson (7) to decrease cell growth of Hela cells. We found that pentadecane-2-one when added in culture medium of the cells, inhibits both cholesterol biosynthesis and cell growth (23). We localized the inhibition at late steps of the process : lanosterol demethylation and lathosterol isomerisation into cholesterol (whereas HMG CoA reductase activity was stimulated by pentadecane-2-one). This allowed us to exclude the possible role of branching pathways and to extend the use of pentadecane-2-one in our studies.

The mammary carcinoma cell line MCF$_7$ has been shown by several groups of workers (15,1) to be hormonally regulated. This cell line appears to be a convenient model system for studying the relationships between cholesterol biosynthesis and cell growth, since the mechanism of hormonal effect on this line is already well understood(15,1).

RESULTS

Cholesterol biosynthesis

a) Kinetic study

The cells were cultured in MEM in the presence of 5 % fetal calf serum which was replaced by steroid-free serum in experiences with estrogens and antiestrogens. Cholesterol biosynthesis activity was evaluated by incorporation of labeled acetic acid into cholesterol, after a detailed analysis of non saponifiable lipids, according to (22).

TABLE 1. Composition (%) of non saponifiable lipids after incorporation of ^{14}C-acetic acid for 1-24 h

Incubation Time	1 h	2 h	4 h	6 h	24 h
%					
Sterones + methylsterols esters	2.3	5.3	4.2	5.2	2.8
C-28, C-29, C-30 sterols	14.8	9.4	6.6	9.7	10.2
n-fatty alcohols	25.5	18.5	28.6	19.8	13.1
C-27 sterols	24.0	37.9	41.9	49.0	67.2
(cholesterol)	(4.9)	(15.4)	(17.5)	(35.8)	(65.5)
lanostenol-aldehyde	3.4	28.8	18.6	16.2	6.7
cholesterol/lathosterol	0.6	1	1.3	6.2	40

The cells cultured in MEM + 5 % fetal calf serum were incubated with $[2-^{14}C]$ sodium acetate for 1 to 24 h. After saponification, the non-saponifiable lipids were analyzed as described in materials and methods(22).

Table 1 shows the composition (in %) of non-saponifiable material after several incubation times. It is mainly composed of metabolites resulting from lanosterol demethylation : C-28, C-29, C-30 sterols, sterones and methyl sterol esters (non polar metabolites), C-27 sterols and bifunctional methylsterols such as lanostenol-aldehyde. The main C-27 sterol identified besides cholesterol is lathosterol.

We can see that C-27 sterol concentration increases with incubation time (and especially cholesterol) whereas other metabolites are disappearing. We have observed the presence of considerable amounts of labeled n-fatty alcohols which arose from reduction of n-fatty acids. This results from a high NADPH-dependent oxido-reductase activity, which is often the case with cancer cells (20).

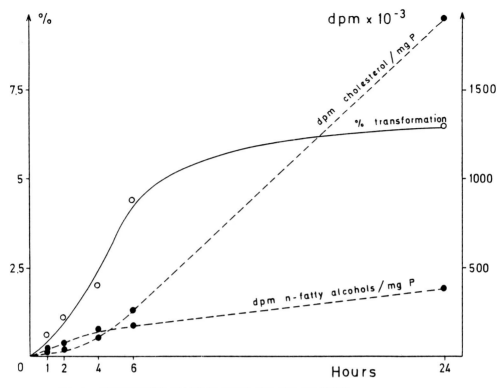

FIG. 1 : <u>TRANSFORMATION OF LABELED ACETIC ACID INTO CHOLESTEROL</u>

The cells growing logarithmically were incubated with $\left[2\text{-}^{14}C\right]$-acetic acid for 1 to 24 h in MEM and the non-saponifiable lipids analyzed after various incubation times.

continuous line : percentage of whole incorporated radioactivity which was transformed into cholesterol.

dotted line : amount of radioactivity (dpm) incorporated into cholesterol and n-fatty acids.

Fig. 1 shows the percentage of incorporated acetic acid which was transformed into cholesterol and the amount of biosynthesized cholesterol and n-fatty alcohols : during the first four hours of incubation, the biosynthesis of n-fatty alcohols was faster than cholesterol biosynthesis, but it soon became slower.

b) <u>Inhibition by pentadecane-2-one</u> : in the two experiments described on table 2 or 3, the cells were cultured for 24 h or 2 h with various concentrations of inhibitor, then pulsed 2 h with labeled acetic acid. The composition of labeled isoprenoid metabolites is given as a %. There is a drastic decrease of C-27 sterols and cholesterol concentrations. Cholesterol inhibition can reach 95 %, but n-fatty alcohol biosynthesis seems to be only slightly modified until the concentration of inhibitor reaches 5.10^{-5} M. At 18.10^{-5}M, cell viability sharply decreased and cholesterol inhibition no longer increased.

TABLE 2. <u>Inhibition of cholesterol biosynthesis by pentadecane-2-one as a function of inhibitor concentration ($0-5.10^{-5}$M)</u>

PENTADECANE-2-ONE	0 (T)	$1.5.10^{-5}$ M	3.10^{-5} M	5.10^{-5} M
%				
Sterones + methylsterols esters	8.9	9.3	11.5	24.8
C-28, C-29, C-30 sterols	23.1	23.1	28.7	36.9
C-27 sterols	67.9	67.6	59.8	38.2
(cholesterol)	(27.7)	(18.8)	(11.6)	(2.4)
dpm x 10^{-3} cholesterol/mgP:	37.2	21.3	15.5	3.9
% inhibition		42.7	58.3	89.5
dpm x 10^{-3} n - fatty alcohols/mgP	56.3	49.3	38.9	56.5

The cells were cultured for 24h with various concentrations of inhibitor and pulsed for 2h with ^{14}C-sodium acetate. The non saponifiable lipids were extracted and analyzed as described in materials and methods **(22)**. The composition of labeled isoprenoid metabolites is given in %.

TABLE 3. <u>Inhibition of cholesterol biosynthesis by pentadecane-2-one as a function of inhibitor concentration ($4.5-18.10^{-5}$M)</u>

PENTADECANE-2-ONE	0 (T)	$4.5.10^{-5}$M	9.10^{-5} M	18.10^{-5} M
%				
Sterones + methylsterols esters	7.3	56.4	82.9	86.9
C-28, C-29, C-30 sterols	10.6	7.6	6.4	3.4
C-27 sterols	82.1	36.0	10.7	9.7
Cholesterol	27.2	6.6.	2.4	2.6
% inhibition of cholesterol		80	9 4	95
dpm x10^{-3}n-fatty alcohols/mgP	178.0	88.0	65.0	60.0
C-27 sterols/methylsterol	4.5	0.6	0.1	0.1
cholesterol/lathosterol	1.7	0.4	0.45	0.6

The cells were cultured for 2 h with various concentrations of inhibitor and pulsed for 2 H with $[2 - ^{14}C]$-sodium acetate. The non saponifiable lipids were analyzed. The composition of labeled isoprenoid metabolites is given in %.

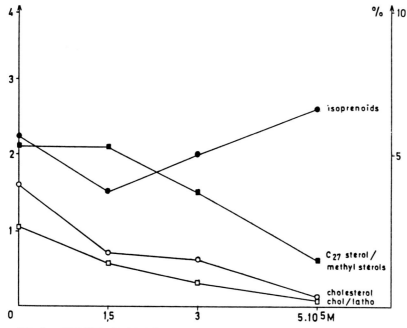

FIG. 2 : INHIBITION OF CHOLESTEROL BIOSYNTHESIS BY PENTADECANE-2-ONE AS A
FUNCTION OF CONCENTRATION

        The cells growing logarithmically were cultured for 22 h in the
presence of pentadecane-2-one (+ 5 % DCC) and the non-saponifiable lipids
analyzed, after a two hours pulse of $[2-^{14}C]$-acetic acid.
  —0—0— : percentage of whole incorporated radioactivity which was transformed
              into cholesterol.
  —0—0— : percentage of whole incorporated radioactivity which was transformed
              into isoprenoid metabolites.
  –▢–▢– : cholesterol/lathosterol.
  –■–■– : C-27 sterols/methylsterols.
              ("methylsterols" include also sterones and methylsterol esters).

     Fig. 2 gives some informations about the mechanism of
pentadecane-2-one effect on cholesterol biosynthesis : the
ratios C-27 sterols/methylsterols and cholesterol/latho-
sterol decreased with increasing concentration of inhibitor. This means that the inhibition occurs at lanosterol
demethylation and lathosterol isomerisation into cholesterol, i-e at late steps of the biosynthetic process. As the
amount of total isoprenoid metabolites did not decrease,
we can conclude that HMGCoA reductase was little or not
modified. This was confirmed by a direct measurement of
the reductase activity, as shown in Table 4.

     Fig. 3 shows inhibition of cholesterol biosynthesis as
a function of culture time with the inhibitor, as a concentration of $4.5.10^{-5}$. The inhibition is already high (80 %
after 3 h) and reaches 90 % after 60 h culture with inhibitor ; the ratios C-27 sterols/methyl sterols and choleste-
rol/lathosterol sharply decrease.

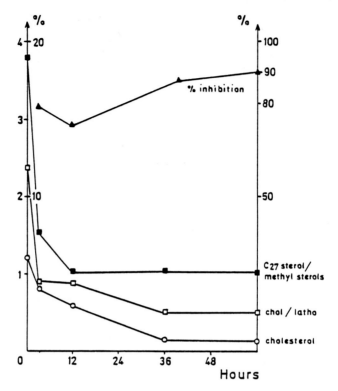

FIG. 3 : <u>INHIBITION OF CHOLESTEROL BIOSYNTHESIS BY PENTADECANE-2-ONE AS A
FUNCTION OF TIME</u>

       The cells growing logarithmically were cultured for 3-60 hours in
the presence of $4.5.10^5$M pentadecane-2-one, and the non-saponifiable lipids
analyzed, after a two hours pulse with $[2-^{14}C]$-acetic acid.

—0—0— : percentage of whole incorporated radioactivity which was transformed
        into cholesterol.

—□—□— : cholesterol/lathosterol

—■—■— : C-27 sterols/methylsterols

—▲—▲— : cholesterol inhibition (%)

TABLE 4. <u>Effect of pentadecane-2-one on HMG CoA reductase
activity</u> (after 24 h incubation with 5.10^{-5}M
inhibitor)

	CONTROL	INHIBITOR
dpm x 10^{-3} isoprenoids	133.5	118.5
HMG CoA reductase pm/min/mgP	170	160
dpm x 10^{-3} cholesterol/mgP	16.6	4.1
inhibition (%)		75
C-27 sterols/methylsterols	2.2	1.6
cholesterol/lathosterol	0.9	0.6

Inhibition of cell growth by pentadecane-2-one

Fig. 4 shows a growth experiment in the presence of
4.5.10^{-5}M pentadecane-2-one + 5 % steroid-free serum (DCC).
We can see an inhibition of about 50 %, and a partial rescue with 5.10^{-8}M estradiol.

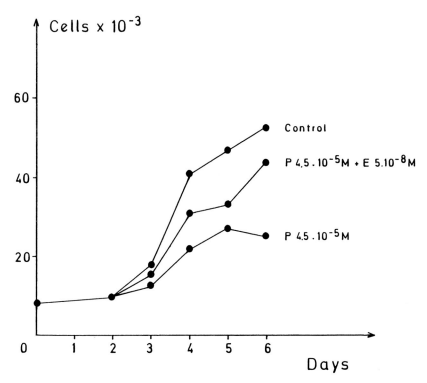

FIG. 4 : <u>INHIBITION OF CELL GROWTH WITH PENTADECANE-2-ONE</u>

The cells were cultured in MEM + 5 % dextran-coated charcoal
serum (DCC), in the presence of 4.5 10^{-5}M pentadecane-2-one or 4.5 10^{-5}M
pentadecane-2-one + 5.10^{-8}M estradiol.

Effect of estradiol and tamoxifen
on cholesterol biosynthesis

The effect of estrogens and anti-estrogens on growth of
CMF$_7$ cells has been studied by several groups of authors
(15,1).
The effect of estradiol on cholesterol biosynthesis was
assayed in 3 experiments, and that of tamoxifen in 2 experiments, in various conditions of serum (5 and 2 %) and
effector concentration, (E : 5.10^{-8}M, 10^{-9}M, Tam : 10^{-7}M,
5.10^{-7}M) between 0 and 48 h of culture.
Fig. 5 shows the variation of cholesterol and total
isoprenoid metabolites : cholesterol as well as isoprenoids

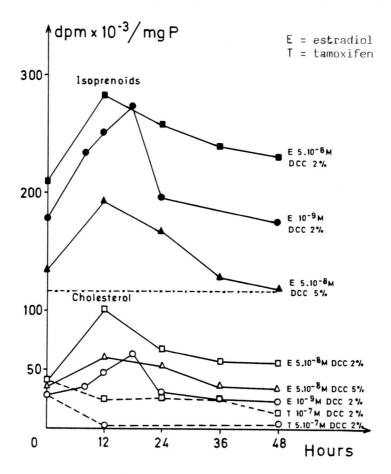

FIGS. 5 to 7: EFFECT OF ESTRADIOL AND TAMOXIFEN ON CHOLESTEROL
               SYNTHESIS

  The cells were cultured in MEM + 2 or 5% DCC, in the presence of
estradiol (5.10^{-8}M or 10^{-9}M) or tamoxifen (5.10^{-7}M or 10^{-7}M) for 0 to
48 h. Non-saponifiable lipids were analyzed after a two hours pulse
with $[2-^{14}C]$-acetic acid.

FIG. 5: Incorporation of radioactivity into cholesterol (-o-o-) and
         isoprenoids (-•-•-).

  biosynthesis are stimulated by estradiol, but cholesterol
stimulation is considerably higher ($\simeq 100$ %) than isoprenoid stimulation ($\simeq 20$ %). In 2 experiments, the stimulation shows a maximum between 12 and 24 h of culture in the
presence of estradiol. In a third experiment ($E.10^{-9}$M, 2%
DCC), the maximum was localized at 18 h.
  Tamoxifen strongly inhibits cholesterol production :
inhibition is already complete after 12 h of culture with
5.10^{-7}M tamoxifen.
  The variations of the ratios cholesterol/lathosterol
(shown in Fig. 6) and C-27 sterol/methylsterols (shown in
Fig. 7) are in agreement with post HMG CoA stimulation by

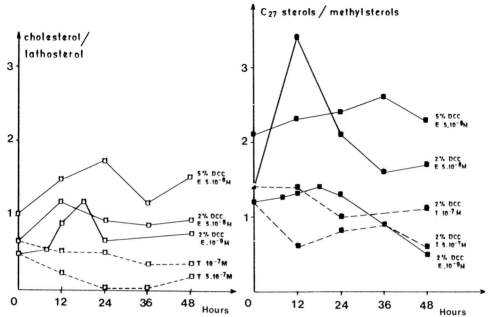

FIG. 6: Cholesterol/lathosterol.   FIG. 7:   C-27 sterols/methylsterols.

estradiol and post HMG CoA inhibition by tamoxifen, at the
steps of lanosterol demethylation and lathosterol isomerisation to cholesterol.

DISCUSSION AND CONCLUSION

The cholesterol necessary for membrane structure is
normally supplied to the cell by the light density lipo-
proteins (LDL) which (after internalisation) inhibit HMGCoA
reductase activity. Recently several groups of authors
culturing various types of cells in the presence of the
physiological constituent LDL reached to a similar conclusion concerning the existence of a tight linkage between
HMGCoA reductase activity and cell division (2, 10, 24, 25).
In our study, cholesterol biosynthesis inhibition by
2 different inhibitors occurs at late steps of the process :
it thus seems very probable that the crucial metabolite
involved in cell growth is cholesterol itself. Both the
inhibition and stimulation of cholesterol biosynthesis pre-
ceed the effect of cell growth. This suggests that cholesterol biosynthesis could be an early step of the estrogenic
and anti-estrogenic effect on cell growth.
Existence of two pools of cellular cholesterol has been
described by Lange and d'Allessandro (13) and it seems now
obvious that cellular needs in cholesterol (even in non
steroidogenic cells) are not only structural. Recently
Cornell et al (4) have shown that cholesterol plays a role
in phospholipids biosynthesis. Our results strongly suggest that a specific pool of endogenously synthesized
cholesterol is necessary to support cell growth. They give
a new insight on the role of post-HMG CoA regulations in
this complex phenomenon.

REFERENCES

1. Coezy, E., Borgna, J.L., Rochefort, H. (1982) : Canc. Res., 42 : 317-323.
2. Cohen, D.C., Massoglia, S.L. and Gospodarowicz, D. (1982) J. Biol. Chem., 257 : 9429-9437.
3. Cornell, R., Grove, G.L., Rothblatt and Horwitz, A.F. (1977) : Exp. Cell. Res., 109 : 299-307.
4. Cornell, B.R., Goldfine, H. (1983) : Biochem. Biophys. Acta, 750 : 504-520.
5. Faust, J.R., Goldstein, J.L. and Brown, M.S. (1979) : Arch. Biochem. Biophys., 192 : 86-99.
6. Faust, J.R., Brown, M.S. and Goldstein, J.L. (1980) : J. Biol. Chem., 255 : 6546-6548.
7. Gilbertson, J.R., Fletcher, R.D., Kawalek, J.C. and Demcisak, B. (1976) : Lipids, 11 : 172-178.
8. Goldstein, J.L., Hegelson, J.A. and Brown, M. (1979) : Chem., 255 : 5403-5409.
9. Habenicht, A.J., Glomset, J.A. and Ross, R. (1980) : J. Biol. Chem., 255 : 5134-5140.
10. Heiniger, H.J. and Marshall, D. (1982) : Proc. Natl. Acad. Sci. U.SA., 79 : 3823-3827.
11. Janus, M.J. and Kandutsch, A.A. (1979) : J. Biol. Chem., 254 : 8442-8446.
12. Kandutsch, A.A. and Chen, H.W. (1977) : J. Biol. Chem., 252 : 409-415.
13. Lange, Y. and d'Alessandro, S. (1978) : J. Sup. Structure, 8-391.
14. Liljeqvist, L., Gürtler, J. and Blomstrand, R. (1973) : Acta Chem. Scand., 27 : 197-208.
15. Lippman, M., Bolan, G., Huff, K. (1976) : Canc. Res., 36 : 4535-4601.
16. Namburidi, A., Subramanian, R. and Rudney, H. (1980) : J. Biol. Chem., 255 : 5894-5899.
17. Perkins, S.L., Ledin, S.F. and Stubbs, J.D. (1982) : Biochem. Biophys. Acta, 711 : 83-89.
18. Pratt, H.P., Fitzgerald, P.A. and Saxon, A. (1977) : Cell. Immunology, 32 : 160-170.
19. Quesney-Huneeus, V., Wiley, M.L. and Siperstein, M. (1979) : Proc. Natl. Acad. Sci. U.S.A., 76 : 5056-5060.
20. Snyder, F. and Snyder, E. (1975) : Progr. Biochem. Pharmacol., 10 : 1-14 (Karger, Basel).
21. Tabacik, C., Astruc, M., Laporte, M., Descomps, B. and Crastes de Paulet, A. (1979) : Biochem. Biophys. Res. Comm., 88 : 706-712.
22. Tabacik, C., Aliau, S., Serrou, B. and Crastes de Paulet, A. (1981) : Biochem. Biophys. Res. Comm., 101 : 1087-1095.
23. Tabacik, C., Aliau, S., Devillier, C. and Sultan, S. (1983) : 24th Intern. Conf. on the Biochem. of Lipids, Toulouse (France).
24. Volpe, J.J., Obert, K.A. (1981) : J. Biol. Chem., 256 : 2016-2021.
25. Witte, L.D., Cornicelli, J.A., Miller, R.W. and Goodman, D.S. (1982) : J. Biol. Chem., 257 : 5392-5401.

Progress in Cancer Research and Therapy,
Vol. 31, edited by F. Bresciani, et al.
Raven Press, New York © 1984.

Steroid Binding and Cytotoxicity in Cultured Human Pancreatic Carcinomas

*Chris Benz, **Israel Wiznitzer, and **Constance Benz

*Cancer Research Institute, University of California, San Francisco, California 94143; and **Department of Medicine, Yale University School of Medicine, New Haven, Connecticut 06510*

The presence of sex steroid receptors has correlated with endocrine responsiveness in a variety of human tumors including breast, prostate, endometrial and ovarian carcinomas (12). Other human tumors including renal cell, melanoma, meningioma, sarcoma, colorectal, hepatoma, and most recently, pancreatic carcinoma, have been reported to contain such receptors (5,11), but endocrine therapy of these tumors has either never been attempted or has not been adequately correlated with receptor content (6,9).

Several clinical studies have suggested that combined chemo-endocrine therapy may improve the clinical response rate in women with estrogen receptor (ER) positive breast cancer (1,8,13). Furthermore, in vitro studies using ER-positive human breast cancer cells have shown that the antimetabolite 5-fluorouracil (FUra) can act synergistically in combination with the antiestrogen tamoxifen (TAM) (2,3). FUra is considered the single most active drug available for treatment of pancreatic carcinoma, yet its overall response rate is less than 30% (15). Thus, if the endocrine responsiveness of pancreatic cancer can be established, it is possible that chemo-endocrine therapy may dramatically improve the prognosis for 95% of patients who would otherwise die from this neoplasm within five years of diagnosis.

TUMOR CELL LINES

Four human pancreatic carcinoma cell lines were compared with two ER-positive human mammary carcinoma lines (MCF-7 and T-47-D) for the presence of specific estradiol (E_2) binding and sensitivity in vitro to E_2, TAM, and progesterone (Pg). Growth inhibition by FUra or endocrine agent, as measured in a monolayer clonogenic assay (4), was recorded as either the mean percent of control growth or the 25% inhibitory dose, ID_{25}. Specific E_2 binding, measured by the whole cell assay of Shafie and Brooks (10), was analyzed by Scatchard plot to determine binding capacity (fmol/10^6 cells) and binding affinity, K_d (nM). The pancreatic tumor lines included COLO-357 (7), MIA PaCa (14), RWP-1 and RWP-2 (courtesy of Michael Turner, Roger Williams General Hospital, Providence, RI).

CHEMO-ENDOCRINE SENSITIVITY

Since FUra is considered first-line chemotherapy for pancreatic cancer, in vitro responsiveness to this antimetabolite was measured and compared with endocrine sensitivity. COLO-357, derived from an untreated metastatic deposit

223

of a well-differentiated pancreatic adenocarcinoma (7), was exposed to varying concentrations of FUra over 6 hr. It is known that the serum half-life of FUra after a single bolus injection is less than 20 min, thus a 6 hr exposure period in vitro likely overestimates the actual C x T relationship of FUra in vivo. Nevertheless, Table 1 shows that significant inhibition of COLO-357 growth could only be achieved by exposure to FUra at concentrations in excess of 10 μM.

TABLE 1. COLO-357 Growth Inhibition by FUra

μM FUra (6 hr)	Mean % of Control Growth ($\pm$ SD)
0	100 $\pm$ 5
0.1	85 $\pm$ 11
1.0	90 $\pm$ 15
10.0	71 $\pm$ 14
100.0	1 $\pm$ 1
1000.0	0.1 $\pm$ 0

These tumor cells were grown in medium containing 10% fetal calf serum. To determine their in vitro sensitivity to endocrine agents, identical culture conditions were employed. The endocrine agents TAM, E_2 and Pg were administered continuously to COLO-357 cells; the serum-supplemented medium was not stripped of endogenous steroids in an effort to simulate in vivo

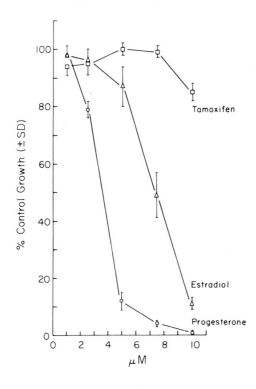

FIG. 1.

Growth inhibition of COLO-357 cells was measured in a monolayer clonogenic assay as previously described (4). Tamoxifen, estradiol and progesterone were added 24 hr after plating cells in serum-supplemented medium. Colonies were counted on day 6 and results were recorded as the percent of control colony growth.

treatment conditions. Figure 1 shows that E_2 and Pg were able to inhibit COLO-357 growth in dose-dependent fashions. In comparison to FUra, E_2 and Pg were growth inhibitory at concentrations 2- to 5-fold lower than equitoxic doses of the antimetabolite. TAM, on the other hand, produced only minimal inhibition of COLO-357 growth at concentrations $\leq$ 10 μM.

SPECIFIC ESTRADIOL BINDING

For measurement of specific E_2 binding, the serum-supplemented medium was rinsed off and replaced by serum-free medium. The monolayer cells were then incubated ($37°C$ x 1 hr) with varying concentrations of (^{3}H)-E_2 $\pm$ 100-fold excess diethylstilbestrol. Scatchard analysis of the specific E_2 binding in COLO-357 cells is shown in Figure 2. The number of calculated binding sites in COLO-357 cells (12 fmol/10^6 cells) was about one-third the number of binding sites determined for MCF-7 (35 fmol/10^6 cells) and T-47-D (37 fmol/10^6 cells) cells. Possibly of greater significance, the binding affinity of COLO-357 cells was found to be 5- to 10-fold lower than that calculated for the mammary carcinoma cells.

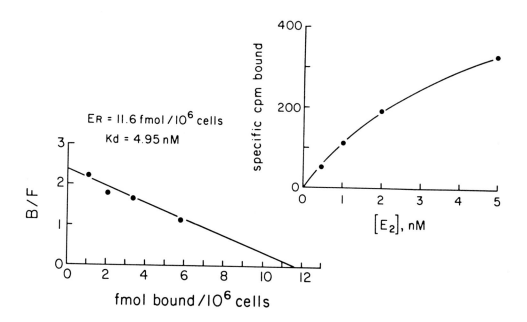

FIG. 2. Specific estradiol (E_2) binding of monolayer COLO-357 cells was measured in serum-free medium ($37°C$ x 1 hr) by the method of Shafie and Brooks (10). Estrogen receptor (ER) capacity (fmol/10^6 cells) and affinity (K_d) were determined by Scatchard analysis, as shown.

BINDING AFFINITY AND ENDOCRINE SENSITIVITY

When the mean ID_{25} dose of TAM was compared for COLO-357, MCF-7 and T-47-D cells, a positive rank order correlation with specific E_2 binding was apparent (Table 2). The more avidly binding MCF-7 cells were also more sensitive to TAM by an order of magnitude difference over the COLO-357 cells.

TABLE 2. Tamoxifen Sensitivity and E_2 Binding Affinity

Cell Line	ID_{25} TAM	K_d specific E_2 binding
MCF-7	<1µM	0.1 nM
T-47-D	2µM	1 nM
COLO-357	10µM	5 nM

The other three pancreatic tumor cell lines were similarly assayed for endocrine responsiveness and specific E_2 binding. Table 3 shows that a rather variable pattern of sensitivity to TAM, E_2 and Pg was observed. Each of the four pancreatic tumors could be growth-inhibited by at least one endocrine agent administered at a concentration < 5 µM. TAM sensitivity, per se, showed a less than perfect correlation with binding affinity (K_d), and overall (TAM, E_2 and Pg) endocrine sensitivity appeared to correlate well with E_2 binding affinity. The number of E_2 binding sites did not correlate with overall endocrine sensitivity, although an inverse relationship with E_2 growth inhibition was noted (Table 3) and the significance of this latter observation is uncertain.

TABLE 3. Endocrine Sensitivity and ER in Pancreatic Carcinomas

Cell Line	ID_{25} (µM)			ER	
	P_g	E_2	TAM	(fmol/10^6 cells)	K_d(nM)
M1A PaCa	0.5	5.0	2.0	5	1.1
COLO-357	2.0	7.0	10.0	12	5.0
RWP-1	5.0	>10.0	3.0	32	8.2
RWP-2	>10.0	9.0	5.0	15	9.2

SYNERGISTIC INTERACTIONS

In view of the cytotoxic synergy demonstrated between TAM and FUra in MCF-7 and T-47-D mammary carcinoma cells (9,10), we attempted to extend these observations to other endocrine agents and other endocrine-responsive tumors. Table 4 shows the growth-inhibiting effects of combining two mildly toxic doses of FUra with either TAM, E_2 or Pg in COLO-357. The ratios of observed/expected percent clonal growth (O/E) were used to indicate additive (O/E = 1.0 $\pm$ 0.2), antagonistic (O/E > 1.0), or synergistic (O/E < 1.0) interactions. As shown in Table 4, all the chemo-endocrine combinations were synergistic. Pg + FUra resulted in the greatest synergistic interaction with O/E values $\leq$ 0.2.

TABLE 4. Chemo-Endocrine Synergy in COLO-357

	% Control Growth	TAM (10µM)	E_2 (5µM)	(2.5µM)	Pg (5µM)
µM FURA					
0	100%	86%	85%	44%	8%
15	91%	61%	25%	8%	1%
20	79%	43%	26%	7%	<1%
O/E[a]		.78	.32	.2	.1
		.63	.39	.2	<.1

[a] Observed/expected (O/E) clonal growth: <1.0 $\pm$ .2 = synergism, >1.0 = antagonism

SUMMARY AND CONCLUSIONS

Four human pancreatic carcinoma cell lines were found to bind specifically in culture to (^3H)-E_2. When compared to two ER-positive mammary carcinoma cell lines, the total number of binding sites in the pancreatic tumor cells were similar, but their binding affinities were reduced with K_d's ranging between 1 nM - 9 nM. All of the pancreatic tumors were growth inhibited in vitro by Pg, E_2 or TAM at concentrations 2- to 5-fold less than that required by FUra to produce an equitoxic effect. Administration of FUra in combination with growth-inhibiting doses of Pg, E_2 or TAM resulted in synergistic cytotoxicity, and Pg + FUra showed the greatest synergistic interaction. These in vitro studies support the need for clinical trials to assess the value of endocrine or chemo-endocrine therapy in human pancreatic carcinoma.

ACKNOWLEDGMENTS

This work was supported by grants CA 36769 and CA 36773 from the National Cancer Institute and grant CH-235 from the American Cancer Society.

REFERENCES

1. Allegra, J.C., Woodcock, T.M., Richman, S.P., Bland, K.I. and Wittliff, J.L. (1982): Breast Cancer Res. Treat., 2: 93-99.
2. Benz, C. and Cadman, E. (1983): In: Biochemical and Biological Markers of Neoplastic Transformation, edited by P. Chandra, pp. 381-390. Plenum Publishing, New York.
3. Benz, C., Cadman, E., Gwin, J., Wu, T., Amara, J., Eisenfeld, A. and Dannies, P. (1983): Cancer Res. (in press).
4. Benz, C., Schoenberg, M., Choti, M. and Cadman, E. (1980): J. Clin. Invest., 66: 1162-1165.
5. Greenway, B., Igbal, M., Johnson, P. and Williams, R. (1981): Br. Med. J., 283: 751-753.
6. Leake, R., Laing, L., Calman, K. and Macbeth, F. (1980): Cancer Treat. Rep., 64: 797-799.
7. Morgan, R.T., Woods, L.K., Moore, G.E., Quinn, L.A., McGavran, L. and Gordon, S.E. (1980): Int. J. Cancer, 25: 591-598.
8. Mouridsen, H., Palshof, T., Engelsman, E. and Silvester, R. (1980): In: Breast Cancer -- Experimental and Clinical Aspects, edited by H. Mourisden and T. Palshof, pp. 119-123. Pergamon Press, Oxford.
9. Patterson, J. and Battersby, L. (1980): Cancer Treat. Rep., 64: 775-778.
10. Shafie, S. and Brooks, S. (1977): Cancer Res., 37: 792-799.
11. Stedman, K., Moore, G. and Morgan, R. (1980): Arch. Surg., 115: 244-248.
12. Stoll, B.A. (1979): The Practitioner, 222: 211-217.
13. Wada, T., Koyama, H. and Terasawa, T. (1981): Breast Cancer Res. Treat., 1: 53-58.
14. Yunis, A., Arimura, G. and Russin, D. (1977): Int. J. Cancer, 19: 128-135.
15. Zimmerman, S.E., Smith, F.P. and Schein, P.S. (1981): Cancer, 47: 1724-1728.

Progress in Cancer Research and Therapy,
Vol. 31, edited by F. Bresciani, et al.
Raven Press, New York © 1984.

Glucocorticoid Receptors: *In Vitro*–Clinical Correlations in Human Leukemia and Lymphoma

*Clara D. Bloomfield, **Nikki J. Holbrook, **Allan U. Munck,
‡Carol M. Foster, ‡Howard Eisen, and †Kendall A. Smith

*Section of Medical Oncology, Department of Medicine, University of Minnesota,
Minneapolis, Minnesota 55455; Departments of **Physiology and †Medicine,
Dartmouth Medical School, Hanover, New Hampshire 03755; and ‡Laboratory of
Developmental Pharmacology, National Institute of Child Health and Human
Development, Bethesda, Maryland 20205

Glucocorticoids are routinely used in some adult hematologic malignancies, but not in others. They are included in almost all combination chemotherapy regimens for acute lymphoblastic leukemia (ALL) and in many for malignant lymphoma (ML); however, they are relatively infrequently used for acute nonlymphocytic leukemia (ANLL) and chronic lymphocytic leukemia (CLL). Their antitumor effectiveness correlates only modestly with their use, since significant antitumor effect is seen in only approximately 50% of ML, 35-40% of ALL and <15% of ANLL and CLL. However, side effects of glucocorticoid therapy are seen in almost all patients; these are often quite severe in an elderly group of patients, such as those with adult hematologic malignancies. Consequently, <u>in vitro</u> tests that would rapidly identify before treatment those patients likely to benefit from steroids would be of considerable use clinically.

Most if not all physiologic and pharmacologic actions of glucocorticoids appear to be initiated through glucocorticoid receptors, protein molecules that the hormone encounters after traversing the cell membrane, and with which it initially forms complexes that are found in the cytosol after cell disruption (24). Through a poorly understood process, the cytosolic complexes become "activated", giving rise to complexes with affinity for DNA that are rapidly bound to the nucleus. It appears that the nuclear-bound complexes stimulate formation of mRNAs for particular effector proteins that are then responsible for the effects of the hormones in the cell.

Consequently, we have undertaken a series of studies in adults with various leukemias and lymphomas which have as their major objective the determination of the utility of analyzing glucocorticoid receptors in tumor cells to identify pretreatment those patients likely to respond to glucocorticoid. The current results from some of these studies are summarized in this paper.

METHODOLOGY
Summary of Studies

Results from the following sets of studies in adults with ANLL, ALL,

ML and CLL are summarized in this paper: (1) glucocorticoid receptor levels in tumor cells; (2) analysis by rapid DNA-DEAE mini-column chromatography of activated and nonactivated cytoplasmic glucocorticoid-receptor complexes; (3) molecular weight analysis by SDS-PAGE of the glucocorticoid receptor; (4) in vitro glucocorticoid assays and antitumor response to glucocorticoid therapy in ML and; (5) sequential studies of tumor receptor number in ML.

Patients

Different populations were studied in the different experiments as indicated below. All patients, however, were adults ($\geq$16 years of age) and all gave informed consent. All patients from whom malignant cells were obtained for study had leukemia (ANLL,ALL or CLL) or lymphoma. Patients were diagnosed as having leukemia on the basis of bone marrow aspiration and trephine biopsies and as having ML on the basis of lymph node or other tumor mass histology using standard criteria. Cases of ANLL and ALL were categorized according to the FAB classification based on the cytology and cytochemical reactivity of their neoplastic cells (1). Cases of ML were classified histologically according to the International Working Formulation for Clinical Usage (25).

Preparation and Handling of Tissues

In patients with ML, involved lymph nodes or other tumor masses served as the source of neoplastic cells. Different portions of the same tissue were used to obtain sections for histology, cryostat sections for immunologic analysis and single cell suspensions. Part of the same cell suspension was utilized for glucocorticoid studies and immunologic (lymphocyte surface marker) analysis. Lymph nodes were classified immunologically as B-lymphomas or T-lymphomas using previously defined criteria (11). The biopsy specimens were classified histologically and immunologically without knowledge of the in vitro glucocorticoid data. The majority of specimens studied contained at least 70% malignant cells as determined by immunologic analysis (3).

In patients with leukemia, bone marrow or blood were the source of tissue studied. Different portions of the same sample were used for morphology, immunologic analysis and in vitro glucocorticoid assays. Specimens sampled always contained a minimum of 50% malignant cells. Malignant cells were identified on the basis of cytology and cytochemistry in ANLL and on the basis of morphology and lymphocyte surface markers in ALL and CLL. For the in vitro glucocorticoid assays, the samples were diluted at least 1:5 in RPMI 1640 medium and cultured for 24 hours at ambient temperatures. The mononuclear cell population of the suspension was then separated by Ficoll-Hypaque gradient centrifugation and studied for glucocorticoid receptors. The enriched mononuclear cell preparation usually yielded more than 80% of the desired malignant cells as determined by cytologic analysis.

Glucocorticoid Receptors and In Vitro Glucocorticoid Sensitivity

The methods used for determining receptor sites per cell have been previously detailed (8). Briefly, cells were incubated with a near saturating concentration (40nM) of [^{3}H]dexamethasone (SA 35Ci/mol, New

England Nuclear, Boston, MA) with (B) and without (A) an excess of unlabelled dexamethasone (2µM) for 30 minutes at 37°C. The cell suspension was then cooled to 3°C. Cytoplasmic receptors were determined by lysing the cells with a rapid dilution into hypotonic $MgCl_2$ (1.5mM) containing dextran-coated charcoal to adsorb free glucocorticoid. After centrifugation an aliquot of the released cytosol was removed and counted by liquid scintillation. Nuclear receptor sites were determined similarly by lysing cells in hypotonic $MgCl_2$. The released nuclei were then pelleted, the supernatant removed, and the nuclear pellet counted.

For both nuclear and cytoplasmic binding, receptor binding in counts per minute (cpm) was calculated by subtracting the bound cpm obtained from incubation (B) (which estimates nonsaturable binding) from the cpm obtained from incubation (A), corrected for differences in the radioactive-steroid concentrations in the 2 incubations. These cpm were converted to bound steroid molecules per cell. Receptor sites per cell were calculated from these values by extrapolating to infinite steroid concentrations, assuming a Kd=10nMol/l of dexamethasone for the glucocorticoid receptor (8). Total receptor sites per cell were calculated as the sum of the cytoplasmic and nuclear receptor sites per cell.

In vitro sensitivity to glucocorticoids was measured by studying the effects of dexamethasone on incorporation of radiolabeled leucine, uridine, and thymidine (32). Cells ($1x10^6$/ml) were incubated in quadruplicate without and with 100nM dexamethasone for 20h at 37°C. Radiolabeled leucine, uridine, and thymidine were then added and the incubation was continued for 4h. The cells were then harvested on glass-fiber filter-paper, and isotope incorporation was determined by liquid scintillation counting. Results for in vitro sensitivity studies have been expressed as percent change from the values obtained when cells were incubated without dexamethasone.

DNA-DEAE Mini-column Chromatography for Separation of Activated and Nonactivated Cytoplasmic Glucocorticoid Receptor Complexes and Mero-Receptors

Details of these methods have been published elsewhere (15). In brief, glucocorticoid-receptor complexes were formed by incubating intact cells with approximately 30nM [^{3}H]triamcinolone acetonide ([^{3}H]TA) for about 2 hours at 0°C, a procedure that yields mainly nonactivated complexes. Cells were lysed at 0°C in 1.5mM $MgCl_2$ containing dextran-coated charcoal, and the broken-cell suspension was centrifuged to give the cytosols used for the experiments described. Cell-free activation was accomplished by warming cytosols to 25°C for 15 minutes. Cytosols were then run through mini-columns with 10mM tris buffer containing 10mM sodium molybdate (pH 7.8). As previously described (15), the mini-columns are 3 small columns in 1-ml plastic syringes connected in series. The top one contains DNA-cellulose, the next DEAE-cellulose, and the bottom one hydroxylapatite (HAP). When a cytosol is passed through the columns, activated complexes are retained with high efficiency by the DNA column, nonactivated complexes by the DEAE column, and mero-receptor and other complexes that do not bind to DNA or DEAE are retained on the HAP column. Each column bed is then assayed for radioactivity as a single sample. In this paper results are expressed as percent in each of these 3 forms.

SDS-PAGE of [³H] Dexamethasone-21-Mesylate Covalently Labeled Glucocorticoid Receptors

Our methods have been previously described in detail (9). In brief, intact neoplastic cells were labeled with 100nM [³H] dexamethasone mesylate (DM) with or without 100 fold molar excess of triamcinolone acetonide (TA). They were then incubated for 1 hour at 4°C. The cells were then broken by freezing followed by rapid thawing in buffer containing 20mM sodium molybdate. Cytosol was immediately treated with SDS buffer to minimize receptor degradation. Samples were applied to gel lanes on SDS gels prepared by the technique of Laemmli (18).

Statistical Methods

Differences between groups were evaluated for significance at the p=0.05 level or less. Differences in percentages for discrete variables were tested with the Pearson chi-square statistic correcting for continuity in 2x2 tables. Differences in continuous variables between groups were tested with the Mann-Whitney test.

RESULTS

Glucocorticoid Receptor Levels in Tumor Cells from Untreated Adults with ANLL, ALL, CLL and Lymphoma

Tumor total glucocorticoid receptor levels from the first 140 untreated adults studied are shown in Figure 1 and Table 1 by type of disease. All patients had measurable numbers of receptors but receptor levels tended to be higher in acute leukemia than in CLL or ML. In all 4 diseases, there was a wide range in receptor level (3,4,7).

To determine if this wide range in receptor level correlated with morphologic subtypes within diseases, we compared receptor levels among the FAB classes in ANLL and ALL and among the groups of the International Working Formulation for Clinical Usage in lymphoma. No significant differences in receptor level were identified in ANLL among M1 to M5 nor in ALL between L1 and L2 (7,4). No cases of M6 or L3 were

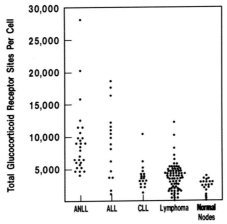

FIG. 1. Glucocorticoid receptor levels by disease in tumor cells from untreated adults with leukemia or lymphoma.

TABLE 1. Tumor glucocorticoid receptors in leukemia and lymphoma

Diagnosis	No. pts.	Total Receptor Sites/Cell	
		Median	Range
ANLL	33	8305	4273-28,393
ALL	16	9332	1348-18,697
CLL	18	3524	1877-10,480
Lymphoma	73	3440	87-12,919

studied. Similarly, no significant differences in total receptor level in ML were seen among histologic class (Figure 2). In all morphologic subgroups in which adequate numbers of cases were studied, there were wide ranges in receptor level.

Receptor levels among detailed immunologic phenotypes defined by monoclonal antibodies have not yet been analyzed. However, when adult ALL was classified as T (E^+, SIg^-) or non-T, non-B (E^-, SIg^-) there was not a significant difference in receptor level (4). Similarly, there was no significant difference between B-ML (CIg^+ and/or SIg^+, T^-) and T-ML (CIg^-, SIg^-, T^+).

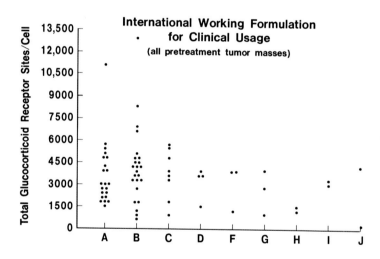

FIG. 2. Glucocorticoid receptor levels by International Working Formulation subgroups. A-ML, small lymphocytic; B-ML, follicular small cleaved cell; C-ML, follicular mixed small cleaved and large cell; D-ML, follicular predominantly large cell; F-ML, diffuse, mixed small and large cell; G-ML, diffuse, large cell; H-ML, large cell immunoblastic; I-ML, lymphoblastic; J-ML, small non-cleaved cell.

Analysis of Activated and Nonactivated Cytoplasmic Glucocorticoid-Receptor Complexes by Rapid DNA-DEAE Mini-column Chromatography

A possible reason for failure of patients to respond to glucocorticoid therapy is that the neoplastic cells have abnormal forms of the glucocorticoid receptor. Defects in the receptor have been described in murine and human lymphoma and leukemia cell lines (27, 33) and have recently been suggested in human leukemia (21). One way of studying if the receptor is biologically abnormal is to evaluate if activated cytoplasmic glucocorticoid-receptor complexes are formed and whether they are present in normal amounts.

Glucocorticoid-receptor complexes in cytosols from normal lymphoid cells incubated with [³H]-labeled glucocorticoid can be resolved into three different components, their relative amounts depending on the incubation conditions (15). Two of these correspond to the well-established activated and nonactivated forms (23). The third appears similar to the mero-receptor complex (28). Mero-receptor is a small fragment which has been shown to be produced by proteolytic cleavage of larger receptor forms in cell-free systems. Whether it has any physiological relevance is unclear. We have used our rapid mini-column chromatographic procedure for separating these three complexes based on their differential affinities for DNA, DEAE, and HAP (15), to examine the relative proportion of complexes in cytosols from neoplastic cells of patients with leukemia and lymphoma (13,14). A major advantage of this technique is the rapidity of the mini-column separation procedure (5-10 minutes, compared to hours by conventional methods) which drastically diminishes the time during which degradation of complexes can take place. Furthermore, since the columns can be prepared and run simultaneously in large numbers, they afford the opportunity for experiments requiring analysis of many samples.

The percentage of cytosolic glucocorticoid-receptor complexes in each form following cell free activation at 25° for 15 minutes in neoplastic cells from 35 patients with various leukemias and lymphomas is shown in Table 2. Results are compared to those obtained with peripheral lymphocytes from 5 healthy volunteers. As shown, activated receptor complexes were seen in all diseases studied. However, cytosols from cells of untreated ANLL patients had decreased amounts of activated complexes and more mero-receptor compared to other leukemias and lymphomas.

TABLE 2. Cytosolic glucocorticoid-receptor complexes[a]

	% in Each Cytosolic Form (mean)				
	ANLL (n=16)	ALL (n=4)	CLL (n=9)	ML (n=6)	Lymphs Normal (n=5)
Activated	31	53	55	61	51
Nonactivated	17	19	30	23	24
Mero-receptor	52	27	15	15	25

[a]Cell-free activation at 25° for 15 minutes

Although results from CLL and ML patients were quite homogeneous, there was a wide range in results in acute leukemia, especially ANLL. Thus, we correlated these results with the FAB classification in ANLL. Sufficient numbers of cases were present to study M1, M2 and M4. As can be seen in Table 3, less activated complex and more mero-receptor were seen in myeloid (M1, M2) than in monocytic (M4) leukemias. Interestingly, these results are similar to those obtained with normal peripheral granulocytes and monocytes (14), and suggest that the differences in stability of cytosolic complexes for different ANLL specimens reflect the differentiation state of the malignant cell.

Our data suggested that all cases of ANLL could form activated receptor, but that under the conditions used to activate, ANLL cytosolic receptors were rapidly degraded to mero-receptor (14). An

TABLE 3. Cytoplasmic glucocorticoid-receptor complexes in untreated ANLL by FAB[a]

| | % in Each Cytosolic Form (mean) | | |
	Activated	Nonactivated	Mero
ANLL			
M1 (n=4)	14	18	67
M2 (n=5)	19	13	67
M4 (n=6)	52	19	29
Normal			
Granulocytes (n=3)	6	13	81
Monocytes (n=2)	45	26	29

[a]Cell free activation at 25° for 15 minutes

obvious explanation for this kind of result is that ANLL cells contain high levels of receptor-degrading enzymes, which are absent from cells that do not form mero-receptor such as those from CLL patients. In fact, Sherman et al. have shown the presence of an enzyme in rat kidney cytosols capable of converting complexes in rat liver cytosols to mero-receptor (29), and similarly Vedeckis has shown that addition of mouse liver cytosol to AtT-20 cell cytosol results in fragmentation of the otherwise stable AtT-20 complexes (36). In the present study we performed mixing experiments between labile ANLL cells and stable CLL cells (Figure 3). Aliquots of cells from ANLL and CLL patients, one labeled with [^{3}H]TA, and the other treated with the same concentrations of TA to control for any possible hormone effects, were mixed and then broken to yield a mixed cytosol. The cytosol was analyzed with mini-columns before and after warming to 25°C. The first two mixtures in Figure 3 ([^{3}H]TA-ANLL+TA-ANLL and [^{3}H]TA-CLL+TA-CLL) are controls. They show that, as in Table 2, warming to 25°C causes much more mero-receptor formation in cytosols from ANLL cells than from CLL cells.

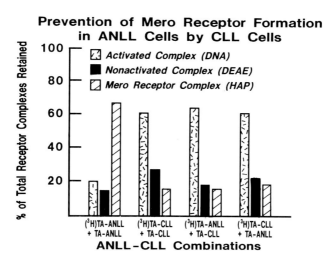

FIG.3. Distribution of receptor complexes in warmed cytosols of mixed ANLL and CLL cell preparations.

The third and fourth mixtures shown in Figure 3 are designed to test the standard interpretation, according to which the presence of cytosol from ANLL cells in both these systems should cause the [^{3}H]TA-labeled receptors to be degraded to mero-receptor. In neither case, however, does this happen. ANLL cells did not cause formation of mero-receptor in cytosols from CLL cells (exp. 4, [^{3}H]TA-CLL+TA-ANLL, Figure 3). Moreover, CLL cells prevented formation of mero-receptors in cytosols from ANLL cells (exp. 3, [^{3}H]TA-ANLL+TA-CLL, Figure 3), and normal amounts of activated complex were found in these ANLL cells. In other experiments, we showed that this protective activity was dependent on the number of CLL cells added to the cell mixture (14). Thus, we conclude that the reason for formation of mero-receptor in ANLL cytosols is not simply a high content of proteolytic enzymes, but rather a lack of an endogenous factor(s) (protease inhibitor) capable of inhibiting mero-receptor formation. Most importantly, although it has been reported that receptors from ANLL cells appear abnormal (21), we could find no evidence from our experiments that mero-receptors or other abnormal cytoplasmic glucocorticoid-receptor complexes were present in intact ANLL cells (or in other leukemia or lymphoma cells) under normal conditions.

Molecular Weight Analysis by SDS-PAGE of the Glucocorticoid Receptor in Human Leukemia and Lymphoma

An alternate way in which an abnormal form of the glucocorticoid receptor might be detected is by its molecular weight. However, study of the molecular weight of the receptor has been difficult, because until recently, glucocorticoid receptors in lymphoid cells have only been detectable by use of radiolabeled steroids (such as dexamethasone) which form non-covalent steroid-receptor complexes that dissociate readily. We have recently developed a technique that uses [^{3}H]dexamethasone-21-mesylate ([^{3}H]DM) to label covalently the glucocorticoid receptor in human lymphoid cells (9,10); this allows the use of analytical procedures such as SDS-PAGE, allowing reliable molecular weight determinations.

Glucocorticoid receptors from neoplastic cells from 2 patients with ANLL, 3 with ALL, 3 with CLL and 3 with ML have been labeled covalently with [^{3}H]DM and analyzed by SDS-PAGE in the manner previously described (9). In all cases an $Mr=95,000$ protein moiety was labeled covalently; labeling was inhibited by excess glucocorticoid (triamcinolone acetonide) (Figs. 4 & 5). This is consistent with previous reports of the molecular weight of the glucocorticoid receptor in human circulating mononuclear cells from normal volunteers, EBV-transformed B-cells obtained from normal donors (35), human cell lines (5,34) and rat thymocytes and liver (9,10). This 95,000 moiety appears to represent the reduced denatured fundamental unit of the glucocorticoid receptor. Under non-denaturing conditions the native or nonactivated glucocorticoid receptor is apparently much larger and may consist of a multimer of receptor subunits or a complex with other nonreceptor proteins (15,26,37).

In most of the leukemia and lymphoma specimens, smaller labeled moieties were also detected which showed saturable binding ($M_r \cong 75,000$, 57,000, 45,000, 35,000 and 31,000) (see example in Fig. 5). These moieties probably represent proteolytic fragments of the $M_r \cong 95,000$

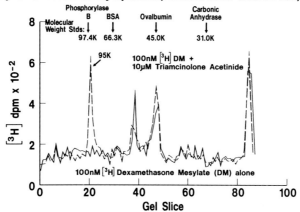

FIG. 4. [³H]DM labeling of glucocorticoid receptor as analyzed by SDS-PAGE. Gel lanes contain proteins from 40µl of sample. Intact lymphoma cells from a lymph node of a patient with follicular small cleaved cell lymphoma were labeled with 100nM [³H]DM alone (- -) or in combination with 10µM TA (—).

receptor subunit. It is known that the glucocorticoid receptor is unstable in some human leukemic cell cytosols (7,14). In our present assay, proteolysis could certainly occur during the limited, but definite, exposure to cell free conditions. We are currently evaluating techniques to denature cells directly in an effort to minimize formation of smaller labeled proteins.

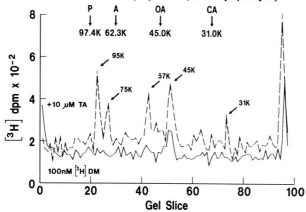

FIG. 5. Intact lymphoma cells from a lymph node of a patient with ML small lymphocytic were labeled with 100nM [³H]DM alone (- -) or in combination with 10µM TA (—).

In Vitro Glucocorticoid Assays and Antitumor Response to Glucocorticoid Therapy

As indicated initially, the major goal of our studies has been to determine if in vitro studies of tumor glucocorticoid receptors could be used to predict antitumor response to glucocorticoid therapy. The studies described so far indicated that all human leukemias and lymphomas have glucocorticoid receptors and that these appear to be biologically normal. The only in vitro tumor glucocorticoid assays that we have studied that appeared promising for predicting response were receptor number and in vitro sensitivity. The fact that the range in receptor number per cell varied widely within a given disease, and that this number was not explained by morphologic or immunologic subtype of the disease, suggested that receptor number in particular might predict response. To test this directly we studied a group of patients with malignant lymphoma.

To clearly determine if an in vitro glucocorticoid assay predicts antitumor response, one needs to be able to administer glucocorticoid as a single-agent for a period of time sufficient to obtain an antitumor response. Among adults with leukemia or lymphoma this is most readily done in ML. Newly diagnosed patients with acute leukemia cannot ethically be routinely treated for more than a few days with glucocorticoid alone. Similarly, since patients with CLL rarely respond to glucocorticoid it is difficult to justify exposing them routinely to the toxicity of steroid therapy. However, glucocorticoids are included in almost all chemotherapy regimens for lymphoma and these patients tend to have slowly progressive disease so that two weeks of single agent steroid therapy is readily tolerated. Moreover, since approximately 50% of patients have significant antitumor effect, but toxicity occurs in up to 90% (22), there is a clear need for developing a way to predict which patients will respond to glucocorticoid therapy.

We have studied 47 adults with a diagnosis of B-cell ML. Thirty-nine patients were first studied at diagnosis and 8 at relapse. Four had received prior glucocorticoid therapy; these patients had been off steroids for a minimum of 6 weeks when in vitro studies were performed. This was done since our previous studies have shown that in vivo glucocorticoid administration causes a fall in receptor level in neoplastic cells from patients with ANLL, ALL, CLL and ML, as well as in circulating lymphocytes from normal volunteers, which may persist for as long as 17 days after stopping glucocorticoid therapy (30,31).

The study protocol consisted of first obtaining informed consent in writing from each patient (2). Then each patient underwent biopsy of an involved lymph node for pathologic examination and in vitro glucocorticoid studies. Following biopsy, each patient was treated with dexamethasone at a dose of 4mg every 6 hours. Single agent glucocorticoid therapy was administered for a minimum of 5 days, since that is the duration of glucocorticoid treatment in most combination chemotherapy regimens for ML. In 39 of the 47 patients glucocorticoid alone was continued for at least 2 weeks.

Antitumor response to dexamethasone was measured by a single investigator who had no knowledge of the results of the in vitro glucocorticoid studies. At the end of single-agent glucocorticoid therapy patients were classified as responders, mixed responders or nonresponders. They were scored as responders if they had a partial remission defined as at least a 50% reduction in all measurable tumor and had developed no new disease. In a few patients, all tumor masses decreased by at least 50%, but this was accompanied by an increase in the number of circulating lymphoma cells. These patients were classified as mixed responders. Patients who demonstrated less than a 50% decrease of all tumor masses or developed any new mass were classified as nonresponders.

TABLE 4. Clinical characteristics of lymphoma patients according to response to glucocorticoid therapy

	Response to Glucocorticoid Therapy		
	Remission	Mixed	None
Number of Patients	22	6	19
Sex	12:10	4:2	16:3
Median Age (yrs)	63	48	61
Diagnosis (IWF)			
Small lymph (A)	23%	0	42%
Foll. sm. cleaved (B)	55%	50%	37%
Other follicular (C,D)	14%	33%	10%
Other diffuse (F,G,H,J)	9%	17%	10%
Treatment Status at Study			
Newly diagnosed	91%	83%	74%
Prior glucocorticoid	0	1	3
Disease Extent at Study			
"Stage" I-IIIA	13%	0	26%
"Stage" IVA	55%	50%	47%
"Stage" IIIB-IVB	32%	50%	26%
Blood involvement	9%	83%	26%

Of the 47 patients treated with single-agent glucocorticoid therapy, 22 (47%) achieved a partial remission, 6 (13%) had a mixed response and 19 (40%) demonstrated no significant antitumor effect. Clinical and histological characteristics of these 3 patient groups are shown in Table 4. The only significant difference among groups was that the mixed responders more frequently had blood involvement at diagnosis. Nonresponders tended to more frequently be male and more often had diffuse lymphoma. Patients in all three response groups received single-agent glucocorticoid therapy for comparable periods of time (median 14 days).

The results of the in vitro glucocorticoid studies for the 3 response groups are summarized in Table 5 and Figure 6. Median total glucocorticoid receptor sites per cell were 4031 for patients who achieved a partial remission,4024 for patients who had a mixed response and 2049 for the nonresponders. Receptors were significantly higher in responders than nonresponders ($p<.002$). The median inhibition of thymidine incorporation was also significantly greater in responders than nonresponders (23% vs. 9%, $p=.02$). Significant differences between responders and nonresponders were not seen in dexamethasone inhibition of radiolabeled leucine or uridine incorporation.

No pretreatment clinical characteristics could be used to predict those patients who would respond to glucocorticoid therapy. However, using total glucocorticoid receptor levels we could accurately predict

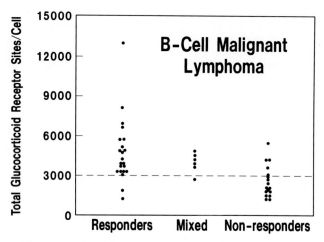

FIG. 6. Glucocorticoid receptor levels by clinical response to dexamethasone therapy.

response in 37 (82%) of 45 patients. Among 30 patients with nodal tumor receptor levels of more than 3000 sites per cell, 25 (83%) demonstrated more than a 50% decrease in nodal mass. Similarly among 15 patients with nodal tumor receptor number of less than 3000, only 3 (20%) so responded.

TABLE 5. Correlation of in vitro glucocorticoid studies with response to glucocorticoid therapy in B-cell lymphoma

| | Response to Glucocorticoid Therapy | | | p^a |
	Remission	Mixed	None	
Number of patients	22	6	19	
Glucocorticoid Receptors (sites/cell)^c				
Cytoplasmic	937	999 (.01)^b	549	.002
Nuclear	3067	2411 (.07)	1500	.002
Total	4031	4024 (.01)	2049	.0006
Glucocorticoid Inhibition of Isotope Incorporation (%)^c				
Leucine	27	29	17	NS
Uridine	35	32	22	.06
Thymidine	23	28	9	.02

^{a}P value for response groups: remission vs. none
^{b}P value for response group: mixed vs. none
^{c}Values are medians

Sequential Studies of Tumor Receptors

Little is known regarding the development of resistance to glucocorticoid therapy. It is generally thought that patients who have previously received glucocorticoid are less likely to respond to such therapy at relapse, though little data are available to evaluate this hypothesis. Among our 4 patients described above who had previously received glucocorticoid therapy, when retreated with dexamethasone as a

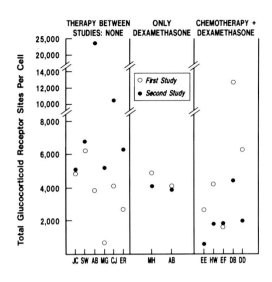

FIG. 7. Effect of therapy on changes in tumor glucocorticoid receptor levels in patients with malignant lymphoma.

single-agent 3 failed to respond and one had a mixed response. To determine if patients at relapse might have cells with fewer receptors, and thus a lower response rate, we have initiated a study of sequential analysis of glucocorticoid receptors from involved lymph nodes in ML.

To date we have studied 12 patients. Time between studies was more than 3 months in 11 of these patients. All had been off steroids at least 3 months at the time of the second study. Therapy between studies consisted of no treatment in 6 patients, dexamethasone alone in 2 patients and chemotherapy and dexamethasone in 5 patients.

As shown in Figure 7, receptor level remained constant or increased in the patients who received no steroid. Receptor levels fell slightly at relapse in both patients who received only steroids between studies. However, receptor levels fell dramatically in 4 of the 5 patients who received chemotherapy and steroid. Receptor levels in these 4 patients were 22 to 43% of initial levels. These preliminary data suggest that glucocorticoid therapy, especially in combination with other agents, may result in selection of neoplastic cells with lower numbers of receptors. This selection of cells with lower levels of receptor may be one explanation for the development of glucocorticoid resistance in patients with ML.

DISCUSSION

The studies summarized here suggest that neoplastic cells from all adult leukemias and lymphomas have measurable numbers of glucocorticoid receptors when studied pretreatment with appropriate assays. Similar results have been obtained by others in childhood as well as adult hematologic neoplasms (6,12,19,20). Whether the numbers of receptors per cell are similar to those found in the nonneoplastic state is unknown. Until we know the corresponding nonneoplastic cell in which malignant transformation occurs it is impossible to perform the appropriate comparisons. Compared to normal mature lymphocytes such as are found in nonneoplastic lymph nodes, the numbers of receptors in ALL, ML and CLL are higher (3,4,7), but these neoplasms appear to consist of cells with markers of much less differentiation, and glucocorticoid receptors in normal less differentiated human lymphoid cells have not been measured. There is currently little reason to suspect that the number of receptors is abnormal in neoplastic cells.

All leukemias and lymphomas that we have studied have demonstrated a wide range in numbers of receptor sites per cell. This range was not predicted by standard morphologic classification. It was also not predicted by broad immunologic class. However, in childhood ALL, studies utilizing more precise immunologic phenotyping suggest that B-ALL has lower numbers of receptors than T-ALL, and T-ALL lower numbers than common-ALL (6,19). Detailed immunologic phenotyping with the many monoclonal antibodies now available against lymphoid and myeloid differentiation antigens, may allow us to sort out the broad range in receptor level among morphologic classes as we better define the stage of differentiation of the malignant cell.

All our studies to date suggest that the glucocorticoid receptor in human ANLL, ALL, CLL and ML is biologically normal. In all diseases the receptor appears to be of normal size and activate normally. Consequently,it currently appears unlikely that studies of receptor size or state of activation of cytoplasmic glucocorticoid-receptor complexes will be useful for predicting response to glucocorticoid therapy.

Receptor number in B-cell malignant lymphoma has correlated with response to glucocorticoid therapy. Similar results have been reported in ALL (4,12,17,20). The reason for this is unknown. Certainly high receptor levels per se do not predict for response to glucocorticoid therapy. Receptor levels are generally high in ANLL, but response to glucocorticoid therapy is infrequent. Among B-cell lymphomas, for unexplained reasons, receptor number appears to identify a cell which is sensitive to glucocorticoid treatment. The antiproliferative effects of glucocorticoids are poorly understood and require further study. Among B-cell lymphomas it is possible that there is a simple relationship between receptor number and clinical response, but even here it is probable that the relationship is complex.

It has been suggested that glucocorticoid receptor level is an independent prognostic factor for predicting first remission duration and/or survival in childhood ALL (6,19). We have not found this to be the case in adult lymphoma (data not shown). Since essentially all children with ALL receive glucocorticoids, it is impossible to determine if receptor level predicts remission or survival independent of glucocorticoid administration and response. Glucocorticoids remain an important therapeutic agent in childhood ALL and a correlation between receptor number and response to glucocorticoid could explain the correlation of receptor level with remission duration and survival.

In a small number of patients with lymphoma studied sequentially, we have found that tumor receptors at relapse are usually lower in patients who have previously received glucocorticoid therapy, especially in combination with other chemotherapeutic agents. These data suggest that glucocorticoid therapy may result in selection of lymphoma cells with lower numbers of receptors. They also suggest that chemotherapy, in addition to glucocorticoid, may accelerate the process. Similar results have been found in vitro in cell lines but these are the first data to indicate that such may also be true in patients (16). These data also suggest that it may be especially important to study receptors in patients at relapse before retreating them with glucocorticoid. It is of interest that of the four patients who had received previous glucocorticoid therapy in whom we correlated clinical response to glucocorticoid therapy with receptor levels, none of them achieved a partial remission upon retreatment. However, more patients must be studied to confirm our preliminary results. Moreover, it needs to be determined if patients initially sensitive in vivo to glucocorticoid become resistant in vivo when tumor receptor levels fall.

To date we have correlated tumor receptor levels only with response to single agent glucocorticoid therapy in lymphoma. Whether these results will be translatable to combination chemotherapy regimens which include glucocorticoid or to other diseases requires further study. If such is the case then determination of tumor glucocorticoid receptor level may become a necessary part of the evaluation of patients with lymphomas or leukemias, just as estrogen receptor analyses are required in patients with breast cancer.

ACKNOWLEDGEMENTS

This research was supported in part by Public Health Service grants CA-26273 and CA-17323, American Cancer Society grant no. CH-167 and the Coleman Leukemia Research Fund.

REFERENCES

1. Bennett, J.M., Catovsky, D., Daniel, M.-T., Flandrin, G.,Galton, D.A.G., Gralnick, H.R., and Sultan, C. (1976): Br. J. Haematol.,33:451-458.
2. Bloomfield, C.D., Smith, K.A.,Peterson, B.A., Hildebrandt, L., Zaleskas, J., Gajl-Peczalska, K.J., Frizzera, G., and Munck, A.(1980): Lancet, i:952-956.
3. Bloomfield, C.D., Smith, K.A., Peterson, B.A., Gajl-Peczalska, K.J., and Munck, A.U. (1981): J. Steroid Biochem., 15:275-284.
4. Bloomfield, C.D., Smith, K.A., Peterson, B.A., and Munck, A. (1981): Cancer Res., 41:4857-4860.
5. Cidlowski, J.A., Richon, V. (1983): Proc 65th Annual Meeting of the Endocrine Society, San Antonio, TX, (abstract) p. 227.
6. Costlow, M.E., Ching-Hon, P., and Dahl, G.V. (1982): Cancer Res., 42:4801-4806.
7. Crabtree, G.R., Bloomfield, C.D., Smith, K.A., McKenna, R.W., Peterson, B.A., Hildebrandt, L., and Munck, A.(1981): Cancer Res., 41:4853-4856.
8. Crabtree, G.R., Smith, K.A., and Munck, A.(1981): In: The Leukemic Cell, edited by D. Catovsky, pp. 252-269. Churchill Livingstone, London.
9. Foster, C.M., Eisen, H.J., and Bloomfield, C.D. (1983): Cancer Res., 43:5273-5277.
10. Eisen, H.J., Schleenbaker, R.E., and Simons, S.S. (1981): J.Biol.Chem., 256:12920-12925.
11. Gajl-Peczalska, K.J., Bloomfield, C.D., Frizzera, G., Kersey, J.H., and Lebien, T.W. (1982): In: Diversity of Phenotypes of non-Hodgkin's Malignant Lymphoma, edited by E.Vitetta, pp.63-67. Academic Press, New York.
12. Ho, A.D., Hunstein, W., Ganeshaguru, K., Hoffbrand, A.V., Brandeis, W.E., and Denk, B. (1982): Leuk. Res., 6:1-8.
13. Holbrook, N.J., Bloomfield, C.D., and Munck, A. (1983): Cancer Res., 43:4478-4482.

14. Holbrook, N.J., Bloomfield, C.D., and Munck, A. (1984): Cancer Res., 44:407–414.
15. Holbrook, N.J., Bodwell, J.E., Jeffries, M., and Munck, A. (1983): J. Biol. Chem., 258:6477–6485.
16. Huet-Minkowski, M., Gasson, J.C., and Bourgeois, S. (1981): Cancer Res., 41:4540–4546.
17. Iacobelli, S., Marchetti, P., de Rossi, G., and Mastrangelo, R.(1983): J. Steroid Biochem., 19:40s.
18. Laemmli, U.K. (1970): Nature, 277:680–685.
19. Lippman, M.E., Yarbro, G.K., and Leventhal, B.G. (1978): Cancer Res., 38:4251–4356.
20. Mastrangelo, R., Malandrino, R., Riccardi, R., Longo, P., Ranelletti, F.O., and Iacobelli, S. (1980): Blood, 56:1036–1040.
21. McCaffrey, R., Lillquist, A., and Bell, R. (1982): Blood, 59:393–400.
22. McClean, J.W., Kiely-Grandbois, K., Hurd, D.D., Peterson, B.A., and Bloomfield, C.D. (1983). Proc. Am. Soc. Clin. Oncol., 2:217.
23. Munck, A., and Foley, R. (1979): Nature, 278:752–754.
24. Munck, A, and Leung, K. (1977): In: Receptors and Mechanism of Action of Steroid Hormones Part II, edited by J. R. Pasqualini, pp. 311–397. Marcel Dekker, New York.
25. The Non-Hodgkin's Lymphoma Pathologic Classification Project (1982): Cancer, 49:2112–2135.
26. Raaka, B.M., and Samuels, H.H. (1983): J. Biol. Chem., 258:417–425.
27. Schmidt, T.J., Harmon, J.M., and Thompson, E.B. (1980): Nature, 286:507–510.
28. Sherman, M.R., Pickering, L.A., Rollwagen, F.M., and Miller, L.K. (1978): Federation Proc., 37:167–173.
29. Sherman, M.R., Moran, M.C., Tudzon, F.B., and Stephens, Y.-W. (1983): J. Biol. Chem., 258(17):10366–10377.
30. Shipman, G.F., Bloomfield, C.D., Smith, K.A., Peterson, B.A., and Munck,A. (1981): Blood, 58:1198–1202.
31. Shipman, G., Bloomfield, C.D., Gajl-Peczalska, J.J., Munck, A., and Smith, K.A. (1983): Blood, 61:1086–1090.
32. Smith, K.A., Crabtree, G.R., Kennedy, S.J., and Munck, A.U. (1977): Nature, 267:523–525.
33. Stevens, J., and Stevens, Y.W. (1979): Cancer Res., 33:4011–4021.
34. Thompson, E.B., Zawydiwski, R., Brower, S.T., Eisen, H.J., Simons, S.S., Schmidt, T.J., Schlechte, J.A., Moore, D.E., Norman, M.R., and Harmon, J.M. (in press): In: Nobel Symposium No. 57 Steroid Hormone Receptors: Structure and Function. Elsevier Press, Stockholm.
35. Tomita, M., Benor, S., Chrousos, G.P., Brandon, D.B., Foster, C.M., Taylor, S., and Lipsett, M.B. (1983): Proc. 65th Annual Meeting of the Endocrine Society, San Antonio, TX, p. 261.
36. Vedeckis, W.V. (1983): Biochem., 22:1975–1983.
37. Vedeckis, W.V. (1983): Biochem., 22:1983–1989.

Progress in Cancer Research and Therapy,
Vol. 31, edited by F. Bresciani, et al.
Raven Press, New York © 1984.

Functional Domains in Wild-Type and Variant Glucocorticoid Receptors of Lymphoid Cells

Ulrich Gehring

Institut für Biologische Chemie, Universität Heidelberg, D-6900 Heidelberg, Federal Republic of Germany

Mouse lymphoma cells in continuous culture have been used amongst other cell types to study steroid hormone action. Various cell lines respond to glucocorticoids by growth inhibition which is followed by cell death in some lines. This type of cellular response can quite easily be used to select for unresponsive cell variants which then can be compared to the wild-type in an attempt to find out more details about the mechanism of hormone action. In the case of the S49.1 line it turned out that all the resistant variants characterized in some detail have defects of one type or another in the hormone specific receptors (6, 7, 15, 2o, 24).

Most of the glucocorticoid resistant variants of S49.1 cells have greatly reduced or virtually undetectable steroid binding activity. However, two types of variants have been obtained in which hormone binding is normal but the interaction of the receptor-glucocorticoid complexes with cell nuclei, chromatin, or DNA is abnormal. In the "nuclear transfer deficient" (nt$^-$) type the receptors are defective in nuclear binding. In the phenotype of "increased nuclear binding" (nt^i) the receptor-hormone complexes show increased nuclear binding and abnormally high affinity for DNA. The isolation of these resistant variants with receptor defects points to the qualitative importance of intact receptors for the physiological hormone response to occur. The quantitative role of receptors for cellular responsiveness has been emphasized by the isolation of cell variants of decreased glucocorticoid sensitivity which have been shown to contain significantly decreased receptor levels (11).

The present paper summarizes experiments with wild-type, nt$^-$, and nt^i receptors of S49.1 lymphoma cells which were carried out in order to obtain a better understanding of the function and structure of these receptors. In these experiments four different methods were used: DNA-cellulose chromatography, photoaffinity labeling with a radioactive glucocorticoid, mild proteolysis of native receptors with

various endoproteinases, and reaction with monoclonal antibodies. The data are discussed in view of a domain model
for the glucocorticoid receptor.

BINDING OF RECEPTOR-GLUCOCORTICOID COMPLEXES TO NUCLEI AND
DNA

The nt^- and nt^i variants mentioned above were detected
first amongst clones of glucocorticoid resistant S49.1 cells
because of abnormal distribution of receptor complexes between cytoplasm and a crude nuclear fraction (16). Similar
differences in nuclear binding were also seen in cell-free
incubations of isolated nuclei with steroid-treated cytosols
in which the origin of the cytosol rather than that of the
nuclei determined the extent of nuclear binding (7, 9). Decreased and increased nuclear binding in nt^- and nt^i variants, respectively, are reflected by decreased and increased
binding to deproteinized DNA. This is particularly obvious
when unfractionated DNA is adsorbed to cellulose and the
receptor complexes are chromatographed on this type of
affinity matrix (24). As summarized in Table 1, wild-type
receptor complexes reluted from DNA-cellulose with about
180 mM salt while nt^- and nt^i receptor complexes required
lower (70 to 90 mM) and higher (210 to 230 mM) salt concentrations, respectively.

TABLE 1. DNA-cellulose chromatography[a]

Receptor type	KCl concentration required for elution (mM)	
	native	after chymotrypsin
wild-type	175	236
nt^- type (clone 22R)	75	129
nt^- type (clone 83R)	86	87
nt^i type (clone 55R)	225	229
nt^i type (clone 143R)	210	209

[a]Cytosol receptor complexes with [^{3}H]triamcinolone acetonide were activated and chromatographed on DNA-cellulose
(prepared from unfractionated calf thymus DNA) either prior to
or after treatment with α-chymotrypsin. (Data from ref. 10).

These differences in chromatographic behaviour reflect
differences in the affinities to DNA of these variant receptor types (1, 24).

PHOTOAFFINITY LABELING OF RECEPTORS

Affinity labeling of steroid hormone receptors has in recent years become a valuable analytical tool since it allows
one to determine the polypeptide molecular weights of receptors under denaturing conditions (for a review, see ref. 17).
Crude receptor preparations can be used since after removal
of excess free ligand the hormone is only bound to specific

receptor sites and consequently only these are covalently
tagged. Since steroids containing α,β-unsaturated ketone
structures can be excited by long wavelength UV light (2)
we have used the high-affinity glucocorticoid,triamcinolone
acetonide in radiolabeled form to investigate receptors of
lymphoma cells (4, 10).

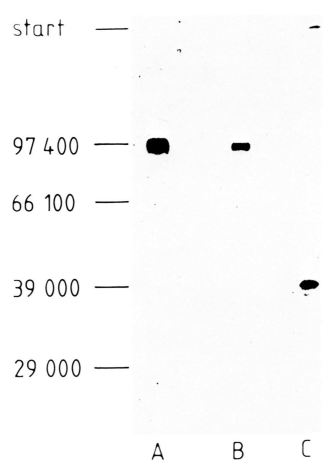

FIG. 1. <u>SDS gel electrophoresis of photoaffinity labeled receptors</u>.
Cytosol receptor complexes with [³H] triamcinolone acetonide were subjected to
photolabeling and subsequent gel electrophoresis. Fluorography was used to detect
radiolabeled bands. (A) S49.1 wild-type;
(B) S49.1 nt⁻ (clone 83R); (C) S49.1 nt¹
(clone 55R). (Data modified from ref. 10).

Figure 1 shows the fluorogram after gel electrophoresis in sodium dodecylsulfate. A single steroid-labeled band of molecular weight 94 000 ± 5000 was obtained with wild-type and nt⁻ receptors. Variant receptors of the nt^i type, however, yielded a major labeled band of molecular weight 40 000 ± 2000 and, in addition, in some experiments a minor band of about 37 000. The data are summarized in Table 2 for wild-type S49.1 cells and two independent cellular clones of both the nt⁻ and nt^i variant types. It is interesting to note that the same steroid-labeled polypeptide molecular weight was observed whether the wild-type receptor of lymphoma cells was in the activated state or stabilized in the non-activated form (4).

TABLE 2. Molecular weights of receptor types[a]

Receptor type	Molecular weight of steroid-labeled receptor polypeptide		
	native	after chymotrypsin	after trypsin
wild-type	94 700	38 000	29 000 and 27 000
nt⁻ type (clone 22R)	94 000	37 400	29 000 and 27 300
nt⁻ type (clone 83R)	94 000	37 400	
nt^i type (clone 55R)	40 300	39 000	29 200 and 27 400
nt^i type (clone 143R)	40 800	41 000	

[a]Cytosol receptor complexes with[³H]triamcinolone acetonide were subjected to photolabeling and subsequent SDS gel electrophoresis. Treatment with chymotrypsin (10 µg/ml, 5 min.) or trypsin (20 µg/ml, 30 min.) was after photolabeling. (Data from ref. 10).

PROTEOLYSIS OF RECEPTOR-GLUCOCORTICOID COMPLEXES

Partial proteolysis with α-chymotrypsin of wild-type receptors of mouse lymphomas (1, 18) and rat liver (23) has previously been shown to create receptor forms with abnormal DNA binding properties. This can best be demonstrated by use of DNA-cellulose chromatography. Figure 2 shows an experiment in which the wild-type receptor of lymphoma cells was exposed to α-chymotrypsin under mild conditions and subsequently chromatographed on DNA-cellulose. The treated complex required about 230 mM salt for elution as compared to 180 mM if not exposed to the enzyme. This increased affinity for DNA corresponds to that of native nt^i receptors (Table 1). Chymotrypsin treatment of nt⁻ receptors either did not change the affinity for DNA or produced a slight increase depending on the cell clone (Table 1). By contrast, α-chymotrypsin did not further increase the DNA affinity of nt^i variant receptors (Table 1).

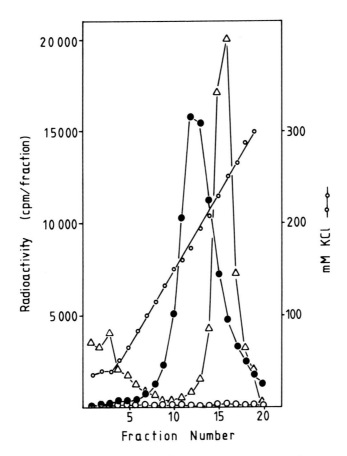

FIG. 2. DNA-cellulose chromatography.
S49.1 wild-type cytosol receptor complexes with [^{3}H]triamcinolone acetonide were activated at 20° and chromatographed on DNA-cellulose either
in the native state (●) or following
a 10 min. treatment with 10 µg/ml
α-chymotrypsin (Δ) or a 30 min.
treatment with 20 µg/ml trypsin (o).
(Data modified from ref. 4, 10).

Chymotrypsin treated wild-type and variant receptors were
also subjected to photoaffinity labeling and subsequent SDS
gel electrophoresis (Figure 3). With wild-type and nt$^-$ receptors, steroid-labeled polypeptides of molecular weight
38 000 were obtained while there was no change in the size
of nt^i receptors (Figure 3, Table 2).

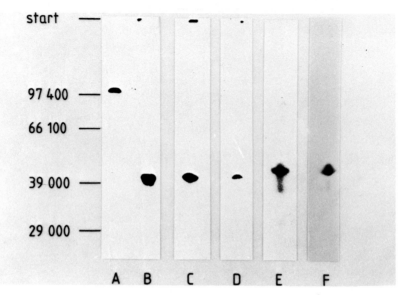

FIG. 3. <u>SDS gel electrophoresis of chymotrypsin-treated receptors</u>.
Cytosol receptor complexes with [^{3}H]triamcinolone acetonide were subjected to photolabeling followed by a 5 min.
treatment with 10 µg/ml α-chymotrypsin.   (A) Control of
S49.1 wild-type without chymotrypsin treatment; (B) S49.1
wild-type; (C) S49.1 nt$^-$ (clone 22R); (D) S49.1 nt$^-$ (clone
83R); (E) S49.1 nt^i (clone 55R); (F) S49.1 nt^i (clone 143R).

Partial proteolysis of wild-type, nt$^-$, and nt^i receptors
with trypsin yielded steroid-labeled polypeptides of molecular weights of about 38 000, 29 000, and 27 000 (Table 2).
The 38 000 fragment, however, was seen only under very mild
conditions and was readily further degraded to the smaller
receptor fragments (10). The tryptic receptor fragments of
27 000 to 29 000 which still carry the steroid label were
not able to bind to DNA as was shown by DNA-cellulose chromatography (Figure 2). These fragments correspond to the
so-called mero-receptors (12). It is interesting to note
that similar receptor fragments were also generated by a
lysine-specific protease but not by an arginine-specific
enzyme (10).

REACTION WITH ANTIBODIES

Monoclonal antibodies directed against the native rat
liver glucocorticoid receptor have recently been described
(22). Some of these were used with wild-type and variant

receptors of S49.1 mouse lymphoma cells (Table 3). The antibodies reacted both with wild-type and nt⁻ receptors but not with nt^i receptors. Interestingly, one of the antibodies bound slightly better to nt⁻ receptors than to the wildtype.

TABLE 3. Reaction with antibodies[a]

Receptor type	Binding of receptors to antibodies (%)	
	mab 49 (IgG)	mab 57 (IgM)
wild-type	47	21
nt⁻ type (clone 22R)	59	18
nt⁻ type (clone 83R)	54	22
nt^i type (clone 55R)	0	0
nt^i type (clone 143R)	1	1

[a]Cytosol receptor complexes with [^{3}H] triamcinolone acetonide were activated at 20° and subsequently incubated at 0° over night with excess monoclonal antibodies. In a second step,complexes were incubated with rabbit anti-mouse immunoglobulins coupled to Sepharose, extensively washed, and the amount of bound steroid determined. (Data from ref. 8).

DOMAIN MODEL

The data summarized here suggest a molecular model for the wild-type glucocorticoid receptor. Within the polypeptide chain of molecular weight 94 000 the receptor contains three functionally distinct domains: one for hormone binding, one for nuclear interaction, and a third domain which is involved in modulating nuclear interaction or DNA binding of the receptor-steroid complex. The domain model is presented in Figure 4.

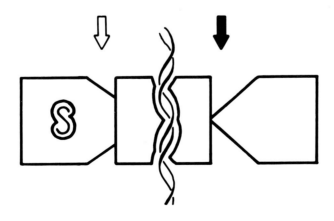

FIG. 4. Domain model

The function of the modulation domain is to alter the receptor-hormone complex in such a way that the biologically relevant acceptor sites in chromatin are recognized and the
expression of specific genes is regulated. The modulation
domain can therefore be regarded as "specifier domain" (21);
this is why the model of Figure 4 shows it as an arrow-like
structure. If the modulation domain is missing from the receptor molecule as is the case in nt^i variants the receptor-
hormone complex might bind too tightly to chromatin such
that it has no chance to find the appropriate gene loci
which need to be regulated. The modulation domain can easily
be removed from the wild-type receptor by proteolysis for
example with chymotrypsin. Even though the molecular weights
of the residual receptor structure and of the nt^i receptor
are not quite the same (Table 2) they appear to be functionally identical since both have increased affinity to DNA
and require the same abnormally high salt concentration to
elute from DNA-cellulose (Table 1).

In the graphic presentation of the receptor model (Figure
4) the three domains are shown as blocks of about equal size.
In reality, however, the sizes of these domains appear to
be quite different. The size of the modulation domain is
expected to be about 55 000 and that of the steroid and
nuclear binding domains together about 40 000. Even though
trypsin and other proteases cleave the 40 000 molecular
weight polypeptide to steroid binding fragments of 27 000 -
29 000 it might not be justified to conclude that the nuclear interaction domain is strictly localized within a polypeptide region of about 10 000 molecular weight. The proteases might cleave off or destroy some of the essential
parts of the nuclear binding domain while leaving others
intact. Therefore, the functional domains of the receptor
molecule may partially overlap in ways which are not obvious
from Figure 4. Also it should be mentioned that the sequential order of these domains along the 94 000 molecular
weight polypeptide of the wild-type receptor is unknown.
It is clear, however, that the modulation domain is located
distal to the cluster of steroid and nuclear binding domains
since this part of the molecule can be cleaved off under
conditions which leave the other two domains linked.

The model in Figure 4 also indicates the areas of the
receptor polypeptide which join the functional domains. The
linker between the modulation domain and the remainder of the
molecule is indicated by a closed arrow; it appears to be
some kind of a hinge region in the receptor molecule. It is
especially sensitive to proteases and can easily be cleaved
by chymotrypsin, trypsin and probably various other proteases including endogeneous cellular enzymes. The other linker, indicated by an open arrow, is apparently somewhat less
accessible to proteases but can be split, for example, by
trypsin.

The modulation domain appears to contain the main antigenic determinants of wild-type glucocorticoid receptors.
Antisera against the highly purified rat liver receptor did
not react with the steroid labeled chymotryptic receptor

fragments of rat liver or P1798 mouse lymphoma (5, 13, 14).
The cleaved off immunoreactive fragment, however, could be
recovered by gel filtration as a separate entity of high
molecular weight (3, 14). This finding supports the view
that chymotrypsin acts at a hinge region of the molecule
rather than cleaving the modulation domain into many fragments. The receptor of the glucocorticoid resistant P1798
mouse lymphoma which is of the nt^i type and has a polypeptide molecular weight of 40 000 (10) was not bound by the
polyclonal antibodies (19). Similarly, monoclonal antibodies directed against the rat liver glucocorticoid receptor
did not react with nt^i variant receptors of S49.1 cells
while they bound wild-type and nt^- receptors (Table 3). In
a recent study the nt^i type variant of the P1798 lymphoma
was used to search for the immunoreactive fragment in cell
extracts (14), however, it was not detected.

As to the cellular origin of nt^i variant receptors there
are several possible explanations: (I) a deletion mutation
in the receptor gene might lead to an abridged polypeptide
from which the modulation domain is missing; (II) a nonsense
mutation might cause premature protein chain termination;
(III) substitution of an amino acid in the hinge region of
the molecule might render it particularly susceptible to
intracellular proteolysis. The latter possibility appears
unlikely in view of the fact that no immunoreactive receptor
material was found in nt^i cells (14). Also the overexpres-
sion of an endogeneous protease that degrades the receptor
can be ruled out because hybrids of nt^i cells with either
wild-type or nt^- cells contain two distinct receptor types
(6, 24). Unfortunately we cannot at present distinguish
between alternatives (I) and (II).

The three functional domains disclosed for the wild-type
glucocorticoid receptor are probably not unique to this receptor type. It is likely that the same kind of domain
structure as outlined in Figure 4 is also present in receptors for other steroid hormones.

REFERENCES

1. Andreasen, P.A., and Gehring, U. (1981): Eur. J. Biochem.,
     120:443-449.
2. Benisek, W.F. (1977): Methods Enzymol. 46:469-479.
3. Carlstedt-Duke, J., Okret, S., Wrange, Ö., and Gustafs-
     son, J-Å. (1982): Proc. Natl. Acad. Sci. USA, 79:
     4260-4264.
4. Dellweg, H.-G., Hotz, A., Mugele, K., and Gehring, U.
     (1982): EMBO J., 1:285-289.
5. Eisen, H.J. (1982): In: Biochemical Actions of Hormones,
     edited by G. Litwack, Vol. IX, pp. 255-270. Academic
     Press, New York.
6. Gehring, U. (1980): In: Biochemical Actions of Hormones,
     edited by G. Litwack, Vol. VII, pp. 205-232. Academic
     Press, New York.
7. Gehring, U. (1980): In: Hormones and Cancer, edited by
     S. Iacobelli, H.R. Lindner, R.J.B. King, and M.E.

Lippman, pp. 79-88. Raven Press, New York.
8. Gehring, U. (1983): J. Steroid Biochem., 19:475-482.
9. Gehring, U., and Tomkins, G.M. (1974): Cell, 3:301-306.
10. Gehring, U., and Hotz, A. (1983): Biochemistry, 22:4013-4018.
11. Gehring, U., Ulrich, J., and Segnitz, B. (1982): Mol. Cell. Endocrinol., 28:605-611.
12. Miller, L.K. (1980): In: Biochemical Actions of Hormones, edited by G. Litwack, Vol. VII, pp. 233-243. Academic Press, New York.
13. Okret, S., Carlstedt-Duke, J., Wrange, Ö., Carlström, K., and Gustafsson, J.-Å. (1981): Biochim. Biophys. Acta, 677:205-219.
14. Okret, S., Stevens, Y.-W., Carlstedt-Duke, J., Wrange, Ö., Gustafsson, J.-Å., and Stevens, J. (1983): Cancer Res., 43:3127-3131.
15. Pfahl, M., Kelleher, R.J., and Bourgeois, S. (1978): Mol. Cell. Endocrinol., 10:193-207.
16. Sibley, C.H., and Tomkins, G.M. (1974): Cell, 2:221-227.
17. Simons, S.S., and Thompson, E.B. (1982): In: Biochemical Actions of Hormones, edited by G. Litwack, Vol. IX, 221-254. Academic Press, New York.
18. Stevens, J., and Stevens, Y.-M. (1981): Cancer Res., 41:125-133.
19. Stevens, J., Eisen, H.J., Stevens, Y.-W., Haubenstock, H., Rosenthal, R.L., and Artishevsky, A. (1981): Cancer Res., 41:134-137.
20. Stevens, J., Stevens, Y.-W., and Haubenstock, H. (1983): In: Biochemical Actions of Hormones, edited by G. Litwack, Vol. X, pp. 383-446. Academic Press, New York.
21. Vedeckis, W.V. (1983): Biochemistry, 22:1975-1983.
22. Westphal, H.M., Moldenhauer, G., and Beato, M. (1982): EMBO J., 1:1467-1471.
23. Wrange, Ö., and Gustafsson, J.-Å. (1978): J. Biol. Chem., 253:856-865.
24. Yamamoto, K.R., Gehring, U., Stampfer, M.R., and Sibley, C.H. (1976): Recent Progr. Horm. Res., 32:3-32.

Progress in Cancer Research and Therapy,
Vol. 31, edited by F. Bresciani, et al.
Raven Press, New York © 1984.

Glucocorticoid Sensitivity and Resistance in the NALM-6 Human Leukaemic Lymphoblast Cell Line

Philip A. Bell and Christopher N. Jones

Tenovus Institute for Cancer Research, Welsh National School of Medicine, Heath Park, Cardiff CF4 4XX, Wales, United Kingdom

Permanent cell lines established from neoplastic lymphoid cells represent valuable model systems for the analysis of the therapeutically important growth-inhibitory and cytotoxic effects of glucocorticoids and of the processes leading to steroid resistance in leukaemia and lymphoma. Studies with such cell lines may also illuminate the relationships between steroid responsiveness and differentiation status, for normal as well as neoplastic cells, since leukaemic cells can be classified in terms of their cell lineage affiliation and maturation status and they retain many of the phenotypic characteristics of their normal counterparts at a corresponding stage of differentiation (8,9).

A number of murine thymic lymphoma cell lines have been used for the genetic analysis of glucocorticoid action and for the study of steroid resistance (5,7), but only one steroid-sensitive human lymphoid cell line, CCRF-CEM, derived from a patient with acute lymphoblastic leukaemia (ALL), has been investigated in depth (4,10,15). In CEM cells, as in almost all of the murine cell lines that have been studied, steroid resistance appears to arise as a result of rare genetic (mutational) events; these are predominantly if not exclusively associated with glucocorticoid receptor defects (5,7,17). However, the behaviour of these cell lines may not necessarily be representative of that of the majority of cases of human ALL. CEM cells have an immunological phenotype characteristic of immature T lymphocytes (9,13), as do thymic lymphoma cell lines from the mouse; this phenotype is associated only with a minor subcategory of human ALL (8). Accordingly, we have begun to investigate the glucocorticoid responsiveness of a number of human leukaemic lymphoblast cell lines representative of other categories of ALL. Cells from one of the lines studied, NALM-6, a pre-B cell line (12-14), display a novel pattern of glucocorticoid sensitivity and resistance.

MATERIALS AND METHODS

NALM-6 cells were obtained from Dr. M.F. Greaves, Imperial Cancer Research Fund Laboratories, London, and were maintained in logarithmic growth in stationary suspension culture at 37°C in RPMI 1640 tissue

culture medium supplemented with 5% foetal calf serum; experiments were
initiated with cells at 10^5/ml in fresh medium. Details of experimental
procedures for cell counting, the determination of ^{3}H-thymidine incorporation and the estimation of DNA fragmentation and release from cells
prelabelled with ^{14}C-thymidine have been reported previously (3,4).
Glucocorticoid receptor levels were determined with ^{3}H-dexamethasone
using a whole-cell receptor assay (2).

RESULTS AND DISCUSSION

   NALM-6 cells have the phenotype of the pre-B cell variant of common
ALL; they express the common ALL and HLA-DR antigens, are terminal
deoxynucleotidyltransferase-positive and possess cytoplasmic but not
surface membrane immunoglobulin (12-14). Glucocorticoid receptors
could readily be detected in these cells using a whole-cell assay; the
concentration of specific, saturable binding sites for ^{3}H-dexamethasone
was 9580 ± 970 sites/cell, with an equilibrium dissociation constant of
13.0 ± 1.8 nM at 37^{0}C. In addition, the cells were responsive to glucocorticoids, as noted earlier by Ralph (16). Dexamethasone inhibited the
incorporation of ^{3}H-thymidine by the cells in a time- and concentration-
dependent manner, as shown in Fig. 1. Half-maximal inhibition was produced by approx. 10 nM dexamethasone, and 1 µM dexamethasone produced
total inhibition of incorporation after 4 days of treatment, in absolute
as well as relative terms. Inhibition of ^{3}H-thymidine incorporation
was glucocorticoid-specific (results not shown) and by all of the generally accepted criteria appeared to represent a glucocorticoid receptor-
mediated effect that was exerted in a uniform manner on the entire cell
population.

   As anticipated from these results, treatment of NALM-6 cells with
1 µM dexamethasone resulted in the inhibition of cell growth; cell num-

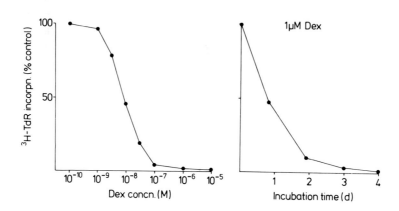

FIG. 1.   Concentration-dependence of the effect of dexamethasone on
^{3}H-thymidine incorporation by NALM-6 cells, 70-72h after steroid addition
(left panel); time-course of the effect of 1 µM dexamethasone on ^{3}H-
thymidine incorporation, determined by pulse-labelling for 2h (right
panel).

bers reached a maximum 2d after steroid addition and then began to decline (Fig. 2). They did not continue to decline, however, but reached
a minimum after 4d and remained constant thereafter. Cell viability,
determined by nigrosine dye exclusion, declined between 1 and 4d after
steroid addition and then stabilized, so that a substantial proportion
of the cells remained viable for a prolonged period (Fig. 2). No mitoses
were evident among the cells of this persistent population, and they
were smaller than untreated cells and had a more restricted size distribution. Thus, all of the cells appeared to be growth-inhibited by
the steroid, but only a proportion of them were killed. The growth-
arrested cells were capable of resuming growth after being washed free
of steroid and transferred to fresh medium; further addition of dexamethasone to the fresh medium prevented this resumption of growth.
These results suggest that growth inhibition is a direct, reversible
action.

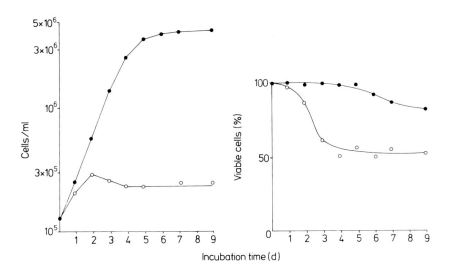

FIG. 2.   Effect of 1 µM dexamethasone on the growth (left panel) and
viability (right panel) of NALM-6 cells. Solid symbols, untreated cells;
open symbols, steroid-treated cells.

The resistance of a substantial fraction of the cells to steroid-
induced killing was confirmed by measurement of the release of labelled
DNA fragments from cells prelabelled with ^{14}C-thymidine for 24h. The
endonucleolytic cleavage of chromatin and the release of fragmented DNA
from the dying cells are characteristic features of the cytotoxic actions
of glucocorticoids and certain other agents on lymphoid cells (18,19).
Virtually complete release of ^{14}C-DNA from steroid-sensitive CEM-C7 cells
is observed after treatment with 1 µM dexamethasone for 4d (4), but
exposure of NALM-6 cells to the same concentration led only to the partial release of ^{14}C-DNA. Net release of ^{14}C-DNA in response to 1 µM
dexamethasone amounted to approx. 30% of the total, and occurred predomi-

nantly during the first 3 days of treatment, as shown in Fig. 3. In contrast, exposure to 5 mM butyrate, another agent that is cytotoxic for immature lymphoid cells (3), led to near complete DNA fragmentation and release (Fig. 3). Additional experiments established that 1 μM dexamethasone did produce maximal, though incomplete, DNA damage.

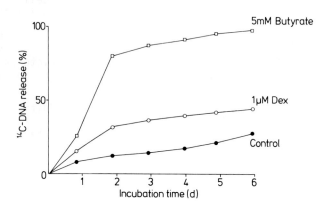

FIG. 3.   Effects of 1 μM dexamethasone or 5 mM butyrate on the release of ^{14}C-DNA fragments from NALM-6 cells.

     This pronounced disparity between the extent of the growth-inhibitory and cytotoxic actions of dexamethasone could have been due to heterogeneity within the NALM-6 cell line, and so sublines of NALM-6 were isolated by cloning and subsequent recloning at limiting dilution. All of the clonally derived sublines that were investigated responded to dexamethasone in a manner similar to that of the parent line; although there were variations in the proportion of cells killed and in the final plateau concentration of cells, they all showed the mixed response of complete growth inhibition and partial killing. No sublines showing exclusively cytotoxic or growth-inhibitory responses were identified, and so we conclude that the mixed response is an inherent feature of clonally derived NALM-6 cells. It is interesting to note that leukaemic cell lines established from mice infected with Abelson leukaemia virus respond to glucocorticoid treatment in what may be a similar manner (11); like NALM-6, these too are pre-B cell lines.
     The mechanisms underlying the heterogeneous response of NALM-6 cells to dexamethasone and other glucocorticoids are presumably of epigenetic origin, and remain to be elucidated. The cytotoxic response to glucocorticoids appears to be a differentiation-linked response that is expressed only in immature lymphoid cells (1), so it is possible that the mixed response shown by NALM-6 cells reflects the outcome of kinetic competition between cell killing and a process of conversion of the cells to a state where they are growth-inhibited but not killed - i.e., differentiation. In this respect it is noteworthy that treatment of NALM-6 cells with the tumour-promoting phorbol ester, 12-O-tetradecanoyl-phorbol-13-acetate (TPA), induced total resistance to both the growth-inhibitory and cytotoxic actions of dexamethasone, as shown in Fig. 4. This phorbol ester has been shown to induce some degree of differentiation

in a number of leukaemic cell lines (6). Steroid resistance did not
appear to be a consequence of the lowered growth rate of TPA-treated
cells, since cells whose growth rate had been reduced to a similar extent
by serum deprivation remained steroid-responsive (Fig. 4). The change
in phenotype induced by TPA treatment was modest; reactivity of the
cells with an antiserum to terminal deoxynucleotidyltransferase was markedly reduced, but the expression of all other markers was unchanged.

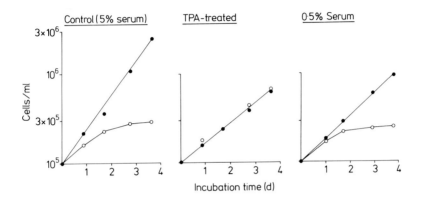

FIG. 4.   Effect of 1 μM dexamethasone on the growth of untreated
NALM-6 cells (left panel), cells treated with 10 ng/ml of TPA (centre
panel), or cells grown in 0.5% serum (right panel). Solid symbols,
control cells; open symbols, steroid-treated cells.

CONCLUSIONS

The studies reported here have demonstrated that cells of the NALM-6
human leukaemic lymphoblast cell line can become resistant to the cytotoxic and growth-inhibitory actions of glucocorticoids by mechanisms that
appear to be of non-mutational origin. Clearly, it will be important to
determine whether these processes are operative to any significant extent
in human leukaemia, and whether they can account for the occurrence of
steroid resistance in any patients. A process that leads to growth inhibition without cell killing would not only limit the effectiveness of
glucocorticoid therapy but would also prevent proliferation-dependent
cytotoxic agents from exerting their full effects, and would provide a
reservoir of malignant cells capable of resuming growth on the cessation
of chemotherapy. Unlike a mutational mode of resistance, however, such
a process is potentially reversible.

ACKNOWLEDGEMENTS

We are grateful to Dr. M.F. Greaves for providing the NALM-6 cell
lines and performing the analyses of immunological markers, and to
Dr. R.M. Gledhill (King's College Hospital Medical School, London) for
cloning the cells. We thank the Tenovus Organization for continuing
financial support.

REFERENCES

1. Bell, P.A. (1981): In: Mechanisms of Steroid Action, edited by G.P. Lewis, and M. Ginsburg, pp.75-84. Macmillan, London.
2. Bell, P.A., Greaves, M.F., Sloman, J.C., Thompson, E.N., and Whittaker, J.A. (1983): J. Steroid Biochem., 19: 851-855.
3. Bell, P.A., and Jones, C.N. (1982): Biochem. Biophys. Res. Commun., 104: 1202-1208.
4. Borthwick, N.M., and Bell, P.A. (1982): Eur. J. Cancer Clin. Oncol., 18: 1093-1098.
5. Bourgeois, S., and Newby, R.F. (1980): In: Hormones and Cancer, Progress in Cancer Research and Therapy, Vol. 14, edited by S. Iacobelli, R.J.B. King, H.R. Lindner, and M.E. Lippman, pp.67-77. Raven Press, New York.
6. Delia, D., Greaves, M.F., Newman, R.A., Sutherland, D.R., Minowada, J., Kung, P., and Goldstein, G. (1982): Int. J. Cancer, 29: 23-31.
7. Gehring, U. (1980): In: Hormones and Cancer, Progress in Cancer Research and Therapy, Vol. 14, edited by S. Iacobelli, R.J.B. King, H.R. Lindner, and M.E. Lippman, pp.79-98. Raven Press, New York.
8. Greaves, M.F. (1981): Cancer Res., 41: 4752-4766.
9. Greaves, M.F., and Janossy, G. (1978): Biochim. Biophys. Acta, 516: 193-230.
10. Harmon, J.M., Norman, M.R., Fowlkes, B.J., and Thompson, E.B. (1979): J. Cell Physiol., 98: 267-278.
11. Harris, A.W., and Baxter, J.D. (1979): In: Glucocorticoid Hormone Action, edited by J.D. Baxter and G.G. Rousseau, pp.423-448. Springer-Verlag, Berlin.
12. Hurwitz, R., Hozier, J., LeBien, T., Minowada, J., Gajl-Peczalska, G., Kubonishi, I., and Kersey, J. (1979): Int. J. Cancer, 23: 174-180.
13. Minowada, J., Janossy, G., Greaves, M.F., Tsubota, T., Srivastava B.I.S., Morikawa, S., and Tatsumi, E. (1978): J. Natl. Cancer Inst., 60: 1269-1277.
14. Minowada, J., Oshimura, M., Abe, S., Greaves, M.F., Janossy, G., and Sandberg, A.A. (1978): Proc. Am. Assoc. Cancer Res., 19: 109 (Abstract 434).
15. Norman, M.R., and Thompson, E.B. (1977): Cancer Res., 37: 3785-3790.
16. Ralph, P. (1979): Immunol. Rev., 48: 107-121.
17. Schmidt, T.J., Harmon, J.M., and Thompson, E.B. (1980): Nature, 286: 507-510.
18. Thomas, N., Edwards, J.L., and Bell, P.A. (1983): J. Steroid Biochem., 18: 519-524.
19. Wyllie, A.H. (1980): Nature, 284: 555-556.

Progress in Cancer Research and Therapy,
Vol. 31, edited by F. Bresciani, et al.
Raven Press, New York © 1984.

Cellular and Molecular Events Regulated by Androgens in the S115 Mouse Mammary Tumour Cell Line

P.D. Darbre, S.A. Curtis, and R.J.B. King

Imperial Cancer Research Fund, London WC2A 3PX, England

Steroid hormones regulate the growth of many normal and tumour cells, but the detailed mechanism is still unclear. The early events, involving binding of steroid to its specific receptor within the cell, have been studied extensively (7), and more recently, molecular studies have defined regions in the DNA which bind to the receptor molecules (2, 13, 18, 21, 31). However, later events remain within an unknown 'black box'. We have attempted to define specific post-receptor events which are regulated by androgens in breast tumour cells, looking at both the cellular and molecular level.

Our model system has involved the use of the S115 mammary tumour cell line derived from the androgen-dependent Shionogi 115 mouse mammary carcinoma (17). When this cell line is cultured continuously in the presence of testosterone (+A cells), it exhibits a positive proliferative response to androgen (22). Growth of these cells is responsive to but not dependent on androgens and after several weeks of culture in the absence of testosterone, the cells become unresponsive to androgens (-A cells) (23, 28). This loss of response is not accompanied by major changes in receptor levels (15, 16) suggesting that post-receptor event(s) are involved.

CELLULAR EVENTS

Removal of testosterone from +A cells results in changes within 1-3 days, including a reduced growth rate (15), an increased density regulation (28) and a dramatic change from fibroblastic to epithelial morphology (6, 30). The cells become more sensitive to certain growth stimuli, such as serum concentration, (28) and develop an increased dependence on anchorage to the substrate for growth (29), including loss of ability to grow in suspension culture (30). In addition, marked changes occur in the cell membrane and cytoskeletal structure. Specific focal adhesions appear between cell and substrate, there is an increase of cell surface fibronectin, and intracellular actin becomes organized into well-defined microfilament bundles (4, 29). Based on these phenotypic changes in vitro, it has been suggested that in this cell line, androgens control a change between a normal (- testosterone) and a transformed (+ testosterone) phenotype. Thus, these cells provide a model for studying both steroid-controlled development of transformed characteristics and the loss of steroid hormone sensitivity.

MOLECULAR EVENTS

In view of the well-documented involvement of mouse mammary tumour virus (MMTV) in the development of mammary carcinomas in the mouse, it was considered possible that viral elements might play a role in this change of phenotype in the S115 cell line. No virus particles have been detected yet in the S115 cells (29) but have been identified in the Shionogi tumour (1). However, absence of exogenous virus units is not critical in that most inbred strains of mice contain also endogenous, inherited MMTV sequences (24) and it could be these latter units that are involved. Furthermore, glucocorticoids control the expression of MMTV (20, 31), and although androgens or oestrogens had not to date been shown to play any role, the involvement of some steroid hormones made it at least interesting to study MMTV in the S115 cells. Thus we have sought to characterize MMTV-related sequences and their expression in the S115 cells.

<u>Proviral Copies in S115 DNA</u>

Proviral MMTV DNA contains at least three genes, <u>gal</u>, <u>pol</u> and <u>env</u>, which are bounded at both ends by long terminal repeat segments (LTR) (3, 9). As yet, no oncogene has been defined in this virus, but from sequencing studies (9, 10, 11) and <u>in vitro</u> translation (8), an open reading frame (orf) has been found within the LTR which has coding potential for an additional protein(s).

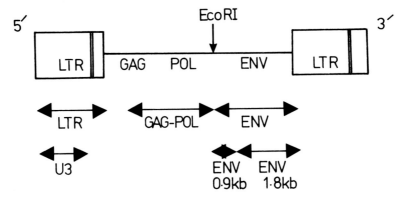

FIG. 1. Restriction map of MMTV proviral DNA from the exogenous strain of GR mice.

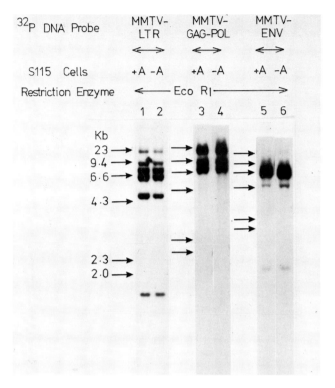

FIG. 2. Restriction enzyme analysis of proviral MMTV sequences in the
DNA of S115 cells. Positions of the molecular weight markers are
indicated by arrows.

The characterization of MMTV sequences in the S115 cells has relied
on restriction enzyme digestion and Southern blotting, using the DNA
probes as indicated in Fig. 1. The detailed methods used have been
described previously (5). The restriction enzyme Eco RI cleaves the
proviral DNA once, generating two fragments both of which contain LTR
sequences but only the 5' fragment contains gag-pol sequences and only
the 3' fragment contains env sequences. Fig. 2 shows Eco RI digests of
DNA from both androgen maintained (+A) and androgen deprived (-A) cells
hybridized to three different probes. The S115 cells contained MMTV-
related sequences and no difference was noted in proviral copies between
the +A and -A cells.

Expression of Proviral Copies - Androgen Control

Although no gross difference was found in the proviral copies present
in the +A and -A cells, distinct differences were found in terms of the
RNA present. Characterization of RNA sequences related to MMTV was
carried out by gel electrophoresis and Northern blotting, the details of
which have been published elsewhere (5). Fig. 3 shows a Northern blot
of RNA from +A and -A cells which was probed with the LTR probe. RNA
was found only in the androgen-maintained (+A) and not in the long-term

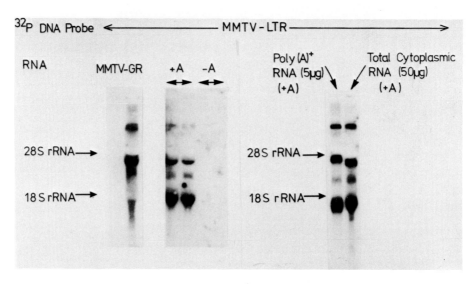

FIG. 3. Analysis of MMTV-LTR-related RNA in both +A and -A S115 cells.

androgen-deprived (-A) cells. The +A cells produced at least 4 RNA
species and these are compared in Fig. 3 to the RNA produced in mink
lung cells infected with the exogenous GR strain of MMTV. The major
species of RNA in the +A cells was of 16S, although 35S, 24S and 20S RNA
was also found. However, this contrasted to the pattern of RNA in the
MMTV-infected cells where the 16S RNA was barely detectable. Fig. 3
shows that these LTR-related RNAs were all polyadenylated and therefore
unlikely to represent non-specific hybridization to ribosomal RNA.
Furthermore, it is known that gross RNA levels per S115 cell are
unaffected by androgens (14), indicating that the difference between
+A and -A cell RNA is a specific effect.
    The extent of homology of these different RNAs in the +A cells with
different parts of the MMTV genome was examined (Fig. 4). The 35S RNA
hybridized to all the probes, suggesting that it was the full-length
MMTV transcript. The 24S RNA contained only LTR and env sequences,
indicating it to be the spliced env message. However, the 16S RNA was
only detected strongly by the LTR and U3 probes and weakly by the 1.8 Kb
region of the env gene. This indicated that it lacked the entire gag-
pol and 0.9 Kb env regions and presumably part of the 1.8 Kb env region
also. It is thus possible that this 16S RNA could be the spliced
message encoding the orf protein. A similar RNA has been characterized
recently from other mouse strains (25, 27).
    A time-course of loss of these MMTV-LTR-related RNAs from +A cells
during androgen withdrawal (-T) (Fig. 5) revealed loss of RNA after 6
days and complete disappearance by 7-9 weeks. Recovery of RNA during
re-addition of androgen (+T) can also be achieved (Fig. 5). Withdrawal
of androgen for 5 days followed by re-addition for 1 day restored RNA
levels, as did withdrawal for 6 weeks followed by re-addition for 1
week.

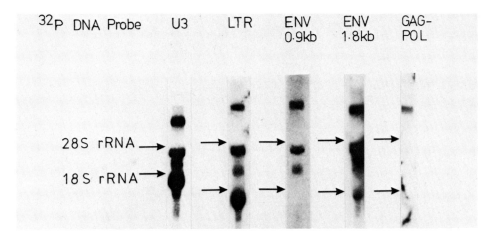

FIG. 4. Homology of S115 RNA to different parts of proviral MMTV

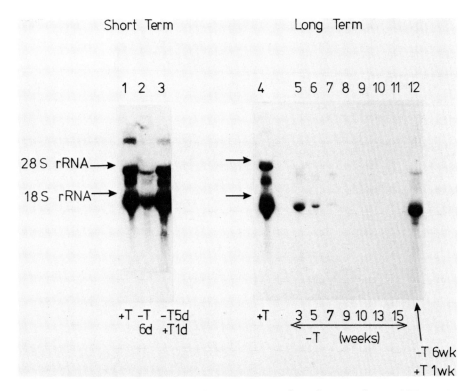

FIG. 5. Androgen sensitivity of MMTV-LTR-related RNA of +A S115 cells

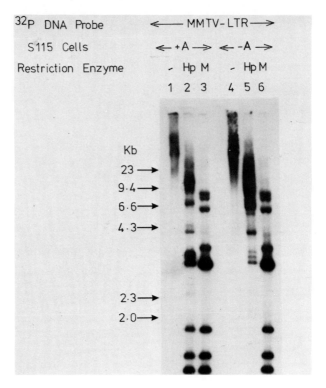

FIG. 6. Methylation patterns of proviral sequences in the DNA of +A and -A S115 cells.

Expression of Proviral Copies - Glucocorticoid Control

As the synthetic glucocorticoid, dexamethasone, is known to stimulate MMTV proviral transcription, we studied how it might interact with androgens to affect levels of MMTV-related RNAs in the S115 cells. Addition of dexamethasone to +A cells did not alter the RNA present and did not stimulate any RNA production in the -A cells. An increase in LTR-related RNA was found when dexamethasone was tested in +A cells which had been deprived of testosterone for 1 to 4 weeks (5).

Role of DNA Methylation in Proviral Transcription

In view of the suggested role of DNA methylation in gene expression (12, 19), DNA methylation was studied in the proviral copies of +A and -A S115 cells to see if lack of RNA in the -A cells was accompanied by any alteration in methylation patterns. DNA methylation patterns can be studied using the isoschizomeric restriction enzymes Hpa II and Msp I. These enzymes cut unmethylated DNA at the same sites but differ in their sensitivity to cytosine methylation (26). Fig.6 shows DNA from +A and -A cells either undigested or digested with Hpa II or Msp I. The resulting Southern blots were probed with the LTR probe. Since the two enzymes cut both +A and -A DNA into different fragments, it appeared that both DNA samples were methylated to some extent. If either DNA had been totally unmethylated, identical patterns would have been seen with both enzymes. However, comparison of the enzymes patterns between the +A and -A DNA did reveal differences in the extent of methylation. Similar patterns were found with the enzyme Msp I but different patterns were seen with Hpa II, indicating that -A cell DNA is more extensively methylated at certain Hpa II-sensitive sites than is +A DNA.

CONCLUSIONS

1) We have demonstrated the presence in S115 cells of DNA sequences homologous to mouse mammary tumour virus.

2) MMTV-related m-RNA is found in S115 cells only when grown in the long-term presence of androgen. Experiments on short-term withdrawal and re-addition of androgen have demonstrated further the androgen-sensitivity of this RNA.

3) The major 16S m-RNA in S115 cells is predominantly derived from the LTR and may code for the putative orf protein(s).

4) Dexamethasone alone will increase the RNA in short-term androgen-deprived +A cells but not in -A cells or in testosterone-stimulated +A cells.

5) Prolonged culture in the absence of androgen results not only in loss of MMTV-related RNA but also in an increase in methylation of certain MMTV-related sequences in the DNA.

These results have implications relevant to the mechanism of steroid hormone action and in particular on the progression of tumour cells from steroid-sensitivity to insensitivity. Further studies on the relationship between the phenotypic changes observed in the S115 cells, viral RNA and DNA methylation should provide much useful information.

ACKNOWLEDGEMENTS

We thank Drs. Clive Dickson and Gordon Peters for providing the cloned MMTV DNA used in these studies and for their help.

REFERENCES

1. Bellocci, M., Malorni, W., Natoli, C., Quintarelli, G., and Sica, G. (1983): *J. Steroid Biochem. Suppl.*, 19:595.
2. Chandler, V.L., Maler, B.A., and Yamamoto, K.R. (1983): *Cell*, 33:489-499.
3. Cohen, J.C., Majors, J.E., and Varmus, H.E. (1979): *J. Virol.*, 32:483-496.
4. Couchman, J.R., Yates, J., King, R.J.B., and Badley, R.A. (1981): *Cancer Res.*, 41:263-269.
5. Darbre, P., Dickson, C., Peters, G., Page, M., Curtis, S., and King, R.J.B. (1983): *Nature*, 303:431-433.
6. Desmond, W.J., Wolbers, S.J., and Sato, G. (1976): *Cell*, 8:79-86.
7. DeSombre, E.R. (1982): *Clinics in Oncology*, 1:191-213.
8. Dickson, C., Smith, R., and Peters, G. (1981): *Nature*, 291:511-513.
9. Donehower, L.A., Huang, A.L., and Hager, G.L. (1981): *J. Virol.*, 37:226-238.

10. Donehower, L.A., Fleurdelys, B., and Hager, G.L. (1983): *J. Virol.*, 45:941-949.
11. Fasel, N., Pearson, K., Buetti, E., and Diggelmann, H. (1982): *EMBO J.*, 1:3-7.
12. Felsenfeld, G., and McGhee, J. (1982): *Nature*, 296:602-603.
13. Geisse, S., Scheidereit, C., Westphal, H.M., Hynes, N.E., Groner, B., and Beato, M. (1982): *EMBO J.*, 1:1613-1619.
14. Jagus, R. (1979): *Expl. Cell Res.*, 118:115-125.
15. King, R.J.B., Cambray, G.J., and Robinson, J.H. (1976): *J. Steroid Biochem.*, 7:869-873.
16. King, R.J.B., Cambray, G.J., Jagus-Smith, R., Robinson, J.H., and Smith, J.A. (1976): In: *Receptors and Mechanisms of Steroid Hormones*, edited by J.R. Pasqualini, pp.215-261. Marcel Dekker, New York.
17. Minesita, T., and Yamaguchi, K. (1965): *Cancer Res.*, 25:1168-1175.
18. Mulvihill, E.R., LePennec, J.P., and Chambon, P. (1982): *Cell.*, 24:621-632.
19. Razin, A., and Riggs, A.D. (1980): *Science*, 210:604-610.
20. Ringold, G.M. (1979): *Biochim. biophys. Acta*, 560:487-508.
21. Scheidereit, C., Geisse, S., Westphal, H.M., and Beato, M. (1983): *Nature*, 304:749-752.
22. Smith, J.A., and King, R.J.B. (1972): *Expl. Cell Res.*, 73:351-359.
23. Stanley, E.R., Palmer, R.E., and Sohn, U. (1977): *Cell*, 10:35-44.
24. Traina, V.L., Taylor, B.A., and Cohen, J.C. (1981): *J. Virol.*, 40:735-744.
25. Van Ooyen, A.J.J., Michalides, R.J.A.M., and Nusse, R. (1983): *J. Virol.*, 46:362-370.
26. Waalwijk, C., and Flavell, R.A. (1978): *Nucleic Acids Res.*, 5:4631-4641.
27. Wheeler, D.A., Butel, J.S., Medina, D., Cardiff, R.D., and Hager, G.L. (1983): *J. Virol.*, 46:42-49.
28. Yates, J., and King, R.J.B. (1978): *Cancer Res.*, 38:4135-4137.
29. Yates, J., Couchman, J.R., and King, R.J.B. (1980): In: *Hormones and Cancer*, edited by Iacobelli *et al.*, pp.31-39. Raven Press, New York.
30. Yates, J., and King, R.J.B. (1981): *Cancer Res.*, 41:258-262.
31. Other chapters in this book.

Progress in Cancer Research and Therapy,
Vol. 31, edited by F. Bresciani, et al.
Raven Press, New York © 1984.

Combined Cytotoxic and Endocrine Therapy in Breast Cancer

*,† Carsten Rose and *Henning T. Mouridsen

*Department of Oncology I, The Finsen Institute; and †The Fibiger Laboratory, DK-2100 Copenhagen, Denmark

During the early 7o's it became established that the use of multible drug cytotoxic therapy leads to higher rates of response than those obtained by endocrine treatment of advanced breast cancer. Irrespective of combinations and schedules of the different cytotoxic drugs, response rates of 5o-7o% were achieved. However, the realization that cure cannot be accomplished in advanced breast cancer by this rather toxic treatment has reinforced the use of endocrine therapy either in combination with cytotoxic drugs or as single modality therapy. Furthermore, the use of hormonal manipulation as first line therapy is justified since there is a close correlation between the content of estrogen and progesterone receptors in breast cancer and the hormone responsiveness of the tumor. Utilizing this knowledge of the receptor status of the tissue, it is possible to select a group of patients for endocrine therapies where response rates are comparable to those obtained by cytotoxic treatment (48).

However, since the modes of action and spectra of toxicities for cytotoxic and endocrine therapies are different, and since experimental, pathological, and clinical data substantiate the concept that mammary tumors are heterogeneous, it is attractive to explore new approaches if combining cytotoxic and endocrine treatment for advanced breast cancer in order to improve the rate of response and to be able to substantially prolong survival without an increased treatment related morbidity.

RATIONALE FOR COMBINED THERAPY

Tumor heterogeneity

It is well known that mammary tumors differ greatly with respect to both inter- and intratumor morphology (19,21). Using flow-cytometry, it has been shown that clones of tumor cells with different DNA content are found within the same human mammary carcinoma (7,79). Perhaps even more important neoplastic subpopulations have been demonstrated to exhibit different growth behaviour and different functional properties. Dexter and co-workers (18) were able to isolate cell-sublines from a spontaneously developed mammary adenocarcinoma in mice that differed both in morphology and with respect to growth properties such as in vitro doubling time, cloning efficiency and tumorigenicity. Not surprisingly, Heppner et al (3o) could demonstrate that these cell-lines exhibited different sensitivities to various drugs and drug scheduling.

Experimental mouse mammary tumors (9,71,72) seem to contain both hormone dependent and hormone independent tumor cells with corresponding high and low levels of estrogen and progesterone receptors.

Human tumors have also been shown to variate intra-tumorally with regard to estrogen receptors (69). Allegra and co-workers (2) found that although the receptor pattern were identical in 85% of simultaneously examined metastatic sites, receptor status following hormone therapy shifted from being receptor positive to receptor negative. This finding could indicate heterogeneity in the original estrogen receptor pattern and is generally in agreement with the experimental observation, that hormonedependent GR-mouse mammary tumors allowed to regress completely upon hormone withdrawal all exhibit spontaneous regrowth at a later point of time (lo). As a consequence of their previous finding of heterogeneity within the GR-tumor, Sluyser et al. (73) treated tumor-bearing animals with a combination of cyclophosphamide and tamoxifen and observed that this combined treatment resulted in an additive inhibition of tumor growth.

Clinical evidence for independent action of cytotoxic
and endocrine therapy.

Is it beyond the scope of this review to present data for the many obvious biological, biochemical, and pharmacological differencies in modes of action and toxicities between cytotoxic and endocrine therapies. How endocrine manipulations lead to regression of hormone dependent tumors is far from known (28) but arrest of growth and subsequent cell-lysis are major events during the course of tumor regression. Cytotoxic therapy generally leads to an interruption in replication of DNA and is thought to be most active in tumors with a high growth fraction. Thus, a possible pharmacodynamic antagonism of the two treatment modalities is conceivable.

Goldie et al. (27) have analyzed the rationale for the repetitive use of non-cross resistant cytotoxic therapy by a mathematical model and further developed this model by which they could substantiate the claim that use of concurrent cytotoxic and endocrine therapy achieves the greatest probability of cure when adjuvant therapy is employed in treatment of breast cancer (26). Basic assumptions in this model are that cytotoxic and endocrine therapies act independently, and that the two modalities are non-cross resistant. It therefore seems important both conceptually and clinically to investigate whether these two basic conditions are valid.

Table 1 shows the response to endocrine therapy with tamoxifen in relation to the estrogen receptor status of either the primary tumor or a metastasis. Although different assay techniques and cut-off values have been used, estrogen receptor status seems to be a good predictor of response to endocrine therapy. Because an inverse correlation has been demonstrated between a low labeling endex and a high content of estrogen receptors in breast carcinomas (49,7o), Lippman and associates (4o) examined whether estrogen receptor status was related to response to cytotoxic therapy.

Table 1.   RESPONSE TO TAMOXIFEN IN RELATION TO ER-STATUS

Ref.	Cut-off limit fmol/mg cyt.prot.	Responders/Total ER-positive	ER-negative
Rose 82	1o	12/24	2/14
Stewart 8o	-	7/18	o/5
Ingle 81	-	5/11	-
Beex 81	5	7/13	o/7
Nagai 8o	-	4/7	2/7
Mattsson 8o	1o	6/9	-
Morgan 82	1o	1o/15	o/3
Lipton 82	1o	1o/18	-
Mouridsen 8o	2o	6/12	1/9
Mouridsen 79	2o	7/11	2/9
Tormey 82	-	7/23	o/7
Ingle 82	3	5/13	o/7
Glick 81	1o	29/48	-
Bezwoda 82	3	15/24	-
Rubens 82	5	4/24	o/12
Total		13o/27o	7/73
%		5o	1o
95% C.L.,%		44-56	4-19

Their data (table 2) suggested, that the absence of estrogen receptors predicted a favourable response to cytotoxic treatment. However, examining pooled data from the literature, it is not obvious, that any such correlation exists (table 2) since response to cytotoxic treatment is in the range of 5o% for both estrogen receptor positive and negative patients.

The data in table 3a and 3b from 9 randomized clinical trials in advanced breast cancer (all fulfilling the criteria stated below) demonstrate, that there is considerable cross sensitivity and nearly a complete cross resistance between tamoxifen treatment and different additive and inhibitive endocrine modalities. In contrast, an analysis of data concerning cross sensitivity and non-cross resistance between endocrine and cytotoxic therapy shows response rates to second line cytotoxic therapy of about 6o% in both responders and non-responders to various forms of endocrine therapy (table 4).

Table 2.   RESPONSE TO CYTOTOXIC THERAPY IN RELATION TO ER–STATUS

Ref.	Cut–off limit fmol/mg cyt.prot.	Responders/Total ER–positive	ER–negative
Lippman 78	1o	3/25	34/48
v.Maillot 8o	15	26/51	15/5o
Kiang 8o	3 or 4	17/19	9/21
Hilf 8o	1o	11/22	15/22
Jonat 8o	2o	14/23	1o/3o
Nomura 8o	2	7/16	6/31
Rosenbaum 8o	1o	12/16	6/14
Rubens 8o	5	2o/33	8/14
Samal 8o	3 or 4	28/36	28/45
Young 8o	6	6/9	8/2o
Manni 8o	–	1o/17	9/18
Cocconi 83	3	6/13	5/7
Total		16o/28o	155/317
%		57	49
95% C.L., %		52–64	44–55

It appears from table 5, that response rates of 25-35% can be obtained when endocrine therapy follows multiple drug cytotoxic treatment irrespective of response to the first treatment.

Although the compiled data originate from retrospective analysis, the impression that response to first line endocrine therapy predicts a response to subsequent endocrine therapy appears to be valid. On the contrary, the response to cytotoxic therapy following endocrine therapy or visa versa seems unaffected by the response to the first treatment modality. Thus, the idea of independent action and non-cross resistance between endocrine and cytotoxic therapies is conceivable.

Lippman recently (42) questioned whether the simultaneous combination of the two different treatment approaches should continue or not. We will in the following review the available clinical data on combined cytotoxic-endocrine treatment of advanced breast cancer.

Criteria of selection

The clinical trials reviewed have met the following criteria:
1. the trials should be randomized and prospective.
2. a maximum of 2o patients in each treatment group.
3. statements of response criteria compatible with the UICC criteria (78).
4. information about response, duration of response, survival, dominant site of disease, side effects etc. must be given.

Table 3a.   CROSS SENSITIVITY TO SECOND–LINE ENDOCRINE THERAPY

Ref.	2. line drug	Cross sensitivity (CR+PR)/R	(%)	95% C.L., %
Stewart 8o	DES	2/5	(4o)	5-85
Ingle 81	DES	5/11	(46)	17-77
Beex 81	EE$_2$	1/3	(33)	1-91
Mattsson 8o	MPA	4/4	(1oo)	4o-1oo
Ingle 82	MEG	2/6	(33)	4-78
Smith 81	AG+H	4/6	(67)	22-96
Harvey 82	AG+H	4/9	(44)	14-79
Ingle 82	AG+H	1/4	(25)	1-81
Total		23/48	(48)	33-63

R: Responders to Tamoxifen.

5. the articles must have been written in English, French or German to be considered.
Exceptions have been made for two phase II trials in view of their theoretical importance (3,59).

Table 3b.   NON–CROSS RESISTANCE TO SECOND–LINE ENDOCRINE THERAPY

Ref.	2. line drug	Non-cross resistance (CR+PR)/NR	(%)	95% C.L., %
Stewart 8o	DES	1/1o	(1o)	o-45
Ingle 81	DES	4/22	(18)	5-4o
Beex 81	EE$_2$	o/2	(o)	o-84
Westerberg 8o	FLU	1/1o	(1o)	o-45
Mattsson 8o	MPA	2/6	(33)	4-78
Ingle 82	MEG	o/1o	(o)	o-31
Smith 81	AG+H	5/34	(15)	5-31
Harvey 82	AG+H	1/14	(7)	o-34
Ingle 82	AG+H	o/7	(o)	o-41
Total		14/115	(12)	7-2o

NR: Non-responders to Tamoxifen.

Table 4.   ENDOCRINE THERAPY FOLLOWED BY CYTOTOXIC THERAPY

Ref.	1. line treat- ment	Response rate (CR+PR)/N	2. line treat- ment	Cross sensiti- vity (CR+PR)/R	Non-cross resistance (CR+PR)/NR
Legha 80	ET	53/136	CT	37/53	56/83
Manni 80	ET	27/66	CT	2o/27	25/39
Kiang 81	DES	12/27	CF	3/6	3/3
Tormey 82	ET	11/27	DA	5/11	1o/16
Bezwoda 82	TAM	15/24	CMF	1/7	2/9
Cavalli 83	Ox/TAM	37/199	CT	16/37	84/162
Mouridsen 83b	ET	8/25	MTXT	4/8	8/17
Total	ET	163/5o4	CT	86/149	188/329
%		32		58	57
95%C.L.,%		28–36		49–65	53–63

R = responders to ET as 1. line therapy.

NR= non-responders to ET as 1. line therapy.

Table 5.   CYTOTOXIC THERAPY FOLLOWED BY ENDOCRINE THERAPY

Ref.	1. line treat- ment	Response rate (CR+PR)/N	2. line treat- ment	Cross sensiti- vity (CR+PR)/R	Non-cross resistance (CR+PR)/NR
Cocconi 82	CMF	–	CMF+TAM	7/16	5/23
Rose 83	CT	3o/78	ET	9/3o	12/48
Total	CT	3o/78	ET	16/46	17/71
%		39		35	24
95% C.L., %		28–5o		21–5o	15–36

Table 6.   ENDOCRINE THERAPY OF ADVANCED BREAST CANCER

Ablative	Oophorectomy
	Adrenalectomy
	Hypophysectomy
Inhibitive	Danazol
	LHRH-analogues
	Aminoglutethimide
	Δ^1-Testololactone
	Trilostane
Additive	Estrogens
	Androgens
	Progestins
	Glucocorticoids
Competitive	Anti-estrogens
	Anti-androgens

COMBINATIONS OF CYTOTOXIC AND ENDOCRINE THERAPY

The various forms of endocrine treatment in advanced breast cancer can be divided into four groups according to their mode of biological action as shown in table 6. Cytotoxic therapy as either single agent or in multiple drug combinations, has been combined with ablative, additive, or competitive endocrine modalities. Furthermore, the combination of cytotoxic and endocrine therapies have been applied either simultaneously, sequentially or alternatingly. Although they are used extensively in combination with various different cytotoxic treatments, glucocorticoids have been omitted from this review. In the following sections we will also briefly mention how the mode of action of the different endocrine modalities might influence their combination with cytotoxic drugs.

Combined cytotoxic and ablative therapy

The rationale for the use of the ablative endocrine procedures is that steroid hormones promote growth of some mammary tumor cells. Thus, a decrease in the concentration of these hormones is assumed to induce tumor regression in a manner similar to that seen in hormone dependent tumor in GR-mice. Tumor regression in these animals deprived of estrogen and progesterone appears to result from a decrease in the tumor cell production rate while the cell-loss rate remains constant (35). In addition, the growth fraction is also reduced in these animals (by a factor of 3), indicating that steroid hormones stimulate the growth of these tumor by enhancing the growth fraction.

In the clinical situation it appears from table 7a that the combined effect of oophorectomy and cytotoxic therapy has been evaluated against ablation alone in 3 randomized trials.
The response rate to oophorectomy ranges from 18-27%. The addition of cytotoxic drugs increased the rate of response in all 3 studies. Furthermore, Brunner et al. (11) also found a therapeutic benefit using the combined approach compared with multiple drug cytotoxic therapy alone. Although the median values for response duration and survival were higher for the combined endocrine cytotoxic therapy in all 4 trials, a statistically significant prolongation of the response duration was observed only in the ECOG-study (2o). This can be partly explained by

Table 7a.   SIMULTANEOUS CYTOTOXIC AND ABLATIVE ENDOCRINE THERAPY

Ref.	Treatment	Response Rate (CR+PR)/N	%	Response duration (days)	Survival (days)
Brunner 77	CMFVP	1o/23	44	234	396
	CMFVP+Ox	14/19	74	285	597
Ahmann 77	Ox	7/26	27	119^{X}	616
	Ox+CFP	1o/26	39	371^{X}	917
Falkson 79	Ox	7/38	18	15o	9oo
	Ox+C	35/54	65	48o	69o
	Ox+VPCMF	38/53	72	51o	78o
Cavalli 83	Ox	12/54	22	–	63o
	Ox+CT	25/55	46	–	759

^{X}Time to progression.

the fact (table 7b) that in 3 of the 4 trials the cytotoxic therapy
was applied sequentially. In each study the cumulated response rate
tended to be the same for the different treatment groups.
This was also seen to be the case in the trial performed by Nemoto et al.
(55) whose initial goal was to compare adrenalectomy, single drug therapy (adriamycin) and a combination of prednisone and cytotoxic agents
(cyclophosphamide + 5-FU). The study also examined the importance of
the sequence of the 3 modalities, since patients relapsing in the different treatment arms were given the other therapies as second and third
line treatments. Although the response rate to the first treatment sche-
dule was nearly identical in all 3 study arms, the survival was slightly better in those patients starting with the cytotoxic therapy. The

Table 7b.   SEQUENTIAL CYTOTOXIC AND ABLATIVE ENDOCRINE THERAPY

Ref.	1. line treat- ment	Response rate (CR+PR)/N	%	2. line treat- ment	Response rate (CR+PR)/N	%	Survival (days)
Ahmann 77	Ox	7/26	27	CFP	4/19	21	616
	Ox+CFP	1o/26	39	–	–	–	917
Falkson 79	Ox	7/38	18	VPCMF	16/32	5o	9oo
	Ox+C	35/54	65	–	–	–	69o
	Ox+VPCMF	38/53	72	–	–	–	78o
Cavalli 83	Ox	12/54	22	CT	11/54	2o	63o
	Ox+CT	25/55	46	–	–	–	759

Table 8a.   CYTOTOXIC AND ADDITIVE ENDOCRINE TREATMENT

Ref.	Treatment	Response rate (CR+PR)/N	%	Response duration (days)	Survival (days)
Brunner 77	CMFVP	26/48	54	318	576
	CMFVP+DES	3o/48	63	252	8o1
Kiang 81	DES	12/27	44	-	-
	DES+CF	32/48	67	-	-
Goldenberg 75	TESTOL	8/4o	2o	75o	-
	F	2/35	6	45o	-
	TESTOL+F	5/36	14	45o	-
Cole 73	C	7/3o	23	186	-
	NAND	o/26	o	-	-
	C+NAND	1/22	5	24o	-
Lloyd 79	AC+CALUST.	13/2o	65	645	7o5
	AC	19/36	53	345	4o5

amount of data on the importance of the scheduling of oophorectomy in premenopausal patients is limited, and studies based on estrogen receptor status are obviously needed in order to define how this effective endocrine treatment modality can be utilized in combied therapy.

Combined cytotoxic and additive therapy

The mode of action underlying the paradoxical effect of additive treatment with pharmacological doses of steroid hormones such as estrogens, androgens and progestins in tumor growth is largely unknown. Nevertheless, cytotoxic drugs have been combined with all three classes of sex steroid hormones. The additive effect of DES (table 8a) has been tested in two trials and resulted in higher response rates than either cytotoxic (11) or estrogen therapy (38) alone.
In the latter study, patients were stratified according to ER-status, and the therapeutic benefit in the combined group was observed even within the estrogen receptor positive group (87 vs. 64%). The survival data from this trial are difficult to interpret, since they have been divided into too many subsets.

Synthetic androgens have been added to cytotoxic agents in three trials (16,25,44) all of which are small. A beneficial effect of the combined treatment on rate of response, duration of remission and survival was only found when calusterone was administered together with low-dose adriamycin and cyclophosphamide (44).

Progestins, expecially in very high doses, have been used extensively in recent years for treatment of advanced breast cancer in spite of the fact that neither the optimal dose nor route of administration has been fully elucidated. Cytotoxic therapy and treatment with progestins (table 8b) has been combined in four trials, three of which included adriamycin. Almost all the patients in two of the studies (11,65) had received prior endocrine treatment, but this can hardly explain the observed antagonistic effect of the combined therapy with

Table 8b.   CYTOTOXIC AND ADDITIVE ENDOCRINE TREATMENT

Ref.	Treatment	Response rate (CR+PR)/N %		Response duration (days)	Survival (days)
Brunner 77	CMFVP	23/37	63	3oo	684
	CMFVP+MPA	2o/38	53	267	543
Rubens 78	AV/CMF+Plac	2o/33	61	266	45o
	AV/CMF+NEA	19/36	53	266	24o
Della Cuna 83	FAC	22/4o	55	27o	48o
	FAC+MPAim	3o/4o	75	57o	84o
	FAC+MPAp.o.	26/4o	65	39o	66o
Pellegrini 82	VAC	42/87	48	–	–
	VAC+MPAim	46/92	5o	–	–
Goldenberg 73	Ch	8/82	1o	36o	27o
	Ch+P	18/87	21	21o	27o
	HC+TIT	1o/86	12	33o	27o

regard to rate of response, response duration, and survival. However, in another study (17) the intramuscular administration of MPA as opposed to the oral one, increased the duration of response and survival whereas the response rates were similar.

In conclusion, results of combined cytotoxic and additive endocrine therapy are inconsistent, and some of the findings even indicate an antagonistic effect. However, the number of patients in each trial is rather small, and treatment stratification according to estrogen receptor status has taken place in only one of the studies. It is therefore difficult to reject the rationale for combined hormone and cytotoxic therapy on the basis of these data.

Combined cytotoxic and competitive endocrine therapy

The primary step in the action of the anti-estrogen tamoxifen is a competition with estradiol for binding to the cytoplasmic estrogen receptor, rendering the tumor cells insensitive to circulating levels of estrogens. At the chromatin level, the mechanism of action of tamoxifen is complex, but ultimately leads to a partial block of the cell-cycle in the early G_1-phase and a decrease in proportion of cells in the S-phase as demonstrated in the human breast cancer cell-line MCF-7 (58).

Tamoxifen has been given in combination with cytotoxic therapy in simultaneous, sequential or alternating modes. Simultaneous use of tamoxifen and non-adriamycin containing regimens has been evaluated in four trials. In three of these, a higher rate of response was observed in the combined treatment group (table 9a). Two identical studies where tamoxifen was combined with CMF both demonstrated an increase in response rate and more important an increase in the number of patients achieving a complete remission (table 1o). This trend is most pronounced in the EORTC study (53a) in which prolongation of the duration of re-

Table 9a.   SIMULTANEOUS CYTOTOXIC AND COMPETITIVE ENDOCRINE THERAPY. TAMOXIFEN.

Ref.	Treatment	Response rate (CR+PR)/N	%	Response duration (days)	Time to PD (days)	Survival (days)
Galmarini 81	CFVb	35/64	55	–	–	–
	CFVb+TAM	46/69	67	–	–	–
Clavel 82	TAM+DROST	1o/34	29	294	–	7oo
	CMF	4/3o	13	154	–	85o
	CMF+TAM+DROST	9/34	27	3o8	–	6oo
Cocconi 83	CMF	36/71	51	329	168	777
	CMF+TAM	46/62	74	357	336	546
Mouridsen 83a	CMF	51/1o5	49	378	27o	623
	CMF+TAM	86/115	75	574	48o	735

sponse, the time to progression, and survival is observed. In the study by Cocconi and co-workers (15) more than half of the patients initially receiving only CMF were later treated with both CMF and tamoxifen, which makes a direct comparison of the survival data between the two studies difficult. Even when tamoxifen is part of an adriamycin containing regimen (table 9b), combined cytotocix and endocrine therapy seems superior. The demonstrated differencies in response rates are only significant, however, in the studies by Tormey (76) and Pouillart (61). With

Table 1o.   TAMOXIFEN IN COMBINATION WITH CMF

Ref.		N	CR N	CR %	CR + PR N	CR + PR %
Cocconi 83	CMF	71	6	8	36	51
	CMF+TAM	62	8	13	46	74
Mouridsen 83a	CMF	1o5	21	2o	51	49
	CMF+TAM	115	36	31	86	75
Total	CMF	176	27	15	87	49
	CMF+TAM	177	44	25	132	75

% increase in CR + PR   53%

% increase in CR   67%

Table 9b. SIMULTANEOUS CYTOTOXIC AND COMPETITIVE ENDOCRINE THERAPY.
TAMOXIFEN.

Ref.	Treatment	Response rate (CR+PR)/N	%	Response duration (days)	Time to PD (days)	Survival (days)
Arraztoa 81	CAF–CMF	46/54	85	–	–	–
	CAF–CMF+TAM	5o/58	86	–	–	–
Tormey 82	DA	16/55	29	16o	11o	27o
	DA+TAM	34/67	5o	28o	17o	34o
Pouillart 82	CAFV	38/59	64	39o	–	39o
	CAFV+TAM	43/54	8o	42o	–	48o
	CAFV+TAM+NET	37/46	8o	51o	–	48o
Boccardo 82	CMFV/AC	8/2o	4o	–	45o	–
	CMFV/AC+TAM	15/2o	75	–	6oo	–

regard to the non-adriamycin containing regimens, the available data on
duration of response, time to treatment failure, and survival favour
combined cytotoxic endocrine therapy while the survival advantage is
not statistically significant.

Table 9c. SEQUENTIAL CYTOTOXIC AND COMPETITIVE ENDOCRINE THERAPY.
TAMOXIFEN.

Ref.	1. line treatment	Response rate (CR+PR)/N	%	2. line treatment	Response rate (CR+PR)/N	%	Survival (days)
Glick 81	TAM	43/88	49	TAM	28/33	85	–
				TAM+CMF	25/29	87	–
				CMF(PD only)	–	–	–
Bezwoda 82	TAM	15/24	63	CMF	3/9	33	513
	TAM+CMF	17/26	65	–	–	–	531
Cocconi 83	CMF	36/71	51	CMF+TAM	12/39	31	777
	CMF+TAM	46/62	74	–	–	–	546
Cavalli 83	TAM	25/145	17	CHEMO	23/145	16	825
	TAM+CHEMO	6o/152	4o	–	–	–	711

The question of sequential cytotoxic and tamoxifen therapy has been addressed in four trials (table 9c). Glick and co-workers (23) found equal rates of remission of about 85% among 88 patients, all of whom were first treated with tamoxifen for 12 weeks, and thereafter randomized to continue either with tamoxifen alone or a combination of tamoxifen and CMF. All patients had either estrogen receptor positive or estrogen receptor unknown tumors, thus explaining the high rate of response of 44% during the first 12 weeks of therapy. Fifty-two receptor positive patients were treated with either tamoxifen or tamoxifen plus CMF in the study by Bezwoda et al. (6). The addition of cytotoxic therapy to tamoxifen treatment in this selected group of patients did not increase either the rate of remission or median time of survival above that obtained with tamoxifen alone. In a large trial performed by the Swiss-group (12) 297 patients were randomized to either treatment with tamoxifen or to tamoxifen in combination with one of three different cytotoxic regimens depending on the cooperative groups own definition of the aggressiveness of the disease. The group of patients initially treated with tamoxifen alone were subsequently treated with cytotoxic therapy, and the cumulated response rate and the survival in these patients were similar to those observed with the combined therapy. The treatment was given irrespective of estrogen receptor status; but even so, a remission rate of 17% in those patients first treated with tamoxifen alone is rather low and difficult to interpret.

Alternating or repetitive use of cytotoxic and endocrine therapy has been proposed (42,57) as an approach by which non-dividing cells could be recruited and thereby optimize the effect of the cytotoxic drugs (table 9d). In a still ongoing randomized trial Lippman and co-workers (41) have tried to recruit cells into the S-phase by a short pulse of the estrogen Primarin subsequent to treatment with tamoxifen on day 2-6. Cyclophosphamide and adriamycin are administered on day 1, and in order to exploit possible synchronization, 5-FU and methotrexate are given immediately following the Primarin stimulation. The data presented so far from this trial reveal no differences in rate of response or time to progression and survival was only extended in the group of responders treated with cytotoxic and endocrine therapy.

In a phase II trial (3), 35 patients were treated with tamoxifen for lo days followed by Primarin for 4 days. Methotrexate and 5-FU were then given on day 14 in order to utilize the presumed cell-cycle specific effect of these two drugs. A remarkably high rate of remission of 69% was obtained by this rather non-toxic regimen. The EORTC Breast Cancer Cooperative Group is currently evaluating the same concept of estrogen recruitment (59) in a phase II trial where 55 patients so far have been treated continously with aminogluthetimide and hydrocortisone (plus oophorectomy in pre-menopausal patients) with courses of FAC every three weeks. Each course is preceded by oral administration of ethinyl estradiol. A response rate of 71% has been achieved. Thus, the available clinical data on the simultaneous use of cytotoxic and tamoxifen therapy suggest an additive effect in terms of response rates, whereas the data regarding survival is conflicting. The sequential use of tamoxifen in cytotoxic therapy as well as the alternating approach aimed at increasing tumor-cell kill is theoretically attractive but has to be further elucidated in phase III trials.

Table 9d.   ALTERNATING CYTOTOXIC AND ENDOCRINE THERAPY

Ref.	N	CR+PR (%)	Treatment	Schedule (days)
Lippman 82	9o	6o	TAM PRIMARIN	
			CYT ADM 5-FU MTX	
		62	CYT ADM 5-FU MTX	
Allegra 83	29	72	TAM PRIMARIN	
			MTX 5-FU LEUCOVERIN	
Paridaens 83	55	71	AG+H(Ox) EE$_2$ CYT ADM $\longrightarrow$ MTX 5-FU	

DISCUSSION

Various endocrine treatment modalities in combination with cytotoxic therapy has been compared to each treatment modality alone in only 25 randomized trials with at least 2o patients in each treatment, arm. Our current understanding of how to utilize combined endocrine- and cytotoxic therapy is, therefore, based upon the treatment of a total of about 3ooo patients. Needless to say, this is only a very small fraction of the total number of women with recurrent disease, and this pronounced selection of patients for clinical trials may also explain the inconsistence of the data presented in this review. In addition the small number of patients and inadequate data on long term survival in many of the clinical trials prohibit valid statistical analysis.

Although the biological rationale for the combined therapy appears sound in theory, an additive effect has been demonstrated in only some of the experimental clinical trials. In this respect combination of cytotoxic therapy with either oophorectomy or tamoxifen seems to be best elucidated. In these studies an increase in the response rate in the order of what can be expected on the basis of the assumption of independent biological actions of the two treatment modalities is observed.

Recent trials have been based upon our present understanding of tumor cell kinetics that have been explored through basic research. It seems obvious that more knowledge about the biology and the diversity of mammary carcinomas has to be gained both in the laboratory and in the clinic before rational stratification can provide the basis for prospective clinical trials in unselected patient populations. Furthermore, in the evaluation of the clinical data it is imperative to look beyond the short-term effects of the therapy and to analyze the complete course of the disease from its diagnosis and until death. Hopefully, future approaches for such trials will include an evaluation of the role of endocrine pertubation of cell-cycle kinetics and of the effectiveness of a reduction of the tumor cell burden by endocrine therapy prior to the initiation of the cytotoxic therapy.

ACKNOWLEDGMENT

Our thanks to Susan M. Thorpe for constructive criticism.

ABBREVIATION

AG: aminoglutethimide
A: adriamycin
CALUST: calusterone
Ch: chlorambucil
C: cyclophosphamide
CYT: cyclophosphamide
CT: cytotoxic therapy
D: dibromudulcitol
DES: diethylstilbestrol
DROST: drostanolone
EE_2: ethinylestradiol
ER: estrogenreceptor
ET: endocrine therapy
F: 5-FU
FLU: fluoxymesterone
H: hydrocortisone
HC: hydrocortisone

M: methotrexate
MTX: methotrexate
MEG: megestrolacetate
MPA: medroxyprogesteroneacetate
MTXT: mitoxantrone
NAND: nandrolone
NEA: norethisteroneacetate
NET: norethisterone
Ox: oophorectomy
P: prednisone
Plac: placebo
TAM: tamoxifen
TESTOL: testololactone
TIT: triiodothyronine
V: vincristine
Vb: vinblastin

REFERENCES

1. Ahmann, D.L., O'Conell, M.J., Hahn, R.G., Bisel, H.F., Lee, R.A. and Edmonson, J.H. (1977): New Engl.J.Med. 297: 356-36o.
2. Allegra, J.C., Barlock, A., Huff, K.K. and Lippman, M.E. (198o): Cancer 45: 792-794.
3. Allegra, J.C. (1983): Seminars Oncology lo (2): 23-28.
4. Arraztoa, J., Ramirez, G. (1981) ASCO, C 4ol: 435.
5. Beex, L., Pieters, G., Smals, A., Koenders, A., Benraad, T. and Kloppenborg, P. (1981). Cancer Treat. Rep. 65: 179-185.
6. Bezwoda, W.R., Derman, D., De Moor, N.G., Lange, M. and Levin, J. (1982): Cancer 5o: 2747-275o.
7. Bichel, P., Skovgaard Poulsen, H. and Andersen, J. (1982): Cancer 5o: 1771-1774.
8. Boccardo, F., Rubagotti, A., and Rosso, R. (1982): In: The Role of Tamoxifen in Breast Cancer, edited by S. Iacobelli et al., pp. 73-84, Raven Press.

9. Briand, P., Thorpe, S.M. and Daehnfeldt, J.L. (1979): Acta Path.
    Microbiol. Scand. Sect. A. 87: 427-436.
lo. Briand, P., Rose, C. and Thorpe, S.M. (1982): Eur.J.Cancer Clin.Oncol.
    18: 1391-1393.
11. Brunner, K.W., Sonntag, R.W., Alberto, P., Senn, H.J., Martz, G.,
    Obrecht, P. and Maurice, P. (1977). Cancer 39: 2923-2933.
12. Cavalli, F., Beer, M., Martz, G., Jungi, W.F., Alberto, P., Obrecht,
    J.P., Mermillod, B. and Brunner, K.W. (1983). Brit.Med.J. 286:5-8.
13. Clavel, B., Cappelaere, J.P., Guerin, J., Klein, T., Pommatau, E.
    and Berlie, J. (1982). Sem.Hôp.Paris 58: 1919-1923.
14. Cocconi, G., De Lisi, V., Boni, C., Magnani, P., Bertusi, M., Ravai-
    oli, A. and Giovannetti, E. (1982). In: The Role of Tamoxifen in
    Breast Cancer, edited by S. Iacobelli et al. pp. 35-43, Raven Press.
15. Cocconi, G., De Lisi, V., Boni, C., Mori, P., Malacarne, P., Amadori,
    D. and Giovanelli, E. (1983). Cancer 51: 581-588.
16. Cole, M.P., Todd, I.D.H. and Wilkinson, P.M. (1973). Br.J.Cancer 27:
    396-399.
17. Robustelli Della Cuna, G., Cuzzoni, Q., Pretti, P. and Bernardo, G.
    (1983). In: Role of Medroxyprogesterone in Endocrine Related Tumors.
    vol. II., edited by L. Campio, G. Robustelli Della Cuna and R.W.
    Taylor, pp. 131-14o, Raven Press.
18. Dexter, D.L., Kowalski, H.L., Blacer, B.A., Fligiel, Z., Vogel, R.
    and Heppner, G.H. (1978): Cancer Res. 38: 3174-3181.
19. Dunn, T. (1959) In: Physiopathology of Cancer, edited by F. Homburger
    and N.H. Fishman, pp. 38-84, Paul B. Hoeber, New York.
2o. Falkson, G., Falkson, H.C., Glidewell, O., Weinberg, V., Leone, L.
    and Hollnad, J.F. (1979): Cancer 43: 2215-2222.
21. Fisher, E.D. (1977) In : Breast Cancer, edited by W.L. McGuire, pp.
    43-123, Churchill Livingstone, New York.
22. Galmarini, F., Santos, R., Bruno, R., Cases, O., Chiesa, J., Bertac-
    chini, C., D'Auria, A. and Dominguez, E. UICC Conf.Clin.Oncol.
    (1981): o3-o359.
23. Glick, J.H., Creech, R.H., Torri, S., Holroyde, C., Brodovsky, H.,
    Catalono, R.B. and Varano, M. (1981). Breast Cancer Res. Treat. 1:
    59-68.
24. Goldenberg, I.S., McMahan, C.A., Escher, G.C., Volk, H., Ansfield,
    F.J. and Olson, K.B. (1973): Cancer 31: 66o-663.
25. Goldenberg, I.S., Sedransk, N., Volk, H., Segaloff, A., Kelley, R.M.
    and Haines, C.R. (1975): Cancer 36: 3o8-31o.
26. Goldie, J.H., Bruchowsky, N., Coldman, A.J. and Gudauskas, G.A.
    (1981): Canadian J.Surg. 24: 29o-293.
27. Goldie, J.H., Coldman, A.J. and Gudauskas, G.A. (1982): Cancer
    Treat.Rep. 66: 439-449.
28. Gullino. P.M.: In: Breast Cancer, edited by W.L. McGuire (1979) pp.
    51-77, Plenum Medical, New York.
29. Harvey, H.A., Lipton, A., White, D.S., Santen, R.J., Boucher, A.E.,
    Shafik, A.S., Dixon, R.J. and members of the central Pennsylvania
    Oncology Group (1982) Cancer Research 42: 3451s-3453s.
3o. Heppner, G.H., Dexter, D.L., DeNucci, T., Miller, L.R. and Calabresi,
    P. (1978). Cancer Res. 38: 3758-3763.
31. Hilf, R., Feldstein, M.L., Savlov, E.D., Gibson, S.L. and Seneca, B.
    (198o): Cancer 46: 2797-28oo.
32. Ingle, J.N., Ahmann, D.L., Green, S.J., Edmonson, J.H., Bisel, H.F.,
    Kvols, L.K., Nichols, W.C., Creagan, E.T., Hahn, R.G., Rubin, J.
    and Frytak, S. (1981): New Engl. J. Med. 3o4: 16-23.

33. Ingle, J.N., Ahman, D.L., Green, S.J., Edmonson, J.H., Creagan, E.T., Hahn, R.G., Rubin, J. (1982) Am.J.Clin.Oncol. 5: 155-16o.

34. Ingle, J.N., Green, S.J., Ahmann. D.L., Edmonson, J.H., Nichols, W.C. Frytak, S. and Rubin, J. (1982). Cancer Research 42: 346ls-3467s.

35. Janik, P., Briand, P. and Hartmann, N.R. (1975): Cancer Research 35: 3698-37o4.

36. Jonat, W., Maass, H., Stolzenbach, G. and Trams, G. (198o). Cancer 46: 28o9-2813.

37. Kiang, D.T., Frenning, D.H., Gay, J., Goldman, A.I. and Kennedy, B.J. (198o): Cancer 46: 2814-2817.

38. Kiang, D.T., Frenning, D.H., Gay, J., Goldman. A.I. and Kennedy, B.J. (1981): Cancer 47: 452-456.

39. Legha, S.S., Buzdar, A.U., Smith, T.L., Swenerton, K.D., Hortobagyi, G.N. and Blumenschein, G.R. (198o): Cancer 46: 438-445.

4o. Lippman, M.E., Allegra, J.C., Brad Thompson, E., Simon, R., Barlock, A., Green, L., Huff, K.K., Do, H.M.T., Aitken, S.C. and Warren, R. (1978): New Engl.J.Med. 298: 1223-1228.

41. Lippman, M.E., Cassidy, J., Wesley, M., Young, R.C. (1982): ASCO C-3o5.

42. Lippman, M.E. (1983). Breast Cancer Research and Treatment 3: 117-127.

43. Lipton, A., Harvey, H.A., Santen, R.J., Boucher, A., White, D., Bernath, A., Dixon, R., Richard, G. and Shafik, A. (1982): Cancer Research 42: 3434s-3436s.

44. Lloyd, R., Jones, S.E. and Salmon, S.E. (1979): Cancer 43: 6o-65.

45. von Maillot, K., Gentsch, H.H. and Gunselmann (198o): J.Cancer Res. Clin.Oncol. 98: 3o1-313.

46. Manni, A., Trujillo, J.E. and Pearson, O.H. (198o). Cancer Treat. Rep. 64: 111-116.

47. Mattsson, W. (198o) In : Role of Medroxyprogesterone in Endocrine-Related Tumors, edited by Iacobelli, S. and A. Di Marco, pp. 65-71, Raven Press.

48. McGuire, W.L. (1978): Seminars Oncol. 5 (4): 428-433.

49. Meyer, J.S., Rao, B.R., Stevens, S.C. and White, W.L. (1977): Cancer 4o: 229o-2298.

5o. Morgan, L.R. and Donley, P.J. (1981) Rev. Endocrine-related cancer, suppl. 9: 3o1-318.

51. Mouridsen, H.T., Ellemann, K., Mattsson, W., Palshof, T., Daehnfeldt, J.L. and Rose, C. (1979): Cancer Treat.Rep. 63: 171-175.

52. Mouridsen, H.T., Salimtschik, M., Dombernowsky, P., Gelshøj, K., Palshof, T., Rørth, M., Daehnfeldt, J.L. and Rose, C. (198o); In: Breast Cancer, edited by H.T. Mouridsen and T. Palshof, pp. 1o7-11o, Pergamon Press, Oxford.

53a.Mouridsen, H.T., Rose, C., Engelsman, E., Sylvester, R., and Rotmensz, N. (1983) Eur.J.Cancer. Submitted.

53b.Mouridsen, H.T., Rose, C., Oosterom, A., Nooi, M. (1983): Cancer Treat.Rev. In press.

54. Nagai, R. and Kumaoka, S. (198o). Clin. Eval. 8: 321-352.

55. Nemoto, T., Rosner, D., Diaz, R., Dao, T., Sponzo, R., Cunningham, T., Horton, J. and Simon, R. (1978): Cancer 41: 2o73-2o77.

56. Nomura, Y., Yamagata, J., Takenaka, K. and Tashiro, H. (198o) Cancer 46: 288o-2883.

57. Osborne, C.K. (1981) Breast Cancer Research and Treatment 1: 121-123.

58. Osborne, C.K., Boldt, D.H., Clark, G.M. and Trent, J.M. (1983): Cancer Research 43: 3583-3585.

59. Paridaens, R., Blonk van der Wijst, J., Julien, J.P., Ferrazzi, E., Clarysse, A., Heuson, J.C., Sylvester, R. and Rotmensz, N. (1983): 3rd. Breast Cancer Working Conf. p. 1.1o. Amsterdam.

6o. Pellegrini, A., Robustelli Della Cuna, G., Estevez, R., Luchina, A., Da Silva Neto, J.B., Lira Puerto, V., Cortes-Funes, H. and Arraztoa, J. (1982): Proc. 13th International Cancer Congress: 1629, Seattle, USA.

61. Pouillart, P., Palangie, T., Jouve, M., Garcia-Giralt, E., Asselain, B., Magdelenat, H. (1981): Rev. Endocr. Rel.Cancer, suppl. 9:439-453.

62. Rose, C., Theilade, K., Boesen, E., Salimtschik, M., Dombernowsky, P. Brünner, N., Kjær, M. and Mouridsen, H.T. (1982) Breast Cancer Research and Treatment 2: 395-4oo.

63. Rose, C., Kamby, C. and Mouridsen, H.T. (1983) Unpublished data.

64. Rosenbaum, C., Marsland, T.A., Stolbach, L.L., Raam, S. and Cohen, J.L. (198o): Cancer 46: 2919-2921.

65. Rubens, R.D., Begent, R.H.J., Knight, R., Sezton, S.A. and Hayward, J.L. (1978): Cancer 42: 168o-1686.

66. Rubens, R.D. and Hayward, J.L. (198o): Cancer 46: 2922-2924.

67. Rubens, R.D. (1981): Rev. Endocr. Rel. Cancer, suppl. 1o: 29-37.

68. Samal, B.A., Brooks, S.C., Cummings, G., Franco, L., Hire, E.A., Martino, S., Singhakowinta, A., Vaitkevicius, V.K. (198o): Cancer 46: 2925-2927.

69. Silfverswärd, C., Skoog, L., Humla, S., Gustafsson, S.A. and Nordenskjöld, B. (198o): Europ.J.Cancer 16: 59-65.

7o. Silvistrini, R., Daidone, M.G. and Gentili, C. (1981) In: Commentaries on Research in Breast Disease, edited by R.D. Bulbrook and D.J. Taylor, pp. 1-4o, Allan R. Liss, New York.

71. Sluyser, M. and Van Nie, R. (1974): Cancer Research 34: 3253-3257.

72. Sluyser, M., Evers, S.G. and DeGoeij, C.C.J. (1976) Nature 263: 386-389.

73. Sluyser, M., De Goeij, C.C.J. and Evers, S.G. (1981): Europ.J.Cancer 17: 155-159.

74. Smith, I.E., Harris, A.L., Morgan, M., Ford, H.T., Gazet, J-C., Harmer, C.L., White, H., Parsons, C.A., Villardo, A., Walsh, G., McKinna, J.A. (1981): Br.Med.J. 283: 1432-1433.

75. Stewart, H.J., Forrest, A.P.M., Gunn, J.M., Hamilton, T., Langlands, A.O., McFadyen, I.J. and Roberts, M.M. (198o) In: H.T. Mouridsen and T. Palshof (eds.) Breast Cancer, pp. 83-88, Pergamon Press, Oxford.

76. Tormey, D.C., Falkson, G., Crowley, J., Falkson. H.C., Voelkel, J., Davis, T.E. (1982): Am.J.Clin.Oncol. 5: 33-39.

77. Tormey, D.C., Lippman, M.E., Edwards, B.K. and Cassidy, J.G. (1983): Ann.Intern.Med. 98: 139-144.

78. UICC. Hayward, J.L., Carbone, P.P., Heuson, J-C, Kumaoma, S., Segaloff, A. and Rubens, R.D. (1977): Europ.J.Cancer 13: 89-94.

79. Vindeløv, L., Thorpe, S., Rasmussen, B.B., Christensen, I.J. and Rose, C. (1982). The Scandinavian Breast Cancer Symposium, Abstract 14.

8o. Westerberg, H. (198o): Cancer Treat.Rep. 64: 117-121.

81. Young, P.C.M., Ehrlich, C.E. and Einhorn, L.H. (198o): Cancer 46: 2961-2963.

Progress in Cancer Research and Therapy,
Vol. 31, edited by F. Bresciani, et al.
Raven Press, New York © 1984.

Combination Chemo-Hormonal Therapy in Patients with Stage IV Breast Cancer

Joseph C. Allegra and Thomas T. Kubota

University of Louisville School of Medicine and James Graham Brown Cancer Center, Louisville, Kentucky 40292

Metastatic breast cancer is a common disease. It is estimated that approximately 270,000 women are currently alive with Stage IV disease in the United States. For many years, hormonal therapy has been the mainstay of early treatment of metastatic breast cancer; however, if one randomly selects patients for treatment with the various types of hormonal manipulation, only about 30% of unselected patients will obtain an objective response to the hormonal therapy (4,5). Over the past five years, estrogen receptors have been extremely valuable in predicting tumor response, and therefore, useful in selecting patients for hormonal manipulation. If a tumor contains significant quantities of estrogen receptor in its cytoplasm, the likelihood of objective response to treatment with hormones increases to approximately 50 to 60% (6,8,9). More important, it is also known that if a breast tumor does not contain significant amounts of estrogen receptor protein, the likelihood of an objective response to an endocrine manipulation is less than 10%.

Combination chemotherapy also yields response rates in the range of 50 to 60% with acceptable toxicity. Patients with estrogen receptor negative tumors who are not candidates for hormonal manipulation are characteristically treated even at first recurrence with cytotoxic chemotherapy.

One of the obvious problems with the treatment of Stage IV breast carcinoma, either with hormonal therapy or with cytotoxic chemotherapy, is that all of the objective remissions are partial remissions. This, by definition, implies that the measurable tumor has decreased in size by at least 50%, yet not totally disappeared. There are few complete remissions using either modality of therapy. The attainment of complete remissions in the treatment of any solid tumor, and specifically in the treatment of Stage IV breast carcinoma, is important since cure is not a reasonable objective until one can attain complete remissions in a high percentage of patients.

One aspect of breast tumor biology which may be involved in our inability to attain complete remissions in breast cancer could be heterogeneity. It is known that estrogen receptor positive tumors contain predominantly estrogen receptor positive cells, but also contain cells which lack these receptors. Likewise, estrogen receptor negative tumors contain great numbers of cells lacking the estrogen receptor but also contain some cells possessing estrogen receptor. In

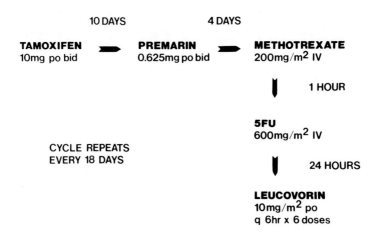

FIGURE I. Combination chemo-hormonal therapy utilizing synchronization and stimulation of tumor cells.

order to attack these divergent populations of cells, clinical invest-igators have, over the past five years, empirically designed combina-tions of hormone therapy and chemotherapy aimed at killing the estro-gen receptor positive component of the tumor and the rapidly dividing estrogen receptor negative component. Thus far, these types of com-bination chemo-hormonal therapy regimens have yielded slightly higher overall remission rates, but no significant increase in complete remission (10).

The question then arises concerning how else one could manipulate tumor cells utilizing both hormonal therapy and chemotherapy in an attempt to induce a higher complete remission rate? Figure I illus-trates a schema which utilizes the concepts of synchronization and stimulation of tumor cells. In this concept, endocrine therapy is uti-lized to synchronize tumor cells which are then rescued by a second hormonal manipulation.

The rescue aspect of this schema is an attempt to increase the number of cells in the S phase of the cell cycle. The cells are then subsequently treated with S phase-specific cytotoxic chemotherapy in an attempt to further enhance cell kill. This type of clinical trial schema was based on laboratory observations. Lippman et al. (7) have studied the effects of estrogens and anti-estrogens on growth of human breast cancer cells in great detail. Those investigators showed in a human breast cancer cell model in long term tissue culture that estro-gen stimulates the growth of human mammary carcinoma, whereas the anti-estrogen, tamoxifen, inhibits growth. The tamoxifen growth inhibition can be "rescued" by physiologic concentrations of an estro-gen. They observed a marked rise in thymidine incorporation in the rescued cells to levels exceeding both control and estrogen-stimulated values in the early periods of estradiol rescue of tamoxifen. These data suggest that cells were arrested by anti-estrogen in a uniform stage of the cell cycle. They postulated that when estradiol addition reversed the tamoxifen inhibition, a larger proportion of the cells entered the DNA synthetic phase of the cell cycle and the nucleoside incorporation increased dramatically.

The combination chemo-hormonal therapy schema in Figure I is therefore based upon the observations that breast cancers exhibit cellular heterogeneity with regard to estrogen receptor status, and that hormonal therapy and chemotherapy have different mechanisms of action and of toxicity, and further that cell cyle specific agents are most effective against rapidly dividing cells. It is the hope that utilizing hormones and chemotherapy in this manner may result in a better response when compared to either therapy alone.

MATERIALS AND METHODS

Fifty-one patients with histologically documented, measurable adenocarcinoma of the breast, referred to the Division of Medical Oncology at the University of Louisville between July 1980 and July 1983 were entered into this clinical trial. Eligibility criteria for entry into this study included histologically confirmed metastatic breast cancer, measurable disease, serum creatinine less than 1.5 mg/dl, and/or a creatinine clearance greater than 60ml/min, Karnofsky performance status of 50 or better, and an expected survival of over 2 mo. All patients were treated without regard to their ER status. Patients were ineligible if they had received prior tamoxifen therapy; however, all forms of prior chemotherapy and other forms of hormonal therapy did not make a patient ineligible for this clinical trial provided that they were off this therapy for 4 wk prior to entering the study and had fully recovered from the toxic effects of the prior therapy. Prior radiation therapy was also acceptable provided nontreated lesions existed for measurement. The protocol contained no age or menopausal restrictions.

Their median age was 56 years, with a range of 30-78 years. Forty patients were postmenopausal and 11 premenopausal. Their median Karnofsky performance status was 90, with a range of 70-100. Their median disease-free interval was 18 mo, with a range of 0-16 years.

Twenty-nine of the patients, or 57%, had tumors that were ER-positive, sixteen were ER-negative, and six had tumors of unknown ER status. All of the ER assays were performed using a sucrose density gradient technique (11) on a multipoint titration assay with coated charcoal (12). ER status was determined by biopsy of metastatic tissue prior to therapy in the majority of cases. A cutoff valve for positivity was chosen at 10^{-15} mole/mg of cytoplasmic protein.

With respect to dominant site of disease, the majority of the patients had soft-tissue dominant metastases and only one-third had visceral dominant metastases.

The treatment schema for this Phase II clinical trial is illustrated in Figure I. Patients with metastatic breast cancer were administered tamoxifen in a dosage of 10 mg orally twice a day. They received tamoxifen for 10 days. The tamoxifen was then discontinued and the patients received Premarin, a conjugated estrogen, in a dosage of 0.625 mg orally twice a day. The Premarin was continued for 4 days. On the fourth day of Premarin therapy the patients received methotrexate fluorouracil 200mg/m^2 iv, followed in 1 hr by 5-fluorouracil 600 mg/m^2 iv. Twenty-four hours later the patients were rescued with leucovorin orally at 10 mg/m^2 every 6 hr for six doses. The treatment cycle was repeated every 18 days.

In all cases, assessment of response was performed using standardized response criteria (1). In brief, a complete remission was defined as the clinical disappearance of all detectable disease. This included healing of all bone lesions and a return of the patient to a premorbid performance status. A partial remission was defined as a 50% decrease in the product of perpendicular diameters of all measurable disease and no evidence of new lesions. The duration of remission was calculated from the beginning of therapy.

RESULTS

Fifty-one patients have been entered into this Phase II clinical trial and fifty patients are currently evaluable for response. One patient is too early to evaluate. The overall response rate is 64%. The complete remission rate is 40% with twenty of the fifty evaluable patients attaining a complete remission. The partial remission rate was 24% and 22% of the patients had stable disease. Only 7 patients (14%) have had immediate progression of their disease. The median duration of remission is, at the present time, 12 months.

Of the 32 responders, ten (10) had visceral dominant disease, twenty had non-visceral dominant disease, and two had bone dominant disease.

Patients with visceral dominant disease had a response rate of 59% whereas the response rate of soft tissue metastases was 74%. Bone dominant disease had the lowest response rate at 33%.

The response rate in estrogen receptor positive tumors was 62% (18/29) and 60% in estrogen receptor negative tumors (9/15). Five of six estrogen receptor unknown tumors responded.

The number of sites of metastatic disease did not influence response rate. Patients with only 1 site of disease had a response rate of 66%, whereas patients with 3 or more sites had a response rate of 71%.

DISCUSSION

The preliminary results of this combination chemo-hormonal therapy regimen in patients with metastatic breast cancer are presented as a model of the transition from basic laboratory observations to design of treatment regimens. This treatment regimen utilizing tamoxifen, Premarin, methotrexate, and 5-fluorouracil has a clear-cut biochemical rationale and takes advantage of the known biochemical heterogeneity of breast tumors with respect to ER status. The regimen is designed to set up rapidly dividing cells for cell kill by cell cycle-specific cytotoxic agents.

This combination is clearly effective. Our overall remission rate is 64%, but more important, our complete remission rate is high at 40%. As stated previously, other therapies utilizing hormones, chemotherapy, or combinations of hormones and chemotherapy have not shown any increase in the frequency of complete remissons (2). Gewirtz and Cadman, (3) utilizing sequential methotrexate and 5-fluorouracil without tamoxifen and Premarin, reported a 53% response rate (9 of 17 patients). Five of these patients had a complete remission (29%). As in our study, non-visceral dominant disease had the highest response rates, although one complete remission was reported in bone and one in liver.

It is important to note that the patient characteristics of our group of patients are very favorable. Their Karnofsky performance status is excellent at 90, and their dominant site of disease is non-visceral. This differs markedly from standard chemotherapy trials in which 50-60% of patients have visceral-dominant disease (10). Our patient population is such that the majority of the patients in this study were treated with this combination chemo-hormonal therapy regimen at the time of first recurrence, and therefore exhibit less visceral-dominant disease than a patient population that has experienced prior hormonal therapy or chemotherapy.

It is important to note that our regimen has minimal toxicity. Both hematologic and non-hematologic toxicities were mild. This lack of toxicity will allow us to develop additional treatment protocols utilizing new agents with this regimen, forming the nucleus of any new therapeutic designs.

REFERENCES

1. Breast Cancer Task Force Treatment Committee, National Cancer Institute. U.S. Dept. of Health, Education and Welfare Publication No. (NIH) 77-1192, 1977, pp 11-13
2. Carter, SK: Principals of Cancer Treatment. New York, McGraw-Hill, 1981, pp 342-351
3. Gerwitz AM, Cadman E: Cancer 47:2552-2555, 1981
4. Kardinal CG, Donegan WL: Cancer of the Breast (ed 2). Philadelphia, W.B. Saunders, 1979, pp 361-404.
5. Kennedy BJ: Semin Oncol 1:119-126, 1974
6. Legha SS, Davis HL, Muggia FM: Ann Intern Med 88:69-77, 1978
7. Lippman M, Bolan G, Huff AA: Cancer Res 36:4595-4691, 1976
8. McGuire WL: Cancer 36:638-644, 1975
9. McGuire WL, Horwitz KB, Peason OH, et al: Cancer 39:2934-2947, 1977
10. Smalley RV: Principles of Cancer Treatment. New York, McGraw-Hill, pp 327-341, 1981
11. Wittliff, JL: Methods in Cancer Research. New York, Academic Press, pp. 293-354, 1975
12. Wittliff JD, Savlov: Estrogen Receptors in Human Breast Cancer. New York, Raven Press, pp 73-91, 1975

Progress in Cancer Research and Therapy,
Vol. 31, edited by F. Bresciani, et al.
Raven Press, New York © 1984.

Estrogenic Sensitivity and Its Resistance in Normal Murine Mammary Glands

G. Shyamala

Lady Davis Institute for Medical Research, Sir Mortimer B. Davis Jewish General Hospital, Montreal, Quebec, H3T 1E2 Canada

The development and differentiation of normal mammary glands is under multihormonal control involving both steroid and protein hormones (32). Among the steroid hormones, estrogens have been shown to be critical for mammary epithelial cell proliferation (1,22,23). Extensive studies from several laboratories have revealed that the sensitivity of normal mammary tissue to both protein and steroid hormonal stimuli may be profoundly altered in relationship to the ontogeny of mammary epithelium (32,33). In this report studies from our laboratory are described whereby it appears that the estrogenic sensitivity of mammary tissues is also modulated in relationship to mammary development and differentiation.

I. ESTROGENIC RESPONSES IN MAMMARY GLANDS OF CASTRATED VIRGIN MICE

Estrogens elicit several responses in mammary tissues but perhaps the most dramatic and also the most important one is its stimulation of growth. Detailed studies from several laboratories focusing on the molecular mechanisms of estrogen action reveal that the overall responses may be catalogued into two phases; an early inductive phase representing responses occurring prior to increase in DNA synthesis and a later phase of true growth representing DNA synthesis (17). Therefore in these present studies for examining the relationship between estrogenic sensitivity and mammary development and differentiation, we chose three responses to represent both early inductive and later phase of true growth. In castrated virgin mice, as early as one hour after estrogen administration, there is an acceleration of glucose metabolism resulting in a significant increase in mammary glucose oxidation (Fig. 1); this therefore was chosen as a marker for early inductive phase. Beginning at about six hours after estradiol administration, there is an increase in progesterone receptor levels (Fig. 2) which thus serves as an additional marker for the inductive phase. Beginning at approximately twelve hours after estradiol administration, an increase in the rate of mammary DNA synthesis becomes apparent such that, as shown in Fig. 3, at 24 hours after estradiol administration there is a significant increase in the rate of mammary DNA synthesis; thus

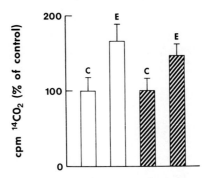

FIG. 1. Effect of estradiol on glucose oxidation in mammary glands and uteri of castrated virgin mice. A single injection of either saline (C) or 3 μg estradiol (E) was given for one hour prior to processing the tissues for glucose oxidation. The data represents mean ± SE for three to five experiments. Control values were: Mammary gland, 75.9 ± 13.6 cpm/mg tissue (□); and uterus, 4656 ± 742 cpm/per uterus (▨) (Shyamala and Ferenczy, 1982).

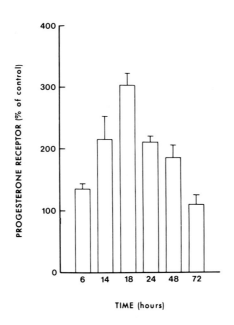

FIG. 2. Temporal relationship between estradiol administration and increase in cytoplasmic mammary progesterone receptor level. Castrated virgin mice were given a single injection of 1 μg of estradiol prior to sacrifice at times indicated. The progesterone receptor levels were assayed by measuring the specific binding of (^{3}H)R5020 in cytoplasmic extracts. Each bar represents the mean ± SE of three to five experiments. Control values for saline injected animals were: 467 fmoles/ mg DNA.

this effect represents the later phase of true growth. Detailed experimental procedures for measuring these estrogenic responses have been described by us previously (11,29).

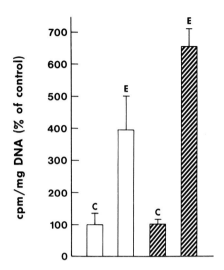

FIG. 3. Effect of estradiol on the rate of DNA synthesis in mammary gland and uterus of castrated virgin mice. A single injection of either saline (C) or estradiol (E) was given for 24 hours prior to processing the tissues for estimating the in vitro incorporation of labelled thymidine into DNA. Control values were: Mammary gland, 2187 ± 733 cpm/mg DNA (□); and uterus, 5062 ± 655 cpm/mg DNA (▨) (Shyamala and Ferenczy, 1982).

Despite the wide documentation that estrogens play a critical role in mammary growth, as yet it is not clear as to whether its action on the breast tissue is mediated directly or indirectly. In particular, it is known that estradiol may stimulate the synthesis and secretion of prolactin by the pituitary cells (20) and also increase prolactin receptors in the mammary glands of mice (26). Therefore it was of importance to ascertain whether the three estrogen responses chosen for our present studies were the result of elevated levels of prolactin accompanying estradiol administration. To this end, the effects of prolactin on mammary glucose oxidation, progesterone receptor-level and rate of DNA synthesis were tested in castrated virgin mice. The results of these experiments indicated that prolactin administration had no significant effect on either mammary glucose oxidation or progesterone receptor level or on the rate of DNA synthesis (Fig. 4).

II. RELATIONSHIP BETWEEN ESTROGENIC SENSITIVITY AND MAMMARY DEVELOPMENT AND DIFFERENTIATION

In our initial studies, to identify the relationship between estrogenic sensitivity and mammary development, progesterone receptor was used as the marker of estrogen action. Since in rodents progesterone is also an important hormone involved in mammary development (32), we felt that in these studies progesterone receptor would serve not only

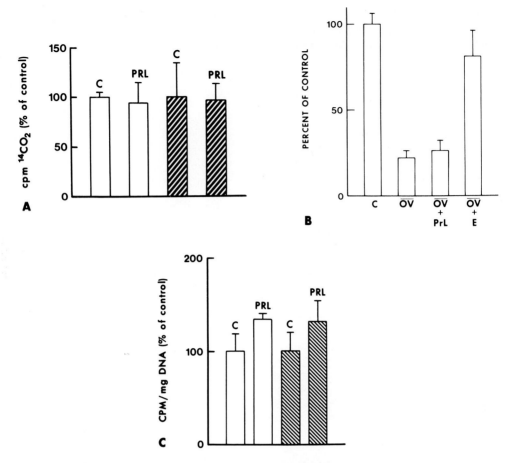

FIG. 4. Effect of prolactin on the estrogenic responses in castrated virgin mice. A single injection of either saline (C) or l mg of ovine prolactin was administered prior to processing the mammary (▢) and uterine (▨) tissues at indicated times.   (A) Glucose oxidation at l h. (B) Progesterone receptor level at 24 h.   (C) Rate of DNA synthesis as measured by *in vitro* incorporation of labelled thymidine into DNA at 24 h.

as a marker of estrogen action but perhaps also yield information regarding the capability of the mammary tissues to respond to progesterone during various stages of development. The relationship between mammary progesterone receptor and mammary development is shown in Fig. 5. As may be seen the progesterone receptor was present in the mammary tissues of virgin, pregnant and postpartum mice but was totally undetectable in the lactating tissue. Also, the levels of progesterone receptor from the tissue of pregnant mice were lower than that in the virgin mice. It is known that (a) pregnancy is accompanied by high serum progesterone levels, (b) during lactation in rodents there is a state of pseudopregnancy (31) also accompanied by high serum progesterone levels, and (c) progesterone can antagonize estrogen mediated increases in progesterone receptor levels (34,35). Therefore, to determine whether the

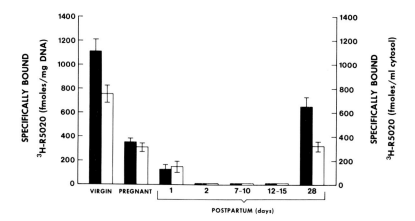

FIG. 5. Relationship between cytoplasmic progesterone receptor levels in mammary glands and different stages of mammary gland development. ■, Data expressed on the basis of DNA; ☐, Data expressed on the basis of milliliters of cytoplasmic extract equivalent to 1 g tissue. Each bar represents the mean ± SE of four to eight separate experiments. In each experiment, mammary glands were pooled from two to four mice. Virgin, adult non-ovariectomized; pregnant, 12-14 days of pregnancy (Haslam and Shyamala, 1979b).

lower levels of mammary progesterone receptor accompanying pregnancy and its absence in mammary tissue during lactation was due to high endogenous levels of progesterone, the effect of estradiol on the progesterone receptor levels in the tissues of castrated pregnant and lactating mice was examined. As shown in Fig. 6, in castrated pregnant mice, estradiol was able to augment the level of mammary progesterone receptor indicating that during this developmental state, the tissue was responsive to estradiol. In contrast, progesterone receptor was still undetectable in the mammary tissues of castrated lactating mice treated with estradiol (Fig. 7). This insensitivity of lactating mammary tissues to estradiol was also apparent with respect to the other two markers of estrogen action. As shown in Fig. 8, in castrated lactating mice there was no estradiol mediated increase in mammary glucose oxidation; similarly estradiol also had no effect on mammary rate of DNA synthesis (Fig. 9). Thus by all criteria of estrogen action chosen for these studies, the mammary glands of lactating mice appeared to be resistant to the action of estradiol.

The non-responsiveness of mammary tissue to estradiol appeared to persist only so long as the glands were secretory since as shown in Fig. 5, at 28 days postpartum, progesterone receptor was detectable in mammary glands and by day 35 postpartum the levels had been restored to that seen in the mammary tissue of virgin mice (Table 1). Similarly, if lactational involution was induced experimentally by pup removal, there was a reappearance of progesterone receptor in mammary tissue (Table 2).

More importantly, this reappearance of progesterone receptor in postpartum mice also appeared to be under estrogenic control. As shown in

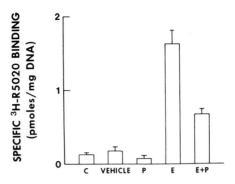

FIG. 6. Effects of estrogen and progesterone on progesterone receptor concentration in mammary gland after 14-16 days of pregnancy. Pregnancies were terminated by ovariectomy and hysterectomy on day 14-16; starting 24 h later, the animals received a further five daily injections of vehicle, or estrogen (E, 1 μg) or progesterone (P, 1 mg) alone or in combinations, as indicated. Controls (C) were assayed at 24 h after ovariectomy and received no other treatment. 24 h after the last injection, cytoplasmic extracts were assayed for specific (^{3}H)R5020 binding. Each value represents the mean $\pm$ SE of three to four experiments (Haslam and Shyamala, 1980).

Table 3, in castrated postpartum mice, the levels of mammary progesterone receptor were considerably lower than that present in the tissues of intact mice (compare with Table 1); however, these levels increased by two fold with a single administration of estradiol. Thus the data revealed that during lactational involution the mammary glands had regained their sensitivity to estrogen.

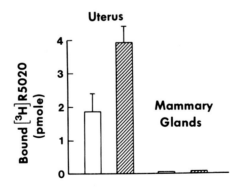

FIG. 7. Effect of estradiol on the amounts of cytoplasmic progesterone receptor in the uterus and mammary glands of castrated lactating mice. Mice were castrated at day 2 of lactation, a single injection of saline (□) or 3 μg of estradiol (▨) was given on day 9 and tissues were assayed at day 10. The results are expressed as means $\pm$ SE for five experiments and represent binding per g of mammary tissue or per uterus (Haslam and Shyamala, 1979a).

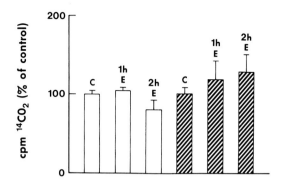

FIG. 8. Effect of estradiol on glucose oxidation in castrated lactating mice. Mice were castrated on day 2 of lactation, a single injection of saline (C) or 3 µg estradiol (E) was given on day 10 of lactation for the times indicated prior to processing the tissues. The data represent the mean $\pm$ SE for five experiments. The values for control (saline-injected) mice were 635 ± 32 cpm $^{14}CO_2$/mg mammary tissue (☐) and 8354 ± 740 cpm $^{14}CO_2$/uterus (▨) (Shyamala and Ferenczy, 1982).

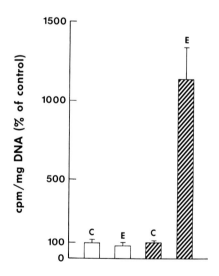

FIG. 9. Effect of estradiol on (^{3}H)thymidine incorporation into DNA in castrated lactating mice. Animals were castrated on day 2 of lactation, injected with either saline (C) or 3 µg estradiol (E) on day 9 of lactation, and tissues were processed on day 10. The incorporation of thymidine into DNA was estimated by in vitro incubation of the tissue. The data represent the mean $\pm$ SE of four experiments. Control data (counts per min/mg DNA) for mammary glands (☐) and uteri (▨) are 3118 ± 648 and 2053 ± 175, respectively (Shyamala and Ferenczy, 1982).

TABLE 1. Reappearance of cytoplasmic progesterone receptor in mammary tissues of postpartum mice

Days postpartum	Progesterone receptor* (fmoles/mg DNA)
28	625 ± 63
35	1490 ± 140
42	1330 ± 125

*Equivalent to the specific binding of (^{3}H)R5020

TABLE 2. Cytoplasmic progesterone receptor levels in mammary tissue during experimentally induced lactational involution (Haslam and Shyamala, 1979b)

No. of days without pups	Progesterone receptor*	
	fmoles/g tissue	fmoles/mg DNA
1	0	0
2	0	0
3	0	0
4	63 ± 37	62 ± 34
5	148 ± 17	125 ± 14
8**	260 ± 20	306 ± 23

*Represents the specifically bound (^{3}H)R5020. Results are expressed as the mean ± SE.
**Day 8 is equivalent to day 15 postpartum. Cytoplasmic extracts of mammary tissues of day 15 postpartum animals kept with their pups contained no detectable progesterone receptor.

TABLE 3. Effect of ovariectomy and estradiol administration on the mammary cytoplasmic progesterone receptor level in postpartum mice

Treatment	Days postpartum	Progesterone receptor* (fmoles/mg DNA)
Saline	28	249 ± 10
Estradiol	28	480 ± 27
Saline	35	331 ± 67
Estradiol	35	675 ± 16

*Represents the specifically bound (^{3}H)R5020. Animals were ovariectomized seven days prior to a single administration of either saline or 3 µg of estradiol for 24 hours. The data represent the mean ± SE of three to five separate experiments.

III. STATUS OF THE ESTROGEN RECEPTOR DURING ESTROGEN-RESPONSIVE AND NON-
RESPONSIVE STATES IN THE MAMMARY GLAND

It is generally believed that one of the reasons for the reduced ability of a target tissue to respond to estradiol may be its altered status

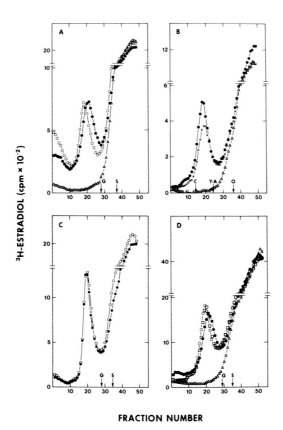

FIG. 10. Sedimentation profiles of cytoplasmic mammary estrogen receptor.
The arrows represent the standards C = catalase, 11.3S; Y-A = yeast alcohol dehydrogenase, 7.6S; G = gammaglobulin, 6.6S; L-A = liver alcohol
dehydrogenase, 5.0S; S = bovine serum albumin, 4.4S; O = ovalbumin, 3.5S.
(A) Cytosol from ovariectomized virgin mice either as is (●,△) or exposed to 10 mM molybdate (O) was incubated with 10 nM (^{3}H)estradiol
alone (O,●) or also with a 100 fold excess of unlabelled estradiol (△)
and centrifuged on gradients in phosphate buffer. (B) Cytosol from intact virgin (✖) or ovariectomized virgin mice (●,△) was incubated
with 2 nM of (^{3}H)estradiol either alone (✖,●) or also with a 100 fold
excess of unlabelled estradiol (△) and centrifuged on gradients in Tris
buffer. (C) Cytosol from ovariectomized virgin mice either as is (●)
or exposed to 10 mM molybdate (O) was incubated with 10 mM of (^{3})estra-
diol and centrifuged on gradients in phosphate buffer with 10 mM molybdate. (D) Cytosol from lactating mice either as is (●,△) or containing
10 mM molybdate (O,□) was incubated with 10 nM of (^{3}H)estradiol either
alone (O,□,●) or also with a 100 fold excess of unlabelled estradiol
(△) and centrifuged on gradients in phosphate buffer only (O,△) or on
gradients with 10 mM molybdate (●,□) (Gaubert et al, 1982).

with respect to estrogen receptor. The cytoplasmic estrogen receptor is present in the mammary glands of both virgin and lactating mice (25,27). In fact, in rodents the level of cytoplasmic estrogen receptor in the mammary glands during lactation may be higher than that found in the glands of virgin mice (8,15,16,19). As shown in Fig. 10 there is also no discernible difference in the molecular form of the cytoplasmic estrogen receptor isolated from the glands of virgin and lactating mice; when appropriate receptor stabilizing agents are used for the assay, the receptor from the glands of both virgin and lactating mice sediment as 8-9S species on sucrose gradients. More importantly, in response to an administration of estradiol, the mammary estrogen receptor in vivo is found to be associated with the nuclear fraction in both the tissues from virgin (25) and lactating mice (27). Thus, the inability of lactating mammary glands to respond to estradiol does not appear to be related to any dramatic differences in the properties of estrogen receptor.

IV. RELATIONSHIP BETWEEN THE MORPHOLOGICAL STATE OF THE MAMMARY TISSUE AND ITS RESPONSIVENESS TO ESTRADIOL

The mammary gland is composed of epithelial, adipose and connective tissues and the relative proportion of each cell type varies according to the developmental state of the gland (32). In these present studies, a histological examination of the mammary glands revealed that there may be a relationship between the composition of the tissue with respect to various cell types and its ability to respond to estradiol. For example as shown in Fig. 11, in the mammary glands of virgin, pregnant and postpartum mice (all of which were responsive to estradiol), there was a predominance of adipose and connective tissue surrounding the epithelium; in contrast, in mammary glands of lactating mice which were nonresponsive to estradiol, the glandular epithelium was predominant. Similarly, when lactational involution had been induced experimentally by pup removal, the emergence of mammary progesterone receptor seen at five days after pup removal (Table 2) was well correlated with the emergence of adipose and connective tissue elements (Fig. 11). This, therefore raised the possibility that the responsiveness of mammary tissue to estradiol or its resistance to this steroid may bear a relationship to the cellular make-up of the tissue. However, during normal development the morphological changes seen in the tissue were always accompanied by changes in the hormonal milieu. We therefore felt that in order to identify whether the morphological state of the tissue was in fact dictating the estrogenic sensitivity, it would be necessary to do the experiments without altering the endogenous hormonal milieu. It is well known (3) that, in addition to an appropriate hormonal milieu, suckling stimulus is essential for lactation to commence in mammary glands. Therefore, by preventing suckling on one side of a lactating mouse by using the technique of unilateral thelectomy (nipple removal), we were able to obtain a fully lactating mammary tissue from nipple-intact glands and non-lactating tissue from the thelectomized glands, while at the same time maintaining the endogenous hormonal milieu as that of lactation. The morphology of the thelectomized mammary glands at seven days postpartum revealed that significant amounts of adipose and connective tissue elements were still surrounding the mammary epithelium while in the contralateral nipple-intact lactating mammary glands, the epithelial cells were predominant (Fig. 12). The effect of estradiol on the thelectomized versus non-thelectomized mammary glands was next exa-

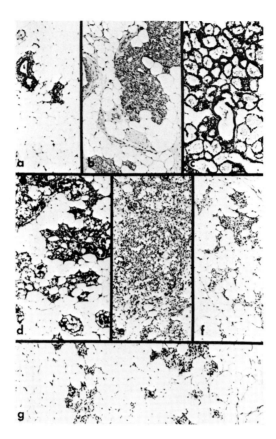

FIG. 11. Histology of mammary glands at different stages of development
and lactational involution. a) Virgin mammary gland with sparse mammary
epithelium and predominance of fat cells (H & E: X125). b) Fourteen-day
pregnant mammary gland. Note increase in number and lobuloalveolar organization of mammary epithelial cells (H & E: X125). c) Twelve day
lactating mammary gland. Note dilation of alveolar lumina and presence
of secretion within lumina (PAS: X125). d) Four day involuted mammary
gland. Note decrease in size of alveolar lumina indicating resorption
of milk constituents (PAS: X125). e) Five day involuted mammary gland.
Note degeneration of lobuloalveolar cells and lymphocytic infiltrations
(H & E: X125). f) Five day involuted mammary gland. Note reduction
in number of mammary epithelial cells, loss of lobuloalveolar organization of the epithelium, and the predominance of fat cells (H & E: X125).
g) Twenty eight day postpartum mammary glands. Note the predominance
of fat cells and loss of lobuloalveolar organization of the mammary epithelial cells indicative of lactational involution (H & E: X125).
(Haslam and Shyamala, 1979b).

mined. As shown in Fig. 13 and 14, while, as expected estradiol was
without any effect on the lactating mammary tissue both with respect to
progesterone level and the rate of DNA synthesis, the thelectomized
glands responded to estradiol with appropriate increases in both progesterone receptor level (Fig. 13) and rate of DNA synthesis (Fig. 14).

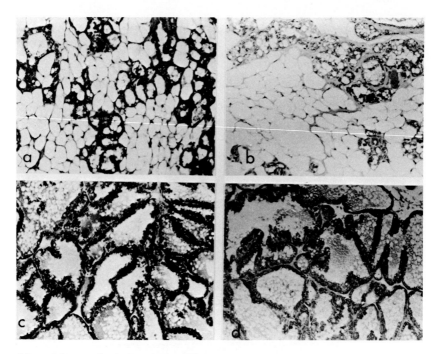

FIG. 12. Effect of thelectomy on mammary glands of postpartum mice.
Thelectomized mammary glands (a) 2 day postpartum and (b) 7 day postpartum. The glands are lobuloalveolar but alveoli have small lumina
indicative of a nonsecretory condition. Contralateral nipple-intact
mammary glands (c) 2 day postpartum and (d) 7 day postpartum. The
alveolar lumina are extensively dilated and secretion filled. Hema-
toxylin and eosin X125 (Haslam and Shyamala, 1980).

V.   AN EVALUATION OF THE MAMMARY FAT PAD AS A POTENTIAL SITE FOR INITIA-
TION OF ESTROGEN ACTION

In the female mouse, the mammary epithelium is embedded in a pad of
adipose and connective tissue commonly known as mammary fat pad; moreover it is the adipose tissue that occupies most of the mass of the mammary gland in a non-pregnant female mouse. In a series of elegant
experiments, DeOme and his co-workers and others (4,7,14,30) have demonstrated that the transplanted mammary epithelium can grow only in the
mammary fat pad. In fact, Faulkin and DeOme (6,7) have suggested that
fat cells may regulate the growth of mammary ductal epithelium in a
sexually mature mouse. Since, as mentioned previously a principal
effect of estrogen on the mammary gland is its impact on growth, it is
conceivable that estrogen may initiate mammary epithelial growth through
processes associated with the mammary adipose and connective tissue.
Moreover, studies characterizing the effects of androgen on embryonic
mammary development reveal that it is the mammary mesenchyme and not the
epithelium which is responsive to androgen (18). In addition, all
changes in the mammary epithelium appear to be secondarily caused by
androgen-activated mesenchymal cells (18). Therefore, by analogy it
appeared that another steroid hormone such as estradiol might also exert
its effect on mammary epithelium by initial interaction with the mesen-

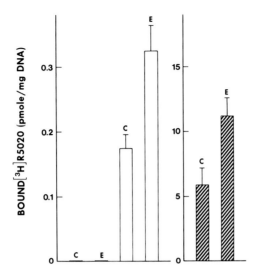

FIG. 13. Effect of estradiol on cytoplasmic progesterone receptor of mammary glands and uterus of unilaterally thelectomized lactators. Two groups of unilaterally thelectomized lactating mice were given a single injection of either saline (C) or 3 µg of·estradiol (E) for 24 h prior to tissue removal. The binding represents specific binding only and is mean ± SE of three to four experiments. (■) Non-thelectomized lactating mammary glands. (□) Thelectomized-nonlactating mammary gland. (▨) Uterus (Shyamala and Haslam, 1980).

chyme; if this were the case receptors for estrogen might be expected to be present in the mammary fat pad.

Therefore we decided to examine whether mammary fat pad devoid of epithelium had estrogen receptors. It is possible to separate the mammary epithelium from adipose and connective tissue in the inguinal mammary glands of 21 day old mice according to the technique described by DeOme et al (4). This mammary fat pad devoid of epithelium is often referred to as the cleared fat pad or de-epithelialized fat pad. As shown in Fig. 15, the cleared fat pad is able to bind (^{3}H)estradiol in a time-dependent and saturable fashion with a high affinity indicating the presence of estrogen receptor. The steroid specificity for the binding of estradiol also appeared to be strictly characteristic of the estrogen receptor (Fig. 15).

The concentration of the receptor in the de-epithelialized gland was estimated to be about 330 ± 22 fmoles/mg DNA while in the intact gland it was found at 720 ± 314 fmoles/mg DNA. However, these figures do not necessarily indicate that in the intact gland of the virgin mouse the estrogen receptors are equally distributed between the fat pad and epithelium. It is known that there is metabolic cooperativity between epithelial cell and adipocytes in mammary tissue and also local glandular factors may influence mammary adipocyte activity (2,5,21); therefore the metabolism of fat pad free of epithelium may be quite different from that containing the epithelium. Nevertheless, the data lend confidence to our hypothesis that the mammary fat pad may be a potential site for the initiation of estrogen action in the mammary tissue. It might also explain why, despite numerous attempts, isolated mammary epithelial cells

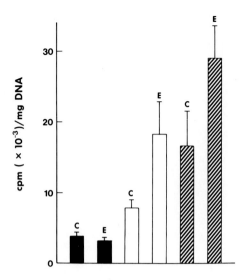

FIG. 14. Effect of estradiol on the in vitro incorporation of (^{3}H)-thymidine into DNA in the mammary glands and uteri of unilaterally thelectomized lactators. Two groups of unilaterally thelectomized lactating mice were given a single injection of either saline (C) or 3 μg estradiol (E) for 24 h before tissue removal and processing. The data represent the mean $\pm$ SE of six experiments. (■) Non-thelectomized lactating mammary glands. (□) Thelectomized nonlactating mammary glands. (▨) Uteri (Shyamala and Ferenczy, 1982).

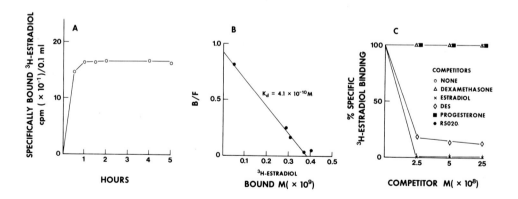

FIG. 15. (A) The time course of the specific binding of (^{3}H)estradiol in cytoplasmic extracts of de-epithelialized mammary fat pad. (B) Saturation analysis of (^{3}H)estradiol binding in cytoplasmic extracts of de-epithelialized mammary fat pad. The data represents the Scatchard plot of specific binding only. (C) The relative effectiveness of various unlabelled steroids to compete for specific (^{3}H)estradiol binding in cytoplasmic extracts of de-epithelialized mammary fat pad (Haslam and Shyamala, 1981).

have so far failed to respond to an estrogen stimulus in vitro.

VI. CONCLUSIONS

The mammary glands of mice respond to estradiol in vivo by several metabolic criteria such as increases in glucose metabolism, progesterone receptor level and rate of DNA synthesis. Furthermore, the estrogenic sensitivity of the mammary tissue as assessed by these various criteria is modulated as a function of development such that the lactating mammary glands appear to be nonresponsive to estradiol. The biological basis for this nonresponsiveness does not appear to reside at the level of altered estrogen receptor status. Rather, a critical evaluation of all our experimental data to date suggests that the mammary adipose and connective tissue elements may play a pivotal role in initiating the action of estradiol in the mammary gland. The possibility that the adipose and connective tissue may indeed play an important role in estrogen action is strengthened by our demonstration of estrogen receptors in the de-epithelialized mammary fat pad.

ACKNOWLEDGEMENTS

These studies were supported by a grant from the National Cancer Institute of Canada. Ms. S. Fraiberg, Ms. C. Lalonde and Mr. D. Saxe assisted in the preparation of the manuscript.

REFERENCES

1. Bresciani, F. (1965): Exp. Cell Res., 38:13-32.
2. Bartley, J.C., Emerman, J.T., and Bissell, M. (1981): Am. J. Physiol., 24(Cell Physiol. 10):C204-208.
3. Cowie, A.T., and Tindall, J.S. (1971): In: The Physiology of Lactation, edited by H. Davson, and A.D.M. Greenfield. Edward Arnold Publication, Ltd., London.
4. DeOme, K.B., Faulkin, L.J., Bern, H.A., and Blair, P.B. (1959): Cancer Res., 19:515-520.
5. Elias, J.J., Pitelka, D.R., and Armstrong, R.C. (1973): Anat. Res., 177:533-548.
6. Faulkin, L.J., and DeOme, K.B. (1958): Cancer Res., 18:51-56.
7. Faulkin, L.J., and DeOme, K.B. (1960): J. Natl. Cancer Inst., 24: 953-969.
8. Gardner, D.G., and Wittliff, J.L. (1973): Biochemistry 12:3090-3096.
9. Gaubert, C-M., Biancucci, S., and Shyamala, G. (1982): Endocrinology, 110:683-685.
10. Haslam, S.Z., and Shyamala, G. (1979a): Biochem. J., 182:127-131.
11. Haslam, S.Z., and Shyamala, G. (1979b): Endocrinology, 105:786-795.
12. Haslam, S.Z., and Shyamala, G. (1980): J. Cell Biol., 86:730-737.
13. Haslam, S.Z., and Shyamala, G. (1981): Endocrinology, 108:825-830.
14. Hoshino, K. (1962): J. Natl. Cancer Inst., 29:835-851.
15. Hseuh, A.J.W., Peck, E.J., Jr., and Clark, J.H. (1973): J. Endocrinol., 58:1-9.
16. Hunt, M.E., and Muldoon, T.G. (1977): J. Steroid Biochem., 8:181-186.
17. Katzenellenbogen, B.S., and Gorski, J. (1975): In: Action of Hormones, edited by G. Litwack, Vol. 3, pp. 137-243. Academic Press, New York.

18. Kratochwil, K., and Schwartz, P. (1976): Proc. Natl. Acad. Sci. US, 73:4041-4044.
19. Leung, B.S., Jack, W.M., and Reiney, C.C. (1976): J. Steroid Biochem., 7:89-95.
20. Lieberman, M.E., Maurer, R.A., and Gorski, J. (1978): Proc. Natl. Acad. Sci. US, 75:5946-5949.
21. Lucas, A., Scopas, C., and Bartley, J.C. (1976): J. Cell Biol., 70:335a.
22. Lyons, W.R., Li, C.H., and Johnson, R.E. (1958): Rec. Progr. Horm. Res., 14:219-248.
23. Nandi, S. (1958): J. Natl. Cancer Inst., 21:1039-1063.
24. Oka, T., Perry, J.W., and Topper, Y.J. (1974): J. Cell Biol., 62:550-556.
25. Puca, G.A., and Bresciani, F. (1969): Endocrinology, 85:1-10.
26. Sheth, N.A., Tickekon, S.S., Ranadive, R.J., and Sheth, A.R. (1978): Mol. Cell. Endocrinol., 12:167-176.
27. Shyamala, G., and Nandi, S. (1972): Endocrinology, 91:861-867.
28. Shyamala, G., and Haslam, S.Z. (1980): In: Perspectives in Steroid Receptor Research, edited by F. Bresciani, pp. 193-216. Raven Press, New York.
29. Shyamala, G., and Ferenczy, A. (1982): Endocrinology, 110:1249-1256.
30. Slavin, B. (1966): Anat. Rec., 154:423.
31. Smith, M.S., and Neill, J.D. (1977): Biol. Reprod., 17:255-261.
32. Topper, Y.J., and Freeman, C.S. (1980): Physiol. Rev., 60:1049-1106.
33. Topper, Y.J. (1980): Adv. Biosci., 25:223-227.
34. Vuhai, M.T., Logeat, F., Warembourg, H., and Milgrom, E. (1977): Ann. N.Y. Acad. Sci., 286:199-209.
35. Walters, M.R., and Clark, J.H. (1979): Endocrinology, 105:382-386.

Progress in Cancer Research and Therapy,
Vol. 31, edited by F. Bresciani, et al.
Raven Press, New York © 1984.

Nuclear Estradiol Receptors and Regression in Human Breast Cancer

Arpad G. Fazekas and John K. MacFarlane

The Montreal General Hospital, University Surgical Clinic, Montreal, Quebec, H3G 1A4 Canada

It has been established that the assay of cytosolic extrogen receptors in human breast cancer greatly improves the selection of patients for endocrine therapy. Success rates of hormonal treatments in patients with positive estrogen receptor tumors generally reach 60% (7,3). More recently the additional measurement of cytosolic progesterone receptors improved response rates to the 75-80% range (8). Still, a sizeable proportion of patients with significant levels of cytosolic hormone receptors fails to benefit from endocrine treatment. Therefore, improvements in the characterization of hormone dependent tumors are likely to increase the accuracy of selection of patients for these manipulations.

According to the theory of estrogen action, the cytosol ER-estradiol complex translocates into the nucleus after undergoing a temperature dependent transformation. We postulated that, in some tumors, this translocation process might be defective (1). Therefore in spite of high estrogen receptor concentrations in the cytosol, the tumor remains hormonally independent.

We demonstrated previously (1) that specific nuclear uptake of ^{3}H estradiol was defective in a significant proportion of ERC rich human breast cancers and that such cases did not respond to endocrine therapy in a small group of 10 patients (6). As a continuation of this study, we present our new data on the simultaneous measurement of cytosolic estrogen and progesterone receptors and specific nuclear uptake of estradiol in a much larger group of tumors, as well as the relationship of these parameters to the clinical responses seen following endocrine manipulation.

MATERIALS AND METHODS

Tumor specimens were obtained from patients with histologically verified cancer of the breast undergoing breast biopsy or mastectomy, and from patients with surgically accessible metastatic disease. Tissues were homogenized in Tris-HCl buffer (0.01 M, pH 7.4, containing 0.0014 M EDTA and 0.5 mM dithiothreitol, TED buffer) in a VIR-Tis-23 homogenizer. Cytosols were obtained by centrifugation of the homogenate at 100,000 g for 1 hr. in an ultracentrifuge. Fresh cytosols were tested immediately for estradiol and progesterone binding.

Radioactive estradiol (2,4,6,7) -$_3$(^{3}H)-estradiol, SA 110 Ci/mmol) and promegestone (17 -methyl-^{3}H) (SA 85.0 Ci/mmol) were purchased from New England Nuclear, Boston, Mass.

ERC was determined using the dextran coated charcoal method. Increasing masses of tritiated estradiol were incubated in duplicate at 4°C for 16 hr. with cytosol aliquots. Non-specific binding was accounted for by preparing the same incubation series with the addition of a 200-fold excess of DES as estrogen competitor. Dissociation constants (k_d) and number of binding sites were calculated by the Scatchard method (10). K_d's obtained were in the 10^{-10} M range and the number of binding sites was calculated as fmol/mg cytosol protein (fmol/mg P). Progesterone receptor was assayed using a similar procedure with Promegestone (17 -methyl-^{3}H), but in a TED buffer containing 10% glycerol.

The nuclear fraction was isolated from the sediment following separation of the cytosol. The sediment was rehomogenized in 5 ml TED buffer in a Potter-Elvehjem type homogenizer, then centrifuged at 2000 g for 10 min at 4°C. The supernatant was discarded and the sediment was rehomogenized again in 5 ml buffer and then filtered through a 100 mesh sieve in order to eliminate fibres of connective tissue. The presence of nuclei was verified by light microscopy in this preparation. Aliquots of this filtrate (0.5 ml/tube), containing the nuclei, were incubated with 10^5 d.p.m. (^{3}H) - estradiol (0.45 pmol/tube), 0.2 ml of cytosol from the same tumor without and with a 100 x excess of nonradioactive DES in triplicates. Incubations were carried out in a Dubnoff metabolic shaker at 30°C for 45 min. After incubation, nuclei were sedimented by centrifugation (2,000 g x 10 min) at 4°C, followed by resuspension in 3 ml TED buffer and a second centrifugation (washing). ERN was extracted from the sediment with 2 ml of 0.4 KCl in TED buffer at 4°C for 1 hr. During this time the tubes were vortexed several times. After extraction, the nuclear pellet was sedimented by centrifugation at 2,000 g x 10 minutes and the supernatant (extract) transferred to scintillation vials and counted for radioactivity. Non specific binding was accounted for by subtracting the values obtained in the parallel experiment performed with DES. ERN was expressed as femtomoles specifically bound estradiol/mg DNA.

RESULTS AND DISCUSSION

It has to be emphasized that our methodology for the assay of ERN significantly differs from methods used by other groups. In our method the washed nuclei are incubated with tritiated estradiol in the presence of cytosol under conditions favouring translocation (4). Estradiol receptors are then subsequently extracted from the nuclei and the specifically bound estradiol is quantitated.

To distinguish our method, it should be named "cytosol-mediated, specific nuclear uptake of estradiol" or shortly "translocation method". However, objections could be justified against the latter term for not measuring purely translocation (direct uptake by ERN without mediating cytosolic receptors certainly takes place). Therefore we prefer to call our method "cytosol-mediated nuclear uptake" or "nuclear estradiol receptor activity".

Both ERC and ERN were assayed in 600 primary and metastatic breast tumors. ERC were classified into 3 groups: Positive (10 > fmol/mgP and up), borderline (3-9 fmol/mgP) and negative (0-2 fmol/mgP). ERN was between 0-746 fmol/mg DNA. Values of ERN between 0 and 19 fmol/mg DNA were arbitrarily regarded as negative and classified as such. This cut off point we regard temporary and is

subject to modification based on future clinical responses. Table 1
shows the correlation of these two receptor groups. It can be seen
that, of 247 cases with significant ERC concentrations, 60 had no or
negligible ERN (24.3%) activity. In the borderline ERC

Table 1 Correlation of ERC and ERN

ERC fmol/mgP	Cases in group	ERN fm/mg DNA 0-19	 20-746	ERN% Negative
10 >	247	60	187	24.3
3 - 9	110	40	70	36.3
0 - 2	243	170	73	70.0

group, the proportion of ERN negatives was higher at 36.3%, while in
the ERC negative it increased further to 70.0%. On the other hand,
there were 73 cases in the ERC negative group with significant nuclear
binding activity, indicating that tumors very poor in cytosolic ER may
have significant nuclear receptor levels. This group could represent
some of the ERC negative tumors that respond to endocrine therapy
(8-10%) in clinical experience (7,6). The occurence of (PgRC) in
connection with ERN was also evaluated. Results obtained in 158
tumors show that a strong positive relationship exists between PgRC
and ERN, with most PgRC positive cases also proving positive for ERN
(74%).
        This supports the theory proposed by Horwitz and McGuire (2) on
the correlation of estrogen and progesterone receptors in breast
cancer. Very similar findings were reported by Romic-Stojkovic and
Gamulin (9) in support of the assumption that induction of PgRC by
estrogen in human breast cancer is mediated by a mechanism involving
nuclear estrogen receptors.
        Since 1977, when our nuclear receptor studies were initiated, we
have been following these patients for their responses to endocrine
treatments. Many of the patients received combined endocrine therapy
and chemotherapy. These were excluded from this analysis. Table 2
shows the responses of 40 patients treated with endocrine therapy
only; including adrenalectomy-oophorectomy, additive therapy with
estrogens or anti-estrogen treatment with tamoxifen or androgens.
Remission was defined as at least a 50% decrease in the size of
measureable lesions, with no evidence of any new lesions, lasting at
least 3 months.

Table 2 Response to Endocrine Therapy as a Function of ERC and ERN

ERC- ERN-	ERC- ERN+	ERC+ ERN-	ERC+ ERN+	ERC+ PgRC+	ERN-	ERN+
0/12	5/5	2/5	18/18	13/15	2/17	23/23
0%	100%	40%	100%	86%	11%	100%

RESPONSE RATE: RESPONDERS/PATIENTS IN GROUP

Essentially all 18 patients with positive ERC and ERN benefited from hormonal treatment, while none of the 12 patients with negative ERC and ERN showed regression. In the mixed results groups, where ERC was negative but ERN positive, all 5 patients responded, while only two out of the five patients with positive ERC but negative ERN responded.

The response rate (100%) found in the doubly positive group is encouraging, since it is better than rates we have previously reported (5) for ERC positive cases (60%). This response rate is also much better than those (77%) reported for ERC and PgRC positive groups (3).

Again, all 23 ERN positives regressed on endocrine therapy, while only 2 of 17 (11%) ERN negatives responded to endocrine treatment. It is of great interest that all the cases (five) with borderline ERC values and positive ERN responded while those with negative ERN did not (three). This suggests that ERN is a more sensitive indication of endocrine dependency than ERC alone or ERC combined with PgRC.

A number of papers were published recently on occupied and unoccupied nuclear estrogen receptors in human breast cancer, but very few data are available relating clinical responses to hormonal treatments. Results published by Laing et al (14) obtained in 32 patients indicated a high remission rate when both cytosolic and nuclear estrogen receptors were present, (RR18/22, 82%) while a very low response rate (1/9) was seen in ERN negative cases. In a subsequent paper, the same authors reported a 71% response rate to endocrine therapy in 42 patients with ER in both the soluble and nuclear fractions (5).

These data, taken together with our results presented here, indicate that the assay of the specific nuclear uptake of estradiol is a better predictor of endocrine dependency than the measurement of cytosolic receptor activity.

REFERENCES

1)   Fazekas, A.G., and MacFarlane, J.K. (1980): J. Steroid Biochem. 13:613-622.

2)   Horwitz, K.B., and McGuire, W.L. (1975): Steroids 25:497-505.

3)   Jensen, E.V., Smith, S., and DeSombre, E.R. (1976): J. Steroid Biochem. 7:911-917.

4)   Laing L., Calman, K.C., Smith, M.G., Smith, D.C., Leake, R.E. (1977): The Lancet 168.

5)   Leake, R.E., Laing, L., Calman, K.C., Macbeth, F.R., Crawford, D., and Smith D.C. (1981): Br. J. Cancer 43: 59-66.

6)   MacFarlane, J.K., Fleiszer, D., Fazekas, A.G. (1980): Cancer 45:2998-3003.

7)   McGuire, W.L., Carbone, P.P., Sears, M.E., and Escher, G.C. (1975): In: Estrogen Receptors in Human Breast Cancer, edited by W.L. McGuire, P.P. Carbone, and E.P. Vollmer, pp. 1-7. Raven Press, New York.

8)   Osborne, C.K., Yochmowitz, M.G., Knight, W.A., McGuire, W.L. (1980): Cancer 46:613-622.

9)   Romic-Stojkovic, R., Gamulin, S. (1980): Cancer Res. 40:4821-4825.

10) Scatchard G. (1949): Ann. N.Y. Acad. Sci. 51:660-672.

Progress in Cancer Research and Therapy,
Vol. 31, edited by F. Bresciani, et al.
Raven Press, New York © 1984.

Growth Hormone Receptors in Human Breast Cancer: Correlation with Oestrogen Receptor Status

*Liam J. Murphy, *Elizabeth Vrhovsek, *Robynne McGinley,
**Leigh C. Murphy, **Robert L. Sutherland, and *Leslie Lazarus

*The Garvan Institute of Medical Research, St. Vincent's Hospital, New South Wales
2010; and **Ludwig Institute for Cancer Research (Sydney Branch), University of
Sydney, New South Wales 2006, Australia

The predictive value of oestrogen receptor (ER) status of breast
tumours in determining those patients likely to respond to endocrine
therapies has been clearly established (5,7) and has encouraged the
search for other hormone receptors in human breast cancer tissue.
While progesterone (8), insulin (4) and lactogenic receptors (1,4,10,
12,15,18) have been demonstrated in human breast cancer biopsies, only
progesterone receptor concentration has been clearly shown to
correlate with ER status (8). The relationship between lactogenic
receptor concentration in breast cancer tissue and ER status has not
been adequately examined. Furthermore the specificity of the
lactogenic receptor in this tissue has not been clearly established
and the frequency of breast cancer biopsies with significant saturable
binding of iodinated ovine prolactin (oPRL), human prolactin (hPRL)
and human growth hormone (hGH) varies considerably even within the one
laboratory where all three ligands were used (1,4,10,12,15,18).

In this study we have investigated the specificity of $[^{125}I]$-hGH
binding sites in cultured human breast cancer cell lines and in
membrane preparations from breast cancer biopies and have demonstrated
that hGH and hPRL are mutually competitive at this receptor site. In
addition a significant correlation between ER and lactogenic receptor
concentration has been demonstrated in both cultured breast cancer
cell lines and breast cancer biopsy specimens.

MATERIALS AND METHODS

Human GH and hPRL were generous gifts from the Human Pituitary
Advisory Committee (Canberra, Australia). Bovine GH was obtained from
Dr M. Sonenberg (New York, NY) while all other hormones used were
generously supplied by the National Pituitary Hormone Program
(Bethesda, MD). Human GH and hPRL were iodinated by the method of
Greenwood et al (3) as described previously (11).

Cell Cultures

A total of 14 cell lines were studied, the sources of which are listed in Table 1. Mycoplasma-free cells were routinely grown as monolayer cultures in RPMI-1640 medium supplemented with 20 mM Hepes, 14 mM sodium bicarbonate, 6 mM L-glutamine, 20 µg/ml gentamicin 10 µg/ml porcine insulin and 10% (v/v) foetal calf serum as previously described (17).

Oestrogen Receptor Analyses

Confluent cell monolayer cultures were harvested with 1 mM EDTA in Dulbecco's phosphate buffered saline and washed with 10 mM Tris-HCl, 1.5 mM EDTA, 0.25 M sucrose buffer, pH 7.4 (TES). The cell pellet was homogenized in TES (3×10^7 cells/ml) using a teflon-glass homogenizer and a crude nuclear pellet was prepared by centrifugation (800 x g for 10 min). This, and all subsequent steps were carried out at 4°. The resulting supernatant was centrifuged at 135,000 x g for 1 hr to give the soluble fraction containing cytosol ER. Nuclear ER was extracted from the washed crude nuclear pellet as previously described (16). Endogenous oestrogens were removed from the extracts by a 30 min incubation with 100 µl/ml of 5% charcoal-0.5% dextran solution. ER concentration was measured in charcoal-dextran treated cell extracts by saturation analysis and data were analysed by the method of Scatchard (13) following correction for non-specific binding.

Breast cancer biopsy specimens were obtained from 31 female patients and stored frozen in liquid nitrogen. The frozen tissue specimens were pulverized using a Braun Mikro-Dismembrator II, added to 5 volumes of ice-cold buffer (20 mM Tris, 3.0 mM Na_2EDTA, 10 mM KH_2PO_4, pH 7.4) and centrifuged for 1 hr at 100,000 x g. ER concentration was measured in this supernatant as described above and the data expressed as fmol/mg protein. Cytosol preparations with an ER concentration of less than 3 fmol/mg protein were considered negative.

Growth Hormone Binding Studies

Binding of $[^{125}I]$-hGH to cell monolayers was measured by incubating 0.1 ng (30,000 cpm) of $[^{125}I]$-hGH with $1 - 5 \times 10^6$ cells in the presence or absence of increasing concentrations of unlabelled hGH for 4 hr at 30° (11). In studies where the binding of $[^{125}I]$-hGH to human breast cancer biopsies was examined, a crude plasma membrane fraction was prepared as follows: the 100,000 x g pellet obtained from preparation of the cytosol for ER assays was homogenized using a Teflon-glass homogenizer in ice cold 0.25 M sucrose and centrifuged at 10,000 x g for 30 min at 4°. The resultant supernatant was centrifuged at 40,000 x g for 40 min at 4° and the pellet was resuspended in 50 mM Tris-HCl buffer, pH 7.4 and washed by recentrifugation. Binding of $[^{125}I]$-hGH was determined by incubating 75 - 100 µg of membrane protein with 0.1 ng of $[^{125}I]$-hGH in 400 µl of binding buffer; 12.5 mM Tris-HCl, 10 mM $CaCl_2$, 0.5% BSA, pH 7.4 for 20 hr at room temperature (18 - 22°). The incubation was terminated by the addition of 2 ml of ice cold binding buffer followed by centrifugation at 1500 x g for 1 hr. The supernatant was decanted and the pellet counted in a NE 1600 gamma counter. All assays were performed in duplicate. Membranes pooled from 30 - 40 breast cancer biopsies were prepared for the study of

specificity of [^{125}I]-hGH binding to breast membranes. Specific binding
of [^{125}I]-hGH to membranes was expressed as the difference in the
percentage of added [^{125}I]-hGH bound in the absence or presence of an
excess of hGH (10^4 ng/ml) per 100 µg of membrane protein. Protein
concentration was measured by the method of Lowry et al. (6) using BSA
as a standard. In assays where different somatogenic and lactogenic
hormones were compared, parallel incubations with and without excess
unlabelled hGH were performed and data were expressed as a fraction of
the maximal specific binding (B/B$_o$).

RESULTS

Breast Cancer Cell Lines

    The specificity of [^{125}I]-hGH binding to the T-47D cell line is
shown in Fig.1. Human PRL was approximately equipotent with hGH in
inhibiting [^{125}I]-hGH binding to saturable binding sites in T-47D cells
while human placental lactogen (hPL) and rat PRL (rPRL) were 3.5% and
1.5% as potent as hGH respectively. Bovine and rabbit GH did not
inhibit [^{125}I]-hGH binding to these high affinity sites. The
specificity of [^{125}I]-hGH binding to MCF 7 and BT-474 cells was

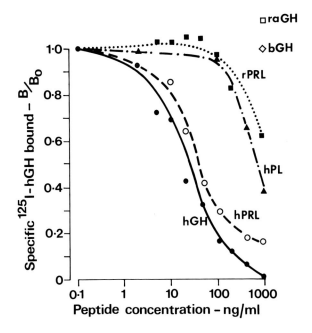

FIG.1 Specificity of [^{125}I]-hGH binding to T-47D cells. Confluent
monolayers, approximately 5×10^6 cells were incubated with 0.1 ng of
[^{125}I]-hGH and increasing concentrations of hGH (●), hPRL (O), hPL
(▲), rPRL (■), bovine GH (◇) or rabbit GH (□) for 4 hr at 30°.
Specific binding is expressed as a fraction of the maximal specific
binding which varied from 2 - 5% of the total radioactivity added.

identical to that described for the T-47D cells. The specificity of
[^{125}I]-hPRL binding to T-47D cells was also examined (Fig.2) and was
found to be similar to that reported by Shiu (14) who demonstrated that
hPRL and hGH were approximately equipotent in inhibiting binding of
[^{125}I]-hPRL to T-47D cells. High affinity (K_a = 0.53 - 2.33 nM^{-1}), low
capacity (330 - 6560 sites/cell) lactogenic receptors were found in all
ER positive cell lines while no specific [^{125}I]-hGH binding to the 4 ER
negative cell lines was detected. The concentration of ER and
lactogenic receptors in each cell line is shown in Table 1. When
considered as a group there was a significant correlation (r = 0.745,
p < 0.001) between ER and lactogenic receptor concentrations in these
breast cancer cell lines.

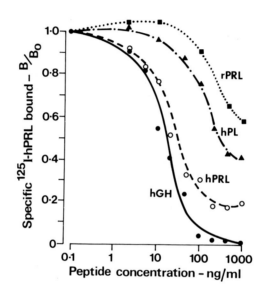

FIG.2. Specificity of [^{125}I]-hPRL binding to T-47D cells. Confluent
monolayers, approximately 5 x 10^6 cells were incubated with 0.1 ng of
[^{125}I]-hPRL and increasing concentrations of hGH (●), hPRL (○), hPL
(▲), or rPRL (■) for 4 hr at 30°. Specific binding is expressed as
a fraction of the maximal specific binding which varied from 2 - 7% of
the total radioactivity added.

Breast Cancer Biopsies

The specificity of binding of [^{125}I]-hGH to the high affinity
binding site in pooled breast cancer membranes was similar to that
described for [^{125}I]-hGH binding to T-47D cells. Human GH, hPRL and
oPRL readily inhibited binding of [^{125}I]-hGH to saturable sites in this
tissue. Human and ovine PRL were marginally less potent, while hPL was
significantly less potent than hGH in inhibiting [^{125}I]-hGH binding to
breast cancer membranes. Bovine GH did not compete with hGH for binding
to this receptor. A similar specificity was observed when [^{125}I]-hPRL
was used as the labelled ligand indicating that hPRL and hGH are

TABLE 1. <u>Oestrogen and lactogenic receptor concentrations in breast cancer cell lines</u>

Cell Line[1]	Lactogenic receptor (sites/cell)	Oestrogen receptor (sites/cell)
MCF 7	4140	9114
MCF 7$_L$	4135	6828
R27	3810	2219
R98	2340	5229
T-47D$_W$	2212	3803
T-47D	6560	4345
MCF 7$_M$	2120	4585
ZR 75-1	4135	2933
BT-474	330	1885
MDA-MB-361	435	2505
MDA-MB-330	not detected	not detected
MDA-MB-231	"	"
MDA-MB-157	"	"
BT-20	"	"

[1] Subscripts have been used to denote different sources of the same cell line. MCF 7 cells were from Dr C.M. McGrath, Michigan Cancer Foundation, Detroit, MCF 7$_L$, R27 and R98 cells were from Dr M.E. Lippman, National Cancer Institute, Bethesda, T-47D$_W$ were from Dr R.H. Whitehead, Ludwig Institute for Cancer Research (Melbourne Branch), MCF 7$_M$ and all other cell lines were supplied by E.G. & G. Mason Research Institute of behalf on the National Cancer Institute Breast Cancer Program Cell Culture Bank.

mutually competitive ligands for the lactogenic receptor in human breast cancer tissue. The mean affinity and concentration derived from Scatchard plots for 8 separate membrane preparations were $K_a = 0.52 \pm 0.09$ (SEM) nM^{-1} and 255 ± 85 fmol/mg protein respectively. The percentage of the added radioactivity bound to individual membrane preparations varied from 10 - 50% of the total radioactivity. A considerable percentage (20 - 60%) of the membrane bound $[^{125}I]$-hGH was not displaced by 10^4 ng/ml hGH and was considered non-specific while specific binding varied between 0 and 12% of the total radioactivity added to the incubation. Approximately 65% (20/31) of the breast cancer biopsy membranes demonstrated significant specific binding of $[^{125}I]$-hGH, that is greater than 1% of the total radioactivity was bound to saturable sites.

Membrane preparations from ER negative tumours demonstrated significantly less specific binding of $[^{125}I]$-hGH than membrane preparations from ER positive tumour biopsies (1.22 ± 0.44 vs. 3.21 ± 0.56% of the total radioactivity added, $p < 0.05$, Wilcoxon) and membrane preparations from breast cancer biopsies with moderately high (101 - 150 fmol/mg protein) or very high (> 150 fmol/mg protein) ER concentrations demonstrated significantly more specific binding of $[^{125}I]$-hGH than tumours with low ER concentrations (< 11 fmol per mg cytosol protein, Fig.3.). A significant correlation between ER concentration and specific $[^{125}I]$-hGH bound was also found with this tumour biopsy material (Fig.4, $r = 0.412$, $p < 0.02$).

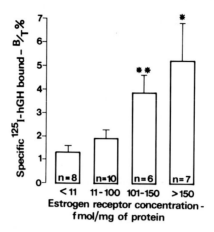

FIG.3. The relationship between specific binding of [^{125}I]-hGH to membrane preparations and oestrogen receptor concentrations in breast cancer biopsies. The 31 breast cancer biopsies were grouped according to the oestrogen receptor concentration expressed as fmol/mg cytosol protein, and the mean ± SEM [^{125}I]-hGH bound per 100 μg of membrane protein was examined. *p < 0.05 and **p < 0.025 difference from tumours with ER concentrations < 11 fmol mg protein.

DISCUSSION

The specificity of the lactogenic receptor in breast cancer tissue is controversial. While Holdaway and Friesen (4) reported that hGH is equipotent with hPRL in displacing [^{125}I]-hPRL, Morgan et al (10) found that hGH did not compete with oPRL for binding to this tissue. In addition, the percentage of tumour biopsies with significant specific binding of iodinated hGH, hPRL and oPRL varies considerably even within the one laboratory (10,12,15,18). In this report we have demonstrated that hGH and hPRL are mutually competitive at the lactogenic receptor site in membrane preparations from breast cancer biopsy specimens and in cultured human breast cancer cell lines.

A significant correlation between ER concentration and specific binding of iodinated hGH to both cultured breast cancer cell lines and breast cancer biopsy tissue has been demonstrated. An absolute relationship between these two parameters is present in cultured breast cancer cell lines, in that ER negative cells are devoid of detectable lactogenic receptor in breast cancer tissue with similar affinity [^{125}I]-hGH is an acceptable ligand for determining lactogenic receptor concentration and affinity. In addition to binding to the lactogenic receptor in breast cancer tissue hGH has been shown to be a potent agonist in this tissue (9). The data reported here for the affinity and concentration of lactogenic receptors in beast cancer cells are in general agreement with those reported by Shiu (14) who used [^{125}I]-hPRL as the ligand.

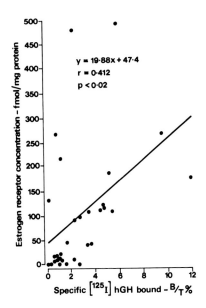

FIG.4. Correlation between oestrogen receptor concentrations and specific [^{125}I]-hGH bound to membrane preparations from individual breast cancer biopsies. A least squares linear regression analysis has been used to determine the relationship between the two parameters. From Murphy et al., submitted for publication.

The ER status of each of the cell lines is similar to that reported elsewhere (2). Since neither MCF 7 nor T-47D cells are thought to be clonally derived it is not surprising that cells from different sources have different ER and lactogenic receptor concentrations.

Significant specific binding of [^{125}I]-hGH (greater than 1% of the added radioactivity) was found in 65% of the 31 breast cancer biopsies examined. This is consistent with data reported by Bonneterre et al. (1) and Stagner et al (15) where significant specific binding of [^{125}I]-hGH was found in 72% and 70% of tumours respectively. In contrast, Turcot-Lemay and Kelly (18) reported that only 12% of tumour biopsies demonstrated significant binding of iodinated hGH while significant binding of iodinated human and ovine prolactin was found in 58% and 30% of biopsies respectively. Since our data suggest that hGH and hPRL bind to the lactogenic receptor in human breast cancer tissue with similar affinities, the observations of Turcot-Lemay and Kelly are difficult to explain. The differences in the percentage of tumour biopsies considered to be lactogenic receptor positive in the published reports may relate to the different assay conditions used, different methods of membrane preparation, the use of MgCl$_2$ to desaturate occupied receptors and the receptor activity of the iodinated hormone used.

A correlation between ER and lactogenic receptor concentrations has been noted in two previous studies (1,15). In both studies iodinated hGH was used as the labelled ligand. In other studies where iodinated human and ovine prolactin have been used no significant correlation was found (4,18). Since we have noted in our laboratory considerable batch to batch variability in the percentage of [^{125}I]-hPRL which is receptor active, it is not surprising that large studies performed over several years using numerous iodinated prolactin preparations have not demonstrated a significant correlation between ER and lactogenic receptor concentration. The significant correlation between ER and lactogenic receptors in breast cancer cell lines and biopsy material reported here suggests that the expression of these two receptors is coupled in mammary tissue. Whilst the most likely explanation for this observation is that ER positive tumours arise from hormonally sensitive cell types which also possess lactogenic receptors, the possibility that oestrogens have a direct effect on lactogenic receptor expression in human breast cancer tissue in a similar manner to the effect of oestrogens on progesterone receptors (8) cannot be excluded. Further studies are needed to evaluate the clinical usefulness of lactogenic receptor determinations in human breast cancer tissue.

REFERENCES

1. Bonneterre, J., Peyrat, J.P.H., Vandewalle, B., Beuscart, R., View, M.C., and Cappelaeke, P. (1982): Eur. J. Cancer Clin. Oncol., 18:1157-1162.
2. Engel, L.W., and Young, N.A. (1978): Cancer Res., 38:4327-4339.
3. Greenwood, F.C., Hunter, W.M., and Glover, J.S. (1963): Biochem. J., 89:114-117.
4. Holdaway, I.M., and Friesen, H.G. (1977): Cancer Res., 37:1946-1952.
5. Jensen, E.V., Block, G.E., Smith, S., Kyser, K., and DeSombre, E. (1971): Natl. Cancer Inst. Monogr., 34:55-70.
6. Lowry, O.H., Rosebrough, N.J., Farr, A., and Randall, R.J. (1951): J. Biol. Chem., 193:265-275.
7. McGuire, W.L. (1973): J. Clin. Invest., 52:73-77.
8. McGuire, W.L., Horwitz, K.B., Pearson, O.H., and Segaloff, A. (1975): Cancer, 39:2934-2947.
9. Malarkey, W.H., Kennedy, M., Allred, L.E., and Milo, G. (1983): J. Clin. Endocrinol. Metab., 56:673-677.
10. Morgan, L., Reggatt, P.R., DeSouza, I., Salih, H., and Hobbs, J.R. (1977): J. Endocrinol., 73:17p-18p.
11. Murphy, L.J., Vrhovsek, E., Sutherland, R.L., and Lazarus, L. (1983): J. Clin. Endocrinol. Metab., in press.
12. Partridge, R.K., and Hahnel, R. (1973): Cancer, 43:643-646.
13. Scatchard, G. (1949): Ann. N.Y. Acad. Sci., 51:660-657.
14. Shiu, R.P.C. (1979): Cancer Res., 39:4381-4386.
15. Stagner, J.I., Jochimsen, R.P., and Sherman, B.M. (1977): Clin. Res., 25:302A.
16. Sutherland, R.L., and Baulieu, E.E. (1976): Eur. J. Biochem., 70:531-541.
17. Sutherland, R.L., Hall, R.E., and Taylor, I.W. (1983): Cancer Res., 43:3998-4006.
18. Turcot-Lemay, L., and Kelly, P. (1982): J. Natl. Cancer Inst., 68:381-383.

Progress in Cancer Research and Therapy,
Vol. 31, edited by F. Bresciani, et al.
Raven Press, New York © 1984.

Prostaglandins and Breast Cancer Without Node Involvement

J.L. Boublil, J.L. Moll, C.M. Lalanne, G. Milano, B.P. Krebs, and M. Namer

Centre Antoine-Lacassagne, 06054 Nice Cedex, France

The prostaglandins are a group of compounds derived enzymatically and non-enzymatically from twenty carbon fatty acids, such as arachidonic acid. During the past twenty years, numerous studies have demonstrated the presence of prostaglandins (PG) in most cells, although the amount and class of PG vary considerably with cell type.

Various malignant tumors are known to produce PG, and in particular breast cancer. In 1977, Bennett et al. (1) reported that malignant breast tumors contain more prostaglandin E (PGE) than benign tumors or normal mammary tissue. The highest PGE levels appear associated with mammary tissues that have metastased to bone. These results have been confirmed by others, including Dowsett (2), Tasjian (3) and Rolland (4). Rolland, Martin et al. have suggested that high PGE production could be used as a marker for the high metastatic potential of the neoplastic cells encountered in breast cancer.

On the basis of this hypothesis, we decided to investigate breast cancer cases with negative lymph nodes. This population is generally considered to have a favorable prognosis, and does not receive any complementary treatment following surgery, yet 25 to 30% of these patients relapse locally or develop metastases in subsequent months or years. Detection of this high risk population would allow such patients to benefit from more optimal treatment.

MATERIALS AND METHODS

Forty women with breast cancer, but without any node involvement, were entered in our study; follow-up for all patients was over five years. Following surgical exeresis of the primary breast tumor, a fragment was immediately taken and placed in liquid nitrogen, then sent to the laboratory.

Prostaglandin E2 (PGE2) concentrations in the cytosol from the primary tumor were measured by a radioimmunoassay. The sensitivity of the method was 2 pg of PGE2. As concerns specificity, the percentage of cross reaction was 3.2% with PGE1 and less than 0.2% with other PG. The cut-off level was 0.5 ng per mg of protein.

Technique

Prostaglandins E2 (PGE2) were extracted from 1 ml of cytosol 105,000 g from surgical specimens of primary breast cancer tumors acidified to pH 3.5. Extraction was performed twice, using 3 ml of a cyclohexane/ethyl acetate mixture (vol/vol). The prostaglandins were then purified on a silicate column and eluted with a benzene/ethyl acetate/methanol mixture (60/40/3).

The reagents employed for the radioimmunoassay included:
- 3HPGE2 commercialized by New England Nuclear (Net 428, specific activity: 100-200 Ci/mmol)
- antisera anti-PGE2 supplied by Institut Pasteur (batch C 79 585)
- cold PGE2 commercialized by SIGMA (ref. P 5640), used for calibration purposes.

RESULTS

Figure 1 is a histogram showing the case distribution of relapses as a function of the PGE2 level. Several remarks are warranted:
- 21 patients had a PGE2 level less than or equal to 0.5 ng/mg protein; none of these patients have relapsed or developed metastases after more than five years
- 12 patients had a concentration between 0.5 and 2 ng/mg protein; 5 have developped metastases and 4 have had local recurrence
- 7 patients had a concentration considerably higher than 2 ng/mg protein; 4 have metastased and 2 others have had local recurrence.
Patients with a high PGE2 concentration in their primary tumor at the time of surgery thus appear at risk for disease evolution.

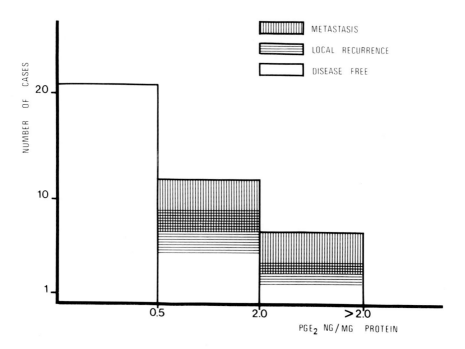

FIG. 1 CASE DISTRIBUTION OF RELAPSES

Table I lists the population of our study, giving the PGE2 concentration in each primary tumor at the time of surgery and prior to any
complementary treatment.

TABLE I STUDY POPULATION

Patient	PGE2 ng/mg protein	Metastases Bone	Metastases Other	Local Recurrence
Vig...	11.3	+ (19)	+ (22) lung	-
Fer...	5.6	+ (16)	-	-
Ven...	5.4	+ (16)	+ (20) brain	+ (11)
Sal...	4.6	-	-	+ (20)
Pan...	3.9	+ (33)	-	-
Fau...	3.7	-	-	-
Tad...	2.5	-	-	-
Zoc...	1.9	-	-	-
Rei...	1.6	-	-	-
Gui...	1.6	-	+ (34) lung	-
Cai...	1.4	-	-	-
Per...	1.3	+ (26)	+ (24) liver	-
Mul...	1.3	-	-	+ (17)
Riv...	1.3	+ (30)	+ (30) brain	-
Col...	1.0	-	-	+ (29)
Aud...	1.0	-	-	-
Arq...	0.9	-	+ (32) liver	+ (23)
Cla...	0.7	-	-	-
Sem...	0.6	+ (47)	-	+ (27)
21 patients $\leq$ 0.50		-	-	-

+ = cases of relapse
- = no recurrence during the over 5-yr followup period
( ) = disease free interval in months

Comparison of the two patient populations, those with a PGE2 level
higher than 0.5 ng/mg protein and those with a PGE2 level lower than
0.5 ng/mg protein, revealed a highly significant difference (p less than
0.001) as concerns the frequency of appearance of visceral metastases
and/or local recurrence. Of the 19 patients with a PGE2 concentration
over 0.5 ng/mg protein, 9 presented metastases, and 7 of these 9 (77.8%)
had bone metastases, either alone or in association with other metastases. It also appears that the higher the PGE2 concentration, the
shorter the free interval. As concerns local recurrences, all were of
a parietal nature except for one instance of axillary node recurrence.
Our overall results can be briefly summarized as follows: (a) when
the PGE2 level was less than or equal to 0.5 ng/mg protein, all patients
were disease free at five years; (b) when the PGE2 level was over 0.5
ng/mg protein, the relapse rate was 63.3% (12/19 patients) and the rate
of metastasis was 47.2% (9/19 patients); (c) for our entire population
of 40 breast cancer patients without node involvement, 12 patients
presented with metastases and/or local recurrence, i.e. 30%, a figure

which is more or less in agreement with other reports published in the literature.

CONCLUSION

Measurement of the PGE2 concentration in the primary breast tumor at the time of surgery might allow detection of a high risk population which could benefit from adjuvant treatment or at least more intensive follow-up. This is especially true for those patients with the highest concentrations. Concomitant analysis of such other prognostic factors as receptors and the Scarff and Bloom grade should allow even better definition of this population.

REFERENCES

1. Bennett, A., McDonald, A.M., Stamford, I.F., Cmarlier, E.M., Simpson, J.S., Zebro, T. (1977): Lancet, ii: 624-626.
2. Dowsett, M., Easty, G.C., Powles, T.J., Easty, D.M., Neville, A.M. (1976): Prostaglandins, 11: 447-460.
3. Tasjian, A.M. (1978): Cancer Res., 38: 4138-4141.
4. Rolland, P.H., Martin, P.M., Jacquemeir, J., Rolland, A.M., Toga, M. (1980): J. Nat. Cancer Inst, 64: 1061-1070.

Progress in Cancer Research and Therapy,
Vol. 31, edited by F. Bresciani, et al.
Raven Press, New York © 1984.

Prolactin and Prolactin Receptors in Human Breast Disease

*M. L'Hermite-Balériaux, *S. Casteels, *A. Vokaer, *C. Loriaux,
**G. Nöel, and *M. L'Hermite

*Service de Gynécologie et d'Obstétrique, FRESERH and U.L.B., Hôpital Brugmann,
1020 Brussels; and **Department of Cancérologie, University of Louvain,
1200 Brussels, Belgium

In 1979 Nagasawa (46) wrote an updated review about prolactin (PRL) and human breast cancer. Since then, no fundamentally new data appeared in the literature that could bring more light about the interrelationships between PRL and human breast cancer. Whereas the role of PRL in experimental animal mammary tumorigenesis is now well established (4, 28, 49, 53, 67) its importance in human breast disease remains to be clarified (61).

The mammary gland is a hormone dependent organ, and the actions of estradiol and progesterone on this organ are now well documented (41,42). The existence of harmonious ovarian cycle function ensures perfect mammary development. Several physiological conditions and external factors that could influence PRL secretion and their possible relation to the development of breast disease are worth consideration.

HUMAN PROLACTIN LEVELS IN BREAST DISEASES

Data have to be considered in the light of several important factors such as age of the patients, hormonal status, whether they have benign or malignant breast disease.

Boyns et al. (5) reported PRL levels to be similar in benign breast disease and breast cancer patients at various stages as in control patients. The data of Jones et al. (27) showed also that the levels of PRL were not significantly different in patients with early breast cancer, when compared to those with benign breast disease.

Several other papers appeared in the literature (20, 30, 49) in which no difference had been found in the PRL levels in breast cancer patients, compared to women matched for age, year of menopause and parity (40).

In the early reports which studied the interrelationships between PRL and breast cancer, only a few (1, 56, 68) mentioned that PRL levels could be elevated. When more elaborate investigations were set up, new data appeared. Rose et al. (57), focusing their attention on the well documented inverse relationship between plasma PRL levels and age, found no correlation between age and PRL levels in breast cancer. But, when patients and controls were classified according to their menopausal status, increased plasma PRL concentrations were found in both premenopausal and postmenopausal breast cancer patients. These data are partly in opposition to the early observation of Franks et al. (18), who showed that premenopausal women had higher PRL levels than postmenopausal women regardless of tumor histology.

Since the greatest amount of PRL is secreted during sleep at night, attempts to evaluate the contribution of PRL in breast disease required studies of the nyctohemeral rhythms of the hormone. Hoff et al. (27) reported decreased PRL levels postoperatively but no major change in these PRL rhythms. On the contrary, Malarkey et al. (35) demonstrated in post-menopausal women with breast cancer a diminished nocturnal PRL peak while premenopausal breast cancer patients, evaluated in the luteal phase of their menstrual cycle, had significantly higher daytime as well as nocturnal PRL concentrations. Wilson et al. (69) did not find abnormal PRL rhythms in postmenopausal women with primary breast cancer. In addition to these data, Tarquini et al. (62) showed that in premenopausal, nulliparous women with benign or malignant breast disease, an abnormal early evening plasma PRL secretion could also be observed.

It is now well established that, in cystic breast disease, PRL levels are also raised (8). Other hormonal abnormalities with respect to steroids can also be observed in women with benign breast disease (29). Considering the ovarian functions in women with benign breast disease, it appears that, in most cases, these patients might have an inadequate corpus luteum function. There is an estradiol versus progesterone inbalance. Increased PRL responsiveness to estrogen may be a characteristic of women with benign breast disease (60). But the question arises, why in certain cases of inadequate luteal function does breast cystic disease appear ?

Since there is a functional relationship between PRL and TSH, the PRL response to TRH was also investigated in breast disease. Ohgo et al. (51) did not find any significant difference in the mean response of plasma PRL following TRH injection in patients with breast cancer, compared with that of normal sujects, but, in the patients with breast cancer and increased basal PRL levels, an exaggerated response of PRL to TRH was observed.

In benign breast cystic disease the TRH-stimulated PRL response was significantly higher in these patients than in controls, indicating clearly that the PRL secreting capacity of the pituitary is increased (54).

Are elevated PRL levels a risk factor ?

Several factors are associated with enhanced risk of breast cancer : early menarche, late age of first term pregnancy, postmenopausal obesity. In none of these situations are abnormal PRL levels found. On the other hand, an abnormal luteal phase evening peak of plasma PRL was observed in women with a family history of breast cancer (31) but the same abnormality was also observed in nulliparous women and in tall and heavy women.
Daughters of women with breast cancer have elevated mean 24 hour PRL levels (22, 32) and a partial resistance of PRL to dopamine suppression (32).

Well established information exists only concerning cystic disease, associated to an increase of the risk of breast cancer by approximatly two to four fold (10, 13).

On the other hand, it is well known that pregnancy, during which very high levels of PRL are encountered, exerts a protective effect on human breast cancer (66).

Until now, no data exist demonstrating that patients with very high PRL levels (pituitary prolactinoma, amenorrhea galactorrhea, drug-induced hyperprolactinemia) might be more at risk to develop breast cancer (6, 7, 16).

TABLE 1. Previous reports of the occurrence of PRL receptors in pathological human breast tissues.

Reference	Pellet used (amount of protein)	Label	Positive if Sp B	Total number M	Total number B	Total of positive (%) M	Total of positive (%) B
Holdaway et al. (24)	100,000 g (500 µg)	h PRL	≥1 %	41	15	8 (20%)	0
Morgan et al. (44)	100,000 g	o PRL	≥0.9 %	55		15 (27%)	
Partridge et al. (52)	15,000 g (200–400 µg)	o PRL	Scatchard	9		3	
Bohnet (2)	100,000 g (500 µg)	h PRL / o PRL	>3 % and N Sp B <3 %	24		5 (21%)	
Di Carlo et al. (11)			≥0.5 %				
Peyrat et al. (55)	105,000 g (400 µg)	hGH / h PRL	≥0.8 %	72	20	35 (49%)	6 (30%)
Bonneterre et al. (3)	105,000 g (400 µg)	hGH / h PRL	≥0.8 %	92		(46%)	
Turcot-Lemay et al. (66)	105,000 g (300 µg)	o PRL / h PRL / hGH	≥1 % / ≥1 % / >1 %	569 / 343 / 95		13 % / 36 % / 1 %	

hGH : human growth hormone; o : ovine
M : malignant; B : benign
Sp B : specific binding; N Sp B : non specific binding

On the other hand, no data exist that patients with disturbed nyctohemeral rhythms, as observed in psychiatric disorders (65), might be
more at risk to develop breast cancer.

PROLACTIN RECEPTORS (PRL-R) IN HUMAN BREAST TUMORS

The initial event of the manifestation of the biological PRL effects
is its binding to a specific receptor at the target cell surface. In
animal species the level of PRL is known to correlate with specific mammary responsiveness. PRL is involved in mammary tumorigenesis and the
PRL-induced responses of the cells are dependent upon PRL-R interactions
(47).   But the number of PRL-R in a particular tissue can also vary with
the hormonal environment of the tissue.   The ability of PRL to stimulate
tumor growth may therefore depend less on serum levels, and more on the
number of receptor sites in the tumor tissue that are able to react
with the hormone. In human breast tumours, the significance of PRL-R
remains to be established, and perhaps will require as much time as
has been necessary to establish the significance of the E-R and Pg-R.
Nagai et al. (45) did not find any correlation between E-R, Pg-R
and PRL levels in 217 breast cancer patients. Only few studies reported
the presence of PRL-R in human breast tumors (Table 1), usually including only a small number of cases; it is only very recently that Turcot-
Lemay et al. (64) reported a serie of 759 cases. However, data remain
controversial, mainly due to the scarcity of available tissue.
The occurrence of PRL-R varied from 10 to 49 %. The differences might
be attributable essentially to differences in labelled hormone (hCG,
oPRL, hPRL), in the conditions of membrane preparation, in the amount
of membrane used in the displacement study, in the incubation conditions.
In order to investigate further these problems, we studied 58 human
breast tumors.

Tissue Processing

The tumoral tissues, freed of fat, were stored in liquid nitrogen.
The frozen tissues were pulverised, and the membranes prepared
according to 3 different protocols (Table 2).

TABLE 2.   Summary of the different conditions used for membrane prepa-
           ration : A : according to Shiu et al. (59); B : according to
           Martin et al. (39); C : according to Bonneterre et al. (3)

	A	B	C
Buffer : Tris (mM)	10	10	20
sucrose	0.3 M	-	-
EDTA (mM)	-	1.5	3
thioglycerol	-	12 mM	-
glycerol	-	10 %	-
dithiotreitol	-	-	1 mM
pH	7.4	7.4	7.8
Centrifugation steps :			
600 - 800 g	10'	-	10'
10,000 - 15,000 g	30'	20'	-
100,000 g	90'	60'	90'

Protocol A refers to the classical membrane preparation technique according to Shiu et al. (59). As membrane reference preparation, the mammary gland tissue from a late pregnant rabbit was treated according to this procedure, and used as control. Protocol B refers to the membrane preparation technique used for the determination of E-R and Pg-R (39). Protocol C refers to the methodology of Bonneterre et al. (3). In the latter case, the 15,000 g centrifugation is omitted and the mitochondrial fraction is thus pelleted with the 100,000 g fraction. The 100,000 g pellet is resuspended in Tris-HCl-25mM, 10 mM MgCl2 buffer(pH : 7.6). The protein concentration is determined by the method of Lowry et al. (34).

Hormones

oPRL (NIADD K - oPRL - I1; AFP 4328 C) was used for iodination and displacement. oPRL was labelled with I^{125} (IMS 300, Amersham, England) by the lactoperoxidase method or the chloramine method. The specific activity varied from 52 to 82 $\mu Ci/\mu g$. The labelled hormone was tested with the reference membrane rabbit mammary gland preparation.

PRL-receptors Assay

The assay was performed according to Shiu et al. (59). The membrane preparations ($\pm$ 400 μg proteins for tumors, 300 μg for rabbit mammary gland) were incubated overnight at room temperature, with 100,000 cpm oPRL, in the presence or absence of excess unlabelled hormone (1 μg oPRL). The final incubation volume was 0.5 ml; the previous Tris HCl buffer was used, containing 0.1 % B.S.A. At the end of the incubation period, 3 ml of ice cold buffer was added and the tubes centrifuged at 1,500 g for 30 min at 4°C. The supernatant was discarded and the tubes counted.

The specific binding (SpB) was calculated as the difference between the radioactivity bound in the absence (total binding) and in the presence of an excess of unlabelled hormone (non specific binding : N SpB); it was then expressed as a percentage of the total radioactivity added.

The membrane preparations of all tumors were tested at least in duplicate. Due to the scarcity of tissue available, no displacement curve could be set up nor Scatchard plot calculated. With the rabbit membrane preparation, 24 experiences were performed : a Ka = 5.7 $\pm$ 2.2 10^{-9}M and N = 45 $\pm$ 12.8 10^{-15}mole/mg protein were found. These data are in agreement with those of Djiane et al. (12). A tumor was considered as positive when the SpB was at least 0.8 %.

Assay for Estradiol Receptors (E-R) and Progesterone Receptors (Pg-R)

In tumors which had been treated according to procedures A and B, E-R and Pg-R were determined by the dextran coated charcoal method (39). In fact, in procedure B, the cytosol was used for steroids receptor determination, and the pellet for PRL-R determination.

The tumors tested according to procedure C, had their E-R and Pg-R determined according to Noël et al. (50). Tumors are considered to be E-R+, Pg-R+ if more than 8.10^{-15}mole/mg protein could be evidenced.

PRL-receptors : Results

The overall results showed that, in the series of 58 tumors presently tested, 14 had a SpB equal to or greater than 0.8 %. The total binding varied between 4.9 to 14.9 % and the N SpB ranged from 4.3 to 13.1 %. Thus, in this series, 25 % were considered to have PRL-R. When the data were analysed according to the membrane preparation technique, out of the 18 tumors treated according to procedure A, 6 (33 %) had PRL-R; out of the 28 tumors treated according to procedure B, only 3 (10 %) had PRL-R, and out of the 12 tumors treated according to procedure C, 5 (41 %) had PRL-R. From these data, although the series is very small, the conditions of the membrane preparation seem to be very important. From previous data (1, 11, 24, 44) percentages of 20 to 30 % of PRL-R positive tumors have been found independently of the label used, of the amount protein put in the assay, and of the definition of the positive cases. Seldom had a distinction been made between benign and malignant tumors. Turcot-Lemay et al (64), using labelled oPRL, found only 13 % of PRL-R positive tumors but they investigated about 569 cases. They observed a different percentage of positive tumors when respectively labelled hGH, hPRL or oPRL were used. The high percentage of positive tumors observed by Bonneterre et al. (3) is very likely essentially due to the different membrane preparation used. The technique they used, desaturation by $MgCl_2$ of the receptors, in order to obtain the total PRL receptors available did not give, in our hands, satisfactory data (33).

In our hands, treatment with $MgCl_2$ led up to 80 % (instead of 30 %) (12) loss of tumoral membrane proteins; furthermore it was quite variable. This could be understood in the light of the fact that breast tumor tissue is heterogeneous.

TABLE 3. Distribution of PRL-R+ and PRL-R- cases according to the presence or absence of E-R and Pg-R. No correlation could be evidenced.

	E-R+		E-R-	
	PgR+	PgR-	PgR+	PgR-
PRL-R + (n = 14)	5	2	4	3
PRL-R - (n = 44)	22	2	1	19

Table 3 summarizes our data comparing the presence of PRL-R to that of steroids-R in the 58 tumors investigated. In 19 tumors (32 %) without PRL-R, no E-R and Pg-R could be evidenced. On the other hand, in 22 cases (37 %) without PRL-R, E-R and Pg-R could be detected. From these data, it can be concluded that PRL-R negative tumors were evenly distributed among the hormone-dependent and hormone-independent tumors. It should be pointed out that in 3 steroid-receptors negative tumors, PRL-R could be evidenced. These results are in agreement with previously published works (55, 64). When Bonneterre et al. (3) did put their positivity threshold for E-R at 50 fmol/mg cytosol proteins, they could find a correlation between E-R and PRL-R. But, to put the limit of positivity at such a high level is open to criticism and the interpretation of these data must thus be regarded with great caution.

It can be concluded that the presence of PRL-R in some human breast cancers is now well established but that their significance remains to be evaluated. It is not clear whether there might be any interest to use preferentially the methodology of Bonneterre et al. (3) : the enrichment of the membrane preparation, in PRL-R present in cellular constituents other than the outer membrane, might lead to an overestimation of the PRL-R. This would probably be the case if indeed PRL is not required beyond its initial binding to its receptor for its action to be attained, as suggested by Edery et al. (15). Prospective studies are now requested in order to correlate the PRL-R status of the tumors to the later evolution of the disease.

There is apparently no correlation, in breast tumor patients, between their circulating PRL levels and the presence of PRL-R. This is in contrast to induced (DMBA or N-nitrosomethylurea) mammary tumors in rats; in these conditions, PRL levels are increased, the tumors appear to be dependent on PRL, and PRL-R are present and subject to hormonal as well as pharmacological modulation (9, 19, 26, 37, 38, 48, 63). Recent data point, in the human, to a possible unfavorable effect of PRL. Thus, Malarkey et al. (36) demonstrated in vitro the positive effect of PRL (as well as of growth hormone) on the growth of dispersed cells from the breast carcinoma of a hyperprolactinemic patient. Holtkamp et al. (25) found a 30 % incidence of hyperprolactinemia in patients with metastatic breast cancer, with the highest incidence in patients with familial type of breast cancer, especially with extremely aggressive disease and short disease free interval. Dowsett et al. (14) found also that postmenopausal breast cancer patients with high PRL levels had a significantly shorter survival.

An early trial of bromocriptine by the EORTC (17) led to the conclusion that inhibition of PRL would have no benefit in the treatment of advanced breast cancer. Nevertheless, Holtkamp et al. (25) just reported that tumors refractory to chemotherapy, in patients with hyperprolactinemia, can be made sensitive again with bromocriptine. Similarly, Grisoli et al. (21) described the spectacular regression (as evaluated by CT scan) of a voluminous brain metastasis during bromocriptine administration. When assessing the results of bromocriptine administration, one should also keep in mind that it does not only modify PRL secretion but also the number of PRL-R (12, 58). It appears too early to conclude as to the effect of bromocriptine as well as to the deleterious effect of hyperprolactinemia on the basis of these sporadic or preliminary data. It must, however, be remembered that bromocriptine does elevate growth hormone in normal women, and that PRL-R can be evidenced by their binding to labeled growth hormone. Finally, animal work by Mittra (43) suggest that the product, which might be important in promoting proliferation of the mammary epithelial cells, is not prolactin itself but a "cleaved" 16 K PRL polypeptide.

ACKNOWLEDGMENTS

Some financial help was obtained from the Fonds Emile Defay (Université Libre de Bruxelles). The skilful secretarial work of Mrs. C. Bekaert is gratefully acknowledged.

REFERENCES

1. Berle, P., and Voigt, K.D. (1972) : Am. J. Obstet. Gynecol., 114: 1101-1102.
2. Bohnet, H.G. (1980) : Arch. Gynecol., 229:333-344.
3. Bonneterre, J., Peyrat, J.Ph., Van de Walle, B., Beuscart, R., Vie, M.C., and Cappelaere, P. (1982) : Eur. J. Cancer Clin. Oncol., 18:1157-1162.
4. Boot, L.M. (1970) : Int. J. Cancer, 5:167-175.
5. Boyns, A.R., Cole, E.N., Griffiths, K., Roberts, M.M., Buchan, R., Wilson, R.G., and Forrest, A.P.M. (1973) : Eur. J. Cancer, 9:99-102.
6. Brown, R.W., Meehan, C., Martin, F.I.R., and Bhathal, P.S. (1982) : Cancer, 50:125-129.
7. Brugmans, J. Verbruggen, F., Dom, J., and Schuermans, V. (1973) : Lancet, ii:502-503.
8. Cole, E.N., Sellwood, R.A., England, P.C., and Griffiths, K. (1977): Eur. J. Cancer, 13:597-603.
9. Costlow, M.E., and McGuire, W.E. (1977) : J. Natl. Cancer Inst., 58:1173-1175.
10. Davis, H.H., Simons, M., and Davis, J.B. (1964) : Cancer, 17:957-978.
11. Di Carlo, R., Muccioli, G., and Di Carlo, F. (1983) : In : Endocrinology of Cystic Breast Disease, edited by Angeli, A., Bradlow, H.L. and L. Dogliotti, pp. 211-218. Raven Press, New-York.
12. Djiane, J., Durand, Ph. and Kelly P.A. (1977) : Endocrinology, 100: 1348-1356.
13. Donelly, P.K., Baker, K.W., Carney, J.A., and Fallon, W.O. (1978) : Mayo Clinic Proc., 50:650-656.
14. Dowsett, M., McGarrick, G.E., Harris, A.L., Coombes, R.C., Smith, I.E., and Jeffcoate, S.L. (1983) : Br. J. Cancer, 47:763-769.
15. Edery, M., Djiane, J., Houdeline, L.M., and Kelly P.A. (1983) : Cancer Res., 43 : 3170-3174.
16. Ettigi, P., Lal, S., and Friesen, H.G. (1973) : Lancet, ii:266-267.
17. European Breast Cancer Group (1972) : Eur. J. Cancer, 8:155-156.
18. Franks, S., Ralphs, D.N.L., Seagroatt, V., and Jacobs, H.S. (1974) : Br. Med. J., 4:320-321.
19. Gibson, S., and Hilf, R. (1979) : Cancer Res., 36:3736-3741.
20. Gorins, A., Netter, A., and L'Hermite, M. (1973) : Annls. Endocrinol. (Paris), 34:601-602.
21. Grisoli, F., Vincentelli, F., Foa, J. Lavail, G., and Salamon, G. (1981) : Lancet, ii:745-746.
22. Henderson, B.E., Gerkins, V., Rosario, I., Casagrande, J., and Pike, M. (1975) : N. Engl. J. Med., 293:790-795.
23. Hoff, J., Hoff-Bardier, M., and Fayard, F. (1978) : J. Gyn. Obst. Biol. Repr., 7:19-30.
24. Holdaway, I.M., and Friesen, H.G. (1977) : Cancer Res., 37:1946-1952.
25. Holtkamp, W., Wander, H.E., von Heyden, D., Rauschecker, H.F., and Nagel, G.A. (1983) : J. Ster. Biochem. 19:suppl.p.:143S.

26. Ip, C., Yip, Ph., and Bernardis, L. (1980) : Cancer Res., 40:374-378.
27. Jones, M.K., Ramsay, I.D., Collins, W.P., and Dyer, G.I. (1977) :
    Eur. J. Cancer, 13:1109-1112.
28. Kim, U., and Furth, J. (1976) : Vitam. and Hormones, 34:107-136.
29. Kuttenn, F., Fournies, S., Sitruk-Ware, R., Martin, P. and Mauvais-
    Jarvis, P. (1983) : In : Endocrinology of Cystic Breast Disease,
    edited by Angeli, A., Bradlow, H.L., and L. Dogliotti, pp. 231-
    252. Raven Press, New-York.
30. Kwa, H.G., De Jong-Bakker, M., Engelsman, E., and Cleton, F.J.(1974)
    Lancet, i:433.
31. Kwa, H.G., and Wang, D.Y. (1977) : Int. J. Cancer, 20:12-14.
32. Levin, Ph., and Malarkey, W.B. (1981) : J. Clin. Endocrinol. Metab.,
    53 : 179-183.
33. L'Hermite-Balériaux, M., and L'Hermite, M. (1983) : In : Receptors
    in growth and reproduction, edited by Saxena, Raven Press,
    New-York. In press.
34. Lowry, O.H., Rosebrough, N.J., Farr, A., and Randall, R.J. (1951) :
    J. Biol. Chem. 193:265-275.
35. Malarkey, W.B., Schroeder, L.L., Stevens, V.C., James, A.G., and
    Lanese, R.R. (1977) : Cancer Res., 37:4650-4654.
36. Malarkey, W.B., Kennedy, M., Albred, L.E., and Milo, G. (1983) : J.
    Clin. Endocrinol. Metab., 56:673-677.
37. Manni, R., Rainieri, J., Arafah, B.M., Finegan, H.M., and Pearson,
    O.H. (1982) : Cancer Res., 42:3492-3495.
38. Manni, R., Rainieri, J., Arafah, B.M., and Pearson, O.H. (1982) : J.
    Endocr., 93:11-16.
39. Martin, P.M., Rolland, P.H., Jacuemier, J., Rolland, A.M., and Toga,
    M. (1978) : Biomedicine, 28:278-287.
40. McFadyen, I.J., Forrest, A.P.M., Prescott, R.J., Golder, M.P.,
    Groom, G.V., Fahmy, D.R., and Griffiths, K. (1976) : Lancet, i:
    1100-1102.
41. McGuire, W.L., Raynaud, J.P., and Beaulieu, E.-E., editors (1975) :
    Estrogen Receptors in Human Breast Cancer. Raven Press, New-York.
42. McGuire, W.L., Raynaud, J.P., and Beaulieu, E.E., editors (1977) :
    Progesterone Receptors in normal and neoplastic tissues. Raven
    Press, New-York.
43. Mittra, I. (1980) : Biochem. Biophys. Res. Commun., 95:1760-1767.
44. Morgan, L., Raggatt, P.R., de Souza, I., Salih, H., and Hobbs, J.R.
    (1977) : J. Endocrinol., 73:17p-18p.
45. Nagai, R., Kataoka, M., Kobayashi, S., Ishihara, K.,Tobioka, N.,
    Nakashima, K., Naruse, M. Saito, K., and Sakuma, S. (1979) :
    Cancer Res., 39:1835-1840.
46. Nagasawa, H. (1979) : Europ. J. Cancer, 15:267-279.
47. Nagasawa, H., Sakai, S., and Banerjee, M.R. (1979) : Life Sciences,
    24:193-208.
48. Nagasawa, H. (1981) : Biomedecine, 34:9-11.
49. Nagasawa, H., and Mori, S., (1981) : Cancer Res., 41:1935-1937.
50. Noël, G., and Maisin, H. (1981) : Arch. Int. Physiol. Biochem., 89:
    B189-190.
51. Ohgo, S., Kato, Y., Chihara, K., and Imura, H. (1976) : Cancer, 37:
    1412-1416.
52. Partridge, R.K., and Hähnel, R. (1979) : Cancer, 43:643-646.
53. Pearson, O.H., Llerena, O., Llerena, L., Molina, A., and Butler, T.
    (1969) : Transactions of the Association of American Physicians,
    82:225-238.
54. Peters, F., Pickardt, C.R., and Breckwoldt, M. (1983) : In :

Endocrinology of Cystic Breast Disease, edited by A. Angeli, Bradlow H.L. and L. Dogliotti, pp. 113-122.

55. Peyrat, J.P., Dewailly, D., Djiane, J. Kelly, P.A., Van de Walle, B., Bonneterre, J., and Lefebvre, J. (1981) : Breast Cancer Res. Treat., 1:369-373.

56. Rolandi, R., Barreca, T., Masturzo, P., Polleri, A., Indiveri, F., and Baralino, A. (1974) : Lancet, ii:845-846.

57. Rose, D.P., and Pruitt, B. (1981) : Cancer, 48:2687-2691.

58. Sheth, N.A., Tikekar, S.S., Ranadive, K.J., and Sheth, A.R. (1978) : Molec. Cell. Endocr., 12:167-176.

59. Shiu, R.P.C., Kelly, P.A., and Friesen, H.G. (1973) : Science, 180: 968-973.

60. Simkin, B. (1983) : Acta Endocrinol. (Kbh),   103, suppl. 256: abstract 301.

61. Smithline, F., Sherman, L., and Kolodny, H.D. (1975) : N. Engl. J. Med., 292:784-792.

62. Tarquini, A., Di Martino, L., Malloci, A., Kwa, H.G., Van der Gugten, A.A., Bulbrook, R.D., and Wang, D.Y. (1978) : Int. J. Cancer, 22: 687-690.

63. Turcot-Lemay, L., and Kelly, P.A. (1980) : Cancer Res., 40:3232-3240.

64. Turcot-Lemay, L., and Kelly, P.A. (1982) : J. Natl. Cancer. Inst., 68:381-383.

65. Van Cauter, E., Linkowski, P., Hoffman, G., Hubain, P., L'Hermite-Balériaux, M., L'Hermite, M., and Mendlewicz, J. (1983) : Acta Endocr., 103, suppl. 256 : 270.

66. Vorherr, H., and Messer, R.H. (1978) : Am. J. Obstet. Gynec., 130: 335-358.

67. Welsch, C., and Nagasawa, H. (1977) : Cancer Res., 37:951-963.

68. Wilson, R.G., Buchan, R., Roberts, M.M., Forrest, A.P.M., Boyns, A.R., Cole, E.N., and Griffiths, K. (1974) : Cancer, 33:1325-1327.

69. Wilson, D.W., Phillips, M.J., Holliday, H.W., Blamey, R.W., Simpson, H.W., Pierrepoint, C.G., Halberg, F., and Griffiths, K. (1983) : Chronobiologia, 10:21-30.

Progress in Cancer Research and Therapy,
Vol. 31, edited by F. Bresciani, et al.
Raven Press, New York © 1984.

Parity and Age Influence Hormonal Risk Factors of Breast Cancer

P.F. Bruning, J.M.G. Bonfrèr, A.A.M. Hart, M. de Jong-Bakker, H.G. Kwa, W. Nooyen, and A.A. Verstraeten

The Netherlands Cancer Institute, 1066 CX Amsterdam, The Netherlands

The role of hormonal abnormalities as risk factors for human breast cancer is still controversial. Prolactin (PRL), "available" estradiol (free E_2), progesterone (P) and weak androgens like dehydroepiandrosterone (DHEA) constitute the main area of interest. Various research groups have failed to demonstrate significant differences in plasma PRL levels in females at putative risk of breast cancer compared to controls. However, Kwa (The Netherlands Cancer Institute) in collaboration with Bulbrook, Hayward, Wang et al (Imperial Cancer Research Fund Laboratories, London) found an abnormal nycthemeral rhythm of plasma PRL in women at risk (4,5). In a cross-sectional study of mothers, sisters and aunts of breast cancer patients they demonstrated a higher plasma PRL level during the early evening hours in the premenopausal unaffected daughters compared to women with no family history. The phenomenon was seen only in the luteal phase of the menstrual cycle. This subtle, but statistically significant abnormality stayed within the range of the normal mean plasma PRL concentration. It was measured in spot samples, i.e. each sample had been taken once from individual women at various times of day and evening. From these cross-sectionally obtained data we concluded that confirmation was needed by a longitudinal study in which abnormal "early evening peaks" of plasma PRL could be demonstrated by taking serial blood samples from the same woman.

Since the plasma concentrations of PRL, but also of various other hormones are known to fluctuate considerably within hours, we have studied the diurnal variation of PRL and steroids of ovarian and adrenal origin by continuous venous sampling. This technique has also yielded information on the area under the concentration-time curve (AUC).

We report here preliminary results with the emphasis on the influence of parity and age on hormonal concentrations in plasma.

METHODS

The investigation concerns four groups of premenopausal women who have been studied during the luteal phase of their menstrual cycle between day 18 and 24 (plasma progesterone at least 10 nmol/l):
1. Group R: women at risk because of at least two first-degree relatives (mother and sister) having breast cancer; 2. Group N: normal women matched for age, parity, socioeconomic status and Quetelet index to women of group R; 3. Group B: women with histologically proven benign

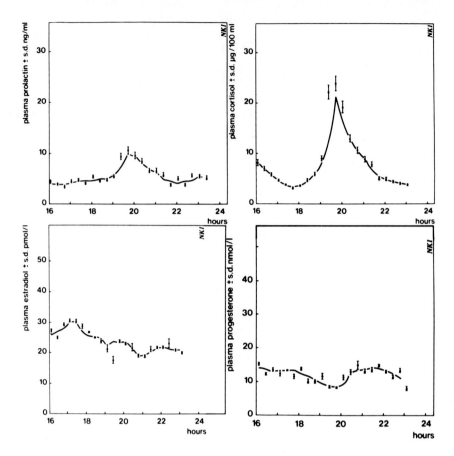

FIG.1. and 2. Typical time-concentration curves for plasma
prolactin, cortisol, estradiol and progesterone
in two premenopausal women during the luteal
phase of their menstrual cycle (between day 18
and 24). Each value represents the mean ± s.d.
from a venous blood sample which was drawn
continuously during a 20 minute interval. The
curves have been obtained by a computerized
smoothing procedure. Data derived from the first
hour after the placement of an indwelling
catheter at 3 p.m. have been omitted.

proliferative breast lesions; and 4. Group C: women curatively treated
for $T_1N_0M_0$ breast cancer more than 6 months ago.
Women taking the contraceptive pill or other drugs and women having abnormal thyroid function were excluded from the study.
Venous blood was continuously drawn by means of a peristaltic pump (LKB)
over 20 minute intervals from 3 till 11 p.m. under standardized conditions. The women were in a comfortable resting position; potential stress
was reduced as much as possible. Hormoneconcentrations in the separate
20 minute samples and in pooled material were measured by radioimmunoassay. PRL determinations were done at 5 plasma dilutions as previously

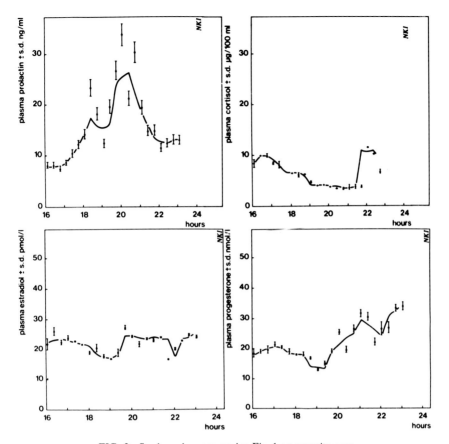

FIG. 2. See legend accompanying Fig. 1 on opposite page.

published (5). Coefficients of intra-assay and inter-assay variation ranged from 3 to 6% and from 9 to 13% respectively, both for PRL and steroid hormones. The average concentration in serial plasma samples was considered representative for the area under the time-concentration curve (AUC), and is represented as such for reasons of convenience. AUC-values are given over the time-period from 4 till 11 p.m. thus excluding the first hour of blood withdrawal when stress could influence the results too much.

Sex hormone binding globulin (SHBG) was measured by a modification of the method of Nisula and Dunn (8), using concanavalin A-sepharose to bind ^{3}H-dihydrotestosterone-saturated SHBG. The coefficient of intra-assay and inter-assay variation were 3.1 to 3.3% and 3.6 to 6.6% respectively, the inter-assay variation being largest at high SHBG values (200 nmol/l DHT). SHBG and DHEA-sulphate were measured in every fourth serial blood sample because of their known long apparent half-life.

RESULTS

In figures 1 and 2 typical individual time-concentration plots are shown. It can be seen that the plasma concentrations of PRL and corti-

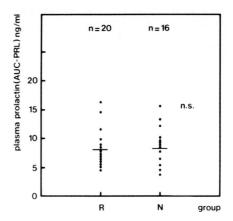

FIG.3. The average plasma concentrations of prolactin (AUC-PRL) between
       4 and 11 p.m. in luteal phase premenopausal women at familial
       risk of breast cancer (group R) were compared with those in
       matched controls (group N). No difference could be demonstrated
       between groups R and N.

sol (F), but also of estradiol (E_2) and progesterone (P) fluctuate
considerably within a few hours time. Androstenedione and dehydroepiandrosterone (DHEA) fluctuated simultaneously with F. The concentrations
of DHEA-sulphate and SHBG were very stable, as expected.
    Transient early evening elevations of PRL have been found in a number
of the women at risk (group R) and of the matched controls (group N).
PRL elevations were sometimes, but not always coincident with elevations
of cortisol.
When the average PRL concentration (AUC-PRL) was considered, no difference was observed between group R and group N(figure 3).

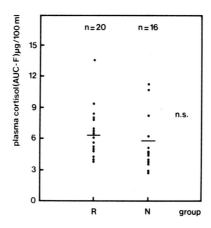

FIG.4. The average plasma concentrations of cortisol (AUC-F) were
       compared as explained in the legend to FIG.3. No difference could
       be demonstrated between groups R and N.

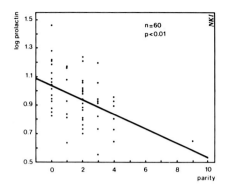

FIG.5. The logarithmic value of the average plasma concentration of
       prolactin (AUC-PRL) and parity (after adjustment for age) in
       60 luteal phase premenopausal women were inversely correlated
       (p < 0.01).

The average cortisol concentration (AUC-F), as an indicator of stress
due to the experimental conditions was very low and similar for both
groups (figure 4.)
   When the influence of parity (adjusted for age) on the plasma concentration of PRL was investigated, it appeared that the two factors were
inversely correlated (p < 0.01), as shown in figure 5.
   No statistical significance could however be reached for prolactin
compared to parity, if the nulliparae were excluded from the regression
analysis. AUC-PRL in the nulliparous group was significantly higher than
in the group of women with children (p <0.002).
AUC-PRL was only weakly correlated with age alone (p = 0.06) when the
whole group was considered. No correlation was found for AUC-PRL and age
in the nulliparous group (mean age 37 years, range 26 to 46 years; n=18.
For AUC-DHEA-sulphate and AUC-DHEA however, a clear inverse correlation
with age was found (p <0.001 and p < 0.01, respectively) as shown in
figures 6 and 7.

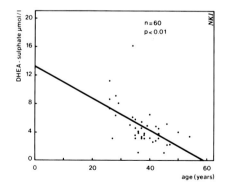

FIG.6. The average plasma concentration of DHEA-sulphate and age (after
       adjustment for parity) in the same individuals as described in
       the legend to figure 5 were inversely correlated (p <0.01).

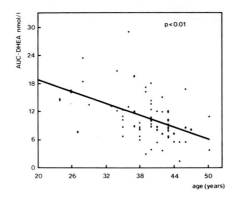

FIG.7. The average plasma concentration of DHEA (AUC-DHEA) and age
(after adjustment for parity) in the same individuals as
described in the legend to figure 5, were inversely correlated
(p <0.01).

No such correlation could be demonstrated for the other steroid
hormones which have been measured, notably androstenedione and andro-
stenediol. Parity was not correlated with DHEA or DHEA-sulphate.
AUC-PRL and AUC-DHEA showed good intraindividual correlation (p < 0.01),
as shown in figure 8.

DISCUSSION

From these preliminary results it may be concluded that the "early
evening peak" of PRL as demonstrated by Kwa in a cross-sectional study
of women at risk of breast cancer because of their family history (4,5),
cannot be used as a marker for individual risk. Such temporary elevations of the PRL-concentration appeared to be by no means specific for
this category and have also been observed in normal matched controls.
Plasma concentrations of PRL showed marked intraindividual fluctuation

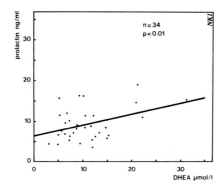

FIG.8. The average plasma concentration of prolactin (AUC-PRL) and
of DHEA (AUC-DHEA) in 34 luteal phase premenopausal women
were correlated (p <0.01)

with time under standardized experimental conditions and maximal exclusion of physical and mental "stress". The low average plasma concentration of cortisol in all groups also hints at a low stress level. Although
some PRL and cortisol elevations were coincidental, others were not,
indicating that unknown factors other than stress may cause a temporary
PRL increase.
Kwa et al (6), using spot sample values obtained from the Guernsey study,
and Rose and Pruitt (9) found an inverse correlation of PRL and premenopausal age. Rose and Pruitt, however, did not consider parity. With our
continuous blood sampling technique, which offers optimal information on
rapidly fluctuating hormone concentrations, we have found only a very
weak correlation between AUC-PRL and premenopausal age. On the other
hand, we could well confirm the Guernsey data, that PRL and parity
(adjusted for age) are inversely correlated in premenopausal women (6).
Kwa et al had observed that PRL values of spot samples from the Guernsey
study when taken between 6 and 10 p.m. decreased with increasing parity.
When the sampling had been done between 1 and 5 p.m. this correlation
was less clear. Moreover the statistical significance of the correlation
dropped considerably when the samples had been taken more than 2 years
after the birthgiving to the last child. When we excluded the nulliparous
women we could not find any correlation between AUC-PRL and parity in
our data. The highly significant difference in AUC-PRL between nulliparous women and women which had one or more children suggests that one
full-term pregnancy is sufficient to decrease plasma PRL. As the AUC-PRL
values were still significantly lower in 35 women which had given birth
to their last child 10 or more years ago, it may be concluded that the
effect of one or more full-term pregnancy on plasma PRL is of long duration. We speculate that this may be caused by a hypothalamic change
which could also have implications for the regulation of other peptide
hormones.
    The difference between the Guernsey data and our own may be regarded
as the consequence of the great variance of spot sample values of PRL
as had to be used in the former experience.
If PRL does promote the development of breast cancer, the decrease of
PRL after birthgiving would at least partially explain the "protection"
which is provided by early and multiple pregnancy (1, 7, 11, 12). The
decrease of DHEA-sulphate and DHEA with age, which we have observed has
also been described by Zumoff et al who used a frequent sampling
technique (14). These findings stress the necessity of age-matched
controls in any study of the plasma concentration of these hormones.
Interestingly, the inverse correlation with premenopausal age could not
be established for other adrenocortical steroids. Parity had no clear
influence on DHEA-sulphate or DHEA. The good intraindividual correlation
between AUC-DHEA and AUC-PRL suggests the possibility that DHEA and
DHEA-sulphate concentrations are not only related to age, but may also
be influenced by PRL. The latter would be in accordance with reports
that DHEA-sulphate has been found to be elevated in hyperprolactinemia
from pituitary adenoma (3, 13). With regard to breast cancer, the observations that DHEA inhibits breast tumor development in mice (10) and
that DHEA and DHEA-sulphate are potent inhibitors of estradiol oxidation
in human endometrium (2) may be relevant.
A decrease of the plasma concentration of DHEA and its sulphate may
cause less protection against breast cancer promoting factors.
    In conclusion: 1. Much controversy on hormones and breast cancer has
resulted from the lack of taking into account that plasma hormones may
fluctuate considerably and unpredictably. Frequent or rather continuous

blood sampling is needed for limited study populations. This holds true for peptide hormones but also for steroids like estradiol and progesterone, the level of which may intraindividually vary over 100 per cent within a few hours under standardized conditions. 2. Decreasing breast cancer risk with parity may be related to a long-lasting decrease of PRL after birthgiving. 3. The inverse correlation of DHEA and DHEA-sulphate with age may imply that a protective hormonal effect against breast cancer gradually abates with increasing age.

ACKNOWLEDGEMENTS

The authors are grateful to M.Buning, A.Eegherdinck, D.Linders, J.van Loon and F.Verhofstadt for their expert technical assistance and to J.H.Schrooten for her excellent secretarial help.

REFERENCES

1. Adami, H.O., A.Rimsten, B.Stenkvist, et.al. (1978). Cancer 41:747-57.
2. Bonney, R.C.,M.J.Reed and V.H.T.James (1983)J.Steroid Bioch.18:59-64.
3. Carter, J.N., J.E.Tyson, G.L.Warne, S.S.McNeilly,C.Fairman and
      H.G.Friesen (1977)J.Clin.Endocrinol.Metab.45:973-80.
4. Kwa, H.G., F.J.Cleton,M.de Jong-Bakker, R.D.Bulbrook,J.L.Hayward
      and D.Y.Wang (1976) Int.J.Cancer 17:441-47.
5. Kwa, H.G. and D.Y.Wang (1977) Int.J.Cancer 20:12-14.
6. Kwa, H.G., F.J.Cleton, R.D.Bulbrook, D.Y.Wang and J.L.Hayward (1981)
      Int.J.Cancer 28:31-34.
7. MacMahon, B., P.Cole, M.Lin, C.R.Lowe, A.P.Mirra,B.Ravnihar,
      E.B.Salter,V.G.Valoras and S.Yuasa (1970) Bull.Wld Hlth Org.43:209-
      21.
8. Nisula, B.C. and J.F.Dunn (1979) Steroids 34:771-91.
9. Rose, D.P. and B.T.Pruitt (1981) Cancer 48:2687-91.
10. Schwartz, A.G.(1979)Cancer Res.39:1129-32.
11. Thein, H. and M.M.Thein (1978)Int.J.Cancer 21:432-37.
12. Tulinius, H., N.Day, G.Johannesson, O.Bjarnason and M.Gonzales
      Cancer 21:724-30.
13. Vermeulen, A., E.Suy and R.Rubens (1977) J.Clin.Endocrinol.Metab.
      44:1222-25.
14. Zumoff,B., R.S.Rosenfeld, G.W.Strain,J.Levin and D.J.Fukushima (1980)
      J.Clin.Endocrinol.Metab.51:330-33.

Progress in Cancer Research and Therapy,
Vol. 31, edited by F. Bresciani, et al.
Raven Press, New York © 1984.

Distribution of Oestradiol in Plasma from Normal Postmenopausal Women and Postmenopausal Women with Breast Cancer

*M.J. Reed, *P.A. Beranek, **Margaret W. Ghilchik, and *V.H.T. James

*Department of Chemical Pathology, St. Mary's Hospital Medical School, London W2; and **Department of Surgery, St. Charles Hospital, London W10, United Kingdom

The failure to find any consistent abnormality in plasma or urinary oestrogen concentrations in postmenopausal women with breast cancer has resulted in an examination of other aspects of oestrogen production, transport and metabolism (4). In a previous study (8) the free fraction of oestradiol (E2) in plasma was measured in a large group of postmenopausal breast cancer patients and the increase in the free fraction of E2 originally reported by Siiteri (9) was confirmed. However, it was concluded from our previous investigation that the difference in the free E2 concentration between normal postmenopausal women and postmenopausal women with breast cancer was very small, although given the length of time required for tumour development, even such a small difference in the free E2 fraction might be important. In the same study a preliminary investigation was carried out of the proportion of E2 bound to albumin and sex hormone binding globulin (SHBG) in plasma from postmenopausal women with benign breast disease or breast cancer. Although no significant difference was found in the distribution of E2 in plasma from the two groups of patients, it was apparent that the concentrations of albumin-bound and SHBG-bound E2 were much greater than the concentration of free E2. In view of the current interest in the availability to target tissues of albumin-bound or SHBG-bound E2, we are examining the distribution of E2 in plasma obtained from postmenopausal women with breast cancer and normal postmenopausal women. The metabolic clearance rates of E2 (MCR-E2) have also been measured in the subjects of the present study and related to SHBG-binding capacity and the distribution of E2. Any differences in either the distribution of E2 or in the relationship of the MCR-E2 to the various factors examined may help in advancing the hypothesis that subjects with breast cancer receive increased exposure to the unopposed action of E2.

Subjects

Eight postmenopausal women with breast cancer and six postmenopausal women who did not have breast cancer have so far been studied. There was no significant difference in the ages, number of years since the menopause, ideal body weights or SHBG-binding capacity between breast cancer and control subjects (Table 1).

TABLE 1.   Subjects ages, number of years since the menopause, ideal body weight, and SHBG-binding capacity

	Age (years)	YPM (years)	IBW (%)	SHBG (μgDHT/100ml)
Normal(n=6)	63.2+11.4[a]	16.3+13.9	100.2+24.7	1.39+0.7
Cancer(n=8)	64.1+11.1	14.3+13.4	104.0+20.3	1.33+0.3

[a] mean $\pm$ S.D.

Plasma samples were obtained and metabolic clearance rate measurements were carried out before surgery. Control subjects were also studied whilst in hospital before undergoing surgery for conditions other than cancer.

Methods

A full description of the methods used in this study has been previously published (4).

Results and Discussion

Several studies have now been carried out to measure the plasma concentration of total unconjugated E2 in plasma from postmenopausal women with cancer, but few investigators have attempted to measure the distribution of oestradiol in plasma. In the present study using a precipitation technique 40.3 $\pm$ 12.6% (mean $\pm$ S.D.) of oestradiol was found to be bound to albumin and 59.7 $\pm$ 13.0% to SHBG in normal postmenopausal women.   These results are in very good agreement with the values reported by Davidson et al. (2).   Further support for the validity of using the precipitation technique to measure the fraction of E2 bound to albumin and calculation of the SHBG-bound E2 fraction comes from the highly significant correlation found between the fraction of SHBG-bound E2 and SHBG-binding capacity as shown in Fig.1.

Total concentration of oestradiol

In the present study the mean plasma concentration of E2 in cancer patients (2.63 $\pm$ 0.65 ng/100ml, mean $\pm$ S.D.) was significantly higher than in control subjects (1.80 $\pm$ 0.48 ng/100ml). This finding contrasts with the results of our previous study (8) where no such difference was detected.   However, in our previous investigation a large proportion of the breast cancer patients were studied some time after the removal of the breast tumour, whereas in the present study E2 concentrations were measured in samples of plasma obtained before surgery.   Drafta et al. (3) and Moore et al. (6) also found significantly increased plasma levels of oestradiol in postmenopausal breast cancer patients, although the levels of E2 reported tended to be much higher than those found in the present investigation.

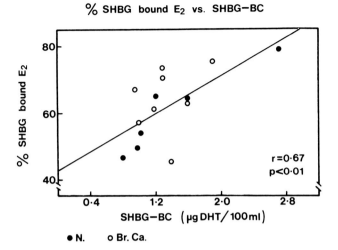

FIG. 1. Correlation between fraction of E2 bound to SHBG
         and SHBG-binding capacity in normal postmenopausal
         women and postmenopausal women with breast cancer

Distribution

Only a small number of subjects have been studied in the present
investigation and no significant difference in the free fraction has so
far been found in cancer patients. As found previously, however, over
50% of the breast cancer patients have a higher free E2 fraction than
the mean value seen in control subjects. The mean values ($\pm$ S.D.) for
the free fraction of E2 in normal and breast cancer patients, together
with the fractions of E2 bound to albumin and SHBG, are shown in Fig.2.
So far, no significant difference has been found in the fractions of E2
bound to albumin or SHBG in normal and cancer subjects.

Oestradiol concentrations

However, as shown in Fig. 3., in addition to a significantly
higher mean concentration of total unconjugated E2 in breast cancer
patients the mean concentrations of free E2 and SHBG-bound E2 were also
significantly increased in cancer patients.
Whereas the difference in the mean concentrations of free E2 in
normal and cancer subjects is only 0.17pg/ml, for SHBG-bound E2 the
difference in mean concentrations is 6.34pg/ml. If, as has been
recently suggested, SHBG-bound E2 is able to enter target tissues
(1,10) the difference in concentrations of SHBG-bound E2 may be of
greater importance in tumour development than the very small difference
in free E2 concentrations.

MCR-E2

Values for the MCR-E2 in postmenopausal women with breast cancer and
control subjects are shown in Fig. 4.

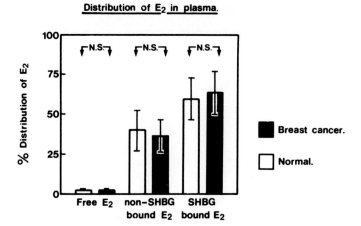

FIG. 2.   Free E2 fractions and fractions of E2 bound to albumin
and SHBG in normal postmenopausal women and postmenopausal women with breast cancer.

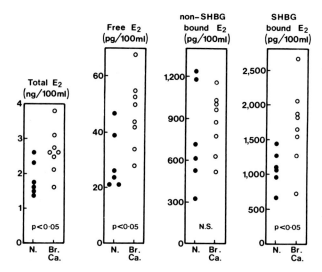

FIG. 3.   Plasma concentrations of unconjugated, free, albumin
bound and SHBG-bound E2 in normal postmenopausal
women and postmenopausal women with breast cancer.

The MCR-E2 was higher than the mean clearance rate in control
subjects in 6 of the 8 cancer patients.   Kirschner et al.   (5) have
previously reported increased oestrogen clearance rates in some postmenopausal breast cancer patients and increased MCR-E2 were also found
in postmenopausal patients with endometrial cancer (4).

A significant correlation was found between the free E2 fraction and
MCR-E2 (r = 0.56, p<0.05).   So far, however, no significant correlation

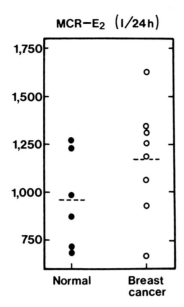

FIG. 4.   MCR-E2 in normal postmenopausal women and postmenopausal
women with breast cancer.

between the albumin-bound E2 fraction and MCR-E2 has been found as might
be expected if this fraction is available for metabolism. The fraction
of E2 bound to SHBG and MCR-E2 appear to be negatively correlated and
this finding is consistent with the concept that SHBG-bound E2 is
protected from metabolism. However, this concept may be too simplistic
(7), as correlations between the concentrations of SHBG-bound E2 and
MCR-E2 for breast cancer patients and normal postmenopausal women
suggest that increased tissue metabolism may also be a component in the
increased clearance rates seen in cancer patients.

It is generally accepted that the MCR of steroids is inversely
related to the affinity of their binding to specific proteins and in
the present study a significant negative correlation (r = -0.59,
p<0.05) was found between SHBG-binding capacity and MCR-E2. A similar
finding was recently reported by Siiteri et al. (10). Although only
a small number of normal and cancer patients have so far been studied in
the present investigation, the results obtained suggest that the
regression lines for normal subjects and cancer patients may differ,
with a similar binding capacity of SHBG being associated with a higher
clearance rate in cancer patients. This is similar to the relationship between SHBG-binding capacity and the free E2 fraction reported by
Moore et al. (6) where for a given level of SHBG, the free fraction of
oestradiol was higher in cancer patients.

Summary and conclusions

The results of the present study have shown that the free fraction of
E2 and MCR-E2 are elevated in about half the number of subjects investigated with breast cancer. A significant increase in the concentration
of free E2 was also found in breast cancer patients, but this increment

was very small compared with the difference in mean concentrations of SHBG-bound E2. From the result of this and our previous study, together with the results of investigations carried out by other groups, there is an increasing amount of evidence for some abnormality in oestrogen binding and clearance in some cancer subjects. As the level of free E2 and clearance rate are directly related, it would appear most likely that there is some abnormality of SHBG or interference with E2 binding to SHBG in cancer patients. Further studies are currently in progress to investigate these possibilities.

ACKNOWLEDGMENT

This work was supported by a grant from the Cancer Research Campaign.

References

1. Bordin, S., and Petra, P.H. (1980): Proc. natn. Acad. Sci. U.S.A., 77:5678-5682.
2. Davidson, B.J., Gambone, J.C., Lagasse, L.D., Castaldo, T.W., Hammond, G.L., Siiteri, P.K., and Judd, H.L. (1981): J. clin. Endocr. Metab., 52:404-408.
3. Drafta, D., Schindler, A.E., Milcu, S.M., Keller, E., Stroe, E., Horodniceanu, E., and Balanescu, I. (1980): J. Steroid Biochem, 13:793-802.
4. James, V.H.T., Reed, M.J., and Folkerd, E.J. (1981): J. Steroid Biochem., 15:235-246.
5. Kirschner, M.A., Cohen, F.B., and Ryan, C. (1978): Cancer Res., 38:4029-4035.
6. Moore, J.W., Clarke, G.M.G., Bulbrook, R.D., Hayward, J.L., Murai, J.T., Hammond, G.L., and Siiteri, P.K. (1982): Int. J. Cancer, 29:17-21.
7. Petra, P.H., Stanczyk, F.Z., Senear, D.F., Namkung, P.C., Novy, M.J., Ross, J.B.A., Turner, E., and Brown, J.A. (1983): J. Steroid Biochem., 19:699-706.
8. Reed, M.J., Cheng, R.W., Dudley, H.A.F., and James, V.H.T. (1983): Cancer Res., 43:3940-3943.
9. Siiteri, P.K. (1981): J. Endocr., 89:119P-129P.
10. Siiteri, P.K., Murai, J.T., Hammond, G.L., Nisker, J.A., Raymoure, W.J., and Kuhn, R.W. (1982): Res. Prog. Horm. Res., 38:457-503.

Progress in Cancer Research and Therapy,
Vol. 31, edited by F. Bresciani, et al.
Raven Press, New York © 1984.

Studies with Mammary Tumours of the Bitch

C.G. Pierrepoint, S.E. Thomas, and C.L. Eaton

Tenovus Institute for Cancer Research, Welsh National School of Medicine, Cardiff, CF4 4XX United Kingdom

The term "model" may be defined as "something that accurately resembles something else". It is probably impossible, in biological terms to meet this definition yet one may apply certain conditions, and that system that complies with the greater number should provide the best model.

The conditions that may be applied to a model for human breast cancer could be (1) The tumours should arise spontaneously, (2) The animal should share as closely as possible the same environment as man, (3) The frequency of occurrence of tumours should be relatively high, (4) The biological behaviour of the tumours should be similar to that in man. This should include histological types, proneness to metastasise, local recurrence following surgery and similar mortality rate, (5) The species-corrected age of incidence should be similar, (6) Possible sparing effects of early reproductive events, (7) Hormonal dependency and finally (8) Early demise to allow the rapid evaluation of differing forms of therapy in delaying this event.

It seems that only the dog and cat share with man, to any marked degree, the propensity for spontaneous mammary tumour development. The incidence in the dog is high, exceeding that for women some three-fold (27). It is certainly true that the pet dog shares the same environment as man and the term "companion animal" is now used to describe it. In order to enjoy this privileged position the dog has had to comply with certain conditions that man has imposed upon himself with regard to reproductive performance. These restrictions on procreation essential to domesticity may have fundamental effects on the mammary gland with age.

The biological behaviour of the canine mammary carcinoma relates closely to that in women. In the latter, the most malignant breast cancer is the infiltrating ductular carcinoma (19) which also occurs with high frequency in the bitch (1,2,25,27). It has been noted that the most outstanding prognostic feature in both species is the mode of growth of the tumour (21).

Recurrence of adenocarcinoma following mastectomy is high (21,22, 23) which emphasises the value of the bitch as a model in the evaluation of therapeutic agents in the prevention of re-growth.

When an age-correction factor is employed (15) the annual age-specific incidence rates for the bitch and woman are virtually identical (27) with the rate of increase declining in the latter at the time of the menopause. Such a reduction is not seen in the bitch which does not undergo an equivalent climacteric.

A hormonal involvement in mammary cancer in both species is widely accepted. Ovariectomy has been shown to reduce the incidence in women

(7,10) whilst in dogs it has been reported (4) that entire bitches have seven times the risk of developing the disease compared with speyed animals. It is also declared (27), that breast disease in the bitch is probably predetermined before the age of 2.5 years. This was related to the number of oestrous cycles she had experienced prior to speying. The risk increasing to 8% and 26% that of the mature entire animal if the animal were allowed to experience one, or two, oestruses respectively before ovariectomy. In women it is accepted that early full-term pregnancy before the age of 20 years, reduces the risk of eventual breast cancer by half compared with women who first become pregnant after the age of 25 years (19). When age-corrected there is a remarkable similarity to the dog.

It is now well-accepted that the steroid hormones achieve their function through a well-defined series of intra-cellular events initiated by the binding of the hormone to specific cytoplasmic receptors followed by the translocation of the resulting complex to the nucleus. Promotion of various transcriptional events results with the synthesis of macromolecules that maintain cell function (11,12,14). Similarly the absence of such receptors would disallow the action of the specified hormone.

It has been known for many years that a proportion of women with breast cancer would respond well to ablative and/or additive endocrine therapy and now, with the relatively recent discovery of steroid receptors in responsive tissue the measurement of these proteins in excised tumour tissue is used as a guide to therapy and as an indicator of prognosis (8,13). Although such forms of therapy in the bitch are at present untried or at least in their very early stages, the canine mammary neoplasms again show close similarities with the human. Receptor proteins for oestrogens have been demonstrated in these tumours (3,5,6, 9,17,24,26).

Table 1 shows the distribution of receptors for oestrogens (ER), progestagens (PR) and androgens (AR) in tumours removed from bitches and classified simply into sarcoma, carcinoma and benign. Those tumours that are included in the benign group are described in the legend. In the series so far investigated there are 21 (6.5%) sarcomas, 158 (48.8%) carcinomas and 144 (44.6%) benign. Almost 70% of the latter group consisted of adenomas and mixed mammary tumours.

It may be seen from Table 1 that somewhat over 50% of the carcinomas possessed oestrogen receptors with a lower incidence in the sarcomas (42.9%). There was also a lower incidence of PR+ (38.1%) and AR+ (47.6%) in the sarcomas than in the group of carcinomas. Some tumours in each of the groups possessed receptors for each of the hormones investigated although a higher proportion of the sarcomas (42.9%) was negative for all three receptors and no sarcoma was found to possess the oestrogen receptor alone.

Comparing our data with those of Raynaud et al. (26) who did not measure the androgen receptor, they found 56% of their benign series had both oestrogen and progestagen receptors out of 50 tumours. In our series of 144 benign lesions there were only 40 (27.8%) that were positive for these two receptors. A similar difference was found in the examination of total malignant tumours 44% (26) and 29.1% in this report. Comparison of ER-PR- in the two series shows very close similarities.

A colony of athymic (nude) immunoincompetent mice has been established in this Institute (29) and the growth characteristics and responsiveness to endocrine therapy of transplanted canine malignant mammary tumours studied. Four such tumours, one, a complex, and two simple

Table 1.

Receptor status of various sub-groups of 323 canine mammary tumours

	Sarcoma	Carcinoma	Benign
	n	n	n
ER+	9(42.9)	88(55.7)	78(54.2)
PR+	8(38.1)	66(41.8)	57(39.6)
AR+	10(47.6)	87(55.1)	75(52.1)
ER+PR+AR+	3(14.3)	35(22.2)	30(20.8)
ER-PR-AR-	9(42.9)	36(22.8)	39(27.1)
ER alone	0(0.0)	16(10.1)	16(11.1)
PR alone	1(4.8)	9(5.7)	6(4.2)
AR alone	1(4.8)	17(10.8)	11(7.6)
Total	21	158	148

The data show the number and percentage ( ) of each tumour type possessing, or not possessing receptors for oestrogens (ER), progestagens (PR) and androgens (AR). The benign group include mixed mammary tumours, hyperplastic lesions, adenomas, papillomas, myo-epitheliomas, fibrosed glands, and inflammatory lesions.

adenocarcinomas and a fibrosarcoma have been studied (29,30). The methods for transplantation and passage have been described elsewhere (29). A prominent feature of their growth was reduction to one half of the latent period by the third passage. The histological appearance remained remarkably constant through serial transplantation with one simple adenocarcinoma becoming slightly more dedifferentiated.

Male and female mice were used as recipients of tumour grafts and the effects, initially, of ovariectomy, orchidectomy and hormone replacement on growth rates of the implants studied. Tumour fragments were implanted subcutaneously on both flanks of entire and ovariectomized female nude mice. Figure 1 shows a much reduced growth rate (significantly different by day 14) in the absence of the ovaries and the restoration to control values by the administration of oestradiol (1µg/day). It is of interest that the same dose of oestradiol administered to entire mice did not increase the rate of growth above that of the controls (Fig. 1).

Figure 2 shows the effect of orchidectomy and testosterone propionate administration on the growth-rate of a complex adenocarcinoma implanted into male nude mice. There is a highly significant (p<0.001) reduction in growth rate, from day 7, of the implants, examined over a 30-day period, in castrated animals. The androgen treatment of these animals produced a growth rate that was not significantly different to the entire controls and again hormone administration did not increase tumour growth in entire animals over that of entire animals receiving the vehicle alone.

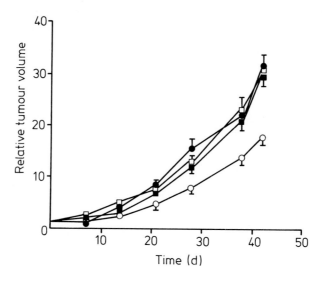

FIG. 1. Growth, at the fifth passage, of a complex adenocarcinoma implanted in nude female mice. Growth is recorded as the volume of the tumour relative to that of the initial implant. Control entire mice ●; ovariectomized mice ○; ovariectomized mice receiving 1µg oestradiol/day □; entire mice receiving 1µg oestradiol/day ■. Growth in the ovariectomized mice receiving vehicle alone (○) is statistically different from the other three treatment groups (p<0.001) at day 21.

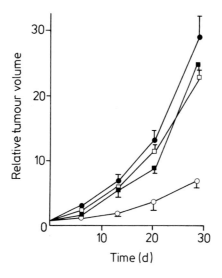

FIG. 2. Growth of a complex adenocarcinoma implanted in nude male mice. Growth is recorded as the volume relative to that of the initial implant. Entire control mice ●; orchidectomized mice ○; orchidectomized mice receiving 50µg testosterone propionate/day □; entire mice receiving 50µg testosterone propionate/day ■. Growth in the orchidectomized mice receiving vehicle alone (○) is statistically different to the other three treatment groups (p<0.001) by day 7.

Figure 3 shows the effect of ovariectomy with and without the administration of the anti-oestrogen, tamoxifen (1-(4-β-dimethylamino-ethoxyphenyl)-1,2-diphenylbut-1-ene) (I.C.I. Ltd., Alderley Edge, Cheshire) on the growth of an adenocarcinoma implanted into nude mice.

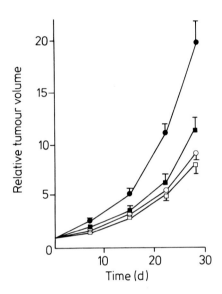

FIG. 3. Growth of a complex adenocarcinoma implanted in nude female mice. Growth is recorded as the volume of the tumour relative to that of the initial implant. Control entire mice, ●; ovariectomized mice, ■; entire mice receiving 50μg tamoxifen/day, ○; ovariectomized mice receiving 50μg tamoxifen/day, □. Growth of the tumour in entire mice receiving the vehicle alone (●) significantly (p<0.001) different to the other three treatment groups at 14 days. Growth of the tumour in ovariectomized mice receiving vehicle alone (■) significantly (p<0.001) different to growth in the ovariectomized mice receiving 50μg tamoxifen/day (□) at 28 days.

As in figure 1 it may be seen there is reduction of growth of the tumour in the absence of the ovaries by day 14 of the experiment. The effect of tamoxifen similarly had a significant (p<0.001) growth reducing effect by day 14 continuing to the end of the experiment it would seem of importance to note that by day 28 there was a reduction in the tumour growth in ovariectomised animals also given tamoxifen compared with that in the mice that were solely ovariectomised and injected with the vehicle. The indications are that circulating oestrogens are still available for partial promotion of growth of the tumours even in the absence of the ovaries. These are probably of adrenal origin or, at least, formed by the peripheral conversion of adrenal androgens.

These findings indicate that some, at least, of canine mammary carcinomas are dependent for full growth on oestrogens and/or androgens and that gonadectomy reduces their growth rate as observed when implanted into nude mice. It has further been shown (28) that DNA-dependent RNA polymerase activity in isolated nuclei from canine mammary tumours was stimulated by cytosol previously incubated with either oestradiol-17β, R5020 (17-methyl-17α,21-dimethyl-19-nor-pregna-4,9-diene-3,20-dione; New England Nuclear, Dreieich, W. Germany) or 5α-dihydrotestosterone only when the tumour contained specific receptors for those steroids. The steroid-cytosol induced effects proved to be dose-dependent.

It is on the basis of such data that a clinical trial has been established in this region to investigate the adjuvant anti-hormone therapy of bitches from which mammary carcinomas have been removed.

It would appear from the evidence cited initially and now with the demonstration of receptors in canine mammary tumours and their hormone dependence and responsiveness that here we have a model that fulfils the criteria listed at the beginning of this paper and this closely resembles breast cancer in women.

ACKNOWLEDGEMENTS

The authors are grateful to the Tenovus Organisation, Cardiff for excellent laboratory facilities and financial support. They also wish to acknowledge the assistance provided by The Clinical Studies Trust Fund Ltd. of the British Small Animal Veterinary Association. The technical skills of Mr. Karl Pettit and Miss Karen Kenvyn are gratefully appreciated.

REFERENCES

1. Bloom, F. (1954). Pathology of the dog and cat. The Genitourinary System with Clinical Considerations. American Veterinary Publications, Evanston, Illinois.
2. Cotchin, E. (1958). J. Comp. Path. 68, 1-22.
3. D'Arville, C.N. & Pierrepoint, C.G. (1979). Europ. J. Cancer 15, 875-883.
4. Dorn, C.R., Taylor, D.O.N., Schneider, B., Hibbard, H.H. & Klauber, M.R. (1968). J. Nat. Cancer Inst. 40, 307-318.
5. Evans, B.A.J., Borthwick, G., Wilson, D.W. & Pierrepoint, C.G. (1977). J. Endocr. 77, 64P-65P.
6. Evans, C.R. & Pierrepoint, C.G. (1975). Vet. Rec. 97, 464-467.
7. Feinleib, M. (1968). J. Nat. Cancer Inst. 41, 315-329.
8. Griffiths, K., Nicholson, R.I., Joyce, B., Morton, M., Campbell, C. & Blamey, R.W. (1983). In: Recent Clinical Developments in Gynecologic Oncology, edited by C. Paul Morrow et al. pp.107-121. Raven Press, New York.
9. Hamilton, J.M., Else, R.W. & Forshaw, P. (1977). Vet. Rec. 101, 258-260.
10. Hirayama, T. & Wynder, E.L. (1962). Cancer 15, 28-38.
11. Jensen, E.V., DeSombre, E.R. & Jungblut, P.W. (1967). In: Endogenous Factors Influencing Host Tumor Balance, edited by R.W. Wissler, T.L. Dao & S. Wood Jr. pp.15-30. University of Chicago Press, Chicago.

12. Jensen, E.V., Jacobson, H.I., Flesher, J.W., Soha, N.N., Gupta, G.N., Smith, S., Colucci, V., Shiplacoff, D., Neumann, H.G., DeSombre, E.R. & Jungblut, P.W. (1966). In: Steroid Dynamics, edited by G. Pincus, T. Nakao and J.F. Tait. pp.133-147, Acad. Press, New York.

13. Jensen, E.V., Smith, S.S. & DeSombre, E.R. (1976). J. Steroid Biochem. 7, 911-917.

14. Jensen, E.V., Suzuki, T., Kawashima, T., Stumpf, W.E., Jungblut, P.W. & DeSombre, E.R. (1968). Proc. Nat. Acad. Sci. USA 59, 632-638.

15. Lebeau, A. (1953). Bul. Acad. Vet. 26, 229-232.

16. Lilienfeld, A.M. (1956) Cancer 9, 927-934.

17. MacEwen, E.G., Patnaik, A.K., Harvey, H.J. & Panko, W.B. (1982). Cancer Res. 42, 2255-2259.

18. MacMahon, B. & Cole, P. (1972). In: Current Problems in the Epidemiology of Cancer, Lymphomas and Leukaemias. Gesselschaft zur Bekampfung der Krebstrandbeiten Nordrhein-Westfaler e.v.

19. MacMahon, B., Cole, P., Lin, T.M., Lowe, C.R., Mirra, A.P., Ravnihar, B., Salber, E.J., Valaoras, V.G. & Yuasa, S. (1970). Bull. Wld. Hlth. Org. 43, 209-221.

20. McDivitt, R.W., Stewart, F.W. & Berg, J.W. (1968). Tumors of the breast. 2nd series, fasc. 2. Washington D.C., Armed Forces Inst. Pathol.

21. Misdorp, W. & Hart, A.A.M. (1976). J. Nat. Cancer Inst. 56, 779-786.

22. Misdorp, W. & Hart, A.A.M. (1979). J. Small Anim. Pract. 20, 395-404.

23. Mitchell, L., de la Iglesia, F.A., Wenkoff, M.S., van Dreumel, A.A. & Lumb, G. (1974) Canad. Vet. J. 15, 131-138.

24. Monson, K.R., Malbica, J.O. & Habben, K. (1977). Amer. J. Vet. Res. 38, 1937-1939.

25. Moulton, J.E., Taylor, D.O.N., Doin, C.R. & Anderson, A.C. (1970). Pathol. Vet. 7, 389-320.

26. Raynaud, J.P., Cotard, M., André, F., Mialot, J.P., Rolland, P.H. & Martin, P.M. (1981). J. Steroid Biochem. 15 201-207.

27. Schneider, R. (1970). Cancer 26, 419-426.

28. Thomas, S.E. & Pierrepoint, C.G. (1983). Europ. J. Cancer Clin. Oncol. 19, 377-382.

29. Thomas, S.E., Thomas, N. & Pierrepoint, C.G. (1983). Europ. J. Cancer Clin. Oncol. 19, 979-987.

30. Thomas, S.E., Thomas, N. & Pierrepoint, C.G. (1983). Europ. J. Cancer Clin. Oncol. 19, 989-994.

*Progress in Cancer Research and Therapy,
Vol. 31,* edited by F. Bresciani, et al.
Raven Press, New York © 1984.

Canine and Feline Mammary Cancers as Animal Models for Hormone-Dependent Human Breast Tumors: Relationships Between Steroid Receptor Profiles and Survival Rates

*A.L. Parodi, *J.P. Mialot, † P.M. Martin, **M. Cotard,
and **J.P. Raynaud

*Ecole Vétérinaire, F-94704 Alfort; **Roussel-Uclaf, F-75007 Paris; and †Faculté
Médecine Nord, F-13326 Marseille, France*

In many countries breast cancer is still the most common malignant disease in women. The progress made during recent years in veterinary oncology has led to considerable interest in animal tumors as models. This is particularly true for mammary tumors in the bitch.

THE CANINE MAMMARY TUMOR MODEL

The mammary tumor incidence rate in bitches is around 200 cases per 100 000, i.e., 3 times higher than the incidence of human breast cancer in the same geographical area (8). Histologically malignant tumors account for up to 50 percent of these tumors.

Several authors give a mean age of 9 to 10 years for the appearance of mammary tumors with a range from 2 to 17 years. The incidence shows a marked rise after 6 years so that, as in women, the majority of tumors occur in the older age group with some in the middle age group (27). No equivalent of the human menopause exists in bitches ; the pattern of changes in the incidence rate in women, which includes a rapid progression until menopause, a break at the menopause, and a slower rise subsequently (30), is unknown in the bitch.

There is no available evidence to suggest that canine mammary cancer is more common in any particular breed or geographical area. There are only a few reports on the familial occurrence of mammary tumors in dogs and there is no evidence, at the present time, that canine mammary tumors are of viral origin.

The incidence of tumors is 2.5 to 3 times greater in the posterior gland (4). It is common for more than one mammary gland to have tumors and these can be of the same or of different histological types.

Mammary tumors in bitches arise both from secretory epithelial cells and myoepithelial cells. According to the World Health Organization classification of tumors and dysplasias of the mammary gland of the dog and cat (14), mammary tumors are classified as "simple" when only one of the cell types is present and as "complex" when both secretory and myoepithelial cells are present. Mesenchymal tumors are less common.

The proportion of carcinoma may vary from 29% to 63% according to the medical status of the bitch (26). The possibility that carcinomas or sarcomas may arise in fibroadenomas or benign mixed tumors is indicated by both histological and epidemiological data (26). Benign tumors may develop from hyperplastic lesions (14). Lungs and locoregional lymphnodes are the commonest sites of metastases.

Steroid Receptor Profiles in Canine Mammary Tumors

Previous studies have demonstrated that canine mammary tumors may contain cytosol estrogen (ER) and progestin (PR) receptors with a comparable incidence to humans (3,5,7,11,13,19,21-23,25,29). Further reports have established the presence of androgen receptor (7,10,21) and, recently, the presence of glucocorticoid and mineralocorticoid cytosol receptors has been evoked (21).

In this study 144 mammary tumors were investigated for the presence of ER and PR by a dextran-coated charcoal adsorption assay (22,29) (Table 1). About 50 percent of these tumors contained both ER and PR on the basis of a cut-off value of 10 fmol/mg protein, whereas 35 percent were receptor negative. The mean concentration of receptor protein was 21.5 fmol/mg protein for ER and 31.5 fmol/mg of protein for PR. There was no significant difference in receptor incidence and levels between benign and malignant tumors.

TABLE 1. Incidence of estrogen and progestin receptors

	ER^+ PR^+		ER^+ PR^-		ER^- PR^+		ER^- PR^-	
Total number (144)	71	(49%)	11	(8%)	11	(8%)	51	(35%)
Benign tumors (50)	28	(56%)	3	(6%)	3	(6%)	16	(32%)
Malignant tumors (87)	38	(44%)	8	(9%)	7	(8%)	34	(39%)
Benign tumors								
Epithelial (25)	14	(56%)	3	(12%)	2	(8%)	6	(24%)
Mixed (25)	14	(56%)	0		1	(4%)	10	(40%)
Malignant tumors								
Carcinomas								
simple type (25)	10	(40%)	2	(8%)	2	(8%)	11	(44%)
complex type (49)	22	(45%)	4	(8%)	3	(6%)	20	(41%)
Mixed tumors[a] (11)	6	(55%)	2	(18%)	2	(18%)	1	(9%
Sarcomas (2)	0		0		0		2	

[a] Carcinosarcomas

At least 40 percent of the epithelial malignant tumors (carcinomas) which constituted 85 percent of the malignant tumors were both ER and PR positive. In this group, no difference was seen in receptor incidence between the simple and complex subtypes, nor were the mean receptor levels different. Only 6 out the 11 carcinosarcomas had both ER and PR. Neither of the two sarcomas was receptor-positive. 56 percent of benign tumors were both ER and PR positive, with no difference between the simple epithelial and complex subtypes.

In a limited number of tumors, androgen (AR), glucocorticoid (GR) and mineralocorticoid (MR) cytosol receptors were also assayed (Table 2)(21).

TABLE 2. Incidence of androgen (AR), glucocorticoid (GR) and mineralocorticoid (MR) receptors

	Receptor concentration (fmol/mg protein)				
	ER	PR	AR	GR	MR
Malignant tumors (n = 19)					
Adenocarcinomas (tubular, simple)	3	1	6	3	3
	5	6	6	3	3
	[38]	[22]	[13]	1	1
	4	5	5	ND	ND
	4	3	9	ND	ND
	[23]	[35]	[18]	ND	ND
Adenocarcinomas (tubular, complex)	[14]	[18]	[13]	ND	ND
	[21]	[30]	8	1	1
	3	6	3	2	2
	3	3	5	ND	ND
	[14]	2	5	[12]	[12]
	2	[10]	3	ND	ND
Adenocarcinoma (papillary, simple)	[10]	7	2	ND	ND
Solid carcinomas	5	6	4	2	2
	0	1	1	0	0
	2	2	3	2	2
	0	6	2	2	2
Fibrosarcoma	0	0	0	0	0
Mixed tumors (Carcinosarcomas)	[21]	5	7	ND	ND
Benign tumors (n = 9)					
Adenomas	8	[11]	[14]	2	2
	4	8	4	ND	ND
Benign mixed tumors	5	2	2	2	2
	9	7	3	1	1
	8	[17]	9	ND	ND
	3	3	3	ND	ND
	9	5	4	ND	ND
	9	7	5	ND	ND
Lobular hyperplasia	[15]	[14]	7	ND	ND

ND = Not determined on account of limited amount of cytosol available

Only 4 out of 28 tumors contained AR. The AR values seemed to be highest in those tumors with high ER and PR values. The GR and MR levels, except for one sample, were at the limit of detection.

These results confirm the presence of steroid ER and PR cytosol receptors in canine mammary tumors. The incidence of ER and PR ($\sim$ 50%) is slightly higher than observed in human breast cancer (5). Conversely, the mean receptor level seems to be lower in bitches than in women. No difference was observed according to the histological type of the tumor.

Steroid Hormone Receptors and Clinical Parameters

No relationship was found between the presence of ER and/or PR and the clinical status of the bitches, i.e., breed, age, genital activity as evaluated by the frequency of gestations, of pseudogestative lactations and of progestin administration (Fig. 1, Table 3). The presence of ER and PR seemed to be more frequent in the smallest tumors, but not significantly so. On the other hand, a significant relationship was found between the number of tumors and the presence of steroid hormone receptors, which were more frequent in multiple (55%) than in single (33%) tumors (22,23, 29).

TABLE 3.   Incidence of steroid hormone receptors according to clinical parameters and tumor characteristics

	$ER^+ PR^+$		$ER^+ PR^-$		$ER^- PR^+$		$ER^- PR^-$	
Number of pregnancies								
None (61)	36	(59%)	2	(3%)	3	(5%)	20	(33%)
One or more (79)	34	(43%)	8	(10%)	8	(10%)	29	(37%)
Unknown (4)	1		1		0		2	
Occurrence of pseudo-pregnancy lactation								
Never (81)	35	(43%)	6	(7.4%)	7	(8.6%)	33	(41%)
Occasionally (22)	15	(68%)	0		2	(9%)	5	(23%)
Regularly (33)	19	(58%)	3	(9%)	2	(6%)	9	(27%)
Unknown (7)	1		1		0		4	
Progestin treatment								
Treated (28)	15	(53.5%)	2	(7%)	1	(3.5%)	10	(36%)
Untreated (112)	54	(48%)	9	(8%)	10	(9%)	39	(35%)
Unknown (4)	2		0		0		2	
Number of tumors								
Single nodule (36)	12	(33%)	2	(6%)	3	(8%)	19	(53%)
Multinodular (108)	59	(55%)	9	(8%)	8	(7%)	32	(30%)
Tumor size (diameter in cm)								
< 5 (57)	34	(60%)	4	(7%)	1	(2%)	18	(31%)
5-10 (59)	26	(44%)	6	(10%)	7	(12%)	20	(34%)
> 10 (29)	10	(34%)	1	(3.5%)	1	(3.5%)	17	(59%)

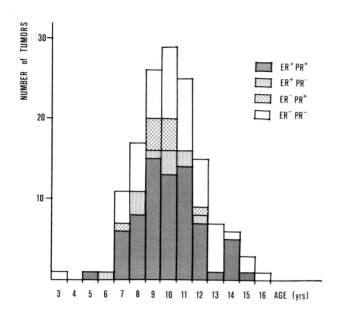

FIG. 1. Incidence of steroid hormone receptors in the bitch according to age.

Steroid Hormone Receptors and Prognosis

Survival rate in women with mammary cancer is known to be higher when the tumor contains steroid hormone receptors (1,6,18). PR has been shown to be a particularly reliable indicator of disease-free interval (20,28). In our study, survival rate was established in 84 bitches, 41 of them with either ER and/or PR levels of 10 fmol/mg protein or above and 43 with low receptor levels (Fig. 2). According to the log rank test, survival was significantly higher in the receptor-rich category (p < 0.001, χ^2 = 13.28 and 13.72 for all cancers and for adenocarcinomas respectively).

In conclusion, canine mammary tumors exhibit many similarities with their human counterpart. Recently-acquired knowledge on the presence of steroid hormone receptors in these tumors indicates that about the same proportion of mammary cancers in dogs and women contain ER and/or PR, and that steroid receptor positivity could be used as an indicator of tumor behavior. However, further studies are necessary to evaluate ER and PR as indicators of hormonal therapy efficiency. If their relevance is confirmed canine mammary cancers (especially adenocarcinomas) would provide an exceptional animal model to test appropriate drugs, doses and administration schedules for hormonal therapy of human breast cancer.

THE FELINE MAMMARY TUMOR MODEL

Mammary carcinoma is somewhat less frequent in cats than in dogs (8) but its histologic features are more similar to those of human carcinoma than are those of either murine or canine mammary carcinoma (24). Although intact female cats have a 7-fold higher relative risk of developing mammary cancer than neutered females (8,15) suggesting some involvement of steroid hormones, feline mammary carcinoma is generally considered a model for cancers less liable to respond to hormone manipulation

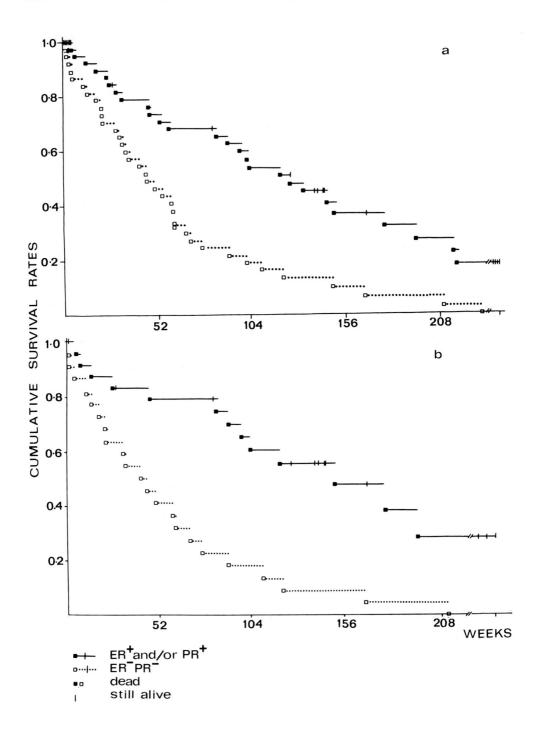

FIG. 2. Cumulative survival rates (a) for all types of canine mammary cancers (p $<$ 0.001, X^2 = 13.28), (b) for canine mammary adenocarcinomas (p $<$ 0.001, X^2 = 13.72).

(15,24). ER was detected in only 2/20 feline mammary carcinomas in one study (12) and in 0/40 samples in another (24). Two more recent studies (9,17) have identified the presence of PR, but neither ER nor AR.

Table 4 gives the results we obtained for feline mammary tumor cytosol (21). ER and/or PR were present in substantial amounts in two malignant tumors (one adenocarcinoma and one solid carcinoma) and in two benign tumors (one adenoma and one lobular hyperplasia). Surprisingly, the highest PR value was found in an adenocarcinoma containing no detectable cytosolic ER in agreement with a report in which none of 7 cytosols had detectable ER whereas all contained PR (17). Thus, feline mammary adenocarcinoma may be representative of the small group of ER$^-$ PR$^+$ human mammary tumors. However, solid carcinomas, benign tumors and maybe to a lesser extent dysplasias, may contain ER. The hormonal pathogenesis (hyperprogesteronism) of benign fibroglandular proliferations of the mammary gland in the cat has already been reported ; these growths regress with ovariectomy (2,16). On the other hand, the very low incidence of ER and PR in carcinoma is to be confronted with the unfortunate prognosis of this disease in the cat (24,31).

TABLE 4. Receptor profiles in mammary tumors of cats

	Receptor concentration (fmol/mg protein)		
	ER	PR	AR
Malignant tumors (n = 9)			
Adenocarcinomas	1	4	ND
(tubular, simple type)	1	0	ND
	3	0.5	[26]
	0	[28]	ND
	0.5	4	10
	4.5	1.5	[13]
	1.5	3	9
Solid carcinomas	3	0.5	ND
	[14]	0	7
Benign tumors and dysplasia (n = 2)			
Adenoma	[31]	[18]	[13]
Lobular hyperplasia	5	[26]	3

ND = Not determined on account of limited amount of cytosol available

Three adenocarcinomas, all ER$^-$PR$^-$, were AR$^+$, a result rather different from that recorded in dogs. The ER$^+$PR$^+$ benign tumor was also AR$^+$. Should this incidence of AR be confirmed in a larger sample of tumors reflecting the overall population, the progression of the disease might be successfully contained by anti-androgen therapy. In only one adenocarcinoma could corticosteroid receptors be assayed. This tumor, rich in AR but low in ER and PR, was found to contain equivalent, and non negligible amounts, of both GR and MR (6 fmol/mg protein).

ACKNOWLEDGEMENTS

This work was supported by an INSERM grant : ATP 58-78-90.

REFERENCES

1. Allegra J.C., Lippman M.E., Simon R., Thompson E.B., Barlock A., Green L., Huff K.K., Do H.M.T., Aitken S. and Warren R. (1979) : Cancer Treat. Rep., 63 : 1271-1277.

2. Allen H.L. (1973) : Vet. Path., 10 : 501-508.

3. André F., Bouton M.M., Cotard M., Martin P.M., Mialot J.P., Secchi J. and Raynaud J.P. (1979) : Cancer Treat. Rep., 63, n° 122 : 1169.

4. Bostock, D.E. (1975) : Eur. J. Cancer, 11 : 389-396.

5. Bronwen, A.J. Evans C.R., Borthwick G., Wilson D.W. and Pierrepoint C.G. (1978) : J. Endocr., 77 : 64-65.

6. Cooke T., George D., Shields R., Maynard P. and Griffiths K. (1979) : Lancet, 1 : 995-997

7. D'Arville C.N. and Pierrepoint C.G. (1979) : Europ. J. Cancer, 15 : 875-883.

8. Dorn C.R., Taylor D.O.N., Frye F.L. and Hibbard H.H. (1968) : J. Natl. Cancer Inst., 40 : 307-318.

9. Elling H. and Ungemach F.R. (1981) : J. Cancer Res. Clin. Oncol., 100 : 325-327.

10. Elling H. and Ungemach F.R. (1983) : J. Cancer Res. Clin. Oncol., 105 : 231-237.

11. Evans C.R. and Pierrepoint C.G. (1975) : Vet. Rec., 13 : 464-467.

12. Hamilton J.M., Else R.W. and Forshaw P. (1976) : Vet. Rec., 99 : 477-479.

13. Hamilton J.M., Else R.W. and Forshaw P. (1977) : Vet. Rec., 101 : 258-260.

14. Hampe J.F. and Misdorp, W. (1974) : Bull. WHO, 50 : 111-133.

15. Hayes H.M. Jr., Milne K.L. and Mandell C.P. (1981) : Vet. Rec., 108 : 476-479.

16. Hinton M. and Gaskell C.J. (1977) : Vet. Rec., 100 : 277-280.

17. Johnston S.D., Hayden D.W., Johnson K.H., Handschin B., Theologides A. and Xiang D.T. (1982) : Cancer Res., Abstract n° 939.

18. Knight W.A., Livingston R.B., Gregory E.J. and McGuire W.L. (1977) : Cancer Res., 37 : 4669-4671.

19. MacEwen E.G., Patnaik A.K., Harvey H.J. and Panko W.B. (1982) : Cancer Res., 42 : 2255-2259.

20. Magdelénat H., Pouillart P., Jouve M., Palangié T., Garcia Giralt E., Bretaudeau B. and Asselain B. (1982) : Breast Cancer Res. Treat., 2 : 195-196.

21. Martin P.M., Cotard M., Mialot J.P., André F. and Raynaud J.P. (in press) : Cancer Chemother. Pharmacol.

22. Mialot J.P., André F., Martin P.M., Cotard M.P. and Raynaud J.P. (1982) : Rec. Med. Vet., 158 : 215-221.

23. Mialot J.P., André F., Martin P.M., Cotard M.P. and Raynaud J.P. (1982) : Rec. Med. Vet., 158 : 513-521.

24. Misdorp W. and Weijer K. (1980) : Am. J. Pathol., 98 : 573-576.

25. Monson K.R., Malbica J.O. and Hubben K. (1977) : Am. J. Vet. Res., 38 : 1937-1939.

26. Moulton J.E., Taylor D.O.N., Dorn C.R. and Anderson A.C. (1970) : Pathol. Vet., 7 : 289-320.

27. Owen L.N. (1979) : Invest. cell Pathol., 2 : 257-275.

28. Pichon M.F., Pallud C., Brunet M. and Milgrom E. (1980) : Cancer Res., 40 : 3357-3360.

29. Raynaud J.P., Cotard M., André F., Mialot J.P., Rolland P.H. and Martin P.M. (1981) : J. steroid Biochem., 15 : 201-207.
30. Seidman H. (1969) : Cancer, 24 : 1355-1378.
31. Weijer K., Head K.W., Misdorp W. and Hampe J.F. (1972) : J. Natl. Cancer Inst., 49 : 1697-1704.

Progress in Cancer Research and Therapy,
Vol. 31, edited by F. Bresciani, et al.
Raven Press, New York © 1984.

Hormonal Receptors in Endometrial Cancer

*D.S. Grosso, *E.A. Surwit, **J.R. Davis, and *C.D. Christian

*Departments of *Obstetrics and Gynecology and **Pathology, University of Arizona Health Sciences Center, Tucson, Arizona 85724*

Adenocarcinoma of the endometrium is now the most frequently occurring gynecological malignancy with an estimated 3700 deaths annually attributable to recurrent or metastatic disease.[1] Progestational agents in the treatment of those patients with advanced disease has proven effective with response rates of 30-40% having been reported.[2,3,4,5] The success of progestational agents in suppressing tumor growth and the apparent involvement of estrogenic hormones in the development of endometrial neoplasia[6] has prompted the investigation of an association between steroid hormone receptor levels and sensitivity to endocrine therapy in gynecologic lesions in a manner analogous to that employed for identification of hormone-dependent mammary carcinomas.[7,8]

In most reported studies of tumor receptor content and hormone dependence, both false positive and false negative cases have been observed. To improve the reliability of the identification of hormone sensitive endometrial tumors, attempts have been made to establish a relationship between receptor status and various pathological correlates. The pathological correlate studied most frequently has been the degree of morphological differentiation of the tumor. However, a consensus has not yet been reached on whether a significant association exists between tumor grade and receptor level.[9,10,11,12,13,14] The methodologies employed for measuring tumor receptor levels vary widely and may contribute in part to the lack of consensus. Since both degree of histological differentiation and receptor levels are related to the sensitivity of endometrial cancers to hormone treatment, the resolution of this controversy is important to understanding the factors which regulate tumor development and growth.

We present here results of an on-going investigation into the involvement of steroid hormones in endometrial carcinoma. The estrogen and progesterone receptor content of endometrial tumors is correlated with the degree of morphological differentiation and to histological type of tumor.

METHODS

Patient Population

Forty-eight consecutive cases of endometrial neoplasia admitted for treatment to the University of Arizona Health Sciences Center were included in this study. Patients' ages ranged from 32-83 years; median age 65 years. Two patients were premenopausal; two cases presented with recurrent disease; and the remainder presented with primary lesions. Long-term treatment with conjugated estrogens (Premarin) for menopausal symptoms was noted in two patients. In one case, the drug was discontinued three years earlier and, in the second, two months prior to surgery. One patient with recurrent disease had received megestrol acetate (Megace) until two months prior to surgery; the other had undergone previous radiation therapy. Histological grading and classification were performed using standard criteria.[15]

Receptor Analysis

Tissues were pulverized in liquid nitrogen and then homogenized in four volumes of THET buffer (5mM Tris-HCl, 5 mM HEPES, 1.5 mM EDTA, 10 mM thioglycerol, pH 8.0 at $4^{O}C$) containing 10% glycerol (THET-10G) with a Polytron homogenizer. The homogenate was centrifuged at 1000 X g for 10 minutes at $4^{O}C$. The supernatant was then centrifuged for 40 minutes at 100,000 X g at $2^{O}C$. Endogenous steroids were removed from the cytosol by treatment with dextran-coated charcoal for 15 minutes at $0^{O}C$ followed by centrifugation.

Receptor analyses were performed with minor modifications as described elsewhere[16,17] using ^{3}H-estradiol or ^{3}H-R5020 for estrogen and progesterone receptors, respectively. Cytosol was incubated for 18 hours at $4^{O}C$ with steroid concentrations of 0.06-8.0 nM in a final assay volume of 0.2 ml. Nonspecific binding was estimated by incubation of a separate set of tubes to which a 100-fold molar excess of diethylstilbestrol for estrogen receptor or progesterone for progesterone receptor had been added. Unbound steroid was removed by addition of 0.5 ml 0.5% Norti A charcoal was removed by centrifugation at 1900 X g at ion for 5 minutes. Bound radioactivity was measured in 0.5 ml aliquots of the supernatant at a tritium counting efficiency of 38%.

Binding parameters B_{max} and K_d were estimated by the graphic method as described by Rosenthal.[18] The criteria for assessing a tumor as positive follows generally the definition of McCarty et al.[14] A tumor was regarded as positive for either receptor if the measured value was equal to or exceeded ten femtomoles/mg of cytosolic protein and exhibited a K_d of less than $10^{-9}M$.

Cytosolic protein analyses were performed by the method of Bradford.[19] Bovine serum albumin was utilized as a standard.

RESULTS

The 48 cases of endometrial neoplasms included in this study were 23 classical adenocarcinomas, 15 adenosquamous carcinomas, two mucinous carcinomas, three clear cell carcinomas, and five papillary carcinomas. Of the 23 adenocarcinomas, 14 were Grade 2 (moderately-differentiated) and nine were Grade 3 (poorly-differentiated) tumors. Five adenosquamous tumors were Grade 3. The absence of Grade 1 (well-differentiated) cancers reflects the referral pattern of the Gynecologic Oncology Division of the University of Arizona.

Estrogen receptor content was determined in 42 of 48 tumors. Progesterone receptor analysis, only, was performed on the remaining six specimens. Progesterone receptor levels were determined in 40 tumors.

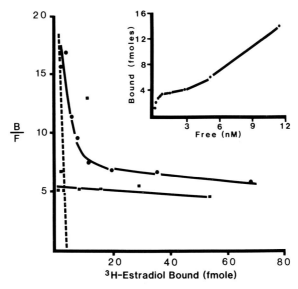

FIG 1. Cytosolic estrogen receptor analysis of an endometrial adeno-carcinoma. Aliquots of cytosol (0.1 mg protein) were incubated in a final volume of 0.2 ml with ^{3}H-estradiol (Total Binding =) or ^{3}H-estradiol plus 100-fold excess of DES (Non-Specific Binding =). Specific Binding = dashed line. K_d = 0.23 nM, B_m = 36 fmoles/mg protein

In 34 of the 48 cases, specimens were of sufficient size to measure both estrogen and progesterone receptor content.

Representative data from saturation analysis of ^{3}H-estradiol and ^{3}H-R5020 binding of cytosols prepared from endometrial adenocarcinomas are shown in Figures 1 and 2, respectively. In nearly all specimens analyzed for this study, non-specific binding compromised a large pro-portion of the total steroid bound. In several instances, estrogen receptor analyses revealed biphasic saturation curves for specific estradiol binding to tumor cytosol (Figure 1), implying the existence of more than one binding protein in these preparations. In an effort to minimize the error introduced by the presence of multiple binding proteins, we have employed the graphical method of Rosenthal[18] for the calculation of binding parameters for high-affinity cytosolic receptors. In contrast to the estrogen receptor analyses, none of the progesterone receptor measurements exhibited biphasic saturation curves.

Overall, 25 of 42 tumors (60%) contained estrogen receptor, and 15 of 40 (37.5%) contained progesterone receptor. The receptor status of the 34 cases in which both receptors were measured is shown in Table 1. Estrogen and progesterone receptors were present in 32% (11/34) of these tumors. Thirty-eight percent (13/34) were negative for both receptors, and 26% (9/34) contained estrogen but not progesterone receptor. One specimen, from a nulli-gravida, four year post-menopausal woman with an earlier history of irregular menses and possible hirsutism exhibited progesterone receptor activity in the absence of estrogen receptor.

The two cases where patients had received premarin were estrogen receptor-positive. One was also progesterone receptor-positive. The specimen from the second patient was of insufficient size to analyze both receptors. The patient with recurrent disease, Grade 3 adeno-

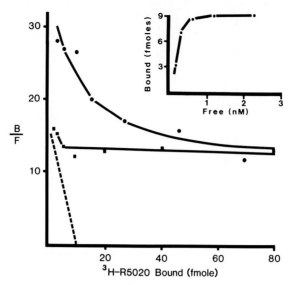

FIG 2. Cytosolic progesterone receptor analysis of an endometrial adenocarcinoma cytosol. Aliquots of cytosol (0.1 mg protein) were incubated
in a final volume of 0.2 ml. Symbols as in Figure 1. K_d = 0.6nM,
B_m = 100 fmoles/mg protein.

carcinoma, undergoing megestrol acetate treatment, had an estrogen
receptor-positive, progesterone receptor-negative tumor.

A strong relationship between histological type of tumor and receptor
status was noted as seen in Table 2. A majority of the adenocarcinomas
were positive for estrogen receptor, 69% (20/29) as compared to 38%
(5/13) of adenosquamous carcinomas. Thirteen of 27 (48%) adenocarcinomas
were progesterone receptor-positive, while only two of 13 (15%) adenosquamous carcinomas contained detectable progesterone receptor, and both
of these were low, i.e., 7.7 and 9.0 fmole/mg protein. High-affinity
estrogen and progestin binding were observed in 43% (10/23) of the adenocarcinomas in contrast to the adenosquamous carcinomas where only one
of eleven contained both receptors. This difference was statistically
significant, p = 0.044, by Fishers Exact Test.

TABLE 1. Receptor status of tumors analyzed for
both estrogen and progesterone receptors.

Receptor	N	%
−ER/−PR	13	38
+ER/−PR[a]	9	26
−ER/+PR[b]	1	3
+ER/+PR[a]	11	32

[a]Includes specimen with ER of 3-10 fmole/mg protein
[b]PR = 7 fmole/mg protein.

TABLE 2. Estrogen and progesterone status according to tumor type.

Tumor Type	Receptor Status					
	$-ER/-PR^a$	$+ER/-PR^a$	$-ER/+PR^a$	$+ER/+PR^a$	$+ER^b$	$+PR^b$
Adenocarcinomas						
Classical	4/16	$5/16^c$	--	$7/16^e$	2/3	$3/4^e$
Clear Cell	1/2	1/2	--	0/2	0/1	--
Mucinous	0/1	0/1	--	1/1	1/1	--
Papillary	1/4	1/4	--	2/4	0/1	--
	6/23	7/23	--	$10/23^d$	3/6	3/4
Adenosquamous	7/11	2/11	1/11	$1/11^{d,e}$	2/2	$0/2^e$

[a]Both estrogen and progesterone receptors analyzed. n/N: n = number in subgroup; N = total number in group.

[b]Estrogen receptor or progesterone receptor only analyzed.

[c]Includes specimen with ER of 3-10 fmole/mg protein.

[d]Difference statistically significant, p = 0.044 by Fishers Exact Test.

[e]Progesterone receptor status in classical adenocarcinoma versus adenosquamous carcinomas, difference statistically insignificant, p=0.04.

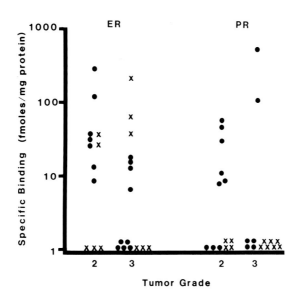

FIG. 3. Distribution of estrogen and progesterone levels by tumor type and grade. See methods for explanation of tumor type and grade. 0 = classical adenocarcinoma, x = adenosquamous carcinoma.

A comparison of the two principal tumor sub-groups, the classical adenocarcinomas and adenosquamous carcinomas, indicates that the difference in progesterone receptor status of the adenocarcinomas and adenosquamous carcinomas was a result of the difference between these sub-groups. Ten of the 20 classical adenocarcinomas exhibited progesterone receptor binding whereas only two of the 13 adenosquamous carcinomas analyzed contained detectable progesterone receptor, p=0.04.

Categorization of the classical adenocarcinomas according to degree of histological differentiation reveals that a greater proportion of Grade 2 tumors (9/10) contained estrogen receptor than did Grade 3 tumors (5/9) (Figure 3). In those tumors with detectable estrogen receptor, the median (25.5 fmoles/mg protein) and mean (57.6 + 28.0; mean + S.E.M.) for the Grade 2 tumors were also greater than for Grade 3 tumors (12.2; 11.3 + 2.8). Similarly, the frequency of progesterone receptor in Grade 2 tumors (7/13) tended to be greater than in Grade 3 tumors (3/7). In contrast to the estrogen receptor, the levels of progesterone receptor in the two Grade 3 tumors were greater than any of the Grade 2 tumors.

Division of adenosquamous carcinomas into receptor positive and receptor negative groups on the basis of histological grade failed to reveal any significant differences. Two of the five Grade 2 tumors and three of the eight Grade 3 tumors contained estrogen receptor. None of the Grade 2 tumors contained detectable progesterone receptor; however, two Grade 3 tumors did contain low levels of receptor (Figure 2).

DISCUSSION

The importance of endocrine influences on neoplastic lesions of the female reproductive tract has long been recognized.[20] The principal agents in this regard are the ovarian steroid hormones. Our understanding of the mechanism by which the ovarian steroids effect tumor development and growth have only recently begun to be understood, spurred by the demonstration of specific receptors for these hormones in the uterus and other organs of the reproductive tract.

Adenocarcinoma of the endometrium has been shown to be hormonally dependent in approximately one-third of cases reported by virtue of its favorable response to endocrine therapeutic modalities.[2,3,4,5] In an analogous manner to mammary cancer,[7] it is believed that hormone-dependent endometrial carcinomas can be identified by their estrogen and progestin receptor content.[10,14,21] Preliminary reports support the putative relationship between receptor content and the effectiveness of hormone therapy in inducing objective remission in endometrial tumors. The efficacy of progestational agents in treating endometrial adenocarcinoma has been reported to be significantly greater in those cases where receptor analyses had demonstrated the presence of progesterone receptors in addition to estrogen receptors.[9,10] Since progesterone receptor synthesis is believed to be under positive estrogen control,[22,23] the presence of both steroid binding proteins within a tumor is highly suggestive of an intact molecular mechanism for the mediation of a hormonal stimulus.

Much of the work in steroid receptor analysis must be viewed in relation to the complexity of the assay system involved. The choice of methodology for measurement of receptors in our study was guided by a concern for obtaining the best estimate of tumor receptor content within the limits of the various available procedures. The clinical significance of accurate estimates of receptor levels has been demonstrated by Heuson[24] who has reported a strong correlation between absolute receptor content of mammary carcinomas and the likelihood of clinical response to endocrine therapy. For these reasons, we have used saturation analysis to determine receptor levels preferentially over sucrose density gradient analysis or one-point assays at a single saturating concentration of steroid. Sucrose gradient analysis generally underestimates total receptor content due to dissociation of steroid from receptor during centrifugation. Single-point assays do not distinguish between high-affinity and low-affinity binding.

Several specimens included in this study exhibited low-affinity estradiol binding in addition to high-affinity receptor binding as exemplified in Figure 1. The failure to account for the contribution of low-affinity binding to that in the high-affinity region will result in an overestimation of the specific high-affinity binding content of the tumor. Using the Rosenthal[18] method for the calculation of binding parameters minimizes the error introduced by the low-affinity components as well as certain systematic errors commonly incurred with other procedures.[25] The range of values for estrogen receptor in our series agrees well with those of Creasman et al[10], Mc Carty et al,[14] and Janne et al[26] and are substantially lower than those reported by Pollow et al[13] and Martin et al.[9]

Low-affinity, displaceable, cytosolic binding of steroid hormones has been reported in both normal[27] and carcinomatous human uterus.[10,12] Recently, the existence of a second estrogen binding protein, referred to as type II receptor having a K_d of approximately 10^{-8}M, has been characterized in the immature rat uterus.[27] The physiological significance of these low-affinity estrogen binding proteins remains to be determined for both normal and neoplastic tissue. It should be noted that favorable clinical responses of either mammary [7,8,24] or endometrial [9,10,14] tumors, as predicted from estrogen receptor measurements, have been established only for the high-affinity binding component. Overestimation of tumor receptor levels resulting from failure to exclude the contribution of low-affinity binding sites could lead to the inappropriate choice of adjuvant therapy in some cases and may obscure correlations between receptor levels and histological, morphological, and clinical criteria.

Recent attempts have been made to relate receptor status to pathological evaluations of recognized prognostic value and response to hormone therapy. The pathological correlate receiving the most attention in this regard has been the degree of morphological differentiation of the tumor. Our data are consistent with previous observations of increasing estrogen receptor levels in those tumors exhibiting a greater degree of morphological differentiation.[10,11,12,14] This correlation has not been universally observed, however, as Pollow et al[13] and Martin et al[9] have reported greater estrogen binding activity in poorly differentiated tumors. A satisfactory explanation for the differences in distribution of estrogen binding among these reports has yet to be provided.

Contrastly, progestin binding has generally been reported to be higher in well-differentiated than in less well-differentiated tumors.[9,12,21] We have not found as marked a differential in progesterone receptor levels in classical adenocarcinomas of different histological grades as have others; however, a trend did appear to be toward a greater frequency of receptor-positive cases in Grade 2 tumors than in Grade 3 tumors.

The correlation between receptor status and degree of differentiation of endometrial carcinomas parallels the relationship between tumor grade and progestin responsiveness noted in early studies of the efficacy of progestins as anti-tumor agents for treatment of this disease.[5,28] The association with a known clinically useful prognostic indicator is important in our attempts to increase our understanding of the molecular mechanisms which mediate the physiological responses to these hormones in malignant tissues. These recent observations provide a basis for the continued investigation of the endocrine regulatory mechanisms which control neoplastic endometrial growth.

An important observation in this study is the infrequent occurrence and low levels of progesterone receptor in the adenosquamous carcinomas. In contrast, nearly 50% of the tumors with more favorable prognosis, i.e., classical adenocarcinomas and mucinous carcinomas, had progesterone receptor present. Based upon this information, one might speculate that adenosquamous carcinomas would be unlikely to respond to endocrine therapy. The lack of receptors may be a significant contributory factor toward the generally recognized[29,30] aggressiveness and poor prognosis of the adenosquamous carcinomas.

REFERENCES

1. Silverberg, E. (1979): Cancer, 29:6.
2. Wentz, W.B. (1964): Obstet. Gynecol., 24:370.
3. Anderson, D.G. (1965): Amer J Obstet Gynecol, 92:87.
4. Kelly, R.M. and Baker, W.H. (1973): Obstet. Gynecol., 25:1190.
5. Wait, R.B. (1973): Obstet. Gynecol., 41:129.
6. Siiteri, P.K. (1978): Cancer Res., 38:4360.
7. McGuire, W.L. and Julian, J.A. (1971): Cancer Res., 31:1440.
8. McGuire, W.L., Pearson, O.H., and Segaloff, A. (1975): In: Human Breast Cancer, edited by W.L. McGuire, P.P. Carbone, and E.P. Vollmer, pp17-30. Raven Press, New York.
9. Martin, P.M., Rolland, P.H., Gammerre, M., et al. (1979) Int. J. Cancer, 23:321.
10. Creasman, W.T., McCarty, K.S., Sr., Barton, T.E., et al, (1980): Obstet. Gynecol., 55:363.
11. Terenius, L., Lindell, A., and Persson, B.H. (1971): Cancer Res., 31:1895.
12. Evans, L.H., Martin, J.D., and Hahnel, K. (1974): Clin. Endocrinol. Metab., 38:23.
13. Pollow, K., Lubbert, H., Boquoi, G., et al. (1975): Endocrinology, 96:319.
14. McCarty, K.S., Jr., Barton, T.K., Fetter, B.F., et al. (1979): Amer. J. Pathol., 96:171.
15. Hendrickson, M.R., and Kempson, R.L. (1980): In: Surgical Pathology of the Uterine Corpus, pp 333-388. Saunders, New York.
16. Schrader, W.T., Smith, K.G., and Coty, W.A. (1976): In: Hormone Action and Molecular Endocrinology, edited by B.W. O'Malley and W.T. Schrader, Texas Health Science Center Printing Office, Houston.
17. Walters, M.R., and Clark, J.H. (1977): J. Steroid Biochem., 8:1137.

18. Rosenthal, H.E. (1967):   Anal. Biochem., 20:525.
19. Bradford, M.M. (1976):   Anal Eiochem, 72:248.
20. Gusberg, S.B. (1967):   Obstet. Gynecol., 30:287.
21. Young, P.C.M., Ehrlich, C.E., and Cleary, R.E. (1976):
    Amer, J. Obstet. Gynecol., 125:353.
22. O'Malley, B.W., Sherman, M., and Toft, D. (1970):   Proc.
    Natl. Acad. Sci., 67:501.
23. Eckert, R.L., and Katzenellenbogen, B.S. (1981):   J.
    Clin. Endocrinol. Metab., 52:699.
24. Heuson, J.C., Longeval, E., Mattheiem, W.H., et al.
    (1976):   Cancer, 39:1971.
25. Braunsberg, H., and Hammond, K.D. (1980):   J. Steroid.
    Biochem., 13:1133-1145.
26. Jänne, O., Kauppila, A., Kontula, K., et al. (1980): In:
    Steroid Receptors and Hormone-Dependent Neoplasia,
    edited by J.L. Wittliff and O. Dapunt, pp 37-44.
    Masson Publishing, New York
27. Smith, R.G., Clarke, S.G., Zalta, E., et al. (1979):
    J. Steroid Biochem., 10:31.
28. Varga, A. and Henriksen, E. (1965):   Obstet. Gynecol.,
    26:656.
29. Silverberg, S.G., Bolin, M.G., and DeGiorgi, L.S. (1972)
    Cancer, 30:1307.
30. Ng, A.B.P., Reagan, J.W., Storaasli, J.P., et al.
    (1973):   Amer. J. Clin. Pathol., 59:765.

Progress in Cancer Research and Therapy,
Vol. 31, edited by F. Bresciani, et al.
Raven Press, New York © 1984.

Endocrine Indicators of Endometrial and Ovarian Tumor Aggressiveness

*R. Vihko, *H. Isotalo, **A. Kauppila, **S. Kivinen,
and *P. Vierikko

Departments of *Clinical Chemistry and **Obstetrics and Gynecology, University
of Oulu, SF-90220 Oulu 22, Finland

A number of observations suggest that determinations of various components of the chain leading to the expression of hormone action in target tissues are useful in certain gynecological malignancies. A great deal of information is available on cytosol estrogen (ERc) and progestin (PRc) receptors, particularly in endometrial carcinoma, and also in ovarian carcinoma. We have recently summarized a number of aspects of ERc and PRc in these diseases (33). Here we will concentrate mostly on the latest findings on ERc and PRc, nuclear estrogen (ERn) and progestin (PRn) receptors and the activities of 17β-hydroxysteroid dehydrogenase (17-HSD) in these two types of malignancies. We will pay special attention to these parameters in the evaluation of tumor aggressiveness.

PATIENTS AND METHODS

Endometrial Carcinoma

The patients and their therapies are described in detail elsewhere (16,18,24). The data on cumulative survival rates are based on the follow-up (up to 36 months) of 61 patients with stage I or II disease and 22 patients with stage III or IV disease. On some occasions, comparisons are made with endometrial specimens from normally cycling fertile-aged women, standardized with respect to the day of the cycle and serum progesterone concentrations (24).

Ovarian Carcinoma

The patients and their therapies are described in detail elsewhere (11,19,32). The data on cumulative survival rates are based on follow-up (up to 36 months) of 18 patients with stage I or II disease and 34 patients with stage III or IV disease.

Methods

Tritiated estradiol-17β and ORG 2058 (16α-ethyl-21-hydroxy-19-nor-4-pregnene-3,20-dione) were used as the labeled ligands in cytosol and nuclear ER and PR measurements, respectively, as described elsewhere (24,32). The activities of 17-HSD were measured essentially as described by Tseng and Gurpide (29).

Statistics

Cumulative survival rates were computed using the product-limit (Kaplan-Meier) method of program 1L (BMDP Statistical Software of 1982, University of California, Los Angeles, CA). The equality of the survival curves was tested using the generalized Savage (Mantel-Cox) test and Breslow's version of the generalized Wilcoxon statistic.

STEROID RECEPTOR DISTRIBUTION AND CONCENTRATIONS IN NORMAL AND CARCINOMATOUS TISSUES

Endometrial Carcinoma

It has been repeatedly shown that normal human endometrium in untreated women always contains ERc and PRc (1, 4,13,24,28,31). The same seems to be true for ERn and PRn (1,24). The great majority of endometrial adenocarcinoma specimens also have significant concentrations of ERc and PRc (summarized in 33). We found that out of 114 endometrial carcinoma specimens, 80 % were simultaneously ERc- and PRc-positive (receptor concentration $>$ 3 or $>$ 6 fmol/mg cytosol protein, respectively), whereas 10 % were both ERc- and PRc-negative (18). Evidence has also accumulated showing that the mean ERc and PRc concentrations are lower in endometrial adenocarcinoma tissue than in normal endometrium (see 24,34).

Nuclear estrogen and progestin receptors also seem to be frequently present in endometrial adenocarcinoma tissue (1, 23,24) and a tendency for higher concentrations in adenocarcinoma tissue than in normal endometrium has been observed (24). In fact, the ratios of cytosol to nuclear ER and PR concentrations were very much higher in normal proliferative endometrium than in endometrial adenocarcinoma (p $\ll$ 0.001 in both cases, ref. 24). The overlap in the PRc/PRn ratio was relatively small, and the nuclear residence of the female sex steroid receptors was especially favored in carcinosarcoma tissue (24).

Ovarian Carcinoma

There is considerable variation in the literature concerning the distribution of ovarian tumors into different categories on the basis of the presence or absence of female sex steroid receptors and on their concentrations.

The results of several recent investigations have confirmed the presence of ERc and PRc in many epithelial (3,6,8,10, 14,27,32) and some sex-cord stromal ovarian malignancies (10,19,32), and the presence of ERn and PRn has also been shown in many types of ovarian malignant tumors (9,10,32). We found significant but low concentrations (mean 8 fmol/mg cytosol protein) of ERc in 57 % of nondiseased ovarian tissues, and close to 30-fold higher concentrations of PRc in the same tissues. The distribution was approximately the same for ERn and PRn, and their mean concentrations were 159 and 1149 sites/cell, respectively (32). There were no major differences between pre-and postmenopausal nondiseased ovaries in the concentrations and distribution of cytosol and nuclear female sex steroid receptors.

Most (74 %) benign epithelial ovarian tumors had significant ($\geq$ 3 fmol/mg cytosol protein) concentrations of ERc, whereas all showed the presence of PRc (in concentrations $\geq$ 6 fmol/mg cytosol protein). Every benign tumor specimen contained ERn and PRn, and their concentrations were significantly higher than in normal ovaries (32). In contrast to this, the concentration of ERc was identical to that in nondiseased ovaries, whereas that of PRc was significantly lower.

ERc was found in 89 % of malignant epithelial ovarian tumors, and its concentration was significantly higher than in normal ovarian tissues and in benign tumors. PRc was also found in the great majority (91 %) of malignant epithelial ovarian tumors, but its concentration was significantly lower than in normal ovarian tissue or benign ovarian tumors. ERn and PRn concentrations were intermediate between those in nondiseased ovaries and benign tumors (32).

It is interesting to observe that there are certain similarities when ERc concentrations are compared in ovarian and breast tissue. The concentration of ERc is very low in normal ovarian (32) and breast (22) tissues, higher concentrations can sometimes be recorded in benign lesions (12,32), whereas the highest ERc concentrations have been measured in malignant tumors of these tissues (22,32). These similarities do not extend to the concentrations of PRc. The concentration of PRc in malignant ovarian tumors is lower than in normal tissues and benign lesions, which is in contrast to the situation prevailing in breast tissue and its tumors.

STEROID RECEPTORS AND CLINICAL STAGE

In evaluation of the interrelationships between steroid receptor concentrations and the generally used prognostic indicators of endometrial and ovarian carcinoma, such as clinical stage and histological grade, we have found it useful to stratify the patient material on the basis of receptor concentrations. We have defined a receptor-rich tumor as having both ERc and PRc in concentrations equal to or higher than 30 fmol/mg cytosol protein, and a receptor-poor tumor is one with one or both cytosol female sex steroid receptors having concentrations of less than this limit (16,19,33).

Endometrial Carcinoma

There is a relationship between cytosol steroid receptor concentrations and the advancement of endometrial carcinoma. Approximately 65 % of tumors at stage I are receptor-rich, and this percentage decreases to 50, 17 and 0 in stages II, III-IV combined, and recurrent and metastatic disease combined, respectively (16,18,33). As seen in Fig. 1, the mean ERc and PRc concentrations are also lowest in stage III-IV disease. However, it is also obvious from this Figure that there is a large overlap in ERc and PRc concentrations in tumors grouped according to the clinical stage of the disease. These data showing that the cytosol steroid receptor concentrations decrease in relation to clinical advancement of the disease are in line with those found in another hormone-associated malignancy, breast carcinoma (22,35). It is therefore very likely that disappearance of hormone dependence takes place during the advancement of endometrial and breast carcinoma, or that the receptor-poor tumors progress more rapidly.

It appears that the potential to invade the myometrium bears a relationship to cytosol steroid receptors. In stage I endometrial carcinoma, PRc concentrations were lower in malignancies clearly infiltrating into the myometrium when compared with PRc levels in superficial lesions. The same tendency was seen in ERc concentrations (16,33).

Ovarian Carcinoma

There were no significant differences in cytosol and nuclear ER and PR concentrations between the four clinical stages of primary epithelial carcinomas (32). However, primary epithelial ovarian carcinomas were more often cytosol receptor-positive (81 % vs. 49 %), and they had higher receptor concentrations than recurrent epithelial ovarian tumors (19).

STEROID RECEPTORS AND HISTOLOGICAL DIFFERENTIATION

Endometrial Carcinoma

In stage I endometrial carcinoma, anaplastic (G3) tumors have a lower frequency of receptor-richness (25 %) than moderately (G2, 62 %) and well (G1, 74 %) differentiated tumors (16). Fig. 2 demonstrates the interrelationships between tumor grade and the concentrations of ERc and PRc. The actual concentrations of these receptors are

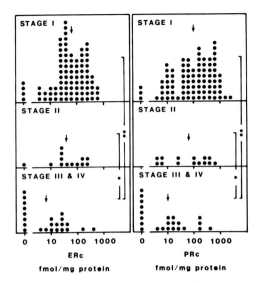

FIG. 1. Histograms representing the frequency distribution
of cytosol estrogen (ERc) and progestin (PRc) receptor concentrations in specimens of endometrial carcinoma grouped
according to clinical stage. Arrows indicate geometric
means. ✳ , p < 0.05; ✳✳, p < 0.01; Student-Newman-Keuls'
test.

significantly lower in G3 tumors than in G1 or G2 tumors.
It is to be observed, however, that there are large overlaps in the concentrations of ERc and PRc in the three
different histological grade categories. Some G3 tumors

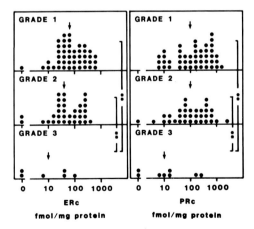

FIG. 2. Histograms representing the frequency distribution
of cytosol estrogen (ERc) and progestin (PRc) receptor concentrations in specimens of stage I endometrial carcinoma
grouped according to histological grade. Arrows indicate
geometric mean. ✳✳, p < 0.01; Student-Newman-Keuls' test.

have relatively high receptor concentrations and some G1
tumors have very low receptor levels. It is therefore very
likely that the two risk factors (low cytosol receptor
concentrations, anaplastic tumor) are at least partly independent.

Ovarian Carcinoma

The reported findings on the possible correlations
between histological grading and ERc and PRc concentrations
in ovarian carcinoma have been inconsistent (3,5,6,19,32).
According to our most recent data (32), PRc concentrations
in serous and mucinous ovarian carcinomas (TABLE 1) are
significantly lower in anaplastic tumors compared with more
differentiated tumors. No such differences were detected
in ERc concentrations and in the concentrations of the
nuclear steroid receptors (TABLE 1).

TABLE 1. Cytosol and nuclear estrogen and progestin receptor concentrations in primary epithelial ovarian carcinomas in relation to
the grade of histological differentiation[a]

Histopatho-logical classification	Grade	ERc	PRc		ERn	PRn
		(fmol/mg cytosol protein)			(sites/cell)	
Serous	G1 + G2	73 + 22[b] (17)[c]	106 + 24 (17)	d	297 + 52 (14)	1919 + 384 (15)
	G3	81 ± 32 (14)	44 ± 19 (14)		213 ± 54 (10)	1398 ± 341 (13)
Mucinous	G1 + G2	16 ± 6 (7)	71 ± 35 (7)	d	738 ± 298 (4)	2743 ± 260 (4)
	G3	35 ± 19 (3)	13 ± 2 (3)		155 ± 28 (2)	2099 ± 1181 (2)
All[f]	G1 + G2	56 ± 15 (27)	101 ± 20 (27)	e	371 ± 76 (20)	2038 ± 292 (21)
	G3	77 ± 25 (18)	37 ± 15 (18)		203 ± 46 (12)	1523 ± 313 (15)

[a]Data from ref. 32; [b]Mean ± SEM; [c]Number of patients; [d]$p < 0.05$;
[e]$p < 0.01$; [f]Four endometrioid lesions included.

STEROID RECEPTORS AND CLINICAL OUTCOME

Endometrial Carcinoma

The upper panel of Fig. 3 shows the cumulative survival
rate of 61 patients with stage I-II endometrial carcinoma.
The patients have been categorized into receptor-rich (41
patients) and receptor-poor (20 patients) on the basis of
ERc- and PRc-concentrations in their tumors. It can be seen
that so far there is no significant difference in the
cumulative survival rates of the two patient categories.

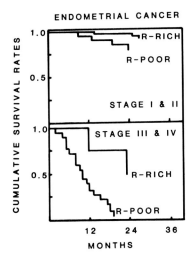

FIG. 3. Cumulative survival rates in stage I-II (upper panel) and stage III-IV (lower panel) endometrial carcinoma. The receptor-rich (R-rich) category is comprised of patients whose primary tumor had both ERc and PRc in concentrations equal to or higher than 30 fmol/mg cytosol protein, and the receptor-poor (R-poor) category is comprised of patients whose tumors had or both receptors present in lower concentrations than this limit.

In contrast to this (lower panel of Fig. 3), there is a significant difference ($p < 0.05$) in the cumulative survival rates of 22 patients with stage III-IV disease in favor of the patients with receptor-rich tumors. At present, it cannot be stated with certainty whether the difference is solely due to the possibility that the receptor-poor tumors are more aggressive, or whether the difference can be related to the better responsiveness of patients with receptor-rich tumors to medroxyprogesterone acetate (100 mg per day), given to all our patients for 24 months following the initial operation. Increasing evidence is accumulating showing a high degree of correlation between the presence of female sex steroid receptors in the tumor prior to treatment and the response to progestin therapy. In a number of studies (summarized in 33) it has been shown that ERc-positive, and more especially, PRc-positive tumors frequently respond to progestin therapy, whereas receptor-negative tumors do not. Concerning combination cytotoxic chemotherapy, it has been shown that after the failure of medroxyprogesterone acetate treatment, patients with receptor-poor tumors respond to cytotoxic chemotherapy more frequently than patients with receptor-rich tumors (17).

Ovarian Carcinoma

The upper panel of Fig. 4 summarizes the cumulative survival rate of 18 patients with stage I-II ovarian car-

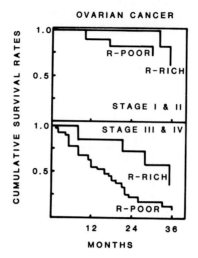

FIG. 4. Cumulative survival rates in stages I-II (upper panel) and stage III-IV (lower panel) ovarian carcinoma. For details, see the legend to FIG. 3.

cinoma. There is no significant difference in the outcome of patients with receptor-rich or receptor-poor tumors during the observation time. This is in contrast to patients with stage III-IV ovarian carcinoma. The patients with receptor-rich tumors have a significantly ($p < 0.05$) larger cumulative survival rate than the patients with receptor-poor tumors. The patients have not received any hormone treatment, and in general there are no differences in the treatment of the two patient categories. It can therefore be concluded that receptor-poor stage III-IV ovarian carcinomas are more aggressive than the corresponding receptor-rich tumors.

The mechanisms behind the greater aggressiveness of receptor-poor ovarian carcinomas compared with receptor-rich are as yet obscure. An increase in the release of proteolytic enzymes has often been associated with biochemical events related to tumor growth and invasion (see e.g. 2,25). We have investigated plasminogen activator activity and ERc and PRc concentrations in normal, benign and malignant tissues of human ovary (11). The mean plasminogen activator activities were significantly higher in malignant than in benign ovarian tumors, and the activities in the latter tissues were again higher than in normal ovarian tissues. However, as is evident from Fig. 5, there were no significant correlations between plasminogen activator activity and cytosol estrogen or progestin receptor concentrations in malignant ovarian tumors. We concluded that the possible female sex steroid dependency of plasminogen activator activity in human ovarian malignancies cannot be demonstrated by cytosol receptor assays alone (11).

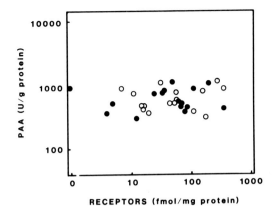

FIG. 5. Relationships between plasminogen activator activities (PAA) in tissue extracts and cytosol estrogen (closed circles) and progestin (open circles) receptor concentrations in malignant ovarian tumors.

17 β-HYDROXYSTEROID DEHYDROGENASE
IN GYNECOLOGICAL MALIGNANCIES

Endometrial Carcinoma

The activity of 17 β-hydroxysteroid dehydrogenase (17-HSD) in the endometrium is stimulated by progestins (20,21, 26,29,30). We did not find any significant differences in the activity of 17-HSD between normal proliferative endometrium and that of adenocarcinoma patients (24). This suggests that the mechanism of progestin action was undisturbed in at least most of these patients. However, because most of our patients were postmenopausal and had low serum progesterone concentrations, the conditions may not have been optimal for detection of disturbances in the expression of 17-HSD activity. In studies using progestin stimulation prior to curettage (7,30,15), it has been observed that the magnitude of the response in 17-HSD activity is very variable in individual patients. This might have relevance for prediction of the responsiveness of endometrial carcinoma patients to progestin administration.

Ovarian Carcinoma

There is only scanty data on 17-HSD activity in ovarian tissues. We found that the activity of this enzyme was relatively low in pre- and postmenopausal normal ovaries, and in benign and malignant ovarian tumors (32). It is not known whether the activity of 17-HSD can be stimulated by progestins in these tissues, as has been shown to be the case in human endometrium. In our patients, the highest mean activities of this enzyme were measured in the group of benign nonepithelial tumors. In addition, in epithelial ovarian malignancies, the activity of this enzyme was significantly higher in stage I disease than in the other stages (32).

CONCLUSIONS

Cytosol estrogen and progestin receptors in endometrial adenocarcinoma specimens are present in lower concentrations than in normal endometrium. In contrast to this, the concentrations of nuclear female sex steroid receptors are higher in malignant than normal tissue. No significant differences were found in the activity of 17β-hydroxysteroid dehydrogenase between these two types of tissue.

The cytosol steroid receptor concentrations decrease in relation to clinical advancement of endometrial carcinoma. In addition, anaplastic malignancies have a lower frequency of receptor-rich tumors than the more differentiated forms. As far as clinical staging and histological differentiation are concerned in relation to cytosol steroid receptor levels, there are large overlaps in the receptor concentrations in the different risk indicator categories of endometrial carcinoma. It is therefore very likely that the different risk indicators (cytosol receptor concentration, clinical stage, histological grade) give data which are additive and independent of each other. The cumulative survival rate in patients with stage III-IV endometrial carcinoma was significantly more favorable in the patients with receptor-rich tumors. The main clinical application of cytosol estrogen and progestin receptor measurements at present is in the categorization of patients with advanced disease into groups which will most likely respond to endocrine treatment or are most likely to benefit from combination cytotoxic chemotherapy.

The great majority of pre- and postmenopausal normal ovaries and benign and malignant ovarian neoplasms contain cytosol and nuclear estrogen and progestin receptors. The ERc concentration was lowest in normal tissues, followed by benign and malignant tumors, whereas the opposite was true of PRc. ERn and PRn concentrations were highest in benign ovarian tumors. There were no significant differences in cytosol and nuclear ER and PR concentrations between the four clinical stages of primary epithelial ovarian carcinomas, whereas the activity of 17β-hydroxysteroid dehydrogenase was significantly higher in stage I disease than in the other stages. Concerning histological differentiation and steroid receptor levels, PRc concentrations in serous and mucinous ovarian carcinomas were significantly lower in anaplastic tumors than in the more differentiated ones. In the group of patients with stage III-IV disease, the patients with receptor-rich tumors had a significantly larger cumulative survival rate than the patients with receptor-poor tumors. The possible need and use of cytosol and nuclear ER and PR measurements, and of 17-HSD activity assays in ovarian diseases needs additional studies.

ACKNOWLEDGMENTS

The investigations from this laboratory summarized above have been supported by The Medical Research Council of The Academy of Finland, and The Finnish Cancer Foundation.

REFERENCES

1. Bayard, F., Damilano, S., Robel, P., and Baulieu, E.-E. (1978): J. Clin. Endocrinol. Metab., 46:635-648.
2. Carter, R.L. (1982): J. Clin. Pathol., 35:1041-1049.
3. Creasman, W.T., Sasso, R.A., Weed, J.C., and McCarty, K.S. (1981): Gynecol. Oncol., 12:319-327.
4. Ehrlich, C.E., Young, P.C.M., and Cleary, R.E. (1981): Am. J. Obstet. Gynecol., 141:539-546.
5. Friedman, M.A., Lagios, M., Markowitz, A., Jones, H., Resser, K., and Hoffman, P. (1979): Clin. Res., 27: 385A.
6. Galli, M.C., De Giovanni, C., Nicoletti, G., Grilli, S., Nanni, P., Prodi, G., Gola, G., Rochetta, R., and Orlandi, C. (1981): Cancer, 47:1297-1302.
7. Gurpide, E. (1981): Cancer, 48:638-641.
8. Holt, J.A., Caputo, A., Kelly, K.M., Greenwald, P., and Chorost, S. (1979): Obstet. Gynecol., 53:50-58.
9. Holt, J.A., Lorincz, M.A., and Hospelhorn, V.D. (1983): J. Steroid Biochem., 18:41-50.
10. Holt, J.A., Lyttle, C.R., Lorincz, M.A., Stern, L.S., Press, M.F., and Herbst, A.L. (1981): J. Natl. Cancer Inst., 67:307-318.
11. Isotalo, H., Tryggvason, K., Vierikko, P., Kauppila, A., and Vihko, R. (1983): Anticancer Res., 3:331-335.
12. Jacquemier, J.D., Rolland, P.H., Vague, D., Lieutaud, R., Spitalier, J.M., and Martin, P.M. (1982): Cancer, 49: 2534-2536.
13. Jänne, O., Kauppila, A., Kontula, K., Syrjälä, P., and Vihko, R. (1979): Int. J. Cancer, 24:545-554.
14. Jänne, O., Kauppila, A., Syrjälä, P., and Vihko, R. (1980): Int. J. Cancer, 25:175-179.
15. Kauppila, A., Isotalo, H., Kivinen, S., Stenbäck, F., and Vihko, R. (1983): Am. J. Obstet. Gynecol., submitted.
16. Kauppila, A., Isotalo, H., Kujansuu, E., and Vihko, R. (1982): Excerpta Med. Internatl. Congr. Ser., 611: 350:359.
17. Kauppila, A., Jänne, O., Kujansuu, E., and Vihko, R. (1980): Cancer, 46:2162-2167.
18. Kauppila, A., Kujansuu, E., and Vihko, R. (1982): Cancer, 50:2157-2162.
19. Kauppila, A., Vierikko, P., Kivinen, S., Stenbäck, F., and Vihko, R. (1983): Obstet. Gynec., 61:320-326.
20. King, R.J.B., Whitehead, M.I., Campbell, S., and Minardi, J. (1979): Cancer Res., 39:1094-1101.
21. Levy, C., Robel, P., Gautray, J.P., De Brux, J., Verma, U., Descomps, B., Baulieu, E.-E., and Eychenne, B. (1980): Am. J. Obstet. Gynecol., 136:646-651.

22. McGuire, W.L., Horwitz, K.B., Pearson, O.H., and Sega-
    loff, A. (1977): Cancer, 39:2934-2947.
23. Mortel, R., Levy, C., Wolff, J.-P., Nicolas, J.-C.,
    Robel, P., and Baulieu, E.-E. (1981): Cancer Res.,
    41:1140-1147.
24. Neumannova, M., Kauppila, A., and Vihko, R. (1983):
    Obstet. Gynec., 61:181-188.
25. Nicholson, G. (1982): Biochim. Biophys. Acta, 695:113-
    176.
26. Pollow, K., Lübbert, H., Boquoi, E., Kreuzer, G., Jeske,
    R., and Pollow, B. (1975): Acta Endocrinol. (Kbh.),
    79:134-145.
27. Schwartz, P.E., LiVolsi, V.A., Hildreth, N., MacLusky,
    N.J., Naftolin, F.N., and Eisenfeld, A.J. (1982):
    Obstet. Gynecol., 59:229-238.
28. Spona, J., Ulm, R., Bieglmayer, C., and Husslein, P.
    (1979): Gynecol. Obstet. Invest., 10:71-80.
29. Tseng, L., and Gurpide, E. (1974): Endocrinology, 94:
    419-423.
30. Tseng, L., Gusberg, S.B., and Gurpide, E. (1977): Ann.
    N.Y. Acad. Sci., 286:190-198.
31. Tsibris, J.C.M., Cazenave, C.R., Cantor, B., Notelovitz,
    M., Kalra, P.S., and Spellacy, W.N. (1978): Am. J.
    Obstet. Gynecol., 132:449-454.
32. Vierikko, P., Kauppila, A., and Vihko, R. (1983): Int.
    J. Cancer, 32:413-422.
33. Vihko, R., Isotalo, H., Kauppila, A., and Vierikko, P.
    (1983): J. Steroid Biochem., 19:827-832.
34. Vihko, R., Jänne, O., and Kauppila, A. (1980): Ann.
    Clin. Res., 12:208-215.
35. Vihko, R., Jänne, O., Kontula, K., and Syrjälä, P.
    (1980): Int. J. Cancer, 26:13-21.

Progress in Cancer Research and Therapy,
Vol. 31, edited by F. Bresciani, et al.
Raven Press, New York © 1984.

Neoplastic Changes in the Human Female Genital Tract Following Intrauterine Exposure to Diethylstilbestrol

Arthur L. Herbst, Marian M. Hubby, and Diane Anderson

Department of Obstetrics and Gynecology, University of Chicago, Pritzker School of Medicine, Chicago, Illinois 60637

More than two decades after the initiation of the use of diethylstilbestrol (DES) for preventing pregnancy losses, seven young women in the Boston area were noted to have a very rare type of vaginal cancer, clear cell adenocarcinoma.[11] In 1971 these seven cases and one additional case were reported with a critical new finding: seven of the eight patients' mothers had received DES during their pregnancies.[12] These cases exceeded the number of cases of clear cell adenocarcinoma in young women previously reported in the world literature. The highly significant correlation between adenocarcinoma and in utero DES exposure was substantiated in other reports of clear cell adenocarcinoma of both the vagina and cervix.[13,14]

To allow for further study of the clinical, epidemiologic, and pathologic aspects of these cases, the Registry for Research on Hormonal Transplacental Carcinogenesis was established in 1971 to provide a centralized data source. All cases of clear cell adenocarcinoma of the vagina and cervix arising in females born since 1940 were sought whether or not there was a history of prenatal DES exposure. The scope of the Registry has subsequently been expanded to include all genital tract tumors occurring in young women with a history of prenatal exposure to any exogenous sex hormone.[1]

Shortly after reports relating vaginal adenocarcinomas to DES exposure, it was recognized that a large proportion of DES-exposed women also had non-neoplastic epithelial changes of the vagina and cervix. These include vaginal adenosis (the presence of columnar epithelium or its mucinous products in the vagina) and cervical ectropion (the

---

[1]Inquiries should be addressed to: Arthur L. Herbst,MD, Registry for Research on Hormonal Transplacental Carcinogenesis, 5841 S. Maryland Ave., Chicago, Illinois 60637. Pathology specimen analyses are carried out under the direction of Robert E. Scully, M.D., Department of Pathology, Massachusetts General Hospital, Boston, Massachusetts 02114

presence of columnar epithelium or its mucinous products within the portio vaginalis of the cervix).

Structural changes of the lower genital tract have also been described which affect some 20% to 40% of DES-exposed women. They have been labelled with such names as "cervical cock's comb" and "vaginal hood". One type consists of a transverse or circumferential ridge around part of the vagina. Such ridges or hoods most often appear in the upper part of the vagina and may obscure the cervix. The cervical "cock's comb" usually appears as an irregular outcropping of the anterior cervical lip. Extensive ectropion can cause the cervix to appear dark pink or red. Circumferential ridges on the cervix may also give the erroneous impression of a pseudopolyp in some cases. The cervical os may be eccentric in location, and hypoplasia of the cervix has also been noted.

EPIDEMIOLOGY OF CLEAR CELL ADENOCARCINOMA

Currently maternal histories are available in 466 cases, and of these 63% had a history of ingestion of DES or a related nonsteroidal estrogen such as dienestrol or hexestrol. In approximately one quarter of the cases there was no documentation available of maternal hormone ingestion. Some of these cases may have had hormone exposure that could not be documented. However, in some cases the maternal history is undoubtedly negative insofar as these cancers did occur very rarely in young females in the pre-DES-era. The remaining cases received treatment for high-risk pregnancy, but the medication used could not be identified.

TABLE 1. Maternal drug exposure histories.

Exposure	Number
Positive for DES, dienestrol or hexestrol	292
Positive for steroidal estrogen, progestins or both	12
Other hormone only (thyroid)	2
Unidentified medication for high-risk pregnancy	43
Negative history	117
	466
History unavailable	29
TOTAL	495

Figure 1 displays the annual occurrence rate of DES-positive cases of clear cell adenocarcinoma of the vagina and cervix by year of diagnosis. The first DES-positive case had been diagnosed in 1961, ten years before the association was established. There is then an increase in the number of cases diagnosed each year well into the 1970s. Insofar as case accessions into the Registry are approximately 80% complete within two years after diagnosis, additional cases can be expected to be accessioned for the years 1981 and especially 1982. It appears that the annual occurrence of these carcinomas may have peaked in the early and mid-1970s, but this is still uncertain. A future decline in the occurrence of these tumors will depend both upon the shape of the age-incidence curve and the degree to which DES usage for pregnancy support decreased after the early and middle 1950s.

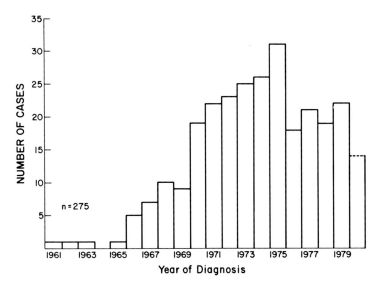

FIG. 1. Occurrence of DES-related clear cell adeno-carcinoma of the vagina and cervix by year of diagnosis.

Currently 262 DES-positive cases accessioned into the Registry have been identified in the United States. However, cases with a positive maternal history have also been identified in Canada, Australia, France, Great Britain, and other countries. Table 2 shows the distribution of birthplaces of DES-positive cases throughout the world. There have been additional cases reported to the Registry with insufficient information to be included here. In general, the occurrence of the tumors has been greatest in areas where DES was more commonly prescribed during pregnancy. On the other hand, in countries such as Denmark where DES and other estrogens were not used for pregnancy support, these tumors have not been noted.

TABLE 2. The birthplace of accessioned DES-positive cases.

Country	Number
United States	262
Canada	5
Australia, New Zealand	4
France	3
Great Britain	3
Europe, other	2
Mexico	1
Belgium	1
Africa	1
	282

The overall risk of vaginal and cervical adenocarcinoma occurring in DES-exposed women is difficult to calculate due to the lack of specific figures on how many mothers actually received DES for pregnancy support. Data published by two major U.S. medical centers indicate that 5% to 10% of their prenatal patients received DES.[15,23] This figure probably estimates the upper limit of DES exposure in the United States during this period. The lower limit of exposure can be derived from the use of DES in the early 1960s, when it was less popular than in the early 1950s. Using these figures, the lower estimate of risk turns out to be that 1% to 2% of women in the United States received DES during their pregnancies from 1951 to 1953.[9] Comparing these data with the knowledge of DES-associated clear cell adenocarcinoma, the risk of developing adenocarcinoma is 0.7 to 1.4 per 1000 exposed females up to the age of 24 years.[16,17] These estimates are consistent with observations made on large groups of DES-exposed females.[22,23,24]

The age-incidence curve of DES-associated clear cell adenocarcinoma shows the peak incidence at about age 19, (figure 2).[10] It is remarkable considering the long latency period of the disease that there should be such a sharp peak incidence over a relatively short time span of 14 to 24 years of age. The sharp rise after age 14 suggests that the onset of adenocarcinoma may be related to the onset of puberty. Definitive figures for occurrence of adenocarcinoma beyond the mid-twenties are not yet available, since most of the patients are only now beginning to approach the age of 30 years. The oldest woman with DES-associated clear cell adenocarcinoma thus far was 33 years of age at the time of diagnosis while the youngest was 7 years old.

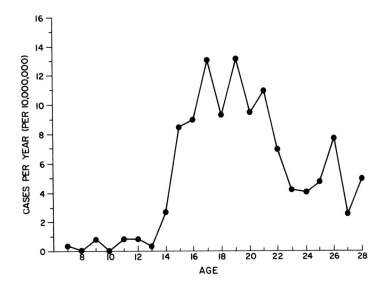

FIG. 2. Incidence of clear cell adenocarcinoma by age at
diagnosis among white females born in the U.S. (Reproduced
with permission of Thieme-Stratton [10])

     The occurrence of clear cell adenocarcinoma in DES-
exposed patients among various birth cohorts for females
in the United States has recently been estimated. In
addition, the occurrence of DES-associated clear cell adenocarcinomas in patients born in 3 year intervals from 1947
to 1960 has also been related to the sale of 25 mg tablets
of DES in the United States by a single drug manufacturer
during that time.[16,17] While there were hundreds of
manufacturers of the drug in the United States during those
years, it was assumed that this manufacturer had a relatively constant share of the market and furthermore that
25 mg tablets sold prior to 1961 were primarily utilized
for pregnancy therapy. In addition, it was assumed that
a tablet manufactured in one year for pregnancy treatment
would relate to a child born the following year. Table 3
shows the comparison of DES sales to the risk of development of clear cell adenocarcinoma in each birth cohort.
The sales of 25 mg tablets for each comparable time interval
correspond extremely closely to the occurrence of clear cell
adenocarcinoma in each birth cohort. The data not only
confirm a parallel relation between the occurrence of DES
usage and the development of clear cell adenocarcinoma, but
also suggest that DES usage for pregnancy support continued
in the United States in the late 1950s and into the early
1960s.

TABLE 3. Comparison of DES by Exposure Index (EI) and
risk of clear cell adenocarcinoma by birth cohort.

Sales year	EI	Relative index[a]	Birth year	Risk of carcinoma[b]	Relative index[a]
1947-1949	0.59	(0.40)	1948-50	2.9	(0.27)
1950-1952	1.49	(1.00)	1951-53	10.8	(1.00)
1953-1955	1.31	(0.89)	1954-56	7.8	(0.72)
1956-1958	1.02	(0.69)	1957-59	6.1[c]	(0.56)
1959-1960	0.71	(0.48)	1960-61	4.6[c]	(0.42)

[a] Sales years 1950 to 1952 and birth years 1951 to 1953
were assigned a value of 1.00 for comparison with
other years
[b] Cases per million population through age 20
[c] Estimated in part
(Reproduced with permission [17])

Further evaluation of the records in which the date the
mother started DES in pregnancy was known precisely revealed that a high proportion began to take DES in early
pregnancy.[17]   Specifically, 80% of the mothers of the
cancer patients had begun treatment in the first 12 weeks
of pregnancy, as opposed to only 50% of a comparable
group of mothers of DES-exposed daughters who did not have
cancer.[24]   These results suggested that the risk of
carcinoma is elevated among DES-exposed females whose
mothers began treatment in early pregnancy. In addition,
vaginal adenosis almost always occurs in patients with
clear cell adenocarcinoma and the time DES was begun during
pregnancy may not have a direct relationship to these
cancers insofar as a similar relationship is known to
exist for vaginal adenosis.

CLINICAL ASPECTS OF CLEAR CELL ADENOCARCINOMA

The staging of adenocarcinoma of the vagina and cervix
has been according to FIGO criteria (Table 4). By this
classification, approximately 60% of the clear cell adenocarcinomas are vaginal and the remainder cervical. If
the tumors are classified by their predominant site, the
ratio would be 70% vaginal and 30% cervical.
The survival of the patients treated for clear cell
adenocarcinoma correlates with the stage of the tumor. The
overall five year survival for stage 1 carcinomas, regardless of mode of therapy, was 87% for carcinomas of the
vagina and 91% for cervical tumors. The overall five year
survival of both stage II vaginal and stage IIa cervical
lesions was approximately 76%. Stage IIb carcinomas had
survival rates of 60% and survival decreased to 37% for
Stage III disease. [18]

TABLE 4.   FIGO staging of vaginal and cervical carcinomas

Carcinoma of the vagina

Stage	
I	Limited to vaginal wall
II	Invades the subvaginal tissues but has not extended to the pelvic wall
III	Reaches the pelvic wall
IV	Extends into the mucosa of the bladder or rectum or outside the true pelvis. If the tumor involves the external os of the cervix, it is classified as cervical and if the vulva is involved it is classified as vulvar.

Carcinoma of the cervix

Stage	
I	Confined to the cervix
IIa	Involves the upper two-thirds of the vagina but has not infiltrated the parametrium
IIb	Involves the upper two-thirds of the vagina with parametrial infiltration but has not reached the pelvic side wall
III	Reaches the pelvic side wall and/or lower one-third of the vagina and/or hydronephrosis or nonfunction of kidney due to tumor
IV	Extends into the mucosa of bladder or rectum or outside true pelvis.

Recently it has been observed that the survival of patients 15 years of age or younger was worse than that of those 19 years of age or older. This difference has been found to reflect the differences in the behavior of the tumor as related to its predominant histologic pattern. The best survival is associated with the so-called "tubulo-cystic pattern", and patients over the age of 19 have a higher incidence of this particular tumor histology in comparison to the younger patients.[17]

NON-MALIGNANT CHANGES ASSOCIATED WITH DES-EXPOSURE

Squamous metaplasia is the transformation of glandular or mucosal epithelium into stratified squamous epithelium and this is found extensively in DES-exposed subjects. It is felt that the squamous metaplasia found in those exposed to DES represents a healing process by which the abnormal vaginal adenosis and cervical ectropion revert to normal squamous epithelium. The changes of adenosis and squamous metaplasia of the vagina have been combined by some workers under the term vaginal epithelial changes.[24]

The extensive transformation zone in areas of vaginal adenosis had prompted some to hypothesize a higher incidence of squamous dysplastic lesions might occur in the DES-

exposed progeny. This larger transformation zone would in
theory provide more surface area of immature metaplastic
epithelium for exposure to potential carcinogens. However, current data do not support the hypothesis that
intraepithelial neoplasia develops more frequently in the
DES-exposed than in non-exposed subjects. Robboy et. al.
(25) found only a 2.1% prevalence rate of dysplasia in a
large series of 1424 patients with in utero DES-exposure.
Furthermore, Robboy and his co-workers found that the
dysplastic changes encountered in DES-exposed progeny were
almost always mild with no prior history of dysplasia and
were slightly more frequent in the cervix than in the
vagina. Severe dysplasia and carcinoma in situ were only
noted in the DES-exposed women specifically referred because of these epithelial changes. In a later publication
based on 4589 young women, squamous cell dysplasia of the
vagina and cervix was detected in 1.8% of DES-exposed
women in the record review groups. [26] The rate in un-
exposed women was actually twice as high.

UPPER GENITAL TRACT CHANGES AND REPRODUCTIVE PERFORMANCE

    In recent years, a number of structural changes of the
upper female genital tract have been described. Several
studies of hysterosalpingograms in DES-exposed women have
been performed. The changes most often associated with
DES exposure are a T-shaped uterine cavity, intrauterine
synechiae, varied irregularities in the shape of the
uterine cavity, and hypoplasia of the uterus itself. Other
studies have employed various methods of evaluating quantitatively the changes in the configuration of the uterine
cavity and have confirmed the overall decrease in size of
the cavity and the relative widening of the lower uterine
segment resulting in the so-called T-shaped uterus. [8]   In
women with lower tract structural abnormalities, 86% had
abnormal hysterosalpingograms; in women with no lower tract
abnormalities, 56% had abnormal hysterosalpingograms. [20]
    Ovarian function and menstrual function in the DES-
exposed women have been studied with inconclusive results.
Whereas some studies report no changes in menstrual function [1], others have suggested a tendency toward menstrual
irregularities.[19]   Current evidence suggests that the
majority of DES-exposed women do not show major derangements
of the hypothalmic-pituitary-gonadal axis.
    Some studies suggest an increased incidence of primary
infertility among a small proportion of those exposed[19];
but other studies have failed to confirm this finding. [2]
Several studies have suggested an increase in pregnancy
wastage.[1,2,19]   This increased fetal loss results mainly
from an increased incidence of miscarriage and premature
labor. There is no evidence for an increased risk of
ectopic pregnancy.[19]
    Since the urinary tract develops in proximity to the
genital tract, the question has arisen as to whether DES-

exposed women show an increased incidence of urinary tract
anomalies. Several studies of intravenous pyelogram data
have been done. The overall incidence of urinary tract
anomalies is in the range of 3% to 5%; duplications of
the collecting system or an absent kidney is the most
common abnormality. The incidence and type of anomalies
found in non-DES-exposed women are similar. [14,21,28]

EMBRYOLOGIC CONSIDERATIONS

The occurrence of lower genital tract anomalies and
clear cell adenocarcinoma following in utero DES exposure
has stimulated further interest in the embryology of the
human vagina. Although still controversial, current
information supports the opinion that in the human both
the Mullerian ducts and the urogenital sinus participate
in the development of the vagina. [5,29] The paired para-
mesonephric, or Mullerian ducts arise as invaginations of
the coelomic epithelium near the urogenital ridge, extend
caudally, and fuse at the urogenital sinus. The Mullerian-
derived glandular epithelium is then replaced by the solid
core of squamous epithelium arising from the vaginal plate.
The vaginal plate then grows cephalad from the urogenital
sinus. The solid core of squamous epithelium canalizes
and forms the permanent lining of the vagina.

The mouse has been a frequently used experimental
animal to study the effect of hormones on the developing
genital tract. In the neonatal mouse the vagina continues
to develop after birth providing an analogy with the intrauterine development of the vagina in humans. By admin-
istering 17B-estradiol or DES to neonatal mice, Forsberg (4)
interfered with the squamous transformation of the columnar epithelium, resulting in the persistence of the Mullerian epithelium in the upper vagina and cervix. [4,6] A pattern of adenosis has been described following neonatal
administration of DES. [7]

In utero exposure to DES in humans may have a similar
effect, i.e. a DES-mediated persistence of glandular
epithelium in the vagina (adenosis). The excess occurrence
of clear cell adenocarcinomas in women with DES exposure
before the 18th week of gestation may be a reflection of
the large volume of ectopic glandular epithelium which
occurs in such patients. Clear cell adenocarcinomas are
intimately related to the tuboendometrial cell of adenosis
and probably arise from atypical tuboendometrial epithelium.[27] The large volume of tuboendometrial epithelium
in patients with DES exposure prior to the 18th week of
intrauterine life may provide a greater substrate for later
development of carcinoma. Estrogens may act as a promoter
in the process of carcinogenesis since the age of incidence
of adenocarcinomas clusters around the time of menarche.
Nevertheless, the mechanism of appearance of these tumors
is not completely understood; approximately 25% of the
adenocarcinomas occur in women without a documented history

of <u>in utero</u> exposure to exogenous estrogens.

In addition to the epithelial changes described, stromal anomalies result in vaginal ridges and structural deformities of the cervix. These structural abnormalities are in turn associated with anomalous development of the Mullerian ducts resulting in abnormal intrauterine contours. Recently, Cuhna (3) has demonstrated that the specific stroma of different levels of the female genital tract have inductive effects that determine the nature of overlying epithelium. This suggests that a primary stromal action of DES could account for both the epithelial abnormalities as well as the connective tissue anomalies often observed in the DES-exposed population.

ACKNOWLEDGMENT

Supported in part by PHS Grant No. 5-RO1-CA-20084 from the National Cancer Institute.

REFERENCES

1. Barnes, A.B. (1979): Fertil. Steril., 32:148-153.
2. Barnes, A.B., Colton, T., Gundersen, J., Noller, K.L., Tilley, B.C., Strama, T., Townsend, D.E., Hatab, P., O'Brien, P.C. (1980): N. Eng. J. Med., 302:609-613.
3. Cuhna, G.R. (1976): Int. Rev. Cytol., 47:137.
4. Forsberg, J.G. (1972): Am. J. Obstet. Gynecol., 113:83-87.
5. Forsberg, J.G. (1973): Am. J. Obstet. Gynecol., 115:1025-1043.
6. Forsberg, J.G. (1975): Am. J. Obstet. Gynecol., 121:101-103.
7. Forsberg, J.G. (1979): National Cancer Institute Monograph, 51:41-56.
8. Haney, A.F., Hammond, C.B., Soules, M.R., Creasman, W.T. (1979): Fertil. Steril., 31:142-146.
9. Heinonen, O.P. (1973): Cancer, 31:573-577.
10. Herbst, A.L. (1981): In Developmental Effects of Diethylstilbestrol (DES) in Pregnancy, edited by A.L. Herbst and H.A. Bern, pp. 63-70, Thieme-Stratton, New York.
11. Herbst, A.L. and Scully, R.E. (1970): Cancer, 25:745-757.
12. Herbst, A.L., Ulfelder, H., and Poskanzer, D.C. (1971): N. Eng. J. Med., 284:878-881.
13. Herbst, A.L., Kurman, R.J., Scully, R.E., and Poskanzer, D.C. (1972): N. Eng. J. Med., 287:1259-1267.
14. Herbst, A.L., Robboy, S.J., Scully, R.E., and Poskanzer, D.C. (1974): Am. J. Obstet. Gynecol., 119:713-724.
15. Herbst, A.L., Poskanzer, D.C., Robboy, S.J., Friedlander, L., and Scully, R.E. (1975): N. Eng. J. Med., 292:334-339.

16. Herbst, A.L., Cole, P., Colton, T., Robboy, S.J., and Scully, R.E. (1977): Am. J. Obstet. Gynecol., 128: 43-50.

17. Herbst, A.L., Cole, P., Norusis, M.J., Welch, W.R. and Scully, R.E. (1979): Am. J. Obstet. Gynecol., 135: 876-883.

18. Herbst. A.L., Norusis, M.J., Rosenow, P.J., Welch, W.R. and Scully, R.E. (1979): Gynecol. Oncol., 7:111-121.

19. Herbst, A.L., Hubby, M.M., Blough, R.R., and Azizi, F. (1980): J. Reprod. Med., 24:62-69.

20. Kaufman, R.H., Binder, G.L., Grey, M.P., and Adam, E. (1977): Am. J. Obstet. Gynecol., 128:51-56.

21. Kaufman, R.H., Adams, E.A., Grey, M.P., and Gerthoffer, E. (1980): Obstet. Gynecol., 56:330-332.

22. Kinlen, L.J., Badaracco, M.A., Moffet, J., Vesey, M.P. (1974): J. Obstet. Gynaecol. Br. Commonw., 81:849-855.

23. Lanier, A.P., Noller, K.L., Decker, D.G., Elveback, L.R. Kurland, L.T. (1973): Mayo Clin. Proc., 48:793-799.

24. O'Brien, P.C., Noller, K.L., Robboy, S.J., Barnes, A.B. Kaufman, R.H., Tilley, B.C., Townsend, D.E. (1979): Obstet. Gynecol., 53:300-308.

25. Robboy, S.J., Keh, P.C., Nickerson, R.J., Helmanis, E.K., Prat, J., Szyfelbein, W.M., Taft, P.D., Barnes, A.B., Scully, R.E., and Welch, W.R. (1978): Obstet. Gynecol., 51:528-535.

26. Robboy, S.J., Szyfelbein, W.M., Goellner, J.R., Kaufman, R.H., Taft, P., Richart, R., Gaffey, T.A., Prat, J., Virata, R., Hatab, P., McGorray, S., Noller, K.L., Townsend, D.E., LaBarthe, D., and Barnes, A.B. (1981): Am. J. Obstet. Gynecol., 140:579-586.

27. Robboy, S.J., Welch, W.R., Young, R.H., Truslow, G.Y., Herbst, A.L., and Scully, R.E. (1982): Obstet. Gynecol., 60:546-551.

28. Smith, O.W., Smith, G. van S., and Hurwitz, D. (1946): Am. J. Obstet. Gynecol., 51:411-415.

29. Ulfelder, H., and Robboy, S.J. (1976): Am. J. Obstet. Gynecol., 126:769-776.

Progress in Cancer Research and Therapy,
Vol. 31, edited by F. Bresciani, et al.
Raven Press, New York © 1984.

Carcinogenic Potential of Estrogens in Some Mammalian Model Systems

Robert H. Purdy

Department of Organic Chemistry, Southwest Foundation for Research and Education, San Antonio, Texas 78284

In 1979, Mortimer B. Lipsett, President of The Endocrine Society and Secretary General of the International Society of Endocrinology, wrote that "There is ample evidence in humans that endocrine-responsive tissues do not develop cancer unless they are stimulated by their growth-promoting hormones" (32). This statement served as the preamble for a conference on Estrogens and Cell Transformation which I organized in Wimberley, Texas, June 5-7, 1983. The objective of this conference was to bring together for the first time in our country a multidisciplinary group of investigators whose present work is related to (a) the metabolic activation of estrogens, (b) the effects of estrogens in in vitro mammalian cell transformation systems, (c) in vivo model systems for investigating estrogens as inducers and promoters of cellular transformation, and (d) cell culture systems for studying nontransformed endometrial and mammary gland cells.

The participants had agreed in advance that the proceedings of this conference would not be published, but serve instead as a stimulus for advancing our knowledge in this area of research, including plans for future studies. It is therefore inappropriate for me to summarize their efforts, which in some cases have been presented at this Congress. However, with the permission of a selected number of investigators, I will describe results in some mammalian model systems that support the concept of a carcinogenic potential for certain estrogens. As Joseph W. Goldzieher and I have stressed, the use of the term potential is most important in this respect, since these efforts are directed toward understanding the mechanism(s) of estrogen-mediated carcinogenesis as a rare event in biological expression, rather than to any direct extrapolation of these results to the frequency of human diseases (48).

ESTROGENS AS MUTAGENS

The Salmonella/mammalian microsome mutagenicity test developed by Ames and coworkers (2) has been used without success so far to detect mutagenic activity of estrogens (14,53,54). A synergistic effect of diethylstilbestrol (DES), a nonmutagen, was reported by Allaben et al. (1) on the mutagenicity of 2-acetylaminofluorene (2-AAF) and N-hydroxyacetylaminofluorene only when a 3-methylcholanthrene (3-MC) induced rat liver S-9 fraction was used in the assays. More recently, Rao et al. (49) reported an enhancement of the mutagenic activity of 2-AAF by the 3-methyl ether of ethynylestradiol (mestranol) using a phenobarbital induced S-9 rat liver activating system. The latter authors did not mention that cleavage of the methyl ether group of this derivative is

required for its hormonal activity, nor did they determine if ethynylestradiol was produced by such cleavage using this microsomal activating
system. It should also be pointed out that estrogens might merely be
acting as inhibitors of the ring hydroxylation of 2-AAF in these assays,
thus inhibiting the detoxification of 2-AAF rather than having a
"co-mutagenic" action on mutational events. A study of the effect of
DES or other estrogens on the metabolism of 2-AAF is required before
such results from Ames assay systems can be considered to be of real
interest.

Clive et al. (7) found that DES (33 μM) caused mutation at the
thymidine-kinase locus of L5178Y mouse lymphoma cells when an Aroclor-
induced rat liver S-9 activating system was used in assays and serum was
omitted from the medium. We have confirmed their results with DES (45)
but have found it as difficult as they did to obtain a reproducible dose
dependence of DES-induced frequency of mutation. A positive effect was
never observed with 25 to 100 μM ethynylestradiol, but 2-hydroxyethynyl-
estradiol produced a significant mutation frequency at 25 and 50 μM concentrations. The data from one such experiment performed without an
added S-9 activating system is shown in Table 1 (Purdy, Meltz, and
Goldzieher; unpublished). The marginal effect observed here led us to
the conclusion that this system could not be effectively utilized for a
comparative study with different estrogens. It is equally important to
point out that a detectable frequency of mutation was not induced by DES
at two loci of Syrian hamster embryo cells (4), nor did DES induce
6-thioguanine resistant mutants of V-79 Chinese hamster cells (5).

TABLE 1. Mutation of L5178Y mouse lymphoma cells

Chemical	Concen-tration	Total Fold Growth (Percent of Control)	Viability (Percent of Control Cloning Efficiency)	Mutation Frequency/ 10^6 Viable Cells	Induced Mutation Frequency (f_i)
				Avg	
Solvent control (DMSO)	0.5%	100	100	46	0
	0.5%			54	49
Ethynyl-estradiol	25 μM	104	100	51	2
	50 μM	106	93	54	5
	100 μM	89	100	46	-3
2-Hydroxy-ethynyl-estradiol	10 μM	106	95	53	4
	25 μM	4	62	151	101*
	50 μM	11	59	156	107*
	100 μM	0.4	--	--	--
MNNG	0.1 μM	12	8	2683	2684*

*Significant at P < 0.01 (7).

Metabolic Activation of DES

DES has been classified as a carcinogen by the International Agency for Research on Cancer on the basis of a positive association between exposure and the occurrence of various cancers in humans, squirrel monkeys, and rodents (62). The association of maternal DES therapy with subsequent vaginal adenocarcinoma in the daughters was reported by Herbst et al. (15). However, as Arthur L. Herbst has pointed out in these proceedings, there are reasons to doubt the classification of DES as a carcinogen or co-carcinogen in these women, since there is a real enigma concerning the 15 to 25% of the cases where changes in the genital tract have been observed, and the less than 0.1% of these daughters who developed malignant tumors. Nevertheless, the CD-1 mouse has been shown to be a useful animal model for studying the transplacental carcinogenicity of DES (35,41). Peroxidase mediated oxidation of DES was proposed by Metzler et al. (40) and Metzler and McLachlan (38) as a pathway for the metabolic activation of DES. More recently, this group demonstrated that the reproductive tract of the CD-1 mouse fetus also has the capacity to oxidatively metabolize DES to Z,Z-dienestrol (34). The finding of oxidative metabolism in this target tissue raises the possibility that such activation may be related to the subsequent expression of DES-induced tumors. The in vitro binding of DES to DNA and protein catalyzed by peroxidases has been demonstrated (8,38,39). Degen et al. (9) have recently provided evidence for the involvement of prostaglandin synthetase in the peroxidative metabolism of DES in Syrian hamster embryo fibroblasts.

Metabolic Activation of Steroidal Estrogens

The key to an understanding of the mutagenic and carcinogenic potential of polycyclic aromatic hydrocarbons is their metabolic activation by microsomal cytochrome P-450 mixed function oxidases. Knowledge of the structures of some of these activated epoxides prompted Soloway and Le Quesne (58) to propose 1,2- and 4,5-epoxides as potential intermediates in the formation of catechol estrogens, the principal metabolites of estrogens in women (11). Subsequently, three of the four possible isomers of this type of intermediate were synthesized in mg amounts in Philip W. Le Quesne's laboratory at Northeastern University for biological investigations (21,47). The mechanism proposed for the P-450 catalyzed formation of 4-hydroxyestradiol is shown in Figure 1. The putative $4\alpha,5\alpha$-arene oxide intermediate (II) in the metabolism of estradiol-17β can either stabilize as the epoxyenone (III) or be converted to 4-hydroxyestradiol (IV) by spontaneous aromatization or enzymatic catalysis. This mechanism is appropriate for tissues where 4-hydroxyestradiol is formed in significant proportion from estradiol, such as in human mammary tumor cells (46) or proliferative human endometrial tissue (51). It is not appropriate for liver tissue where the predominant pathway is 2-hydroxylation.

The principal methods of measuring the formation of pmolar amounts of catechol estrogens involve (a) the radiometric or tritium release assay developed by Fishman (12), (b) the product isolation assay for estrogen 2-/4-hydroxylase activities described by Hersey and Weisz (16), and (c)

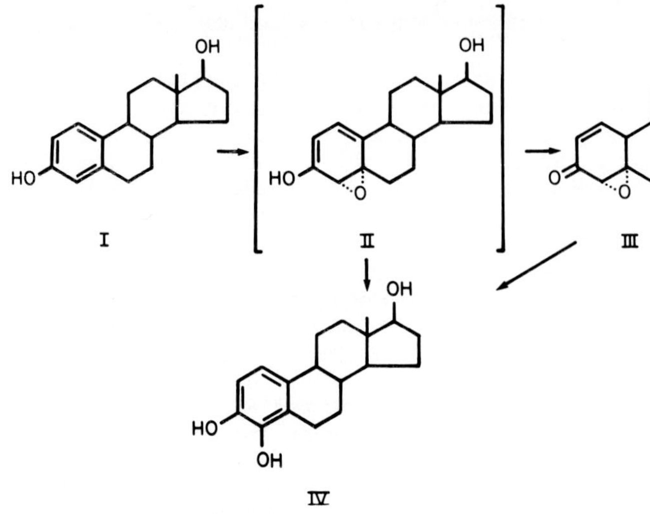

FIG. 1. Postulated metabolic pathways for the formation of 4-hydroxy-estradiol (IV) from estradiol-17β (I). The 4α,5α-arene oxide inter-mediate (II) can spontaneously aromatize to IV or stabilize as the epoxyenone (III).

the radioenzymatic assay developed by Axelrod and his colleagues (42). Since the latter assay is applicable for measuring the rates of catechol estrogen formation from numerous unlabeled estrogens, it is particularly suited for investigations of the rates of metabolic activation of different estrogens in a variety of mammalian model systems. The [³H]-labeled products of this assay with estradiol-17β as substrate are shown in Figure 2. They can be separated by HPLC (46), and relative rates of 2- and 4-hydroxylation of the substrate can be calculated from the profile of the individual products. In cases where the authentic standard monomethyl ethers are unavailable, a mixture of the 2- and 4-hydroxylated metabolites can be prepared by oxidation of the parent estrogen with Fremy's salt by the method of Gelbke et al. (13), and the individual catechol estrogens can be obtained by chromatography. These new catechol estrogens, when incubated with catechol-O-methyltransferase (COMT) and radiolabeled S-adenosyl-L-methionine, provide the necessary labeled reference products for HPLC.

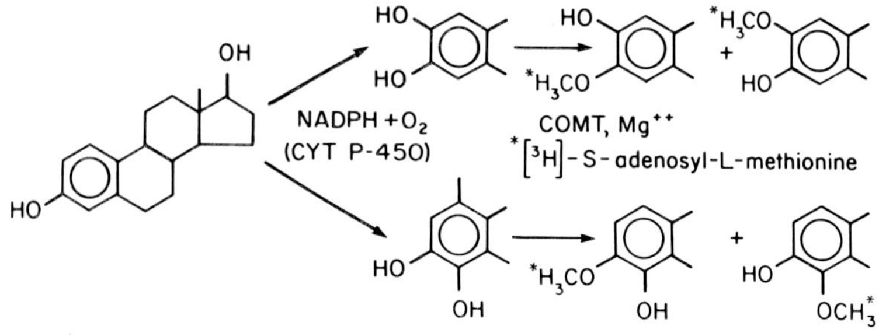

FIG. 2. Radioenzymatic assay for catechol estrogen formation.

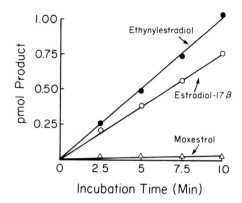

FIG. 3. Radioenzymatic assay of catechol estrogen formation from 50 μM estrogens with microsomes from Balb/c 3T3 cells. The total pmol of the monomethyl ether obtained in the heptane extracts according to the procedure of Purdy et al. (46) is shown as a function of incubation time (min).

The term metabolic activation, in reference to the metabolism of polycyclic aromatic hydrocarbons by P-450 mixed function oxidases, immediately evokes the structures of the proximate and ultimate carcinogenic diol epoxides of the parent hydrocarbons (if they have been determined). Since this sequence has not been established for any estrogen, this term is used here in a more general sense to include formation of (1) an activated epoxide intermediate (such as the 1β,2β-epoxyenone which was trapped in our isolation studies using microsomes from MCF-7 cells; ref. 47) that can be rapidly converted to a catechol estrogen, and/or (2) semiquinones or quinones that are formed by further oxidation of catechol estrogens (reviewed by Ball and Knuppen, ref. 3). A more precise definition of the term metabolic activation as applied to estrogens will necessarily have to await the structural elucidation of DNA adducts whose purification has not yet been described. With this caveat in mind, the relative rates of metabolic activation of three estrogens by microsomes from Balb/c 3T3 cells are illustrated in Figure 3. The products here are the total pmol of monomethyl ethers that have the same retention times by HPLC as the standard reference compounds (46). These data are shown to illustrate the fact that substituents in the C-ring (11β-methoxy group) and D-ring (17α-ethynyl group) can significantly alter the rates of catechol estrogen formation. Raynaud and coworkers first demonstrated that moxestrol is a valuable tag for estrogen receptor-binding sites in human tissues (50). Pharmacokinetic studies have shown moxestrol to have a markedly reduced rate of catechol estrogen formation in vivo (55) as compared with ethynylestradiol. It is known that the introduction of alkyl substituents above the β-face of rings C and D can result in a significant enhancement of hormonal activity. In the case of catechol estrogen formation, however, the 11β-methoxy group apparently produces an unfavorable hydrophobic interaction with the cavity of the P-450 mixed function oxidases that serve as estrogen 2-/4-hydroxylases. A simlar result has been found for 11β-ethylestradiol (44). This circumstance therefore provides us with two examples of estrogens with increased hormonal activity and markedly reduced rates of metabolic activation.

Neoplastic Transformation of Mammalian Cells in Culture by Estrogens

In a study of the transformation of Syrian hamster embryo cells by diverse chemicals, Pienta (43) found that DES (0.37 μM) was positive, whereas ethynylestradiol (170 μM) was negative. This observation was followed by the rigorous investigations of Barrett et al. (4) and McLachlan et al. (36) at the National Institute of Environmental Health Sciences on the transformation of these cells by DES and its analogs. They found no correlation between the estrogenic activity of DES and these analogs and their cell-transforming potency. However, there was a "good association between the metabolic conversion of DES analogs via a peroxidase-mediated oxidative pathway and their ability to induce cell transformation." It was assumed in this work that 3,5,3'5'-tetrafluoro-diethylstilbestrol (TF-DES) could not be metabolized to a catechol due to the presence of fluorine at all four positions ortho to the two phenolic groups. This assumption does not appear to be correct. When we incubated TF-DES with microsomes from Balb/c 3T3 cells or from the rat or primate liver in the radioenzymatic assay for catechol estrogen formation, we obtained [^{3}H]-labeled products whose retention times by HPLC were consistent with the formation of defluorinated catechol monomethyl ethers. Admittedly, our results may not be applicable to the hamster embryo cells used in the investigations at the NIEHS. In this respect, Degen et al. (9) were unable to detect catechol formation when [^{14}C]-labeled DES was added to cultures of Syrian hamster embryo fibroblasts under conditions where DES-induced neoplastic transformation was oberved.

After demonstrating that DES induced neoplastic transformation of the A-31-1-13 subclone of Balb/c 3T3 cells (45,47), and that microsomes from these cells catalyzed the formation of catechol estrogens, we have directed our further efforts to a study of the carcinogenic potential of steroidal estrogens in this mammalian cell model system. This heteroploid subclone was isolated by Kakunaga et al. (18) who demonstrated that it was particularly sensitive to polycyclic aromatic hydrocarbon-induced transformation, in which DNA damage is believed to be the initial step in the action of established carcinogens. In the transformation assay (17) the cells are treated for 72 hr with 5 to 50 μM concentrations of different estrogens. The cells are washed twice with fresh medium and allowed to recover in fresh medium for 24 hr. The cells are then harvested, counted, and plated for the determination of survival (cloning efficiency compared with the controls) and for the subsequent expression of neoplastic transformation (17). The plated cells are refed biweekly for 3 to 4 weeks, then stained and examined for changes in morphology (52). Type III foci refer to areas of transformed cells greater than 2 mm in diameter that consist of piled-up cells with cells overlapping at 30 to 90 degree angles at their periphery. The positive controls are cells treated with 1 μM 3-MC. Cells from several Type III foci appearing after estrogen treatment are transplanted into culture flasks for characterization in terms of their morphology, ability to form aggregates when suspended in medium above an agar base (61), and ability to form multicellular tumor spheroids (64). The final criterion used for neoplastic transformation is the ability of cells from Type III foci to produce fibrosarcomas in NIH nude mice (47).

The data in Table 2 show results for the neoplastic transformation of Balb/c 3T3 cells by the catechol estrogens formed from estradiol-17β, and the three estrogens whose rates of metabolic activation are shown in Figure 3. The results are expressed as the induced frequency (Type III

foci above background/10^4 surviving cells) normalized to 10 μM estrogen
(μM estrogen shown in column 2). The toxicity of 2-hydroxyestradiol
precluded the assay of this catechol at concentrations greater than
5 μM. In both cases the catechols were more potent transforming agents
than was estradiol-17β. The order of the relative rates of metabolic
activation in Figure 3 parallels the normalized frequency of transformation shown in Table 2.

TABLE 2. <u>Neoplastic transformation of Balb/c 3T3 A-31-1-13 subclone
by estrogens</u>

Estrogen	μM	% Survival[a]	Average number of Type III foci above background/10^4 surviving cells/10 μM estrogen
2-Hydroxyestradiol	5	16	8.7
4-Hydroxyestradiol	5	60	5.5
Ethynylestradiol	30	17	2.7
Estradiol-17β	40	23	1.9
Moxestrol	50	96	<0.1

[a]Average cloning efficiency for DMSO controls taken as 100%.

A comparison of the relative rates of catechol estrogen formation
from estradiol-17β and estradiol-17α by microsomes from the Balb/c 3T3
cells used in our transformation assay is shown in Figure 4. The
17α-isomer is the more active substrate, whereas its uterotropic potency
is between 1.5% and 5% of that of estradiol-17β, depending on the
species (20,57). With MCF-7 cells, the estrogenic potency of
estradiol-17α is about 10% of the potency of estradiol-17β (10). The
6α-hydroxyestradiol-17β metabolite of estradiol-17β in Balb/c 3T3 cells
(Purdy, unpublished) is essentially inactive as a substrate of estrogen
2-/4-hydroxylase activity.
  The data in Table 3 provides the relative frequency of neoplastic
transformation found with these estrogens. Estradiol-17α is seen to be

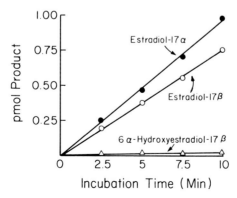

FIG. 4. Radioenzymatic assay of catechol estrogen formation with microsomes from Balb/c 3T3 cells (see Fig. 3).

TABLE 3.   Neoplastic transformation of Balb/c 3T3 A-31-1-13 subclone by estrogens

Estrogen	μM	% Survival[a]	Average number of Type III foci above background/10^4 surviving cells/10 μM estrogen
Estradiol-17α	10	23	13.3
Estradiol-17β	40	17	2.8
6α-Hydroxyestradiol-17β	40	91	<0.1

[a]Average cloning efficiency for DMSO control taken as 100%.

a more potent transforming agent than would be predicted from the relative rates of metabolic activation shown in Figure 4.

To further understand the mechanism involved in the transformation of estrogens, the fluorine probe methodology has been employed. The monofluorinated derivatives 2-fluoro- and 4-fluoroestradiol (Figure 5) were originally prepared in 1968 by Utne et al. (63). Their uterotropic activity has recently been reexamined using chromatographically purified material and has been found in both cases to be very similar to that of estradiol-17β (30,33). In collaboration with Evan H. Appelman at the Argonne National Laboratory we have now synthesized 2,4-difluoroestradiol. Neil J. MacLusky at the Yale University School of Medicine has found that the uterotropic activity of 2,4-difluoroestradiol is similar to that of 2-fluoroestradiol. The 3-fluoro analog of estradiol serves as a control in these studies, since it is not metabolized to a catechol by any of the mammalian microsomes we have tested, or by mushroom tyrosinase.

The relative rates of metabolic activation of estradiol-17β and its fluorinated derivatives by microsomes from our Balb/c 3T3 cells are shown in Figure 6. The unanticipated result that 2,4-difluoroestradiol is a substrate for catechol estrogen formation is supported by data obtained using other P-450 mixed function oxidases, including mushroom

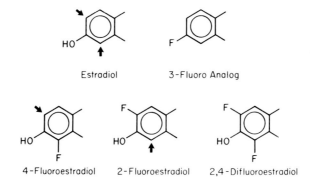

Estradiol   3-Fluoro Analog

4-Fluoroestradiol   2-Fluoroestradiol   2,4-Difluoroestradiol

FIG. 5.   Structures of the A-ring of compounds used in the fluorine probe methodology. The arrows indicate the expected positions of hydroxylation in the radioenzymatic assay of catechol estrogen formation.

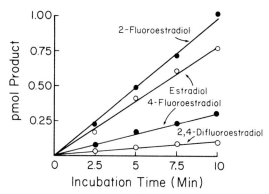

FIG. 6. Radioenzymatic assay of catechol estrogen formation using microsomes from Balb/c 3T3 cells (see Fig. 3).

tyrosinase (Purdy, R.H., unpublished). The HPLC profiles of the [^{3}H]-labeled products from the radioenzymatic assays of 2,4-difluoro-estradiol contained two major peaks with the same retention times as those observed when 4-fluoroestradiol was used as a substrate, and a minor peak with the same retention time as the minor peak obtained when 2-fluoroestradiol was the substrate. Yet HPLC showed that none of these fluorinated substrates were contaminated by detectable amounts of other components. Although this study is not yet complete, our results and those of another laboratory working with rat brain and liver microsomes (Pfeiffer, D. G., Merriam, G. R. and MacLusky, N. J., unpublished) have convinced us that a significant portion of the [^{3}H]-labeled products from radioenzymatic assays with 2-fluoroestradiol as substrate are the defluorinated monomethyl ethers, 2-methoxyestradiol and 2-hydroxy-estradiol 3-methyl ether (Figure 2).

The results for the relative frequency of neoplastic transformation of the above fluorinated estradiol derivatives are shown in Table 4.

Since 2-fluoroestradiol is a more active substrate than 4-fluoro-estradiol or estradiol-17β (Figure 5), and the most potent transforming agent in this group of compounds (Table 4), it might be presumed (without information on the actual products formed from 2-fluoroestradiol) that the 4-hydroxylase pathway is principally involved in the mechanism of neoplastic transformation in this in vitro model system. However our HPLC results described above are not consistent with this conclusion. A similar loss of fluorine has recently been reported by Buening et al. (6) for the P-450 catalyzed oxidation of 6-fluorobenzo[a]pyrene at the

TABLE 4. Neoplastic transformation of Balb/c 3T3 A-31-1-13 subclone by estrogens

Estrogen	µM	% Survival[a]	Average number of Type III foci above background/10^4 surviving cells/10 µM estrogen
2-Fluoroestradiol	25	23	3.8
Estradiol-17β	40	23	1.9
4-Fluoroestradiol	20	34	0.6
2,4-Difluoroestradiol	30	95	0.1

[a]Average cloning efficiency for DMSO control taken as 100%.

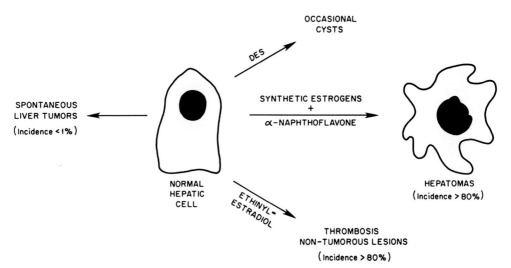

FIG. 7.   Schematic illustration of the induction of hepatomas and liver lesions in Syrian hamsters following treatment with synthetic estrogens.

6-position.   The product, 6α-hydroxybenzo[a]pyrene, was reported to be more active than benzo[a]pyrene in the transformation of Syrian hamster cells in culture (56).   Metabolic defluorination of 6-fluorobenzo[a]-pyrene led Buening et al. (6) in their concluding statement to emphasize "a need for detailed metabolic studies whenever fluorine substitution is used as a probe to assess the role of the substituted position for the carcinogenicity of the parent compound."   Our results support the applicability of their statement to A-ring fluorinated estrogens.

Steroidal estrogens (estrone, estradiol-17β, and estriol) have been found by McLachlan et al. (37) to be weakly active in the Syrian hamster embryo cell model system.   Consistent with results obtained with our Balb/c 3T3 cell system, these investigators at the NIEHS have found that the catechol estrogen metabolites of these steroidal estrogens showed greater activity as transforming agents than their parent estrogens. Their results emphasize the utility of these diploid embryonic cells to also serve as a model system for exploring the mechanism[s] involved in the carcinogenic potential of steroidal estrogens.

In Vivo Model Systems

In 1959, Kirkman found that the hamster kidney is one of the most sensitive tissues with respect to estrogen-mediated carcinogenicity (19).   Although this tissue is not considered to be a typical target organ, it contains estrogen receptors sedimenting at 4S and 8S (22,24). Estrogen treatment also induces a sizeable increase in the progesterone receptor concentration of this tissue (23,26).   Jonathan J. Li and Sara A. Li at the University of Minnesota Medical School found that when α-naphthoflavone (α-NF, an inhibitor of microsomal multisubstrate mono-oxygenases) was incorporated in the diet (0.2%), there was a markedly reduced incidence of renal carcinomas in hamsters treated with DES, compared with similar animals treated with DES alone (25).   The presence of α-NF in the diet did not affect the ability of either DES or estradiol-17β to stimulate the progesterone receptor content of hamster kidneys. An unanticipated result was an 80-100% incidence of multifocal liver tumors in castrated as well as intact male hamsters treated with DES or ethynylestradiol for 10 months and maintained on a diet containing 0.2% α-NF (28). No hepatomas were found in control animals that were similarly treated with α-NF for up to 12 months. These results are summarized in Figure 7. A striking observation in their analysis of the proteins isolated from Syrian hamster hepatic microsomes by SDS polyacrylamide gel electrophoresis was the appearance of a band (5a) in liver microsomes of α-NF treated hamsters which was not altered by concomitant treatment with DES or ethynylestradiol (28). This band is presumed to be a component of the P-450 mixed function oxidases. They have reported that estrogen 2-/4-hydroxylase activity is decreased in kidney but not liver microsomes from α-NF treated hamsters (27).

The Syrian hamster model system offers a unique opportunity to explore the mechanism[s] of estrogen-mediated carcinogenesis in both kidney and liver tissues, since the response of these tissues to estrogens can be dramatically altered by treatment with α-NF. The relative carcinogenic potential of various synthetic and natural estrogens in the Syrian hamster kidney suggests that hormonal activity alone is not sufficient to cause renal tumorigenesis in the hamster (29). Liehr et al. (31) have found that TF-DES treatment resulted in 100% renal tumor incidence after 9.5 months, which was similar to that observed after DES treatment. Again it was assumed that if a catechol pathway was involved in the DES-mediated carcinogenesis, that "fluorination in the ortho positions to the phenolic hydroxyl group was expected to reduce carcinogenic action" of TF-DES. The caveat for this assumption is that it is necessary to obtain relative rates of catechol estrogen formation for DES and TF-DES in the hamster kidney to support the in vivo data. This caveat also applies to results obtained by Liehr (30) for an absence of carcinogenicity of 2-fluoroestradiol in this hamster kidney model system, where the role of metabolic activation was implied in the apparent separation of hormonal activity from the in vivo carcinogenic potential of 2-fluoro- and 4-fluoroestradiol.

CONCLUSIONS

In cultures of the heteroploid A-31-1-13 subclone of Balb/c 3T3 cells and in cultured diploid Syrian hamster embryo cells, both 2- and 4-hydroxyestradiol are more effective than estradiol as inducers of the neoplastic transformation of these cells. These results support the hypothesis that formation of catechol estrogens is involved in the mechanism[s] of estrogen-induced transformation in these in vitro model systems. Using Balb/c 3T3 cells, it has been found that the relative frequency of neoplastic transformation induced by an estrogen or estrogen derivative parallels its relative rate of catechol estrogen formation by the microsomal activating system isolated from large-scale cultures of these cells. This further supports the hypothesis that these catechols are activated metabolites of the parent estrogens.

Results from these in vitro studies with the Balb/c 3T3 cells have provided examples for three of the four possible categories of estrogens shown in Table 5.

TABLE 5. <u>Hormonal activity versus the carcinogenic potential of</u>
<u>estrogens</u>

Hormonally active steroidal estrogens

Carcinogenic Potential: <u>Positive</u>
Examples: Estrone,
Estradiol-17β
Ethynylestradiol

Carcinogenic Potential: <u>Not detected</u>
Examples: 11β-Methoxyestradiol
Moxestrol

Hormonally inactive estrogen derivatives

Carcinogenic Potential: <u>Positive</u>
Examples: [Estradiol-17α]

Carcinogenic Potential: <u>Not detected</u>
Examples: 6α-Hydroxyestradiol
2,4-Dibromoestradiol

Since estradiol-17α must be regarded as a weakly active estrogen, we are now searching for an example of a steroidal estrogen which possesses a detectable carcinogenic potential and is essentially devoid of estrogenic activity. The fact that examples exist for each of the other above categories supports our hypothesis that the carcinogenic potential of an estrogen is related to its relative rate of metabolic activation, rather than to its activity as a hormone.

The Syrian hamster renal and hepatic model systems serve as valuable adjuncts to <u>in vitro</u> culture systems. Results from these <u>in vivo</u> systems provide an opportunity to further correlate the carcinogenic potential of estrogens with their rates of metabolic activation, since the kidney or liver tissues of the exposed animals can be used to measure such relative rates of metabolic activation.

It is anticipated that future efforts will involve the necessary extension of these results to cultured lines of nontransformed human endometrial and mammary epithelial cells. The metabolism of benzo[a]-pyrene by human mammary epithelial cells grown in a serum-free medium is being investigated in detail by Stampfer et al. (59), where DNA adduct formation has been demonstrated. The fact that her group has now been able to induce transformation of such epithelial cells with benzo[a]-pyrene (60) provides a background for examining the carcinogenic potential of estrogens in cells from an estrogen-responsive human tissue which is believed to be at some risk from endogenous estrogens.

ACKNOWLEDGEMENTS

This investigation was supported by grant CA 24629 awarded by the National Cancer Institute, DHHS.

The author is indebted to Mrs. Connie K. Durocher and Mr. Perry H. Moore, Jr., for their excellent work on this program. The author is grateful to Dr. Jean-Pierre Raynaud and Miss Tiiu Ojasoo of Roussel-Uclaf for generous gifts of estrogens and other assistance, and to Mrs. Margaret Rodriguez and Ms. Harriet J. Smith for preparing this manuscript.

The participants in the Wimberley Conference on Estrogens and Cell Transformation are most appreciative for the support provided by the Texas Division of The American Cancer Society, Mead Johnson Pharmaceutical Division, Merrell Dow Pharmaceutical Division, LDC-Milton Roy, New England Nuclear Corp., Ortho Pharmaceutical Corp., Progenics Inc., Roussel Uclaf, G.D. Searle and Co., Steraloids Inc., Stuart Pharmaceuticals, Syntex Laboratories Inc., and Wyeth Laboratories.

REFERENCES

1. Allaben, W. T., Louie, S. C., and Lazear, E. J. (1979): Cancer Lett., 7:109-114.
2. Ames, B. N., McCann, J., and Yamasaki, E. (1975): Mutat. Res., 31:347-363.
3. Ball, P., and Knuppen, R. (1980): Acta Endocrinol. [Suppl.], 232:1-127.
4. Barrett, J. C., Wong, A., and McLachlan, J. A. (1981): Science, 212:1402-1404.
5. Barrett, J. C., McLachlan, J. A., and Elmore, E. (1983): Mutat. Res., 107:427-432.
6. Buening, M. K., Levin, W., Wood, A. W., Chang, R. L., Agranat, I., Rabinovitz, M., Buhler, D. R., Mah, H. D., Hernandez, O., Simpson, R. B., Jerina, D. M., Conney, A. H., Miller, E. C., and Miller, J. A. (1983): J. Natl. Cancer Inst., 71:309-315.
7. Clive, D., Johnson, K. O., Spector, J.F.S., Batson, A. G., and Brown, M.M.M. (1979): Mutat. Res., 59:61-108.
8. Degen, G. H., Eling, T. E., and McLachlan, J. A. (1982): Cancer Res., 42:919-923.
9. Degen, G. H., Wong, A., Eling, T. E., Barrett, J. C., and McLachlan, J. A. (1983): Cancer Res., 43:992-996.
10. Edwards, D. P., and McGuire, W. L. (1980): Endocrinology, 107:884-891.
11. Fishman, J. (1983): In: Catechol Estrogens, edited by G. R. Merriam and M. B. Lipsett, pp. 1-3. Raven Press, New York.
12. Fishman, J. (1983): In: Catechol Estrogens, edited by G. R. Merriam and M. B. Lipsett, pp. 31-36. Raven Press, New York.
13. Gelbke, H. P., Haupt, O., and Knuppen, R. (1973): Steroids, 21:205-218.
14. Glatt, H. R., Metzler, M., and Oesch, F. (1979): Mutat. Res., 67:113-121.
15. Herbst, A. L., Ulfelder, H., and Poskanzer D. C. (1971): N. Engl. J. Med., 284:878-881.
16. Hersey, R. M., and Weisz, J. (1983): In: Catechol Estrogens, edited by G. R. Merriam and M. B. Lipsett, pp. 37-48. Raven Press, New York.
17. Kakunaga, T. (1973): Intl. J. Cancer, 12:463-473.
18. Kakunaga, T., Lo, K.-Y., Leavitt, J., and Ikenaga, M. (1980): Jerusalem Symp. Quantum Chem. Biochem., 13:527-541.
19. Kirkman, H. (1959): Natl. Cancer Inst. Monogr., 1:1-139.

20. Korenman, S. G. (1969): Steroids, 13:163-177.
21. Le Quesne, P. W., Durga, A. V., Subramanyam, V., Soloway, A. H., Hart, R. W., and Purdy, R. H. (1980): J. Med. Chem., 23:239-240.
22. Li, J. J., Talley, D. J., Li, S. A., and Villee, C. A. (1974): Endocrinology, 95:1134-1141.
23. Li, S. A., and Li, J. J. (1978): Endocrinology, 103:2119-2128.
24. Li, J. J., Cuthbertson, T. L., and Li, S. A. (1980): J. Natl. Cancer Inst., 64:795-800.
25. Li, J. J., and Li, S. A. (1981): Proc. Am. Assoc. Cancer Res., 22:11 (44).
26. Li, J. J., and Li, S. A. (1981): Endocrinology, 108:1751-1756.
27. Li, S. A., Klicka, J. K., and Li, J. J. (1983): Endocrine Society, 65th Annual Meeting, San Antonio, TX, Program and Abstracts, p. 312 (925).
28. Li, J. J., and Li, S. A. (1983): Arch. Toxicol., (in press).
29. Li, J. J., Li, S. A., Klicka, J. K., Parsons, J. A., and Lam, L.K.T. (1983): Cancer Res., 43:5200-5204.
30. Liehr, J. G. (1983): Mol. Pharmacol., 23:278-281.
31. Liehr, J. G., Ballatore, A. M., McLachlan, J. A., and Sirbasku, D. A. (1983): Cancer Res., 43:2678-2682.
32. Lipsett, M. B. (1979): J. Natl. Cancer Inst., 43:1967-1981.
33. Longcope, C., Rafkind, I., Arunachalam, T., and Caspi, E. (1983): J. Steroid Biochem., 19:1325-1328.
34. Maydl, R., Newbold, R. R., Metzler, M., and McLachlan, J. A. (1983): Endocrinology, 113:146-151.
35. McLachlan, J. A., Newbold, R. R., and Bullock, B. C. (1980): Cancer Res., 40:3988-3999.
36. McLachlan, J. A., Wong, A., Degen, G. H., and Barrett, J. C. (1982): Cancer Res. 42:3040-3045.
37. McLachlan, J. A., Barrett, J. C., Wong, A., and Degen, G. H. (1983): Cancer Res., (submitted).
38. Metzler, M., and McLachlan, J. A. (1978): Biochem. Biophys. Res. Commun., 85:874-884.
39. Metzler, M., and McLachlan, J. A. (1979): Arch. Toxicol., 2(Suppl.):275-280.
40. Metzler, M., Gottschlich, R., and McLachlan, J. A. (1980): In: Estrogens in the Environment, edited by J. A. McLachlan, pp. 293,302. Raven Press, New York.
41. Newbold, R. R., and McLachlan, J. A. (1982): Cancer Res., 42:2003-2011.
42. Paul, S. M., Purdy, R. H., Hoffman, A. R., and Axelrod, J. (1983): In: Catechol Estrogens, edited by G. R. Merriam and M. B. Lipsett, pp. 83-90. Raven Press, New York.
43. Pienta, R. J. (1980): Chem. Mutagens, 6:175-202.
44. Purdy, R. H. (1983): J. Steroid Biochem., 19:Suppl 46S.
45. Purdy, R. H., Meltz, M. L., Goldzieher, J. W., Goodwin, T. J., and Williams, M. J. (1980): Endocrine Society, 62nd Annual Meeting, Washington, D.C., Program and Abstracts, p. 271 (787).
46. Purdy, R. H., Moore, P. H., Jr., Williams, M. C., Goldzieher, J. W., and Paul, S. M. (1982): FEBS Lett., 138:40-44.
47. Purdy, R. H., Goldzieher, J. W., Le Quesne, P. W., Abdel-Baky, S., Durocher, C. K., Moore, P. H., Jr., and Rhim, J. S. (1983): In: Catechol Estrogens, edited by G. R. Merriam and M. B. Lipsett, pp. 123-140. Raven Press, New York.

48. Purdy, R. H., and Goldzieher, J. W. (1983): In: Intervention in the Aging Process, edited by F. M. Sinex and W. Regelson, Alan R. Liss, Inc., New York, Part 2 (in press).

49. Rao, T. K., Allen, B. E., Cox, J. T., and Epler, J. L. (1983): Toxicol. Appl. Pharmacol., 69:48-54.

50. Raynaud, J. P., Martin, P. M., Bouton, M. -M., and Ojasoo, T. (1978): Cancer Res., 38:3044-3050.

51. Reddy, V.V.R., Hanjani, P., and Rajan, R. (1981): Steroids, 37:195-203.

52. Reznikoff, C. A., Bertram, J. S., Brankow, D. W., and Heidelberger, C. (1973): Cancer Res., 33:3239-3249.

53. Rinkus, S. J., and Legator, M. S. (1980): Chem. Mutagens, 6:365-473.

54. Rudiger, H. W., Haenisch, F., Metzler, M., Oesch, F., and Glatt, H. R. (1979): Nature, 281:392-394.

55. Salmon, J., Coussedière, D., Cousty, C., and Raynaud, J. P. (1983): J. Steroid Biochem., 19:1223-1234.

56. Schechtman, L. M., Lesko, S. A., Lorentzen, R. J., and Ts'o, P. O. P. (1974): Proc. Am. Assoc. Cancer Res., 15:66 (262).

57. Shutt, D. A., and Cox, R. I. (1972): J. Endocrinol., 52:299-310.

58. Soloway, A. H., and Le Quesne, P. W. (1980): J. Theor. Biol. 85:153-163.

59. Stampfer, M.R., Bartholomew, J. C., Smith, H. S., and Bartley, J. C. (1981): Proc. Natl. Acad. Sci. U.S.A., 78:6251-6255.

60. Stampfer, M. R., Ceriani, R., and Bartley, J. (1983): Intl. Assoc. for Breast Cancer Res., Proc., Denver, Colorado, Abst. 130.

61. Steuer, A. F., Rhim, J. S., Hentosh, P. M., and Ting, R. C. (1977): J. Natl. Cancer Inst., 58:917-921.

62. Tomatis, L., Agthe, C., Bartsch, H., Huff, J., Montesano, R., Saracci, R., Walker, E., and Wilbourn, J. (1978): Cancer Res., 38:877-885.

63. Utne, T., Jobson, R. B., and Badson, R. D. (1968): J. Org. Chem., 33:2469-2473.

64. Yuhas, J. M., Li, A. P., Martinez, A. O., and Ladman, A. J. (1977): Cancer Res., 37:3639-3643.

Progress in Cancer Research and Therapy,
Vol. 31, edited by F. Bresciani, et al.
Raven Press, New York © 1984.

Efficacy of Tamoxifen in Endometrial Cancer

*K.D. Swenerton, *K. Chrumka, **A.H.G. Paterson, and *G.C. Jackson

*Cancer Control Agency of British Columbia, Vancouver, V5Z 3J3; and **Provincial Cancer Hospitals Board of Alberta, Edmonton, T6G 1Z2 Canada

Until recently, hormone therapy in endometrial cancer meant the use of progestins in the palliative treatment of advanced disease. Such treatment developed empirically, years before much understanding of hormone physiology evolved (23). The recognition of steroid receptor mechanisms in target tissues (12), and the demonstration that the antiestrogen, tamoxifen, is effective in women with advanced breast cancer (8), offered the possibility of alternative hormone therapies for endometrial cancer (7,9). In 1976, Tisman et al (25) reported subjective improvement in two patients with endometrial cancer treated with tamoxifen.

A pilot study conducted at the Cancer Control Agency of British Columbia during 1978 and 1979 showed tamoxifen to induce complete or partial remission in three of ten women with recurrent endometrial cancer (21). These preliminary data indicated that patients with lower-grade tumours and longer disease-free intervals were more likely to respond. Furthermore, there was a suggestion that cross resistance does not occur between progestins and tamoxifen. As well, such treatment showed remarkably little toxicity, a particular advantage in a group of patients who are often elderly and with coexistent illness which could make them unsuitable for intensive combination chemotherapy.

Encouraged by these results, in December 1979 we embarked in a bi-institutional phase II study to further explore the activity of this drug in women with advanced or recurrent disease. Specifically, the objectives were:

1. To determine the frequency and duration of response,
2. To correlate the response achieved with tamoxifen to that achieved with prior and subsequent hormonal therapy,
3. To define prognostic factors influencing outcome.

Patient entry to this trial was completed in December 1982.

In order to maximize the number of patients available for analysis, this final report summarizes our total experience, including previously published data: a preliminary report (24), the pilot study (21), and an interim report (22).

MATERIALS AND METHODS

Eligibility required a confirmed histologic diagnosis in patients demonstrating progressive disease not suitable for established surgical or radiotherapeutic treatment. All patients had discontinued previous therapy at least four weeks before entering the study and had recovered from prior treatment toxicity. Measurable or evaluable disease had to be present. There were no age or performance status limitations. The technique of pretreatment evaluation has been previously described (21).

Patient performance status was estimated using Eastern Cooperative Oncology Group (ECOG) criteria (15). Tumour steroid receptor data were not available. Histologic material was required for review to determine tumour grade: *Grade I* - highly differentiated adenocarcinoma; *Grade II* - differentiated adenocarcinoma with partially solid areas; *Grade III* - partially solid or entirely undifferentiated carcinoma.

Followup was maintained at four-week intervals to assess patient status, disease extent and response.

To be evaluable for response, patients had to remain on treatment for a minimum of four weeks. Response criteria were based on those suggested by the International Union Against Cancer (11). Additionally, a category of minor response was defined: *minor response* (MR) - $\geq 25\% < 50\%$ decrease (21). The minimum time to progression was one month, the followup interval.

Tamoxifen was administered in an oral dose, 10 mg twice daily and continued indefinitely in patients achieving remission or stable disease status. Patients were removed from study if they developed progressive disease. In each instance, informed consent was obtained.

In an effort to achieve further palliation some patients were subsequently treated with alternative hormone therapy. This consisted of progestin alone (in the form of megestrol acetate, 40 mg four times daily *or* combination therapy (10 mg of tamoxifen twice daily and 40 mg of megestrol acetate four times daily).

RESULTS

Patient Characteristics

A total of 47 patients were enrolled in the pilot and phase II studies. Four patients were ineligible, the diagnosis being unclear in three and evaluable disease not present in another. Of the 43 eligible patients, eight were inevaluable; three never received tamoxifen, in three followup could not be maintained, one received tamoxifen for one week only, and one received simultaneous cytotoxic chemotherapy.

The 35 evaluable patients demonstrated the following pretreatment characteristics: the age of initial diagnosis ranged from 44-74 years, with a median of 62 years. Primary therapy consisted of surgery plus radiotherapy in 19 patients, surgery alone in seven, surgery plus radiotherapy with adjuvant progestins in five, and radiotherapy alone in four. The disease-free interval ranged from no interval to 143 months, with a median of 23 months. All but 13 patients had received prior therapy for recurrent disease. This had included prior progestational therapy in the form of medroxyprogesterone acetate at a continuous oral dose of 100 mg daily in eighteen. Fourteen of the patients had received cytotoxic chemotherapy and eight had received palliative radiotherapy.

Ages at entry into the study ranged from 44 to 87 years, with a median of 66 years. The major site of disease at the beginning of study was pelviabdominal in 14 patients, intrathoracic in 11, and both sites in 10. Patient performance status (ECOG) was 0 in nine patients, 1 in eleven patients, 2 in twelve patients, 3 in three patients, and 4 in none.

Response to Tamoxifen

Overall, two patients achieved CR, six PR, three MR, two stable disease and 22 had disease progression.

In the 11 patients in whom it could be assessed, the time to response ranged from 1½ to 12 months, with a median of two months.

Prognostic Factors

The length of the disease-free interval appeared to predict for response to tamoxifen, as shown in table 1.

TABLE 1. Response (CR + PR + MR) to tamoxifen as a function of disease-free interval (n=35)

	Disease-free interval (years)				
	<1	<2	1-3	>2	>3
Responding fraction of patients	0/13	2/18	4/9	9/17	7/13

Tumour grade also correlated with the likelihood and quality of response as shown in table 2.

TABLE 2. Response to tamoxifen as a function of tumour grade (n=35)

Tumour grade	No. Pts.	CR	PR	MR	STAB	PROG
I	5	0	2	1	0	2
II	12	1	4	1	2	4
III	18	1	0	1	0	16

Patients who had demonstrated a prior response to progestin were also more likely to respond to tamoxifen as shown in table 3.

TABLE 3. Response to tamoxifen as a function of response to prior progestin therapy (n=23)

	No. of patients with	
Response to prior progestin	CR, PR MR	STAB, PROG
Definite objective response	3	2
Equivocal or indeterminate response	2	6
No response	1	9

Table 4 relates the predominant site of metastatic disease and response to tamoxifen. Allowing that patient numbers in each site category are small, response was seen less frequently when disease was present both above and below the diaphragm. This table also depicts the tumour grade for the patients in each of these site categories.

TABLE 4. Response to tamoxifen as a function of predominent site of
disease (n=35)

Site	Responding fractions of patients (CR, PR, MR)	Tumour grade	
		I+II	III
Thoracic	5/11	6	5
Pelviabdominal	5/14	10	4
Both	1/10	1	9

The likelihood of response to tamoxifen was unaffected by patient age,
patient performance status, or whether the patients had received prior
cytotoxic chemotherapy.

Durability of Response

The durability of response, measured by the time to progression, correlates with both tumour grade and disease-free interval as shown in
table 5. This interval ranged widely, for all patients the range was
1-45 months (median 3, mean 6+). For the eleven responding patients the
range was 4-45 months (median 9, mean 14+).

TABLE 5. Time to disease progression as a function of tumour grade and
disease-free interval (n=35)

Tumour grade	Mean time (mos) to disease progression	
	DFI > 2 years	DFI < 2 years
I + II	11+ (13)*	5½ (4)
III	3 (4)	2½ (14)

*number of patients in parentheses.

Subsequent Hormonal Therapy

Eighteen patients, on completing tamoxifen therapy, were then given
further hormonal treatment. This took the form of either megestrol alone
or combined tamoxifen plus megestrol. One women received both, first
megestrol alone, then the combination. Thus, 19 episodes of sequential,
post-tamoxifen, hormonal therapy were administered (Tables 6, 7).

TABLE 6. Response to subsequent tamoxifen-megestrol as a function of
prior tamoxifen response (n=13*)

Response to tamoxifen	Response to tamoxifen + megestrol	
	CR, PR, MR	STAB, PROG
CR, PR, MR	3	3
STAB, PROG	0	6

*one patient too early to assess.

TABLE 7. <u>Response to subsequent megestrol as a function of prior tamoxifen response (n=6)</u>

Response to tamoxifen	Response to megestrol	
	CR, PR, MR	STAB, PROG
CR, PR, MR	1	3
STAB, PROG	0	2

In each instance responders to the sequential treatment had shown a prior response to tamoxifen alone. The time to progression with post-tamoxifen therapy ranged from 5 to more than 10 months, with a median duration of greater than seven months.

Toxicity

With the possible exception of slight nausea in one patient, no incident of toxicity attributable to treatment was observed.

DISCUSSION

Response

Tamoxifen is an effective palliative therapy for certain patients with advanced endometrial cancer. In this series, 11 of 35 women (31%) demonstrated at least a minor objective benefit and 8 of 35 (23%) achieved at least a partial response. This response frequency approximates that seen with progestins which produce objective improvement in one-third (26) and PR in one-sixth (16).

Prognostic factors

The disease-free interval predicted the frequency of response; remissions were three times more frequent in women who demonstrated a disease-free interval greater than three years (7/13 vs 4/22) - a prognostic ratio similar to that of 4:1 found for progestins (16). None of 13 patients with a disease-free interval of less than one year responded to tamoxifen.

Tumour grade predicted outcome. Remissions were five times more frequent in patients with Grade I than Grade III disease (3/5 vs 2/18). This, too, parallels the experience with progestins, where those with well-differentiated tumours responded three times more frequently than those with poorly-differentiated tumours (14). In this, as in most reports, tumour grade was estimated on tissue obtained at primary surgery not on biopsies of metastatic disease. It is possible that metastases are less well differentiated than the primary tumour. Time and clonal evolution may afford a biological advantage to more aggressive, poorly differentiated elements of the tumour (2). Thus estimates of grade based on material obtained at diagnosis could underestimate the virulence of metastatic disease and overestimate the likelihood of hormone response. It is likely that laboratory measurement of hormone receptor function will improve our ability to choose appropriate and effective therapy (2).

A superficial inspection of table 4 suggests that response depends on the predominent site of disease. Response was seen less frequently in those with disease both above and below the diaphragm. However, it can be seen that tumour grade and site are closely related - 9 of 10 tumours situated *both* above and below the diaphragm being Grade III, only 9 of 25 situated *either* pelviabdominally or thoracically being Grade III. It may be that site reflects grade, the more virulent Grade III tumours metastasizing more widely. Therefore, site of disease does not independently predict response to tamoxifen nor to progestins (3,20).

The lack of prognostic influence of patient age, patient performance status and prior cytotoxic chemotherapy is consistent with observations on hormone therapy generally (6).

Durability of Response

The duration of response to tamoxifen was not directly determined in this study, but can be estimated (the time to progression, median nine months, minus the time to response, median two months) to be seven months. This appears to be shorter than the duration of response obtained with progestins (16) and may be, in part, because tamoxifen was given as a secondary hormonal therapy in the majority of our patients.

Subsequent Hormonal Therapy

Some of our patients demonstrated prior responses to progestin, secondary responses to tamoxifen and tertiary responses to either combined tamoxifen and progestin or progestin alone. That sequential hormonal responses can be achieved extends the palliative potential of hormone therapy in this disease. The clinical effectiveness of tamoxifen-progestin therapy was predicted by Sekiya and Takamizawa (19) who showed that these agents have a synergistic inhibitory effect on the colony-forming ability of cells derived from rat uterine adenocarcinoma in vitro. The mechanism of this synergism is unclear, but may be attributed to the induction of increased levels of progesterone receptor by tamoxifen. This effect, potentially re-inducing progestin sensitivity, was described by Robel et al (18) in human endometrial adenocarcinoma tissue in vivo. Tamoxifen has been shown to induce progesterone receptors in patients with endometrial cancer (Allegra et al, 1), but these authors caution that the combination may not be more active than standard single-agents in the primary therapy of this disease.

The observation in one patient that tamoxifen produced a reponse in a tumour unresponsive to progestin (table 3) supports the concept that antiestrogens and progestins exert their effect through separate, albeit functionally interrelated, steroid receptor mechanisms (13).

Comparative Results

A growing number of investigators have reported results using tamoxifen in advanced endometrial carcinoma. These data are summarized in table 8. The individual series are small, but the cumulative data in 91 women suggest an overall response rate of approximately 30% and a complete response rate of approximately 10%. The variability of the responding proportion between studies is considerable and may be, in part, explained by differing prognostic characteristics within the treated groups. For example, Bonte (4) found 9 of 17 women responded. However, only 2 of his 17 patients had undifferentiated tumours while

6 of 17 had well differentiated disease - a very different, prognostically more favourable, population of patients compared to our series.

TABLE 8. Tamoxifen in endometrial cancer

Investigator	No. of Pts	CR	PR	ST
Tisman et al (25)	2	-	-	2
Broens et al (5)	5	1	1	1
Quinn et al (17)	6	1	1	-
Bonte (4)	17	2	7	4
Hald et al (10)	26	4	4	7
Swenerton et al this report	35	2	6	5
Totals	91	10 11%	19 21%	19 21%

CONCLUSION

Tamoxifen now has an established role in the palliative care of certain patients with advanced or recurrent endometrial carcinoma. It provides a nontoxic alternative to progestins and produces objective responses in a similar proportion of patients. Like progestins, the frequency of response to tamoxifen is inversely proportional to tumour grade and proportional to disease-free interval. Not surprisingly, response is more likely in those patients who previously responded to progestins. The durability of response is also greater in those with low grade tumours and longer disease-free intervals.

It has now also been demonstrated that sequential hormonal responses can be achieved, extending the palliative potential of hormone therapy in this disease.

The optimal sequence of hormone therapies has yet to be determined. The intriguing potential for combination hormonal therapy, particularly the use of antiestrogens to induce functional steroid receptors in what otherwise might be hormonally non-responsive disease, remains to be fully explored.

ACKNOWLEDGEMENTS

The authors wish to thank the members of the Division of Gynecologic Oncology of the CCABC for their support and helpful suggestions. Particular gratitude is owed to Lorraine Cho for invaluable assistance with the manuscript.

REFERENCES

1. Allegra, J., Day, T., Carlson, J. and Wittliff, J. (1983): *Am. Soc. Clin. Oncol.*, (abstract), 2:C-562.
2. Benraad, Th.J., Friberg, L.G., Koenders, A.J.M. and Kullanders, S. (1980): *Acta. Obstet. Gynecol. Scand.*, 59:155-159.

3. Bonte, J., Decoster, J.M. Ide, P. and Billiet, G. (1978): *Gynecol. Oncol.*, 6:60-75.

4. Bonte, J., Ide, P., Billiet, G. and Wynants, P. (1981): *Gynecol. Oncol.*, 11:140-616.

5. Broens, J., Mouridsen, H.T. and Soerensen, H.M. (1980): *Cancer Chemother. Pharmacol.*, 4:213.

6. Bruchovsky, N. and Goldie, J.H. (1983): *Drugs and Hormone Resistance in Neoplasia*. CRC Press, Boca Raton.

7. Carbone, P.P. and Carter S.K. (1974): *Gynecol. Oncol.*, 2:348-353.

8. Cole, M.P., Jones, C.T.A. and Todd, I.D.H. (1971): *Br. J. Cancer*, 25:270-275.

9. Donovan, J.F. (1974): *Cancer*, 34, 1587-1592.

10. Hald, I., Pagel, J., Salimtschik, M. and Mouridsen, H.T. (1982): *Rev. Endocr-Rel. Cancer*, 11:43-46.

11. International Union Against Cancer (1977): *Br. J. Cancer*, 35:292.

12. Jensen, E.V., Suzuki, T., Kawashima, T., Strumpf, W.E., Jungblut, P.W. and DeSombre, E.R. (1968): *Proc. Natl. Acad. Sci. USA*. 59:632.

13. Kauppila, A. and Vihko, R. (1981): *Acta. Obstet. Gynecol. Scand.*, 60:589-590.

14. Kohorn, E.I. (1976): *Gynecol. Oncol.*, 4:398-411.

15. Oken, M.M., Creech, R.H., Tormey, D.C., Horton, J., Davis, T.E., McFadden, E.T. and Carbone, P.P. (1982): *Am. J. Clin. Oncol. (CTT)*, 5:649-655.

16. Piver, M.S., Barlow, J.J., Lurain, J.R. and Blumenson, L.E. (1980): *Cancer*, 45:268-272.

17. Quinn, M.A., Campbell, J.J., Murray, R. and Pepperell, R.J. (1981): *Aust. NZ. J. Obstet. Gynaecol.*, 21:226-229.

18. Robel, P., Levy, C., Wolff, J-P, Nicolas, J-C. and Baulieu, E-E. (1979): *C.R. Acad. Sc. Paris*, 287:1353-1356.

19. Sekiya, S. and Takamizawa, H. (1976): *Br. J. Obstet. Gynaecol.*, 83:183-186.

20. Smith, J.P. (1978): *Surg. Clin. North Am.*, 58:201-215.

21. Swenerton, K.D. (1980): *Cancer Treat. Rep.*, 64:805-811.

22. Swenerton, K.D. (1982): *Rev. Endocr-Rel. Cancer*, 11:47-49.

23. Swenerton, K.D. (1982): *Clinics in Oncology*, 1:215-232.

24. Swenerton, K.D., Shaw, D., White, G.W. and Boyes, D.A. (1979): *N. Engl. J. Med.*, 301:105.

25. Tisman, G., Kellon, D.B., Wu, S. and Safire, G.E. (1976): *Clinical Research*, 24:381A.

26. Young, R.C. (1979): In: *Cancer Chemotherapy*, edited by H.M. Pinedo, pp. 361-375, Elsevier, New York.

Progress in Cancer Research and Therapy,
Vol. 31, edited by F. Bresciani, et al.
Raven Press, New York © 1984.

Biochemical Endocrinology of Human Prostatic Tumors

M. Krieg

Department of Clinical Chemistry, Medical Clinic, University of Hamburg, D-2000
Hamburg 20, Federal Republic of Germany

The human benign prostatic hyperplasia (BPH) and prostatic carcinoma (PCA) are the tumors that are the topic of this chapter. Both tumors are very common and their incidence is extremely age-dependent. This is underlined by autopsy findings which demonstrate that BPH is practically non-existent in men younger than 40 years, while in about 85% of men over 80 years a histologically proven BPH is found (13). Also the PCA occurs in only a very small percentage of men who are younger than 40 years, but in about 44% of men older than 80 years (8). Although each BPH or PCA does not gain clinical relevance, still about 50% of patients of an urological department are suffering from these tumors. Moreover, the PCA plays an overwhelming role in male cancer statistics (12): 7.600 deaths per year in the Federal Republic of Germany and 19.000 deaths per year in the U.S.A. are ascribed to PCA. It contributes 8% of all cancer diseases in the male and it is after cancer of the lung and the gastrointestinal tract the third most common cancer of males in the western countries. All these figures make it clear why tremendous efforts are being undertaken to elucidate the still unknown etiology of both human prostatic tumors.

Two fundamental problems complicate human prostatic research at the cellular level. First, sampling and amount of tissue. This point is at once understood when the topography of the prostate is considered. This organ, which normally has the size of a chestnut and the weight of 20 g, is located deep within the urogenital tract. Therefore, sampling of normal prostatic tissue is only possible by transurethral resection or by biopsy via the rectum. Indications for this are practically non-existent. Otherwise, tissue will be available only after prostatectomy, which is in turn rare in cases of PCA or for obtaining normal prostatic tissue. A second point must also be stressed, namely the heterogeneity of the tissue. We know for example that the prostate is composed of an outer and inner zone as well as of stroma and epithelium, compartments which may play completely different roles in the development and maintenance of BPH and PCA (18). Furthermore, heterogeneity is present due to the fact that small areas of normal and diseased prostatic tissue are closely opposed.

ENDOCRINE ENVIRONMENT OF THE HUMAN PROSTATE

It is widely accepted that the fetal and postnatal development of the normal prostate (NPR) is regulated by sexual
steroids (7,37). Furthermore, with respect to the PCA, the
classical papers of Huggins' group (20,21) have shown its
regression after castration or estrogen administration. Finally, concerning the BPH, Moore (35) has reported on its
absence in eunuchs and related cases, and Huggins and Stevens
(19) have shown its regression following castration. These
data suggest that the human prostate is under hormonal control and that androgens and estrogens in particular exert an
exceptional influence on normal and diseased prostatic
tissue.

A first set of studies, devoted to the endocrine control
of human BPH and PCA, was therefore the measurement of the
hormonal environment which may be relevant for prostatic
function, whereby hormones from the testis, adrenal cortex
and pituitary received the most attention. In addition to
the hormones, the plasmatic sex-hormone-binding-globulin
(SHBG) is a potential regulating factor for prostatic function, because it is normally able to bind large amounts of
the circulating androgens and estrogens (4,34,40,42). As it
is well accepted (44,45) that only free, non protein-bound
steroids in plasma enter prostatic cells, the SHBG could indirectly control this steroid uptake. For several years we
have measured hormones and SHBG in blood from patients with
BPH, PCA and from age-matched controls. Through these studies
we hoped to find differences between the three groups with
respect to their blood parameters, and then discuss these
differences as causative factors for the prostatic tumors in
question. Based on our studies (1-3,9) which are more or less
in accordance with the literature (16,45), the following can
be stated: If the BPH group is compared with age-matched controls, no significant difference in testicular and adrenal
steroids, pituitary hormones or in SHBG can be found. The
same holds true if the PCA group is compared with age-matched
controls or if the BPH group is compared with the PCA group.
Hence, there seems to be no specific pattern in the plasmatic
endocrine environment of the human prostate which can be undoubtedly related to BPH or PCA patients, and so far these
studies have not enabled us to link the pathogenesis of prostatic tumors with endocrinological factors. However, as
schematized in Fig. 1, basic problems, underlying this kind
of study, make the aforementioned conclusion less valid. The
above mentioned age dependence and high incidence of BPH and
PCA, ie, the universality of these tumors in aging males,
leads us to question whether we have appropriate age-matched
controls which are absolutely free of neoplasms; this in turn
makes each comparison between a BPH or PCA group with age-
matched controls questionable. However, the endocrine environment of the male, and therefore of the prostate, undoubtedly shows age-dependent changes, eg, a decrease of
androgens (A), and an increase of the estrogen/androgen (E/A)

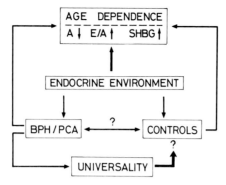

Fig. 1. Scheme of interrelationship between patients with prostatic tumors and age-matched controls. BPH = benign prostatic hyperplasia; PCA = prostatic carcinoma. For further details see text.

ratio and the SHBG level. As long as question marks remain around the age-matched controls due to the universality of prostatic tumors in aging males it cannot be definetely decided whether the age-dependent alterations of the endocrine environment have a pathogenetic significance for the tumors of aging males, or whether these alterations merely reflect the process of aging. Therefore, despite numerous studies it cannot be excluded that the endocrine environment may be of additive or secondary importance to other potential etiological factors with respect to both tumors.

PLASMA VERSUS TISSUE: STEROID AND SHBG LEVELS

From two series of experiments (24,26), in which we simultaneously measured steroids and SHBG in plasma and BPH tissue, mean ratios and correlations were calculated as summarized in Table 1. From the ratios it is evident that 5α-dihydrotestosterone (DHT), estrone and estradiol accumulate in the tissue, as indicated by the figures which are distinctly lower than 1. In contrast, such an accumulation does not

TABLE 1

PARAMETER	RATIO PLASMA/BPH	CORRELATION PLASMA vs BPH	(n)
TESTOSTERONE	14.3	N.S.	(11)
DHT	0.1	N.S.	(13)
ESTRONE	0.5	N.S.	(7)
ESTRADIOL	0.7	N.S.	(11)
SHBG	16.7	P < 0.05	(13)

TABLE 2

RATIO: DHT / TESTOSTERONE

	PLASMA	TISSUE
BPH	0.1	15.0
PCA	0.1	3.3
NPR	0.1	8.0

occur with respect to testosterone and SHBG. Furthermore, based on the correlation between plasma and BPH, no significance was found for steroid levels. Only the SHBG levels were significantly correlated. The data of Table 1 indicate that in the BPH tissue important events take place which regulate the tissue concentration of these steroids; therefore the plasmatic environment appears to be uncoupled. On the contrary, with regard to SHBG the high ratio as well as the significant correlation between plasma and BPH levels, which we have found also for PCA (27), suggest that the cellular SHBG merely reflects the plasmatic contamination of the prostatic tumors. However, it should not be neglected that the SHBG in the tissue itself may be involved in steroid accumulation due to its high binding affinity particularly to DHT. The effectiveness of cellular events involved in steroid accumulation is further substantiated when DHT/testosterone ratios in plasma and prostatic tissue are considered for a BPH, PCA and control group (Table 2), whereby the quotients were derived from our results (2,3,26,28). It should be noted that in 1970 Siiteri and Wilson (41) first demonstrated in their classical paper that the reversal of the quotient in the BPH group is primarily due to an excessive accumulation of DHT in the BPH tissue. The quotients of Table 2 suggest that such an accumulation generally occurs in the human prostate. Furthermore, with regard to the tissue ratios striking differences between BPH, PCA and NPR are found, explainable by differences in androgen metabolism, as we will see later.

STUDIES AT THE CELLULAR LEVEL IN HUMAN PROSTATE

These studies are comprised of the measurement of steroid receptors, steroid metabolism and steroids at the cellular level in NPR, BPH and PCA. Since the human prostate is undoubtedly an androgen dependent organ they have been primarily devoted to androgens. Parallel to these human studies numerous animal experiments, particularly on the rat prostate, have been performed which have led to our present knowledge about the mechanism of androgenic action in target organs (25,32). This chain of events will be briefly reviewed, in order to make the various aspects of human prostatic research understandable.

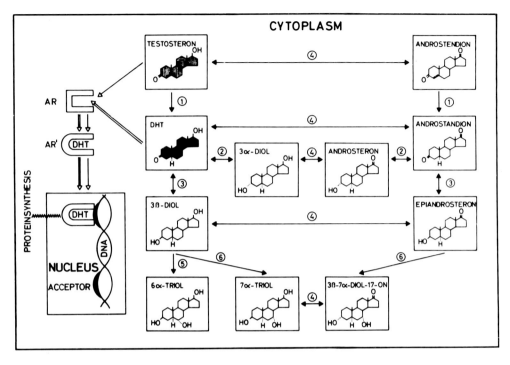

Fig. 2. Scheme of androgen metabolism and androgen-receptor-
interaction at the cellular level of androgenic target
organs. 1 = 5α-reductase (EC 1.3.99.5); 2 = 3α-hydroxysteroid
dehydrogenase (EC 1.1.1.50); 3 = 3β-hydroxysteroid dehydrogenase (EC 1.1.1.51); 4 = 17β-hydroxysteroid oxidoreductase
(EC 1.1.1.63); 5 = 5α-steroid-6α-hydroxylase; 6 = 5α-steroid-
7α-hydroxylase. AR = androgen receptor.

Mechanism of androgenic action

Testosterone, the main circulating androgen, probably enters the cell by passive diffusion. Within the cytoplasm
(Fig. 2) it is irreversibly converted to DHT by 5α-reductase.
Two further enzymes, 3α- and 3β-hydroxysteroid dehydrogenase
(HSDH), reversibly convert DHT to 5α-androstane-3α,17β-diol
(3α-diol) and 5α-androstane-3β,17β-diol (3β-diol), respectively. Still another enzyme, 17β-hydroxysteroid oxidoreductase, metabolizes testosterone to androstenedione; however,
this oxidative pathway is of minor importance. The aforementioned 5α-reductase also converts androstenedione to androstanedione, and the 3α- and 3β-HSDH androstanedione to androsterone and epiandrosterone, respectively. These in turn can
be converted to 3α- and 3β-diol by 17β-hydroxysteroid oxido-
reductase. Endpoints of this pathway of androgens are the
triols (22,36), which are irreversibly formed primarily by
the conversion of 3β-diol. The whole pathway is linked with
the androgen receptor machinery due to the fact that only

TABLE 3

**NUMBER OF RESEARCH GROUPS WHICH HAVE SHOWN
STEROID RECEPTORS IN HUMAN PROSTATE**

	NPR		PCA		BPH	
	C	N	C	N	C	N
AR	6	4	*8	4	*12	*11
ER	2	1	*6	1	*7	1
PR	2	--	4	--	7	1

* containing our group

DHT, and to some extent testosterone, have a high affinity to
the cytosolic androgen receptor (AR). A cytosolic AR-DHT-
complex is then formed which will be translocated into the
nucleus where the androgenic stimulus is transcribed. According to our present knowledge it must be assumed that the androgenic response of the prostate is mediated exclusively by
the selective translocation of the DHT-receptor complex into
the nucleus. The DHT is therefore responsible for the androgenic response, eg, the induction of cell hyperplasia.

Steroid receptors in human prostate

In Table 3 the number of research groups which have independently shown steroid receptors in human prostate between
1975 and 1983 are compiled. Receptor proteins for androgen
(AR), estrogen (ER) and progestin (PR) in the cytosolic (C)
and nuclear fractions (N) of NPR, PCA and BPH are included.
With regard to their binding characteristics, these receptors
are comparable to steroid receptors characterized in classical animal target organs. Table 3 primarily demonstrates that
in the 100.000xg cytosol, and with certain reservations in
the nuclear fraction, of NPR, PCA and BPH, AR, ER and PR are
undoubtedly present. Therefore, in general these figures
allow the assumption that the normal and diseased human prostate is a target organ, particularly for androgens and
estrogens. This would be in accordance with the assumed physiology and pathophysiology of the human prostate. These
steroid receptor studies, ie, their main results and their
relevance to prostatic tumor research, must be considered
separately for NPR, PCA and BPH.

Steroid receptors in NPR.
Concerning the NPR the main results are: First, there are
no significant differences with respect to steroid receptors
in animal target organs like rat prostate. This was found by
us using agargel electrophoresis for receptor assay (29).
Second, there are no significant qualitative or quantitative
differences with respect to steroid receptors in BPH and PCA.
Therefore the results offer no aid to understanding the
pathogenesis of BPH and PCA, and so far a specific pathoge-

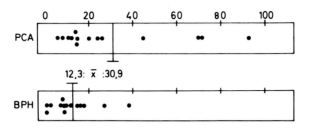

Fig. 3. Cytosolic assayable androgen receptor concentration found in prostatic carcinoma (PCA) and benign prostatic hyperplasia (BPH). For further details see reference no. 27.

netic role of steroid receptors in the human prostate is not discernible.

Steroid receptors in PCA.
Regarding the PCA, the main clinical interest has been focussed on the AR, while the significance of the assayable ER and PR remains completely obscure. Therefore, the summary of results is restricted to the AR. Nearly all studies have revealed a great variation in AR content and a tendency to higher values compared to BPH. This is shown by Fig. 3 in which our results are summarized. A further conclusion is that the predictive role of the AR in evaluating the response to endocrine therapy is uncertain. If one is asking whether the AR in PCA is a prognostic factor for response to therapy, one group is answering "yes" (11,15,33,43), the other "no" (6,10,38,46). In addition, within the "yes" and "no" groups the results are not generally in accordance. At the moment, however, the paper of Ghanadian et al. (15) as well as Trachtenberg and Walsh (43) merit the most attention, because they are best validated methodically. Moreover, both groups independently claim that the nuclear AR content, classified as "rich" or "poor", can play an important predictive role, as the receptor "rich" cases have a significantly longer duration of response to endocrine therapy as well as a longer survival rate. Therefore, these latter findings allow the assumption that the discrimination of the PCA group as AR "rich" or "poor" may be a prognostic factor in terms of evaluating the response to endocrine therapy, in parallel to the ER in the mammary carcinoma.

Steroid receptors in BPH.
The main results and relevance of these studies are only understandable if it is considered that the BPH is composed of fibromuscular stroma and epithelium and that growth and integrity of the epithelium is strongly dependent upon the adjacent stroma (14). Keeping these facts in mind, the data which we have published recently (30) and are summarized in

TABLE 4

STEROID RECEPTORS IN BPH

CYTOSOL	POSITIVE CASES		PERCENTAGE	
	AR	ER	AR	ER
STROMA	12/20	8/19	60	42
EPITHELIUM	11/19	1/20	58	5

AR+ : above 10 fmol/mg protein
ER+ : above 22 fmol/mg protein

Table 4 merit most attention. With regard to the AR we succeeded in demonstrating positive cases in nearly identical
percentages in the cytosol of stroma and epithelium. In contrast, the percentage of the ER positive cases was strikingly
higher in stroma compared to epithelium, in the latter compartment ER could be found only in one single case. The possible relevance of these results is that, in addition to androgens, estrogens via ER may account for the essential role
the stroma plays in the pathogenesis of BPH.

ANDROGEN METABOLISM AND STEROID LEVELS IN HUMAN PROSTATE

With regard to the steroid metabolism in human prostate,
only the metabolism of androgens needs to be considered, because other pathways have only been described sporadicly,
and up to now their significance remains completely obscure.
The various aspects of androgen metabolism and its linkage
via DHT to the receptor machinery has already been introduced
in Fig. 2 and it can be stated that all enzymatic steps have
also been found in the human prostate (45). However, because
of the aforementioned importance which DHT plays in prostatic
function, the measurement of 5α-reductase and $3\alpha(\beta)$-HSDH, the
enzymes primarily involved in the regulation of the tissue
concentration of testosterone, DHT, 3α- and 3β-diol, was of
paramount interest.

Our group has also been interested in this pathway and we
have therefore investigated two crucial questions: First, are
there differences in the reductive pathway of testosterone
between NPR, BPH and PCA and if so, are these differences reflected by endogenous steroid levels? The answer to both
these questions is yes and our results are illustrated in
Table 5. The mean relative enzyme activities of 5α-reductase
and $3\alpha(\beta)$-HSDH have been calculated from in vitro metabolic
results (28). For clarity it must be pointed out that we are
using the term $3\alpha(\beta)$-HSDH, although two different enzymes are
present. However, in pilot studies we found that 3β-diol contributes to less than 15% of the total 5α-androstanediol formation. Therefore the resolution of 3α- and 3β-diol was not
performed in all studies.

The steroid levels in Table 5 are also derived from our

TABLE 5

MEAN RELATIVE ENZYME ACTIVITIES (%) AND STEROID LEVELS (ng/g tissue)

	T	5α-R →	DHT	3α(β)HSDH →	3α(β)-DIOL
NPR (n=3-7)	0.2	100	1.6	100	1.7
BPH (n=11-16)	0.3	151	4.5	83	0.6
PCA (n=3-10)	1.2	24	3.9	44	1.6

studies (28). It must be stressed that we have measured only 3α-diol, although in Table 5 the term 3α(β)-diol is used. To date the actual 3β-diol concentration in the normal and diseased human prostate is unknown. Nevertheless, taking the enzyme activity in the NPR as 100%, the 5α-reductase is significantly higher in BPH and significantly lower in PCA. On the contrary, the 3α(β)-HSDH is highest in the NPR, followed by BPH and PCA. These relative enzyme activities are reflected to a great extent by testosterone (T), DHT and 3α-diol levels, measured radioimmunologically in the same tissue. Due to the rather low 5α-reductase we expect and find a significantly higher T level in PCA than in BPH and NPR. On the other hand, due to the extremely high 5α-reductase and relatively low 3α(β)-HSDH we expect and find significantly higher DHT levels in BPH than in NPR. Finally, in NPR we expect a high concentration of 3α-diol due to the relatively high 3α(β)-HSDH activity; this is clearly shown, the concentration being significantly higher than in BPH. The only finding which does not fulfill our expectations are the comparatively high DHT and 3α-diol levels in PCA for which we have no convincing explanation. In our original publication (28) this point has been thoroughly discussed and related data of other groups have been reviewed extensively.

Keeping our data in mind and considering the literature (17,44,45), the androgen metabolism in the human prostate can be summarized as follows: Concerning the PCA, the metabolism of testosterone is greatly decreased compared to NPR and BPH, however, it must be confessed that the relevance of this finding to the role in the pathogenesis of PCA remains unclear. Concerning the BPH, the metabolism of T is greatly shifted towards DHT as compared to NPR, where the pathway is shifted to 3α-diol. This finding, which has recently been convincingly confirmed (23), may be relevant, as excessive accumulation of DHT - due to an acquired error of androgen metabolism (28) - could induce and/or sustain BPH.

TABLE 6

$$(n=10) \quad K_M \left[\mu M \right] \quad (n=5)$$

5 α − Reductase[*]   3α (ß) − HSDH[°]

Epithelium		
Stroma	0.15 ± 0.08 (SD)	1.5 ± 0.8 (SD)
Whole tissue		

[*] Substrate = Testosterone

[°] ——⫫—— = DHT

STROMAL-EPITHELIAL INTERACTION IN HUMAN BPH

In the foregoing paragraphs it was pointed out that the pathogenesis of BPH is increasingly discussed in the light of a stromal-epithelial interaction. In this regard the favoured assay of ER in the stroma has already been shown (Table 4). In addition, we have measured the 5α-reductase and 3α(ß)-HSDH as well as DHT, estradiol and estrone in epithelium and stroma of BPH and NPR (5,24,30,31).

5α-reductase and 3α(ß)-HSDH in stroma and epithelium

In Table 6 the Michaelis constants (K_M) of the 5α-reductase and 3α(ß)-HSDH are shown. We found that the mean K_M of the 5α-reductase is 10 times lower compared to the K_M of the 3α(ß)-HSDH. Furthermore, we did not find any systematic difference in the K_M's between epithelium and stroma. In addition, we have found identical K_M's in whole BPH tissue. The identical K_M of the 5α-reductase in epithelium and stroma is in contrast to the findings of others (39), who have reported that the K_M of the epithelial fraction is 3-4-fold lower. At the moment an explanation for this discrepancy cannot be given. However, the identical K_M of the 5α-reductase in epithelium and stroma, as illustrated in Table 6, is in accordance with identical inhibition constants which we found when using progesterone, estradiol or estrone as inhibitors for the 5α-reductase in epithelium and stroma (Table 7). There-

TABLE 7

INHIBITION OF TESTOSTERONE−5 α −REDUCTASE

BPH tissue	INHIBITION CONSTANT (μM)		
	Progesterone	Estradiol	Estrone
Whole tissue	0.13	4.3	14.5
Epithelium	0.09	4.8	14.0
Stroma	0.12	2.8	14.5

TABLE 8

V_{max}

[pmol × mg protein^{-1} × hr^{-1}]

	5α – Reductase		3α(ß) – HSDH	
	BPH	NPR	BPH	NPR
Epithelium	66 ± 5 (20)*	42 ± 7 (4)	539 ± 43 (12)	666 ± 131 (5)
Stroma	161 ± 28 (20)	74 ± 9 (4)	436 ± 22 (12)	256 ± 39 (5)
Whole tissue	148 ± 7 (20)	68 ± 10 (3)	526 ± 53 (7)	535 ± 16 (3)

* $\bar{x}$ ± SEM (n)

fore, when calculating the maximal metabolic rates (V_{max}), we used the mean K_M of the 5α-reductase and 3α(ß)-HSDH throughout. The data are summarized in Table 8. Concerning the V_{max} of the 5α-reductase, ie, the maximal conversion rate of testosterone to 5α-reduced metabolites, the BPH stroma possesses about 2.5 times higher activity than BPH epithelium. This difference is less striking in the NPR. Furthermore, compared to the BPH, the 5α-reductase is in general significantly lower in NPR. This leads to a more than 2 times higher 5α-reductase activity in the whole BPH tissue compared to NPR, and apparently this difference between BPH and NPR is predominantly dictated by the high 5α-reductase in BPH stroma. Concerning the V_{max} of 3α(ß)-HSDH, ie, the maximal conversion rate of DHT to 3α- and 3ß-diol, it is remarkable that this enzyme shows a clear tendency to higher values in epithelium compared to the stroma. In addition, comparing BPH and NPR there is in general no significant difference in 3α(ß)-HSDH activity, in contrast to the 5α-reductase. Finally, this series of experiments has revealed that the 3α(ß)-HSDH activity is overall 3-10 times higher than the 5α-reductase. Thus we have the following situation: Per unit protein the human prostate possesses 3-10 times more 3α(ß)-HSDH than 5α-reductase. On the other hand, the K_M of 5α-reductase is on average 10 times lower than of the 3α(ß)-HSDH. Taking both findings, the V_{max} and K_M values, into account, relative metabolic activities can be calculated (31). The results are shown in Fig. 4. Theoretically these ratios of 5α-reduction to 3α(ß)-reduction are indicators of the extent of enzymatically regulated DHT enrichment in the tissue under steady state conditions, ie, whether the primary reaction, the testosterone conversion to DHT, predominates the secondary reaction, the conversion of DHT to 3α- and 3ß-diol, or vice versa. In the epithelium of BPH and NPR ratios of about 1 are found, meaning that enzymatically the epithelium (E) of the normal and diseased prostate might be effectively protected against DHT enrichment. In contrast, the BPH stroma (S) possesses by far the highest ratio, meaning that in the BPH stroma under steady state conditions the highest DHT accumulation occurs. Finally, it is remarkable that the relative

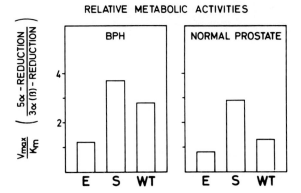

Fig. 4. Relative metabolic activities of 5α- to 3α(ß)-reduction in epithelium (E), stroma (S) and whole tissue (WT) of human benign prostatic hyperplasia (BPH) and normal prostate. The bars represent the mean quotients, which have been calculated as outlined in reference no. 31.

metabolic activity in the whole tissue fraction of BPH is 2 times higher than in the NPR, indicating a 2-fold higher DHT enrichment in the BPH compared to the NPR.

Steroid levels in stroma and epithelium

In a series of experiments (5,24) we have measured radioimmunologically androgens and estrogens in epithelium and

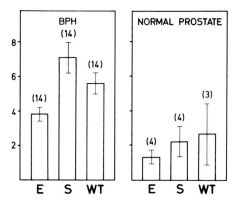

Fig. 5. 5α-dihydrotestosterone (DHT) concentration in nuclei of epithelium (E), stroma (S) and whole tissue (WT) of human benign prostatic hyperplasia (BPH) and normal prostate. After extraction, DHT was quantified by radioimmunoassay. The bars represent the mean ± SEM. The number of prostates examined is shown in brackets. For further details see reference no. 5.

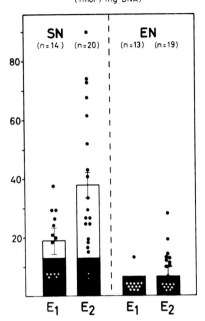

Fig. 6. Estradiol (E_2) and estrone (E_1) concentration in nuclei of stroma (SN) and epithelium (EN) of human benign prostatic hyperplasia, analyzed by radioimmunoassay. The bars represent the mean ± SEM, the solid part of the bars the lower detection limit of the assay.

stroma of BPH, and DHT also in NPR. The data at the nuclear level are shown here. Concerning DHT (Fig. 5), nuclei of BPH stroma possess approximately a 2 times higher concentration than nuclei of the epithelium. Furthermore, in BPH nuclei a higher DHT concentration is generally present than in NPR nuclei. It should be added that the nuclear DHT concentration represents nearly 80% of the total DHT content in the prostate. Particularly with respect to the BPH this distribution of nuclear DHT strongly resembles the distribution of the relative metabolic activities (Fig. 4). Thus we have concluded that the difference in nuclear DHT content between epithelium and stroma of BPH, as well as the overall difference between BPH and NPR, are predominantly dictated by differences in androgen metabolism and that the receptor concentration in the human prostate is always adaquate for translocation of all enzymatically regulated DHT. From this finding, the stroma of BPH becomes the central point of interest. It is the preferential tissue within the BPH for androgenic action.

Moreover, as shown by Fig. 6, we have succeeded in demonstrating for the first time a preferential localization of estrogens, primarily estradiol (E_2), in the stroma nuclei (SN) of BPH, while the epithelial nuclei (EN) contain only small amounts of E_2, the mean being just at the lower detec-

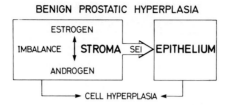

Fig. 7. Scheme of the pathogenesis of the human benign prostatic hyperplasia. SEI = stromal-epithelial interaction.

tion limit of the radioimmunoassay. This finding correlates excellently with the preferential detection of estrogen receptors in BPH stroma although further studies are needed to prove this interrelationship. Nevertheless these data suggest that the BPH stroma is the preferred compartment for not only androgenic, but also for estrogenic action.

Pathogenetic model for human BPH

Compiling the literature (18), the following pathogenetic model for human BPH may be put forward (Fig. 7): In the BPH stroma an imbalance originates between androgens, especially DHT, and estrogens, especially estradiol. It must be stressed that this imbalance originates at the cellular level in the stroma, and is not merely a reflection of plasmatic contaminants. This imbalance then leads to stromal hyperplasia and, due to the aforementioned stromal-epithelial interaction (SEI), to a hyperplasia of the epithelial compartment. The BPH therefore seems to be primarily a stromal and not, as has been widely assumed, an epithelial disease.

CLINICAL RELEVANCE OF PROSTATIC TUMOR RESEARCH

If the high incidence rate and clinical significance of both prostatic tumors are recalled, one question automatically arises, namely what is the clinical relevance of such tumor research for diagnosis and therapy of PCA and BPH? The answer is 2-fold: It is the author's belief that in the case of PCA the androgen receptor assay will attain in the near future a role similar to the estrogen receptor assay for the mammary carcinoma. Hereby the androgen receptor poor cases will be of particular interest because they should be treated at once by an alternative, non-endocrine therapy. Concerning the BPH, so far the biochemical studies are of no value regarding the diagnosis. However, based on the research results, in the near future an alternative to prostatectomy may be an endocrine therapy with 5α-reductase inhibitors or anti-estrogens.

ACKNOWLEDGEMENTS

These studies were supported by the DFG, Sonderforschungs-bereich 34 "Endokrinologie". For secreterial assistance the author thanks Mrs. K. Balmumcu.

REFERENCES

1. Bartsch, W., Steins, P., and Becker, H. (1977): Eur. Urol., 3:47-52.
2. Bartsch, W., Horst, H.-J., Becker H., and Nehse, G. (1977): Acta Endocrinol., 85:650-664.
3. Bartsch, W., Becker, H., Pinkenburg, F.-A., and Krieg, M. (1979): Acta Endocrinol., 90: 727-736.
4. Bartsch, W. (1980): Maturitas, 2:109-118.
5. Bartsch, W., Krieg, M., Becker, H., Mohrmann, J., and Voigt, K.D. (1982): Acta Endocrinol., 100:634-640.
6. Bashirelahi, N., Young, J.D., Sidh, S.M., and Sanefuji, H. (1980): In: Steroid Receptors, Metabolism and Prostatic Cancer, edited by F.H. Schröder, and H.J. de voogt, pp 240-256. Excerpta Medica, Amsterdam.
7. Blacklock, N.J. (1982): In: The Endocrinology of Prostate Tumors, edited by R. Ghanadian, pp 1-13. MTP Press, Lancaster.
8. Chisholm, G.D. and Beynon, L.L. (1982): In: The Endocrinology of Prostate Tumors, edited by R. Ghanadian, pp 241-262. MTP Press, Lancaster.
9. Dennis, M., Horst, H.-J., Krieg, M., and Voigt, K.D. (1977): Acta Endocrinol., 84:207-214.
10. De Voogt, H.J. and Dingjan, P. (1978): Urol. Res., 6:151-158.
11. Ekman, P., Snochowski, M., Zetterberg, A., Högberg, B. and Gustafsson, J.-A. (1979): Cancer, 44:1173-1181.
12. Faul, P. (1982): In: Prostate Cancer, edited by G.H. Jacobi and R. Hohenfellner, pp 57-68. Williams and Wilkins, Baltimore.
13. Franks, L.M. (1954): Ann. R. Coll. Surg., 14:92-106.
14. Franks, L.M., Riddle, P.N., Carbonell, A.W., and Gey, G.O. (1970): J. Pathol., 100:113-119.
15. Ghanadian, R., Auf, G., Williams, G., Davis, A., and Richards, B. (1981): Lancet, 2:1418.
16. Ghanadian, R. (1982): In: The Endocrinology of Prostate Tumors, edited by R. Ghanadian, pp 59-86. MTP Press, Lancaster.
17. Ghanadian, R. and Smith, C.B. (1982): In: The Endocrinology of Prostate Tumors, edited by R. Ghanadian, pp 113-142. MTP Press, Lancaster.
18. Hinman, F., editor (1983): Benign Prostatic Hypertrophy. Springer-Verlag, New York.
19. Huggins, C. and Stevens, R.A. (1940): J. Urol., 43:705-714.
20. Huggins, C. and Hodges, C.V. (1941): Cancer Res., 1:293-297.
21. Huggins, C., Stevens, R., and Hodges, C.V. (1941): Arch. Surg., 43:209-223.
22. Isaacs, J.T., McDermott, I.R., and Coffey, D.S. (1979): Steroids, 33:675-692.
23. Isaacs, J.T., Brendler, C.B., and Walsh, P.C. (1983): J. Clin. Endocrinol. Metab., 56:139-146.
24. Kozak, l., Bartsch, W., Krieg, M., and Voigt, K.D. (1982): Prostate, 3:433-438.

25. Krieg, M. and Voigt, K.D. (1977): Acta Endocrinol.
    [Suppl.], 214:43-89.
26. Krieg, M., Bartsch, W., Herzer, S., Becker, H., and
    Voigt, K.D. (1977): Acta Endocrinol., 86:200-215.
27. Krieg, M., Grobe, I., Voigt, K.D., Altenähr, E., and
    Klosterhalfen, H. (1978): Acta Endocrinol., 88:397-407.
28. Krieg, M., Bartsch, W., Janssen, W., and Voigt, K.D.
    (1979): J. Steroid Biochem., 11:615-624.
29. Krieg, M., Smith, K., and Voigt, K.D. (1980): In:
    Pharmacological Modulation of Steroid Action, edited
    by E. Genazzani, F. DiCarlo, and W.I.P. Mainwaring,
    pp 123-130. Raven Press, New York.
30. Krieg, M., Klötzl, G., Kaufmann, J., and Voigt K.D.
    (1981): Acta Endocrinol., 96:422-432.
31. Krieg, M., Bartsch, W., Thomsen, M., and Voigt, K.D.
    (1983): J. Steroid Biochem., 19:155-161.
32. Mainwaring, W.I.P. (1977): The Mechanism of Action of
    Androgens. Springer-Verlag, New York.
33. Mobbs, B.G., Johnson, J.E., and Connolly, J.G. (1979):
    In: Prostate Cancer and Hormone Receptors, edited by
    G.P. Murphy, and A.A. Sandberg, pp 13-32. Alan R. Liss,
    New York.
34. Moll, G.W. and Rosenfield, R.L. (1979): J. Clin.
    Endocrinol. Metab., 49:730-736.
35. Moore, R.A. (1944): Surgery, 16:152-167.
36. Morfin, R.F., DiStefano, S., Charles, J.-F., and Floch,
    H.H. (1980): J. Steroid Biochem., 12:529-532.
37. Narbaitz, R. (1974): In: Male Accessory Sex Organs.
    Structure and Function in Mammals, edited by D. Brandes,
    pp 3-15. Academic Press, New York.
38. Pfitzenmaier, N., Schmid, W., and Röhl, L. (1980): In:
    Steroid Receptors, Metabolism and Prostatic Cancer,
    edited by F.H. Schröder, and H.J. de Voogt, pp 199-201.
    Excerpta Medica, Amsterdam.
39. Rennie, P.S., Bruchovsky, N., McLoughlin, M.G.,
    Batzold, F.H., and Dunstan-Adams, E.E. (1983):
    J. Steroid Biochem., 19:169-173.
40. Rubens, R., Dhont, M., and Vermeulen, A. (1974):
    J. Clin. Endocrinol. Metab., 39:40-45.
41. Siiteri, P.K. and Wilson, J.D. (1970): J. Clin. Invest.,
    49:1737-1745.
42. Stearns, E.L., Mac Donnell, J.A., Kaufman, B.J.,
    Padua, R., Lucman, T.S., Winter, J.S.D., and Faiman, C.
    (1974): Am. J. Med., 57:761-766.
43. Trachtenberg, J., and Walsh, P.C. (1982): J. Urol.,
    127:466-471.
44. Voigt, K.D., Horst, H.-J., and Krieg, M. (1975): Vitam.
    Horm., 33:417-436.
45. Voigt, K.D., and Krieg, M. (1978): In: Current Topics
    in Experimental Endocrinology, edited by L. Martini, and
    V.H.T. James, pp 173-199. Academic Press, New York.
46. Wagner, R.K., and Schulze, K.H. (1978): Acta Endocrinol.
    [Suppl.], 215:139-140.

Progress in Cancer Research and Therapy,
Vol. 31, edited by F. Bresciani, et al.
Raven Press, New York © 1984.

In Vivo Model for Uptake, Metabolism, and Binding of Androgens in Prostatic Tissue

W. Bartsch, H. Klein, G. Nehse, and K.D. Voigt

Department of Clinical Chemistry, Medical Clinic, University of Hamburg, D-2000 Hamburg 20, Federal Republic of Germany

The endogenous concentration of 5α-dihydrotestosterone (DHT) in the human prostate is regarded as an index of the androgen dependence in prostatic tumors (11). In benign hyperplasia as well as in prostatic carcinoma elevated levels of this androgen have been measured (for review, see (12)). As DHT possesses a high cell proliferative activity in animal experiments (19) and additionally is known to be the natural testosterone metabolite, which predominantly interacts with the androgen receptor system (9), its augmentation in the tissue might be a key event in the disregulation of prostatic growth in these diseases.

From a quantitative aspect, the plasma testosterone level or tissue DHT concentration required for a definitive growth response of the prostate and, perhaps more important, the level to which these constituents must be suppressed for an interruption of prostatic growth stimulation in diseased states is unknown. Although the rat ventral prostate is not an adequate model for prostatic tumors (20), the mechanism of androgen action is similar in various target organs and species. Therefore, model studies of rat ventral prostate might be helpful in defining the mechanism and significance of DHT accumulation in the prostate and its compartments under in vivo conditions for the stimulation of prostatic growth.

In two earlier publications, we characterized the accumulation of DHT in different organs of intact rats (1) and compared the growth response of the prostate with plasma and tissue androgen concentrations following systemic treatment of castrated animals with various doses of testosterone (3). We found a tremendous accumulation of DHT in prostate in comparison to blood and other tissues. A sensitive growth response of the prostate coincided with the DHT accumulation in the tissue, the accumulation being dicussed with respect to a high 5α-reductase activity and a high affinity and capacity of the androgen receptor to retain this metabolite. In continuation of these studies, we focussed our interest on the role of the androgen receptor in accumulating DHT in prostatic cytosol and nuclei under these experimental in vivo conditions.

MATERIALS AND METHODS

Treatment of animals.
Male Wistar rats weighing 340-380 g were used. The animals were castrated on day 1 and treated immediately with testosterone by subdermal
implantation of steroid releasing depots. The depots were prepared from
polydimethylsiloxane tubing. They released testosterone in vitro at a
rate of 6, 60 and 240 µg/24h (3). In 14-day castrated controls ("dose
0"), no depots were implanted. The animals were decapitated on day 15.
In studies with cyproterone acetate (CyAc), this drug was administered
(10 mg s.c. in 0.1 ml sesame oil/benzylbenzoate 3/2, v/v) on day 14, 24h
before decapitation. Determination of the cytosolic androgen receptor by
saturation analysis was performed with rats from which the testosterone
depot was removed 24h before decapitation. In some experiments intact
rats and 24h castrated animals were used.

Determination of DHT in cytosol and nuclei.
Preparation of homogenates, cytosols and purified nuclei as well as
the determination of DHT and testosterone in blood and in various tissue
fractions by RIA were performed as reported earlier (3). Unless otherwise stated, all procedures were performed in an ice bath at 0°C or in a
cold room at 0-4°C.
Dissociation experiments. The cytosol of intact rats was used directly or heated for 1h to 45°C, as indicated. 0.5 ml cytosol and 1.5 ml
dextran coated charcoal suspension (DCC, 0.5% w/v activated charcoal,
0.05% w/v dextran, 0.1% w/v gelatine in buffer I: 50 mM Tris x HCl,
5 mM NaN_3, 1.5 mM $CaCl_2$, pH 7.25) were mixed and rotated overhead
(25 rpm) for the indicated times. After centrifugation (1,000 g, 15 min),
DHT was determined in the supernatant by RIA. As "time-0"-control, the
total DHT content of 0.5 ml cytosol was measured without prior DCC
treatment.
Saturation experiments. Prostate homogenate from 24h castrated animals (0.7 ml) was added to test tubes, in which different amounts of DHT
(0-10 ng) had been evaporated, and was incubated for 2h. Following centrifugation at 100,000 g for 1h, 0.5 ml cytosol was mixed with 1.5 ml
DCC and rotated overhead (25 rpm, 1h), centrifuged (1,000 g, 15 min),
and DHT was determined in the supernatant by RIA.
Determination of "charcoal resistant" DHT (CR-DHT) and CR-DHT-
binding capacity. For the determination of CR-DHT-binding capacity,
0.45 ml prostate homogenate was incubated with 5 ng (38 nM final concentration) DHT for 2h, and centrifuged (100,000 g, 1h). 0.3 ml of the
supernatant was mixed with 0.9 ml of DCC and rotated overhead, as mentioned above. After centrifugation, DHT was measured in the supernatant
by RIA. CR-DHT concentration was determined by the same protocol, omit-
ting the addition of DHT. All determinations were performed in duplicate.

Determination of cytosolic androgen receptor.
The prostates were homogenized in 8 vol of buffer II (buffer I + 10
mM Na_2MoO_4) in a dounce apparatus. Following centrifugation (10,000 g,
10 min) to aliquots of the supernatant different amounts of ^3H-methyl-
trienolone (MT, 1.34-34 nM final conc.) in the same vol. of buffer II
were added, with and without the 100-fold excess of radioinert MT. The
samples were centrifuged (100,000 g, 1h) and maintained in an ice bath
up to 2.5h after the addition of MT. 0.1 ml of the incubated cytosols

was mixed with 0.1 ml protamine sulfate solution (2 mg/ml buffer II).
After 15 min the samples were centrifuged and the supernatant was discarded. The pellets were washed 5 times with 0.9 ml buffer II and the
radioactivity remaining in the pellet was extracted 2x with ethanol and
2x with methylene chloride. The combined extracts were evaporated and
the radioactivity was counted with 42% efficiency. Correction for un-
specific binding was performed by subtracting radioactivity in samples
with 100-fold excess of radioinert MT from those without unlabelled
steroid. The dissociation constant and maximum binding site concentration were determined graphically by Scatchard plots. All determinations
were performed in duplicate.

Miscellaneous. Protein was measured by the biuret reaction and DNA by
the Burton method as reported earlier (2,3). Cyproterone acetate in
plasma was determined by RIA (15), kindly performed by Dr. Düsterberg
(Berlin). Results were analyzed using analysis of variance.

RESULTS

Characterization of methods

In Fig. 1 and Fig. 2 methodological characteristics of
charcoal resistant DHT (CR-DHT) concentration and CR-DHT-
binding capacity are shown. After DCC treatment of cytosol
from intact rats, a time dependent decrease in DHT occurred
within the first 60 min; thereafter, the values remained con-

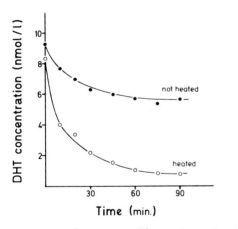 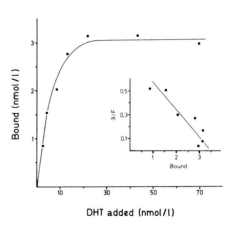

FIG. 1. (Left panel). Dissociation of DHT in prostate cytosol. Prostate
cytosol from intact rats was treated with dextran coated charcoal at 0°C
for the indicated times. After centrifugation, DHT was measured in the
supernatant by RIA. (●) Original cytosol, (o) cytosol heated to 45°C for
1h before adding charcoal.

FIG. 2. (Right panel). Saturation of charcoal resistant binding with
DHT. Prostate homogenate from 24h castrated rats was incubated with the
indicated amounts of DHT at 0°C for 2h. Cytosol was prepared, and was
treated for 1h with dextran coated charcoal. After centrifugation, DHT
was measured in the supernatant by RIA. Insert: transformation of data
according to Scatchard (21).

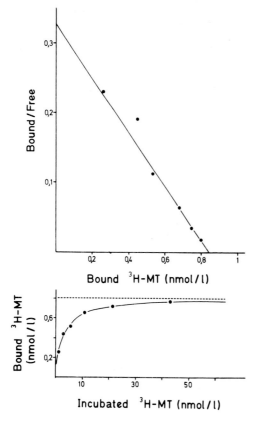

FIG. 3. Determination of cytosolic androgen receptor. Prostate cytosol from 24h castrated rats was incubated with various amounts of ^{3}H-methyltrienolone (MT) in the absence and presence of a 100-fold excess of radioinert MT. The androgen receptor was precipitated with protamine sulfate. Radioactivity was measured in extracts of the precipitates. Bound MT represents the difference in radioactivity of the two parallel experiments. Lower panel: saturation curve, upper panel: transformation according to Scatchard (21).

stant up to 90 min (Fig. 1, upper line). If the cytosol was heated prior to DCC treatment, the decrease in DHT was much more pronounced. The values obtained after 60 min were hardly detectable by the RIA procedure and represent maximally 10% of the initial values (Fig. 1, lower line). In three separate experiments, very similar results were obtained, indicating that a distinct portion of cytosolic DHT is resistant to DCC treatment due to binding to a heat sensitive binding component.

In saturation experiments with cytosol from 24h castrated rats it is demonstrated (Fig. 2) that this binding component is saturable at a low concentration (ca 20 nM) and possesses a high affinity for DHT (K_D in three separate experiments 2-5 nM). From these data, the requirements for our "routine

TABLE 1. Binding of DHT in prostate cytosol.

	CR-DHT[1]	CR-DHT binding-capacity
intact rats	210 ± 25 (11)[2]	167 ± 19 (7)
24h castrated rats	20 ± 3 (4)	113 ± 10 (6)

[1] Charcoal resistant 5α-dihydrotestosterone concentration;
[2] fmol/mg soluble protein ($\bar{x}$±SEM (number of experiments)).

assay" of CR-DHT and CR-DHT-binding capacity, ie, treatment
of cytosol with DCC for 1h without or with prior incubation
with 38 nM (final conc.) of DHT, respectively, were established. Collective values of intact and 24h castrated rats
are given in Tab. 1 and indicate a high degree of saturation
of the binding capacity by DHT in the first condition, and a
large excess of binding capacity over CR-DHT in the second.

With respect to cytosolic androgen receptor determination,
the methodology was evaluated in cytosol from 24h castrated
rats. Again saturation of binding sites with the ligand was
found in the 20 nmolar range (Fig. 3). Scatchard plot analysis revealed a single class of binding sites (Fig. 3, upper
panel). The mean K_D and binding capacity in 8 separate experiments were 1.9 ± 0.9 nM and 107 ± 5 fmol/mg soluble protein, respectively. The latter value is in agreement with
that obtained for CR-DHT-binding capacity (Tab. 1).

Physiological Studies

Plasma testosterone and prostate weight.
As shown in Fig. 4 (left panel), plasma testosterone
values in castrated rats treated for 14 days with testosterone were linearly dependent on the dose administered. 60 µg
testosterone/24h led to values in the "normal range" of intact rats (3). In contrast, relative weight alterations of
the prostate (Fig. 4, right panel) were distinctly more pronounced in the low than in the high dose range. Testosterone
in a dose of 60 µg/24h additionally maintained the prostate
weights in the range of intact rats (3).

DHT in cytosol and nuclei.
In Fig. 5, values of total DHT, CR-DHT and CR-DHT-binding

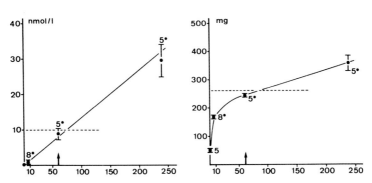

Dose of testosterone (µg/24h)

FIG. 4. Plasma testosterone and prostate weights. Rats were castrated
and treated with testosterone releasing depots for 14d. Left panel:
plasma testosterone measured by RIA, right panel: prostate weights.
Geometric mean values, their standard error and the number of experiments are given. The arrow indicates 60 µg testosterone/24h, the broken
line mean values of intact rats. *) Significantly different from the
next lower dose, P at least < 0.05.

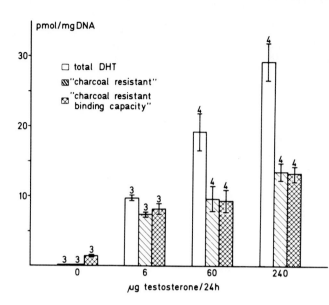

FIG. 5. Total DHT, charcoal resistant DHT and charcoal resistant DHT-binding capacity in prostate cytosol from castrated, testosterone-treated rats, measured by RIA ($\bar{x} \pm$ SEM). Experimental procedure as in Fig. 2, exept that no DHT (charcoal resistant DHT) or 38 nM DHT (charcoal resistant DHT-binding capacity) was added. Total DHT = DHT in original cytosol.

capacity in cytosol of 14d castrated, testosterone-treated rats are given. In 14d castrated controls ("dose 0"), all DHT, (0.20 ± 0.07 pmol/mg DNA, n=3) was charcoal resistant (0.21 ± 0.08, n=3), with an excess of binding capacity (1.41 ± 0.03, n=3). Treatment with 6 µg testosterone/24h already led to significantly (P at least < 0.05) higher values of all three constituents. In this condition, mean CR-DHT accounted for about 90% of CR-DHT-binding capacity and for 76% of total DHT. At higher doses further increases were observed, mainly for total DHT, with less pronounced increases for CR-DHT and

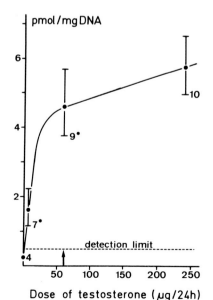

FIG. 6. DHT concentration in prostate nuclei of castrated, testosterone treated rats, measured by RIA. Explanation of symbols see Fig. 4.

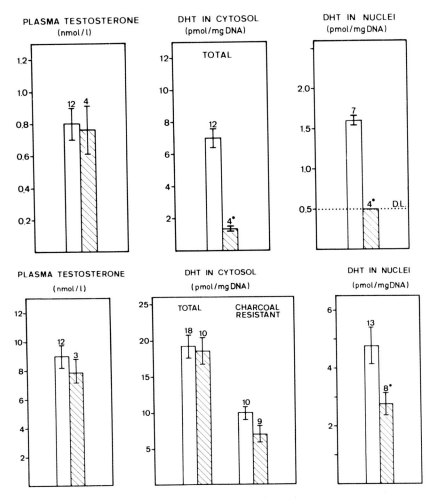

FIG. 7. Influence of cyproterone acetate (CyAc) on testosterone in plasma and on DHT in prostatic cytosol and nuclei. Data represent geometric mean values with their standard error. Open columns: 14d testosterone treated controls, hatched columns: additionally with CyAc (10 mg, 24h) treated rats. *) Significantly different to control, P at least < 0.05, DL = detection limit. Upper panels: testosterone dose 6 µg/24h, lower panels: 60 µg/24h.

CR-DHT-binding capacity. Compared to the next lower dose, these increases were statistically significant (P at least < 0.05) only for total DHT. In the nuclear fractions (Fig.6), significant dose dependent increases in DHT occurred up to the 60 µg/24h dose. Passing to the highest dose, no further increase was observed.

Effect of cyproterone acetate (CyAc) on DHT concentration in cytosol and nuclei.

Following administration of CyAc to testosterone-treated rats, testosterone values in plasma were not affected (Fig.7,

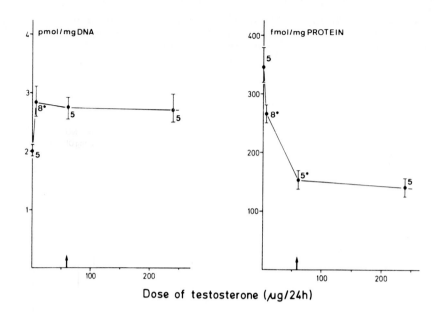

Dose of testosterone (μg/24h)

FIG. 8. Androgen receptor concentration in prostate cytosol from 14d castrated rats, treated for 13d with testosterone. Left panel: data related to the DNA content of homogenates, right panel: values in terms of fmol/mg soluble protein. Explanation of symbols see Fig. 4.

left panels). Following the low testosterone dose (6 μg/24h, Fig. 7, upper panels), mean reduction of total cytosolic DHT was 81%, when compared to testosterone treated controls. This percent reduction was very similar to that of CR-DHT to total DHT in testosterone treated controls (Fig. 5). In nuclei, DHT could not be detected following CyAc treatment.

The decrease in total DHT in cytosol was rather trivial when the same CyAc dose was used in combination with 60 μg testosterone/24h, and was only slightly more pronounced for CR-DHT (Fig. 7, lower panel). The decrease in DHT was most obvious ($P < 0.05$) in the nuclei, although also in this fraction, only a partial reduction was observed. The mean CyAc concentration in plasma at the time of decapitation was 567± 41 nM (n=12) and was similar in rats treated with 10 mg CyAc and 6 or 60 μg testosterone/24h, representing approximately a 600 or 60-fold molar excess over plasma testosterone, respectively.

Androgen receptor in cytosol.
The androgen receptor was measured by saturation analysis with MT after removal of testosterone depots to exclude different degrees of occupation by DHT and different distribution between the cellular compartments. As illustrated in Fig. 8, relative alterations were dependent on the basis for comparison. When the values were expressed in terms of pmol/mg DNA, similar values were obtained in all testosterone

treated groups, whereas significantly lower values were obtained in 14d castrated controls ("dose 0", Fig. 8, left panel). In terms of fmol/mg protein, a dose dependent decrease was obtained, which was most distinct in the low testosterone dose range (Fig. 8, right panel).

DISCUSSION

The determination of cytosolic androgen receptor in conditions in which binding sites are occupied by DHT, eg in intact or castrated, testosterone supplemented rats, requires exchange of bound DHT and radioactive ligands at elevated temperature for a prolonged time period. Due to the lability of the receptor protein, such procedures might lead to an underestimation of the values (4,5,18). To overcome this problem, we measured the amount of DHT which is bound to the androgen receptor directly by RIA. A similar experimental approach was proposed earlier by Blondeau et al. (4).

With respect to CR-DHT concentration in cytosol, the two-phasic dissociation pattern, its heat sensitivity, the saturability at a low DHT concentration, and a K_D in the nmolar range are typical properties of the androgen receptor (13). However, CR-DHT does not allow displacement studies. Thus evaluation of steroid specificity and nonspecific binding are not possible in individual samples. Their evaluation can be performed only indirectly, and we have to discuss to what extent the true receptor bound DHT concentration is overestimated by this method.

From the DHT determinations in heat inactivated cytosols, after DCC treatment a nonspecific contribution of 10% of the initial, total DHT values to CR-DHT might be assumed. In reality, the overestimation should be even lower. This supposition is based on two further observations: (1) In the saturation experiments a clear plateau is observed, even when the DHT concentration is increased 3.5-fold compared to the saturation point. (2) In control experiments (data not shown), in which the protocol of Fig. 2 was used while saturation was performed with ^{3}H-DHT with and without an 100-fold excess of unlabelled DHT, mean nonspecific binding was only 1.3% of the total ^{3}H-DHT concentration. Nevertheless, even assuming an nonspecific contribution of 10% of total DHT to CR-DHT, absolute elevation of CR-DHT values would amount maximally to 23% in cytosol from animals treated with the highest testosterone dose and to a lower percentage in other conditions. Such an overestimation would not affect our main conclusions.

Contrary to the possible overestimation, one has to also to take into account a noticable underestimation of CR-DHT-binding capacity. This assumption is based on data derived from CR-DHT-binding capacity in 14d castrated rat ("dose 0") as compared to the androgen receptor values obtained with the conventional method under the same experimental condition. The higher values, which result in the latter method should be mainly due to the addition of MoO_4^{2-} to buffers used. This substance is known to stabilize the androgen re-

ceptor protein (10,16), which is particularly unstable when
not occupied by its ligand (13). Therefore, we assume especially in the low DHT concentration range a slight overestimation of the percentual occupation by DHT of the androgen
receptor.

Assuming that CR-DHT and CR-DHT-binding capacity reflect
mainly receptor bound DHT and the receptor concentration in
cytosol, the following conclusions can be drawn:

(1) The tremendous accumulation of DHT in cytosol, which
is present particularly under conditions of low plasma androgen is almost exclusively due to binding to and retention by
the androgen receptor.

(2) Saturation of the androgen receptor in cytosol by DHT
in vivo occurs in a low concentration range of plasma testosterone. This conclusion is derived from the finding that
already one tenth of "normal" plasma testosterone leads to
about 90% occupation by DHT of the androgen receptor. Although data on percentage receptor occupation following variation in testosterone substitution have not been reported,
our data are in line with a high degree of receptor saturation by its ligand in intact animals (4,6,8).

(3) The increase in cytosol of DHT bound to the androgen
receptor is accompanied by concommittant alterations of the
DHT concentration in the nuclei and weight alterations of the
prostate, substantiating the functional role of the androgen
receptor in translocating DHT to the nucleus and mediating
androgen dependent processes. The mechanism leading to the
parallel alterations of DHT bound to the androgen receptor
in cytosol and DHT in nuclei is not yet clear. It has been
repeatedly shown (14,17) that an increase in nuclear DHT
receptor complexes occurs simultaneously with a decrease in
the cytoplasmic compartment. Other authors, however, have not
observed any reciprocal behavior of cytosolic and nuclear
androgen receptor (4,6) and it has been suggested that a decrease in cytoplasmic receptor due to translocation might be
overcome by a rapid increase in receptor synthesis (5).

(4) The steroid specificity of DHT accumulation in the
prostate, and thus the involvement of the androgen receptor
is further substantiated by our data following administration
of CyAc. It is thought that this anti-androgen acts via competitive inhibition of DHT-binding to the androgen receptor;
however the CyAc receptor complex is not translocated to the
nucleus (7). With a 600-fold molar excess of CyAc over testosterone in plasma, as obtained by administration with 6 µg
testosterone/24h, indeed similar displacement of the receptor bound portion to total cytosolic DHT was observed. The
simultaneous disappearance of nuclear DHT is again in agreement with the DHT-transporting function of the receptor.

It might be assumed that the 60-fold plasmatic excess of
CyAc compared to testosterone at a higher (60 µg/24h) testosterone dose is not sufficient to achieve complete displacement of DHT. This should be due to the comparatively lower
affinity of the CyAc receptor interaction, which requires a
high excess of this drug over the natural ligand for complete
displacement (22). Furthermore, the relatively weak in vivo

displacement of DHT by CyAc might in part be kinetically controlled.

The observation that a relatively more pronounced decrease in DHT is observed in the nuclear than in the cytoplasmic compartment is of interest. This finding might explain earlier observations (22) that the anti-androgenic action of CyAc is more pronounced than would be expected alone from DHT displacement studies in cytosol. As CyAc treatment was performed in our experiments only for 24h, effects of treatment on prostatic weights could not be measured. A partial reduction of DHT in prostatic nuclei by CyAc has also been reported earlier (7).

(5) The data on cytosolic androgen receptor after depletion of prostatic androgens demonstrate that the androgen receptor per cell (per mg DNA) is not altered by our treatments, although distinct changes in DNA and protein as well as in weight of the prostate are present. The significantly lower receptor value in 14d castrated controls might reflect a relative preponderance of non-androgen responsive cells in the maximally involuted prostate. Therefore, it might be assumed that alterations of the receptor concentration in testosterone-treated animals, as revealed by CR-DHT and CR-DHT-binding capacity are mainly the consequence of rapid androgen influences on intracellular receptor processing, eg synthesis, degradation and translocation.

ACKNOWLEDGEMENTS

This work was supported by the DFG, Sonderforschungsbereich 34 (Endokrinologie). We are grateful to Dr. B. Düsterberg (Berlin) for determination of cyproterone acetate. Furthermore, we thank Mrs. J. Mohrmann for her excellent assistance.

REFERENCES

1. Bartsch, W., Krieg, M. and Voigt, K.D. (1980): J.Steroid Biochem., 13:259-264.
2. Bartsch, W., Krieg, M., Becker, H., Mohrmann, J. and Voigt, K.D. (1982): Acta Endocrinol.(Cobenh.), 100:634-640.
3. Bartsch, W. Knabbe, C. and Voigt, K.D. (1983): J.Steroid Biochem., 19:929-937.
4. Blondeau, J.P., Corpechot, C., Le Goascogne, C., Baulieu, E.E. and Robel, P. (1975): Vit.Horm., 33:61-100.
5. Blondeau, J.P., Baulieu, E.E. and Robel, P. (1982): Endocrinology, 110:1926-1932.
6. Boesel, R.W., Klipper, R.D. and Shain, S.A. (1980): Steroids, 35: 157-177.
7. Callaway, T.W., Bruchovsky, N., Rennie, P.S. and Comeau, T. (1982): Prostate, 3:599-610.
8. Davies, P., Thomas, P. and Griffiths, K. (1977): J.Endocrinol., 74: 393-404.
9. Fang, S. Anderson, K.M. and Liao, S. (1969): J.Biol.Chem., 244: 6584-6595.
10. Gaubert, C.M., Tremblay, R.R. and Dube, j.Y. (1980): J.Steroid Biochem., 13:931-937.

11. Geller, J., Albert, J., de la Vega, D., Loza, D. and Stoeltzing, W. (1978): Cancer Res., 38:4349-4352.

12. Krieg, M., Bartsch, W., Thomsen, M. and Voigt, K.D. (1983): J.Steroid Biochem., 19,:155-161.

13. Krieg, M. and Voigt, K.D. (1977): Acta Endocrinol.(Kobemh.), 85 Suppl.214:43-89.

14. Mainwaring, W.I.P. and Peterken, B.M. (1971): Biochem.J., 125:285-295.

15. Nieuweboer, B and Lübke, K. (1977): Hormone Res., 8:210-218.

16. Noma, K., Nakao, K., Sato, B., Nishizawa, Y., Matsumoto, K. and Yamamura, J. (1980): Endocrinology, 107:1205-1211.

17. Rennie, P.S. and Bruchovsky, N. (1973): J.Biol.Chem., 248:3288-3297.

18. Rennie, P.S. and Bruchovsky, N. (1980): In: Male Accessory Sex Glands, edited by E.Spring-Mills and E.S.E.Hafez, pp 265-287. Elsevier, Amsterdam.

19. Robel, P., Lasnitzki, I. and Baulieu, E.E. (1971): Biochimie, 53: 81-96.

20. Sandberg, A.A., Karr, J.P. and Müntzing, J. (1980): In: Male Accessory Sex Glands, edited by E.Spring-Mills and E.S.E.Hafez, pp 565-608. Elsevier, Amsterdam.

21. Scatchard, G. (1949): Ann.N.Y.Acad.Sci., 51:660-672.

22. Szalay, R., Krieg, M., Schmidt, H. and Voigt, K.D. (1975): Acta Endocrinol.(Kobenh.), 80:592-602.

Progress in Cancer Research and Therapy,
Vol. 31, edited by F. Bresciani, et al.
Raven Press, New York © 1984.

Characterization and Application of PC-82, a Hormone-Dependent, Transplantable Tumor Line, Derived from a Human Prostatic Adenocarcinoma

G.J. van Steenbrugge and F.H. Schroeder

Department of Urology, Erasmus University, 3000 DR Rotterdam, The Netherlands

ABSTRACT

A prostatic tumor line, PC-82, derived from a moderately differentiated adenocarcinoma was maintained for 5 years by serial transplantation on nude mice. The tumor shows a cribriform histology, a slow growth rate, is completely dependent on hormones and secretes immunoreactive prostatic acid phosphatase (PAP). Withdrawal of androgens in PC-82 tumor-bearing mice decreased the tumor volume with $57\pm10\%$ within 6 weeks. Additional treatment with E_2 to castrated animals did not result in a further decrease of the tumor volume in the same period. Administration of androgens (via Silastic implants) simultaneously with tumor transplantation on female and castrated male mice resulted in tumor growth. The level of PAP in the serum of PC-82 tumor-bearing mice was elevated over that in control male nude mice. A correlation was observed between the concentration of PAP in the serum and the tumor burden of the mice. Neither short-term hormonal manipulation nor long-term castration influenced the concentration of PAP in the PC-82 tumor tissue. The properties of this tumor line, especially its hormone-dependence and the secretion of PAP makes this model well comparable with the properties of prostatic cancer in the clinical situation.

INTRODUCTION

Carcinoma of the prostate is one of the most common cancers in the male population. In spite of that, relatively few experimental studies on prostatic carcinoma have been published compared with the number of reports on several other types of cancer. One important reason for this may be the lack of appropriate model systems for prostatic cancer.
In laboratory animals the incidence of prostatic carcinomas is relatively low, although a number of cases have been described during the last few years. Nevertheless, many aspects of human prostatic carcinoma can only be investigated properly by the use of suitable model systems. Perhaps the most important model systems available now have been developed from a spontaneous prostatic carcinoma (R3327) in an aged Copenhagen rat (the Dunning tumor) (6). This tumor gave rise to a variety of lines and sublines with different, and in some cases well defined characteristics,

regarding hormone-sensitivity (7) and metastatic capacity (8). Other animal models that are currently being studied include the sex steroid-induced prostatic carcinoma in the Noble rat (12) which has been studied also after heterotransplantation on nude mice ((2).

A common disadvantage of the models mentioned above is their non-human origin. For that reason several attempts have been made to propagate human tumors in immuno-deficient animals, such as the athymic nude mouse. In vitro cell lines, derived from human prostatic carcinoma, readily induce tumors after injection in nude mice. Thus tumors have been established from the cell lines EB-33 (16), DU-145 (11), PC3 (19) and LNCaP (5). Heterotransplantation of human prostatic carcinomas on nude mice was shown to be successful in only a limited number of cases. Among these only a few appeared to be serially transplantable (13, 9). In our own institution the transplantable line PC-82 was developed (4). The properties of this tumor line (i.e. slow growth rate, hormone dependence and secretion of prostatic acid phosphatase) are well comparable with those of prostatic cancer in the patient (15). In this contribution we report on the characteristics of the PC-82 model and describe some experiments concerning the hormone-dependence (i.e. hormonal manipulation) of this tumor line.

MATERIAL AND METHODS

Tumor Material

The original tumor, a moderately differentiated adenocarcinoma of the prostate, was removed from the patient by total perineal prostatectomy in July 1977. For initial and sequential drafting of the PC-82 tumor tissue, mice of the Balb/c background with an age of 6-12 weeks were used as recipients. Experiments were carried out with nude mice subcutaneously transplanted with tumor tissue. Tumor growth was monitored by (bi)weekly measurement of two perpendicular tumor diameters with calipers. The tumor doubling time was estimated from a semilogarithmic plot of the tumor volume ($T_V = \frac{\pi}{6} (d_1 \times d_2)^{3/2}$) against time. Only tumors with a significant correlation between the measuring points (traject: 50-500 mm^3) were evaluated.

Treatment Of Animals

Treatment (e.g. castration or hormone substitution) was started when tumors were in the experimental phase of growth. Castration of tumor-bearing mice was carried out via the scrotal route under total anaesthesia with chloralhydrate. To prevent daily injection of the nude mice, hormones (i.e. androgens and estrogens) were administered by subcutaneous implantation of Silastic implants (Talas, Zwolle, The Netherlands) packed with crystalline steroid. Using these implants, constant plasma steroid levels in nude mice were reached, which could be maintained for long periods (2-3 months). Installation and removal of implants was carried out under light ether anaesthesia.

Prostatic Acid Phosphatase (PAP)

PAP in extracts of PC-82 tumor tissue and in sera of tumor-bearing mice was immunologically determined according to Vihko and associates (17). In the radioimmunoassay procedure antisera, raised against purified acid phosphatase from the human prostate, were used. As a control, a transplantable, non-prostatic human tumor was analysed. In this tissue PAP was not detectable, indicating the high specificity of the antibody utilized for the determination of PAP in the PC-82 tumors.

Other Procedures

Plasma levels of testosterone and estradiol were estimated using radio-immunoassay procedures. The protein concentrations of the tissue extracts were determined according to Bradford (1), using bovine serum albumin as a standard. DNA in the remaining pellets after tissue homogenization was measured according to the method of Giles and Myers (3) with calf thymus DNA as a standard. Statistical analysis of the data was performed by non-parametric tests (Wilcoxon's test, Spearman's correlation test). Differences were considered statistically significant when a P-value < 0.05 was found.

RESULTS AND DISCUSSION

Characteristics Of The PC-82 Tumor Model

The PC-82 tumor line was initiated by (subcutaneous) transplantation of small tissue fragments, obtained from the patient tumor, on male nude mice. The tumor was shown to be serially transplantable and at the present time (March 1983) it is the 23rd transplant generation. After tissue inoculation followed by a relatively long 'lag-phase', tumors appeared as subcutaneous growing nodules (FIG. 1.).

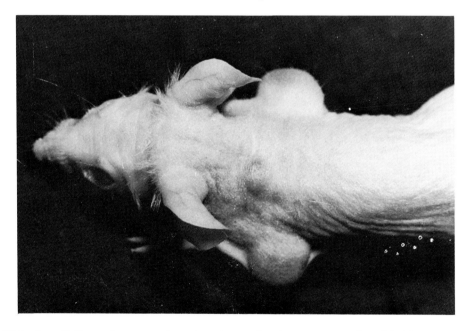

FIG. 1. Male nude mouse bearing two subcutaneous growing PC-82 tumors. Small tumor fragments were grafted on both sides of the shoulder through an incision in the neck of the animal.

The histology of the original tumor is shown in FIG. 2A.

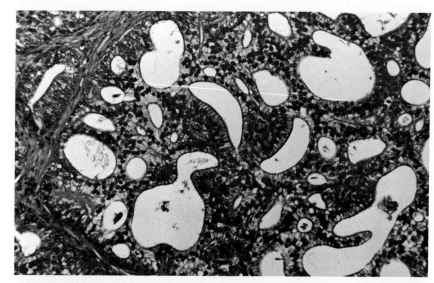

FIG. 2A

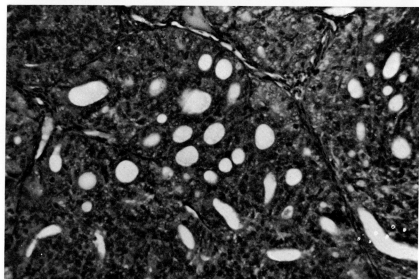

FIG. 2B

FIG. 2A. Histological section of the original patient tumor, graded as
a moderately differentiated adenocarcinoma with a cribriform pattern.
FIG. 2B. Histological section of a PC-82 tumor in the 7th transplant
generation. This tumor mainly consists of epithelial tissue with characteristics comparable with those of the tumor of origin.
(Magnification 125x).

The tumor was graded as being moderately differentiated adenocarcioma of
the cribriform type. FIG. 2B shows the histological pattern of a tumor
grown on the nude mice. This tumor, which closely resembles the original
tumor, also shows the cribriform aspect with many acini. The small stroma
compartment (less than 5 per cent of the total tumor), which was proved

to be derived from the host animal, provides the tumor with supporting
blood vessels, etc. No major alternations in the histological pattern,
which was monitored routinely, were observed during the subsequent mouse
passages.

PC-82 tumor tissue was shown having a slow growth rate. The tumor
doubling time (Td), calculated from growth curves of 45 tumors (grown on
intact male mice) in the 10-14th passage was 18 ± 5 days (mean + S.D.).
The time required to attain a tumor volume of 50 mm3 (Tv-50), i.e. the
tumor 'lag-phase', which was also calculated from these curves was 37 ± 16
days. FIG. 3 shows an example of the growth curve of a tumor in the 15th
passage with a Td of 12 days in the exponential phase of growth.

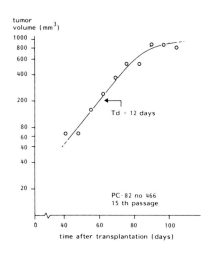

FIG. 3. Representative growth curve of PC-82 tumor in nude mice. The
curve was calculated as described in the section 'Material and Methods'.
A tumor volume of 500 mm3 correlates with a tumor diameter of 1 cm.

After the tumor reached the 500 mm3-point the curve levelled off, indicating the slower growth rate in this phase of growth. Histological examination of tumors passing the 500 mm3-point showed in most cases the
appearance of (central) necrosis, which explained the alternations in
growth pattern of these tumors.

The absence of growth on intact female mice was shown in the first and
several subsequent transplant generations, indicating the androgen dependence of this tumor line. Many experiments were carried out in order to
characterize this important property further (see below).

The tumor secretes prostatic acid phosphatse, which was detectable in
tumor tissue as well as in serum of tumor-bearing animals (see below).

Castration Experiments

Castration of PC-82 tumor-bearing mice resulted in a cessation of
tumor growth in all cases studied so far. In a group of 10 mice, the
tumor volume was decreased with $57\pm27\%$ (mean $\pm$ S.D.) within six weeks
after castration.

A rather extreme example of the response after castration is shown in
FIG 4A. In this experiment, the tumor volume was decreased with 90 per
cent at 40 days after castration. A histological section of this tumor
remaining at 80 days after castration (FIG 4B) shows a degenerating
tumor indicated by hyperchromatic nuclei and clear cytoplasm of the
cells. The main part of the tissue appeared to be fibrotic, while only a
small part kept the original structure.

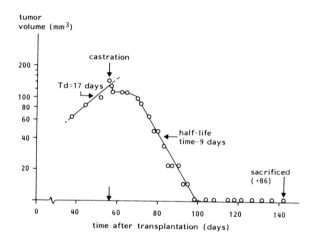

FIG 4A

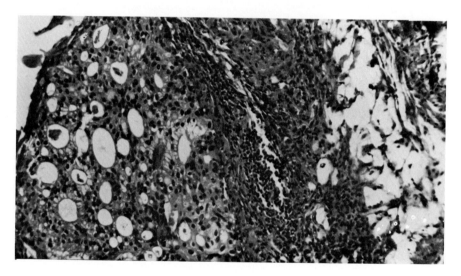

FIG. 4B

FIG 4A. Growth curve of a PC-82 tumor in the 11th passage and the response on castration of the host animal. Castration was carried out when
the tumor had reached a volume of 140 mm³, 56 days after transplantation.
FIG 4B. Histology of this tumor that remained 80 days after castration.
Epithelial tissue with hyperchromatic nuclei and light and vacuolized
cytoplasma. Right part: fibrotic tissue remained after disappearance of
the epithelial part. Note the infiltration of leucocytes in the central
part of this section. (Magnification 125x).

FIG. 5A shows the curve of a tumor with a less pronounced effect after androgen withdrawal. The volume of this tumor was decreased with 40 per cent at 57 days after castration. This tumor also shows degenerative epithelial tissue with flattened cells and pycnotic nuclei (FIG. 5B). However, transplantation of a tumor fragment (at 57 days after castration) on an intact male mouse resulted in regrowth, indicating the presence of viable cells in the tumor.

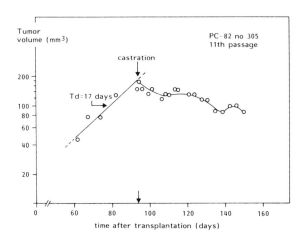

FIG 5A

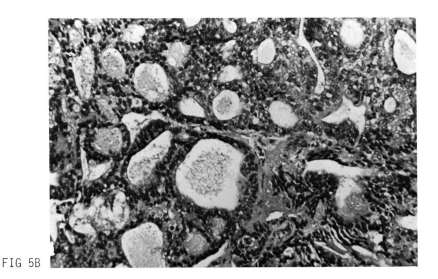

FIG 5B

FIG. 5A. Growth curve of a PC-82 tumor in the 11th passage and the response on castration. Castration was carried out when the tumor had reached a volume of 180 mm^3, 95 days after transplantation. FIG 5B. Histological section of the tumor tissue that remained at 57 days after castration. The original structure was maintained, but with flattened cells and pycnotic nuclei. (Magnification 125x).

In another experiment it was demonstrated that after a long post-castration period (79 days), administration of testosterone (via a Silastic implant) resulted in regrowth of the tumor up to a tumor volume of 1000 mm^3 (FIG. 6).

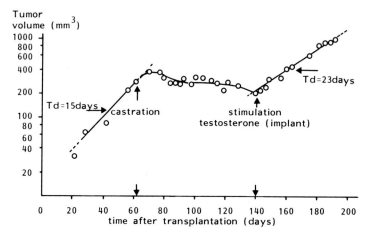

FIG. 6. PC-82 tumor tissue grown on an intact male nude mouse, influence of castration and androgen restimulation. Testosterone was administered by using a Silastic implant. Tumor doubling time before castration and further details are indicated in the figure.

It was concluded that after androgen withdrawal, at least a part of the tumor remained dormant with the possibility to stimulate the growth of the tissue by androgen administration.

In none of the castration experiments performed up to now any hormone-independent growth could be observed. This might indicate that the PC-82 tumor line mainly (or completely) consists of a rather homogeneous population of hormone-responsive tumor cells. If hormone-unresponsive cells are present in the tumor, it would be necessary to extend the post-castration period in order to isolate this hormone-independent clone.

Hormone-Substitution Experiments

As mentioned in the section 'Material and Methods', steroid-containing Silastic implants are very applicable for the long-term administration of hormones in (nude) mice. Constant and physiological levels (8 ng/ml) of testosterone (T) were attained after implantation of castrated male mice with T-implants (length 1,0 cm). (Table 1).

In several mouse transplant-generations the absence of tumor growth on female and castrated male mice was demonstrated. When PC-82 tumor tissue was grafted simultaneously with a T-implant on female mice and on intact and castrated male mice, growth could be demonstrated in at least 85 per cent of the animals. (Table 2).

TABLE 1. Plasma testosterone (T) levels in control and T-implanted male nude mice and male mice after castration and estradiol (E$_2$) implantation.

Group	n	Testosterone (ng/ml)*	Range
Intact controls	16	8.0 $\pm$ 9.7	0.5 - 24.7
T-implant (1,0 cm)	16	8.1 $\pm$ 1.4	5.5 - 10.2
Castration	16	0.14 $\pm$ 0.12	0.03 - 0.26
E2-implant (0,5 cm)	15	1.03 $\pm$ 0.95**	0.23 - 3.9

    *   Values are expressed as mean $\pm$ S.D.

   **   Significantly different from castrated animals (P < 0.01)

TABLE 2. Tumor take and tumor doubling time of PC-82 tumor tissue grown on androgen-substituted castrated and intact male and intact female mice*

Mice	Implant	Number of mice	Tumor take (%)	TV-50** (days)	Tumor doubling time (days)
Intact male	sham	11	85	32 $\pm$ 8	18 $\pm$ 5
Intact male	T	7	100	23 $\pm$ 14	11 $\pm$ 3****
Castrated male	T	5	80	24 $\pm$ 6	14 $\pm$ 5
Intact female	T	7	100	26 $\pm$ 11	12 $\pm$ 3****
Intact male	E$_2$	8	5***	> 65	---

  *   Values expressed as mean $\pm$ S.D.

 **   TV-50: time required to attain a tumor volume of 50 mm^3.

***   Representing one tumor (< 200 mm) at 96 days after transplantation.

**** Significantly different from control group (Wilcoxon test; p< 0.05).

In the substituted groups, the 50 mm^3 tumor volume was attained earlier than in the controls. These differences were statistically not significant, however. (Table 1). The tumor doubling time in the group with hormonally treated intact male and female mice, was significantly shorter than that of tumors grown on intact male mice (p < 0.05). In contrast to the other two T-substituted groups, the tumor take and tumor doubling time in the group with castrated male mice were similar to those in the control male mice. However, in an experiment performed recently with a large group of castrated male mice, T-substitution resulted in a tumor doubling time (12+4 days) that was comparable with those in the intact male and female mice of the present experiment.

The histological picture of all these tumors grown on androgen trea- ted animals did not differ from tumors grown on intact male mice. The mitotic index however, was much higher in tumors of testosterone-treated mice.

It was concluded from these results that the growth rate of PC-82 tumor tissue was increased through the availability of a constant level of testosterone via the Silastic implant. This differs from the situation in the intact male mouse where very large variations of the testosterone levels were found, although the mean plasma level did not differ from those in the substituted group. (Table 2).

Implantation of intact male mice with E_2-implants (length 0.5 cm, used in all further experiments), resulted in supraphysiological plasma levels of 250+50 pg/ml E_2 for periods up to 40 days. In these animals, plasma-T was suppressed to a level of approximately 1 ng/ml (Table 1). However, this level appeared to be still significantly higher compared to that attained after castration.

E_2-implantation simultaneously with tumor grafting prevented the growth of PC-82 tumor tissue almost completely (Table 2). Only one out of 16 tumor transplants resulted in a tumor that exceeded the volume of 50 mm^3. Moreover, this volume was attained after a lag-phase of at least 65 days.

In an additional experiment, PC-82 tumor tissue was grown on T-substi- tuted, castrated male mice. After the tumor had reached the exponential phase of growth, the implants were removed ("castration-like" effect) and partly replaced by an E_2-implant. During the treatment period of 25 days, androgen withdrawal resulted in a decrease of the tumor volume of 50 per cent (Table 3), which was comparable with the results obtained after castration (see previous section). The same results were obtained with the group of mice with E_2-implantation.

TABLE 3. Effect of testosterone withdrawal and of estradiol treatment [*] on PC-82 tumor tissue.

Group	N	$T_V(+)/(-)$ (%)[**]	Range
I Controls	7	+ 100 $\pm$ 28	52 - 134
II "Castration"	6	- 50 $\pm$ 7	45 - 63
III "Castration" + E_2	7	- 50 $\pm$ 10	35 - 65

[*] Treatment period: 25 days

[**] Values are expressed as mean $\pm$ S.D.

Control animals, keeping the T-implant, showed an increase of the tumor volume of 100 per cent during the same treatment period.

From these results it was concluded, that E_2-levels reached with Silastic implantation, only indirectly influenced the take and growth of PC-82 tumor tissue by the suppressive effect on plasma-T levels.

Prostatic Acid Phosphatase (PAP)

The PC-82 tumor secretes immunoreactive PAP. The concentration of PAP in the serum of tumor-bearing mice (73 ± 88 µg/l, n=17), was significantly elevated over that in male control mice (0.5 ± 0.7 µg/l, n=11). A significant correlation (P < 0.001) between the total tumor volume and the level of serum PAP could be demonstrated in a group of 25 intact tumor-bearing male mice (FIG. 7).

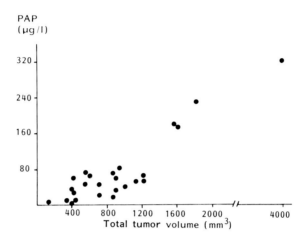

FIG. 7. Relationship between the total tumor volume and the serum concentration of human prostatic acid phosphatase in PC-82 tumor-bearing nude mice (R = 0.73; n = 25; P < 0.001).

Castration of tumor-bearing mice ultimately resulted in a decrease of the mean concentration of PAP in the serum (6.4 ± 8.5 µg/l, n=10), compared to the concentration in untreated animals. This decrease follows the reduction of the tumor volume.

The possible influence of endocrine manipulation on the concentration of PAP in PC-82 tumor tissue was studied. Tumor-bearing animals were left intact, castrated, or treated for a 5-day period with T- or E_2-implantation. The concentration of PAP in the 5-day treated groups was not significantly different from that in the group of intact control mice, either when PAP was based on tissue wet weight or on pellet-DNA (FIG. 8). The significant increase of PAP when expressed per mg DNA in the (short-term) castrated group, could be explained by a significant decrease of the DNA content in this group compared to that in the control group. Even long-term withdrawal of androgens (up to 50 days), did not affect the PAP concentration in the tissue remaining after the treatment period. It was concluded from these data that the concentration of PAP in the PC-82 prostatic tumor tissue is not controlled by androgens, but that the level of PAP in the plasma of tumor-bearing mice is related to the total tumor mass.

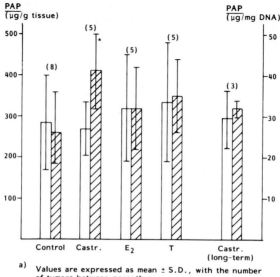

FIG. 8. Concentration of human prostatic acid phosphatase in PC-82 tumor tissue after 5 days of endocrine treatment and after long-term castration. PAP was expressed per g tissue and per mg DNA as indicated.

CONCLUSIONS

The hormone-dependence and the secretion of PAP makes the PC-82 tumor model well comparable with prostatic carcinoma in the clinical situation. The results of the present study and the experiments that will be performed in the (near) future might contribute to our knowledge of hormone-dependent tumor growth. Further studies will be focused on the influence of very low levels of androgens on the growth of prostatic tumor tissue. Although hormone-independent tumor growth could not be observed up till now, this important aspect will be emphasized in the further experimental approach. The possibility to study the effect of several hormones and other (new) treatment modalities on the human prostatic tissue of the PC-82 tumor line, makes this model very applicable.

ACKNOWLEDGEMENTS

We wish to acknowledge the capable assistance of Mrs Marja Groen in attending to many aspects of the nude mice work, Mr Jan-Willem van Dongen for the preparation of the histological sections of the tumors, and Dr. F.H. de Jong (Dept. of Biochemistry II, Erasmus University) for the estimation of steroid levels in plasma of the nude mice.
    This study was supported by the Netherlands Cancer Foundation (KWF) through grant EUR-UR 80-4.

REFERENCES

1. Bradford, M.M. (1976): Anal. Biochem. 72: 248.
2. Drago, J.R. and Gershwin, M.E. (1981): Cancer 47: 55.
3. Giles, K.W. and Mijers, A. (1965): Nature 206: 93.
4. Hoehn, W., Schroeder, F.H., Riemann, J.F., Joebsis, A.C. and Herma- nek, P. (1980): The Prostate I: 95.
5. Horoszewicz, J.S., Leong, S.S., Ming Chu, T., Wajsman, Z.L., Fried- man, M., Papsidero, L., Kim, U., Chai, L.S., Kakati, S., Arya, S. K. and Sandberg, A.A. (1980): In: Models for prostatic cancer, edited by Alan R. Liss, Inc., p.115, New York.
6. Isaacs, J.T., Heston, W.D.W., Weissmann, R.M. and Coffey, D.S.(1978): Cancer Res.: 4353.
7. Isaacs, J.T. and Coffey, D.S. (1979): In: Prostatic cancer, edited by D.S. Coffey and J.T. Isaacs, p. 195, Geneva.
8. Isaacs, J.T., Yu, G.W. and Coffey, D.S. (1981): Invest. Urol. 19: 20.
9. Jones, M.A., Williams, G. and Davies, A.J.S. (1980): J. Roy. Med. 73: 708.
10. Kaighn, M.E., Narayan, K.S., Ohnuki, Y., Lechner, J.F., Jones, L.W. (1979): Invest. Urol. 17: 16.
11. Mickey, D.D., Stone, K.R., Wunderli, H., Mickey, G.H., Vollmer, R.T. and Paulson, D.F. (1977): Cancer Res.: 4049.
12. Noble, R.L. (1980): Cancer Res. 40: 3547.
13. Reid, L.C.M. and Shin, S. (1978): In: The nude mouse in experimen- tal and clinical research, edited by J. Foch and B.C. Giovanella, p. 313, New York.
14. Rivenson, A. and Silverman, J.(1979): Invest. Urol. 16: 468.
15. Romijn, J.C., Oishi, K., van Steenbrugge, G.J., Bolt-de Vries, J. and Schroeder, F.H. (1982): In: Proc. of the 3rd Int. Workshop on nude mice, edited by Gustav Fischer, p. 611, New York.
16. Schroeder, F.H. and Jellinghaus, W.(1978): Nat. Cancer Inst. Monogr. 49: 41.
17. Vihko, P., Kostama, A., Jänne, O., Sajanti, E. and Vihko, R. (1980): Clin. Chem. 26: 1544.

Progress in Cancer Research and Therapy,
Vol. 31, edited by F. Bresciani, et al.
Raven Press, New York © 1984.

Increased Androgen Binding Capacity in Experimental Prostatic Carcinomas Treated with Estrogen

B.G. Mobbs and I.E. Johnson

Department of Surgery, University of Toronto, Toronto, M5S 1A8 Canada

Our previous work on the human prostate has been concerned with the quantitation of androgen receptor, with particular regard to the effect of therapy on AR concentration and cellular distribution. An unexpected finding was that androgen binding capacity was markedly elevated in some patients treated with (DES), particularly if they had also been orchiectomized (8). The elevation of cytosol binding capacity was greatly in excess of the amount expected to occur due to release of AR from the nucleus into the cytosol and/or the freeing of bound cytosol sites due to reduced circulating androgen levels. Because of the difficulty in obtaining sufficient human material to permit characterization of this binding component, it was decided to try to reproduce this phenomenon in the R3327 (Dunning) prostatic adenocarcinoma of the rat. This transplantable tumour has many of the characteristics of human prostatic carcinoma, and has been widely used as a model for the human disease. It has a similar enzyme profile, contains androgen receptor (AR) and estrogen receptor (ER), and growth can be retarded by castration and estrogen treatment. However, a fraction of the cell population is not androgen-sensitive, the tumour therefore eventually relapses from hormonal control and growth is resumed (4).

In our investigation we compared the concentration of high-affinity binding sites for the synthetic androgen methyltrienolone (R1881) in cytosol and nuclear fractions of tumours from untreated control rats with that in tumours from rats which had been treated in a similar way to patients with advanced prostatic carcinoma. The binding was characterized by Scatchard analysis, sucrose density gradient centrifugation (SDGC) and steroid competition studies.

METHODS

Animals and tumours

Copenhagen x Fischer F_1 hybrid rats were obtained from Dr. N. Altman, The Papanicolaou Cancer Research Institute at Miami, Inc., by courtesy of the National Prostatic Cancer Project (D.H.E.W.). The first batch of animals (Group 1) was received already implanted with tumour subcutaneously on each flank: one of these tumours was later excised, minced, and transplanted into a second batch of animals (Group 2). When tumours became palpable, growth was monitored by weekly caliper measurement of the longest diameter and the diameter at right-angles to it. Treatment was begun when the mean diameter reached 1.0-1.5 cm, and tumour size was monitored until the animals were killed.

Treatment

Experimental animals were castrated or treated with the sodium salt of diethylstilbestrol (α, α'-diethylstilbenediol) diphosphate (DESP) in the drinking water at a concentration of 1.6 µg/ml (3). Control animals were left untreated. Intake of DESP was monitored by the use of calibrated water bottles. DESP-treated animals took approximately 10 days to adjust to the treatment, but the overall mean daily intake during the treatment period was 37 ± 16 µg per day ie. approximately equivalent to 8 mg per day in a 70 kg man. The acute effects of treatment were investigated in tumours from animals castrated for 2 days or DESP-treated for 10 days; longer-term effects were investigated in animals castrated for 23-67 days, or DESP-treated for 17-132 days. Control tumours were excised from 0-58 days after reaching 'treatment' size. Two additional treatment regimens were used in the Group 2 animals: some were castrated and put on DESP 28 days later for a further 28 days, and others were treated with DESP for 28 days and then castrated. DESP was discontinued, and the animals were killed 28 days after castration. Before the animals were killed, they were anaesthetized with ether, and blood was drawn from the aorta for serum testosterone assay. Tumours were excised, any necrotic tissue was discarded, and a representative slice was fixed for histological examination. The remainder was rinsed in homogenization buffer, cut into pieces and snap frozen in foil containers in liquid nitrogen, where they were stored until assay (not longer than 10 weeks).

Binding Studies

Isotopes and Chemicals

(^{3}H) methyltrienolone (R1881; SA 87.0 Ci/mmol), (^{3}H) promegestone (R5020; SA 87.0 Ci/mmol), and corresponding radioinert steroids were obtained from New England Nuclear Corp. On arrival the labelled steroids were diluted to 50 µCi/ml in redistilled benzene-ethanol (9:1 v/v) and stored at 0°C for not more than 3 mo. Other unlabelled steroids, DNA standard (sodium salt from salmon testes), protamine sulphate (Grade 1), phenymethylsulfonylfluoride (PMSF), ß-mercaptoethanol, dithiothreitol (DTT) and BSA were obtained from Sigma Chemical Co. (St. Louis, MO); Dextran T70 from Pharmacia (Montreal); charcoal (Norit-A) from Matheson, Coleman and Bell; hydroxylapatite (DNA grade) from Bio-Rad Laboratories (Richmond, CA). The scintillators used were either 5g 2,5-diphenyloxazole (PPO) and 0.1 g p-bis [2-(5-phenyl-oxazolyl]-benzene (POPOP) (New England Nuclear) per 1 of toluene, or PCS (Amersham): toluene (2:1 v/v).

Buffers and solutions

The pH of all buffers was 7.4. Tris: 10mM Tris-HCl; TE: 10mM Tris, 1.5mM EDTA; Buffer A: 10mM Tris, 1.5mM EDTA, 0.5mM ß-mercaptoethanol, 0.1mM PMSF; buffer B: 10mM Tris, 0.25M sucrose, 3mM

MgCl$_2$, 0.1mM PMSF; buffer C: 0.6M KCl in buffer B; buffer D: 10mM
sodium molybdate in buffer A; buffer E: 10mM Tris, 1.5mM EDTA, 1.0mM
DTT, 0.1mM PMSF; buffer F: 10mM sodium molybdate in buffer E; buffer
G: 10% glycerol in buffer F (v/v); DCC: 0.5% charcoal, 0.05%
dextran T70 in buffer A or buffer G, as appropriate; HAP slurry:
washed HAP: 10mM Tris, 50mM KCl 0.7: 1 v/v; Tris-Tween wash: 10mM
Tris-HCl, 1% Tween 80.

Homogenization and tissue fractionation

All tissue handling and assay procedures were carried out at 0-4°
with pre-cooled equipment, glassware and buffer solutions unless
otherwise specified.

Frozen tissue was pulverized in a Thermovac pulverizer (Thermovac
Industries Corp. Copiague, N.Y.) cooled with liquid nitrogen and
then homogenized in buffer A (~100mg/ml) using a Polytron P-10
homogenizer (Brinkman Instruments Inc.) for 2 bursts of 20 s
(setting 3) with a 30 s cooling interval. The homogenate was
centrifuged at 3000g for 10 min to yield a crude nuclear pellet
which was used for nuclear receptor assay, and a crude supernatent
(SN), which was immediately adjusted to contain 10mM molybdate by
the addition of 1/10TH volume of 110mM sodium molybdate in buffer
A. The crude SN was then centrifuged at 145,000g for 1h to separate
the cytosol. An aliquot of cytosol was taken for protein assay (5).

Cytosol assay

Using ^{3}H-R1881 as ligand, cytosol binding sites were assayed at 0°
for 2h in the presence of excess triamcinolone acetonide (TA) and at
15° for 16h. Since TA prevents binding of ^{3}H-R1881 to progesterone
receptor (11), the 0° incubation quantitates free androgen receptor
(AR) sites ie. those not occupied by endogenous androgen only. The
15° incubation permits replacement of endogenously bound androgen by
ligand (exchange) and thus measures total AR sites. Since
progesterone receptor (PgR) is unstable at this temperature, it was
not expected to interfere with the AR exchange assay (10), and TA
was not added to these incubations. The majority of tumours were
assayed under single saturating dose (SSD) conditions using 10nM
^{3}H-R1881 in the presence of 5μM TA ± 1μM R1881 to permit
correction for low affinity binding for the 0°2h assay, and 25nM
^{3}H-R1881 ± 2.5μM R1881 at 2h at 0° followed by 15° 16h, for
the exchange assay. The preliminary incubation in the cold was
carried out to protect unbound sites. Replicate incubations were
carried out at cytosol protein concentrations of 3.0-3.5 mg/ml.
After incubation, receptor-bound steroid was precipitated by the
addition of an equal volume of protamine sulphate (1mg/ml TE
buffer). This was spun down, washed with Tris buffer, and extracted
with methylene chloride at 4° overnight. After evaporation of the
solvent, radioactivity was counted in toluene based scintillator for
20 min or 20K counts.

For Scatchard analysis, the same conditions were used, but ligand
concentrations ranged from 0.1-10nM for free site, and 8-45nM for
cytosol exchange assays. In the latter, prefilling of empty sites
was carried out with 10nM radioinert steroid in the cold. Excess
steroid was removed with DCC, and then the exchange incubation was
carried out.

Nuclear assay

After thorough washing in buffer B, the crude nuclear pellet was resuspended in buffer C, and extracted for 1h at 0° (~ 1 ml buffer/150 mg tissue equivalent). After centrifugation, the pellet was frozen for DNA assay (1). Buffer B, containing ^{3}H-R1881 ± R1881 was added to replicate aliquots of the extract to give a concentration of 25nM ^{3}H-R1881 ± 2.5μM R1881 for SSD assays, or 1-50nM ^{3}H-R1881 ± 100-fold R1881 for Scatchard analysis. Incubation was carried out at 15° for 16h. After cooling in ice, the incubated samples were added to 0.25 ml HAP slurry. Receptor-bound steroid was allowed to adsorb to HAP for 30 min at 0° with vortexing every 10 min. Tris-Tween was added to each tube and the HAP was precipitated by centrifugation. The SN was discarded, and the HAP pellet was washed thoroughly with Tris-Tween to remove all free steroid. Bound steroid was extracted from each HAP pellet with ethanol at room temperature overnight. The extracts were added to toluene scintillator for counting.

Cytosol binding capacity was expressed as fm/mg cytosol protein, and both cytosol and nuclear binding capacity were expressed as fm/mg DNA in the extracted nuclear pellet. Preliminary experiments established that virtually no loss of DNA occurred during pellet preparation from the homogenate, so that homogenate DNA and pellet DNA were equivalent.

Sucrose density gradient centrifugation

For SDGC studies using ^{3}H-R1881, incubation of cytosol and nuclear extracts was carried out as described for the SSD assays. Free steroid was removed from incubated cytosol by incubation with DCC (2 x 5 min) as a pellet (cytosol), or in buffer A to reduce the concentration of KCl in the nuclear extract to 0.15M. After removal of the charcoal, cytosol containing 0.3-1.0 mg protein was applied to duplicate gradients of 5-20% sucrose in buffer D. ^{14}C-labelled γ-globulin and ovalbumin were used as internal markers (7S and 3.6S, respectively). Gradients were spun at 220,000 g_{av} for 3 hr in a vertical (VTi65) rotor and 15 drop fractions were collected into counting vials and counted in 0.25 ml distilled water/10 ml PCS: toluene scintillator. Recovery was 95-103% of the radioactivity applied.

Incubated nuclear extract from untreated tumour was applied to similar gradients. After centrifugation, 15 drop fractions were adsorbed with HAP and washed with Tris/Tween. Radioactivity was extracted with 2.5 ml ethanol and counted in 10 ml toluene scintillator. Recovery was ~ 85% of radioactivity applied.

SDGC studies were also carried out using ^{3}H-R5020 as ligand under conditions which conserve PgR and prevent binding to AR. Homogenization was carried out in buffer E and the crude SN was made 10mM with respect to molybdate. The separated cytosol was made 10% with respect to glycerol in buffer F, and was incubated with 10nM ^{3}H-R5020 in the presence of 1μM cortisol and 50nM 5α-dihydrotestosterone (DHT) ± 1μM R5020 for 2h at 0°. Free steroid was removed with a DCC pellet (15 min) and 0.3 ml aliquots of the separated SN were applied to 5-20% sucrose gradients in buffer G. The gradients were centrifuged and fractionated in the same way as for the ^{3}H-R1881 studies. Recovery was 70-95% of radioactivity applied.

Steroid specificity studies

These were carried out using the same ^{3}H-R1881 concentrations and incubation conditions as for the SSD assays. Competing steroids were added in concentrations 1-100 fold that of the ligand. High affinity binding of ^{3}H-R1881 was defined as that binding competed out by 100-fold radioinert R1881, and relative binding affinity (RBA) was defined as

$$\frac{[R1881]}{[competitor]} \text{ required to reduce high affinity binding by 50\%.}$$

RESULTS

Effect of treatment on animals and tumours

Tumour regression was not observed during treatment, although growth of most tumours stopped or continued at a slower rate for 2-10 wk after initiation of treatment. Tumours in Group 2 animals appeared to be somewhat less sensitive than those in Group 1, with regard to the proportion of tumours whose growth was slowed by treatment and to the length of time before 'relapse'. Serum testosterone levels were variable in untreated animals (mean and range for 10 animals 5.7 (1.9-17.4) nmoles/l), confirming the observation of Grossman et al. (3). In all treated animals serum testosterone was below 1.6 nmoles/l, and in all the longer term castrates and those treated with DESP for more than 20d, the size of the sex accessory glands was markedly reduced.

At the time of excision, some tumours contained cysts filled with clear fluid. Histologically, the tumours contained well-differentiated acini surrounded with stroma which was rather variable in amount and density. At the time of excision, treated tumours did not exhibit marked or consistent histological differences from untreated tumours.

Effect of treatment on ^{3}H-R1881 binding capacity

The results of the SSD assays in the Group 1 tumours are presented in Figure 1, expressed as fm/mg DNA to permit evaluation of cellular distribution of binding sites. Since DNA and cytosol protein yields were approximately 9-12 and 25-40 mg/gm tumour tissue respectively, the cytosol binding per mg DNA is approximately three fold that per mg protein. Values for the dorsolateral prostate (DLP) from an untreated animal are included for comparison. In the DLP, the majority of binding sites for ^{3}H-R1881 were present in the nuclear fraction, and in the cytosol the concentration of sites unoccupied by endogenous androgen (0° + TA) was negligible. In the untreated tumours binding values were quite variable, but the mean concentration present in the nuclei was approximately half that observed in the DLP, and the mean cytosol concentrations were higher in both the 0° and the 15° assay. Nuclear binding was insignificant in all the treated tumours, and mean values for free binding sites were increased relative to those in untreated tumours. The mean concentration of sites assayable at 15° was similar in the untreated and castrated animals, but in some tumours from the DESP treated animals greatly elevated concentrations of ^{3}H-R1881 binding sites were assayable at 15°. The results from the Group 2 animals were similar, except that mean nuclear binding capacity in

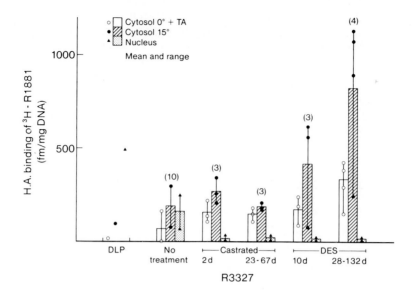

FIG. 1. Binding of ^{3}H-R1881 in cytosol and nuclear fractions of
R3327 tumours assayed under SSD conditions. In the untreated group,
values for individual tumours are omitted, due to lack of space. DLP:
dorsolateral prostate.

untreated tumours was only one-third of that in untreated Group 1
tumours. This was consistent with the binding observed in the 'parent'
tumour used for transplantation and with the somewhat lower sensitivity
to treatment <u>in vivo</u>. Also, elevated binding at 15° was observed in
some tumours from Group 2 animals which had been castrated longer than
4 weeks. Tumours from animals which had been treated with DESP for 4
weeks, followed by castration and sacrifice after a further 4 week had
a similar binding distribution and capacity to acutely (2d) castrated
animals. Tumours from animals which had 4 weeks DESP treatment
beginning 4 weeks after castration showed a similar binding
distribution and capacity to those which had had DESP treatment alone,
with elevated binding at 15°.

Characterization of ^{3}H-R1881 binding

Scatchard analysis

In untreated tumours, Scatchard analysis was carried out using
nuclear and cytosol exchange assays only, owing to the low
concentration of free binding sites. Linear Scatchard plots were
obtained, giving a Kd's of 3.2-7.9nM, and mean Bmax of 247 fm/mg DNA
for the nuclei, and 157 fm/mg protein for the cytosol. Comparison
of the B_{SSD} values for the same tumours showed that the SSD assay
underestimated the Bmax by 7-30%. Linear plots were also obtained
from analysis of free cytosol sites at 0° in treated tumours. Kd's
ranged from 0.08-0.12 nM and Bmax values were virtually identical
with these obtained in SSD assays on the same tumours. In order to
characterize the elevated ^{3}H-R1881 binding sites observed in the

15° assay in the DESP treated tumours, Scatchard analysis was
carried out under exchange assay conditions (Figure 2). Curved
plots were obtained which could be resolved into two components by
the graphic analysis of Rosenthal (9). One component was of high
affinity (Kα ~ 0.5nM) and similar capacity to that observed in
untreated tumour, whereas the other was of much lower affinity (Kd
~ 200nM) and higher capacity (> 500 fm/mg protein). In the 15°
SSD assay, the quantity of high affinity component would have been
overestimated, whereas the lower affinity component would not have
been saturated.

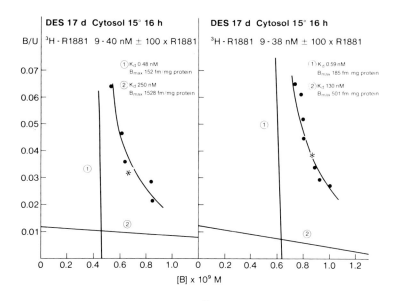

FIG. 2. Scatchard plot analysis of ³H-R1881 binding to cytosol of
DESP-treated R3327 tumours, assayed at 15° in the absence of TA. The
plots have been corrected for nonsaturable binding. Resolution into 2
components was carried out by the method of Rosenthal (9). Asterisks
represent the value at the concentration of ligand used in the SSD
assay.

Sucrose density gradient centrifugation
The results from the SDGC studies were consistent with those from
the Scatchard analysis. Single saturable peaks were observed at ~
4S and ~ 8S in the nuclear extract and cytosol (after exchange
assay) respectively of untreated tumour. A single saturable peak at
~ 8S was also observed in the cytosol of tumour from DESP-treated
animals when incubated under free site conditions (0° + TA) (Figure
3) and in that from a 2-day castrate when assayed under both free
site conditions and at 15°. However in DESP-treated tumours assayed
at 15°, in addition to this peak, there was a considerable amount of
saturable binding distributed in a diffuse way towards the top of
the gradient (Figure 3).

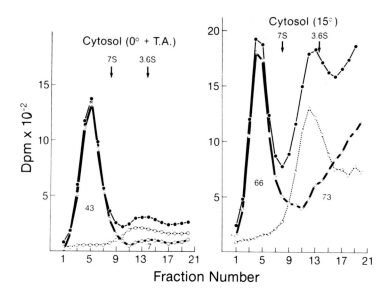

FIG. 3. SDGC analysis of ³H–R1881 binding to cytosol of DESP–
treated tumour, after incubation under free site conditions (left
panel) and at 15° (right panel). Saturable (total–nonsaturable)
binding is represented by the bold line. Figures under the peaks
represent saturable binding expressed as fm/mg protein applied.

Steroid specificity studies

The steroid specificity studies carried out at 15° indicated that
high affinity binding of the ³H–R1881 in the DESP–treated tumours
was qualitatively different from that in untreated tumours. In the
latter, the steroid specificity of this binding was characteristic
of that of an androgen receptor. In order of effectiveness, the RBA
of the competitors used was: R1881 = 1 > DHT = 0.84 > progesterone
= 0.2 > estradiol = DES = 0.02 > R5020, < 0.02 > cortisol < 0.004.
In the DESP–treated tumours, however, the steroid specificity
appeared to have shifted towards that of a progestin–binding
protein. RBA's were: R1881 = 1 > R5020 = 0.43 > norethindrone =
0.27 > cyproterone acetate = 0.11 > DHT = 0.02 > estradiol = 0.01 >
cortisol < 0.004.

Binding of ³H–R5020

SDGC analysis of cytosol from an untreated tumour after incubation
with ³H–R5020 under conditions which conserve PgR and eliminate
binding to AR and glucocorticoid receptor showed a small peak of
saturable binding at ~ 8S. In a parallel analysis on a DESP–
treated tumour, this peak was more than 10–fold larger, and in
addition a smaller peak at ~ 4S was observed (Figure 4).

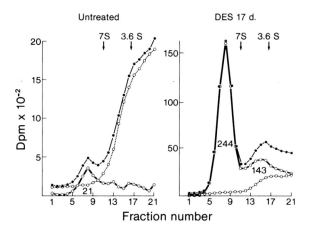

FIG. 4. SDGC analysis of ³H–R5020 binding to cytosol of untreated
and DESP–treated tumours, after incubation under conditions which
conserve PgR. Note the difference in scales on the ordinates. Symbols
as in Fig. 3.

CONCLUSIONS

Some of the effects of treatment on ³H–R1881 binding in the R3327
tumour, viz the reduction in nuclear binding and the increase in
cytosol binding assayable under free site conditions, were expected
consequences of androgen deprivation. This results in release of AR
from the nuclear compartment into the cytosol and 'emptying' of cytosol
sites. However, in addition to these effects, an elevation of binding
at 15° in the absence of TA was observed in some tumours from DESP–
treated animals in both Groups, and also in some long–term castrates in
Group 2. Characterization of the binding under these conditions by
Scatchard analysis and SDGC indicated the presence of two components,
one of which resembled the binding in untreated tumours; the other
appeared to have a lower affinity for ³H–R1881 and was degraded
during SDGC, under conditions suitable for conservation of AR.
Although these conditions were poor for the conservation of PgR, the
steroid specificity of ³H–R1881 binding in DESP–treated tumours at
15° in the absence of TA was more like that of a progestin–binding
protein than that in untreated tumours under the same conditions.
Steriod specificity in untreated tumours was characteristic of that of
AR. Taken together, these results suggested that DESP–treatment
resulted in the appearance of a progestin binding protein, possibly
PgR, which had rather low affinity for R1881 and/or was partially
degraded under the conditions used for AR assay. This conclusion was
supported by SDGC studies using ³H–R5020 as ligand under conditions
which conserve PgR. Saturable binding of ³H–R5020 in the cytosol of
DESP–treated tumour was observed in peaks at ~ 8S and ~ 4S, in
amounts ten–fold that in untreated tumour. Induction of PgR by

estrogen treatment has also been observed in the dog prostate by Dubé
et al. (2). Estrogen receptor has been demonstrated in the prostatic
tissue of several species (reviewed in (7)) and also in the R3327
tumour (6). It seems likely that it is capable of inducing PgR in male
accessory gland tissue and tumours derived from it as well as in female
target organs. However, the observations that we have reported here do
not correspond exactly to those we reported in DESP-treated human
prostatic carcinoma (8). In the latter, the elevated ^{3}H-R1881
binding was due mainly to an increase in free AR sites far greater than
could be accounted for by the effects of reduced circulating
testosterone levels. Nevertheless, we also observed additional
significant amounts of ^{3}H-R1881 binding at 15° in some of the treated
tumours, which were assumed to be due to occupied AR. It is now
apparent that these latter sites may in fact have been due to the
presence of progesterone receptor, and this possibility is now under
investigation.

ACKNOWLEDGEMENTS

This investigation was supported by grant #251 from the Ontario
Cancer Treatment and Research Foundation. Animals were obtained from
Dr. N. Altman, Papanicolaou Cancer Research Institute at Miami, Inc.,
by courtesy of the National Prostatic Cancer Project (D.H.E.W., U.S.)
The sodium salt of diethylstilbestrol diphosphate was kindly supplied
by Frank W. Horner, Ltd., Montreal. The collaboration of Dr. S.
Urbanski in evaluating the histopathology, and Dr. M. d'Costa, for the
serum testosterone radioimmunoassays, is also greatly appreciated. We
thank Ms. J. Thompson and Mrs. S. Parnell for their expert technical
assistance.

REFERENCES

1. Dische Z. (1955): In: The Nucleic Acids, edited by E. Chargaff
    and J.N. Davidson, Edition 1, Vol. 1, p 285-305. Academic
    Press, New York.
2. Dubé, J.Y., Lesage, R., and Tremblay, R.R. (1979): J. Steroid
    Biochem., 10: 459-466.
3. Grossman, H.B., Kleinert, E.L., Herr, H.W., and Whitmore, W.F.
    (1982): The Prostate, 3: 225-229.
4. Isaacs, J.T., Heston, W.D.W., Weissman, R.M., and Coffey, D.S.
    (1978): Cancer Res., 38: 4353-4359.
5. Lowry, O.H., Rosebrough, N.J., Farr, A.L., and Randall, R.G.
    (1951): J. Biol. Chem., 193: 265-275.
6. Markland, F.S., and Lee, L. (1979): J. Steroid Biochem., 10:
    13-20.
7. Mawhinney, M.G., and Neubauer, B.L. (1979): Invest. Urol., 16:
    409-420.
8. Mobbs, B.G., Johnson, I.E., Connolly, J.G., and Thompson, J.
    (1983): J. Steroid Biochem., 19: 1279-1290.
9. Rosenthal, H.E. (1907): Analyt. Biochem., 20: 525-532.
10. Shain, S.A. and Boesel, R.W. (1978): Invest. Urol., 16: 169-174.
11. Zava, D.T., Landrum, B., Horwitz, K.B., and MacGuire, W.L.
    (1979): Endocrinology 104: 1007-1012.

Progress in Cancer Research and Therapy,
Vol. 31, edited by F. Bresciani, et al.
Raven Press, New York © 1984.

Enzymatic and Receptor Systems as Targets for Therapy of Prostatic Cancer

Avery A. Sandberg and Nobuyuki Kadohama

Roswell Park Memorial Institute, Buffalo, New York 14263

The considerations to be discussed have grown out of the observation that though hormonal manipulation may affect the extent of the disease in prostatic cancer, and in some cases remarkably so, it is almost never curative (8). Whether the cancer cells which disappear following hormonal manipulation are extremely sensitive to this approach and recurrence of disease is due to proliferation of other unaffected cells without hormonal dependence or whether recurrence is due to the responsive cells having become resistant to hormonal manipulation, is a question that has not been answered unequivocally. Since in all likelihood prostatic cancers consist of heterogeneous populations of cells (8,37), only some of which are in division or in a metabolic state rendering them sensitive to chemotherapy and/or radiation, we would like to propose a hormonal approach leading to recruitment of non-cycling tumor cells into the proliferative pool with the potential of increasing their chemo- and/or radiosensitivity.

The therapeutic approach promulgated by us in this presentation should be applicable in surgically non-curable cancer of the prostate, especially in the more advanced forms of the disease. Thus, this hypothetical approach may have particular potential in those clinically staged cases found unsuitable for local, curative surgery. Success in advanced prostatic cancer may open possibilities of similar therapeutic regimens in less advanced, surgically non-curable prostatic cancer.

This presentation will address itself to some aspects of hormonally dependent prostatic systems of an intracellular nature whose possible manipulation may have applicability in the treatment of cancer of that gland. However, before discussing these parameters it should be pointed out that the cellular heterogeneity of the normal gland and prostatic cancer, in the latter both genomic and phenotypic (8,37), is undoubtedly associated with a similar heterogeneity of function and histology. Thus, in normal and cancerous prostates, some glands can be shown to be functioning as part of the general secretory activity of the organ, while others appear to be in a resting stage; some cells can be shown to have high acid phosphatase levels, while others seem to be devoid of this enzyme. The very structure of the gland is of a heterogeneous nature, consisting of stroma, epithelium and other elements with many of the physiologic and biochemical characteristics of the cells also showing a similar heterogeneity. For example, most of the 5α-reductase activity and estrogen receptor are present in the stromal cells (7,9,20), whereas the androgen receptor appears to be primarily localized in the

epithelial cells (20).   Thus, in discussing treatment of prostatic
cancer this particular heterogeneity must be taken into consideration
if we are ultimately to treat the disease successfully.   The grade of
histologic differentiation of the cancer is another important aspect,
for the very differentiated tumors tend to resemble the normal gland
biochemically and otherwise, than do the more undifferentiated cancers.
However, heterogeneity of the tumors is also reflected in this area by
the not infrequent lack of correlation between androgen receptor concentration and histologic grade of the tumor (39).   It is possible that
a high proportion of the undifferentiated tumors do not have the endocrine profile characteristic of the more differentiated tumors and this,
of course, would place hormonal manipulation of minimal value in the
treatment of highly undifferentiated tumors, though, as will be discussed later, it is possible that the use of chemotherapy in conjunction
with some hormonal manipulation may have definite value in the therapy
of very undifferentiated cancers.   A caveat to be kept in mind is that
though data obtained in animals can be used in evaluating approaches to
the human gland and its cancers, often these animal glands differ basically from that of the human and not in every case can findings obtained
in animals be applicable to the human condition.   This is true of the
prostate of the rat and dog, though in recent years it has been shown
that the baboon's gland has many similarities to that of the human and
that this primate can serve as an excellent surrogate for performing
experimental studies for extrapolation to the human prostate (35).

We shall address ourselves primarily to two intracellular hormonally
associated systems, i.e., the 5α-reductase system responsible for conversion of testosterone (T) to dihydrotestosterone (DHT) and the androgen receptor for DHT which apparently plays a crucial role in transla-
ting the effects of androgenic hormones in the prostate.
Studies point to the interesting situation in which most of the 5α-
reductase activity is present in the stroma of the gland, while the
androgen receptor is located in the epithelial cells.   On the other hand,
the estrogen receptor (and possibly that for progesterone) is localized
in the stroma, again creating a rather complex situation in which heterogeneity of biochemical pathways is present in the gland.

Emphasis has been placed on the androgen receptor for a number of
reasons (e.g., key role of androgens in the physiology of the prostate,
the high concentrations of the receptor in the gland, correlation with
therapeutic response), though it is certainly not our intent to ignore
other receptors, such as those for estrogens and progestins.   This is
only because the role these latter receptors play in the prostate and
its cancers, and certainly this may turn out to be a crucial one, and
their clinical correlates are much less known than those of the androgen
receptor.   In addition, the interrelationship between the various prostatic receptors under normal and cancerous conditions is still an un-
explored area (30).

Studies in animals, and to some extent in humans receiving estrogen
therapy, have indicated that the 5α-reductase system is dependent on
androgens for its full function (14,22).   Thus, this activity can be
abolished either by orchiectomy or through the administration of estrogens (or LHRH agonists and antagonists) leading to severe suppression
of LH levels and, thus, to cessation of testosterone synthesis by the
testes.   Whether estrogens have a direct effect on the 5α-reductase

system is still a moot point, since most of the cited studies have been performed in vitro utilizing rather large concentrations of estrogens which are unlikely to be present in the gland under in vivo conditions (2,11,23). Inhibition of 5α-reductase activity by chemotherapeutic agents has been used by us as a test system for drugs potentially useful in prostatic cancer; there is little doubt that such inhibition can be induced by some drugs, but this may be a general phenomenon of the activity of the drugs resulting in decreased synthesis of new proteins of which the 5α-reductase system would be one. Nevertheless, significant inhibition of the 5α-reductase system can be induced by certain chemotherapeutic agents (35,38,40).

Control of the androgen receptor system has been less clearly defined than that for 5α-reductase, though it also depends on the action of androgens for its presence and concentration (7,19,27,39). The effects of androgens, particularly of the most powerful one in the prostate, i.e., DHT, are mediated through translocation of the receptor-steroid complex to the nucleus, where functions controlled by androgens are then transcribed into various messenger RNAs and then into proteins. If one of these proteins is the 5α-reductase system or the androgen receptor, then one arrives at a rather circular system in which 5α-reductase and the androgen receptor, which are crucial in converting testosterone to DHT and then in the manifestations of androgenic activity, respectively, are themselves dependent for their integrity on these androgens. In other words, the system is driven by and, therefore, dependent on biologically available free (unbound) testosterone. Thus, manipulation of the systems, either by suppression or activation of the 5α-reductase system and intracellular replacement of the active androgen (DHT) on the receptor by inactive androgens or inert substances, may be useful in those prostatic cancers in which the survival and function of at least a significant proportion of cells is dependent on the androgen associated systems.

At present, the best available stimulator of the 5α-reductase system is testosterone (following its conversion to DHT), though the development of other stimulators with specificity for the prostatic enzyme but lacking the other systemic and side effects of DHT and T may require our attention in the future. A number of steroidal inhibitors (6-methylene derivatives of progesterone, 4-chloro-steroids, substituted 4-aza-4-methyl-androsterone, 4-MA, 16β-ethyl-17β-hydroxy-4-estren-3-one) of 5α-reductase is already available (1,5,6,10,29,42,46,47), as well as steroidal (cyproterone acetate, testolactone) and non-steroidal (flutamide, anandron) competitors for the androgen receptor (24,32). Competitors for the estrogen receptor (tamoxifen) and for the progesterone one (gestrinone-R2323) are also available (24,32).

The relationship between the androgen receptor and those for estrogens and progestins is not clear. In the castrated dog, the administration of estrogens in conjunction with androgens leads to a definitely increased level of androgen receptor, over that seen when the estrogen was not administered (27). The androgen receptor in a system, which though quite different from that of the prostate, i.e., the chick oviduct, is also sensitive to estrogen administration (44). To-date, it is not clear as to what the exact relationship between estrogen administration and the androgen, progestin and estrogen receptors in the human prostate; studies in this area should prove to be of value in interpreting and predicting results obtained on the androgen receptor, particularly in cancerous tissue.

In castrated animals the administration of testosterone or DHT results in a definite increased mitotic activity of the gland, ultimately leading to restoration of its size and function (43). In fact, DHT is probably the key substance necessary for survival of the cells in the prostate. Under normal conditions testosterone is metabolized along the 5α-reductive pathway leading to the production of DHT, the most crucial and powerful androgen in prostatic physiology, with the oxidative system (17β-hydroxysteroid dehydrogenase) leading to the production of androstenedione, a rather weak androgen.   However, it has been shown in cancerous tissue that the ratio of the products of the oxidative and reductive pathways is greatly increased, probably due to much lesser activity of 5α-reductase (12,13,21,28,31,41), though the possibility exists of a definitely increased activity of the oxidative pathway. At present, little is known about the possible effects of the oxygenated steroids in cancer physiology. If such oxygenated steroids play a role in prostatic cancer, advantage could be taken of increasing the 5α-reductase system at the expense of the oxidative one in patients being treated with chemotherapeutic agents and/or ionizing radiation. This hypothesis is based on the premise that cells in division and those replicating their DNA are much more sensitive to chemotherapeutic agents and ionizing radiation than resting cells. Thus, it would appear that for chemotherapy to be effective in prostatic cancer it may be necessary to activate or suppress the 5α-reductase system or the oxidative one in order to have as many cells in the S phase of the cell cycle or in mitosis as is possible. Hence, serious consideration should be given to the concomitant administration of agents of either suppressive or activating nature on the 5α-reductase or oxidative system which can be administered with cytotoxic drugs. The latter would probably have to include a battery of drugs in order to take care of the heterogeneous nature of the cancer cells in prostatic malignancy. Obviously, those cancers in which the activity of either the reductive or oxidative pathway is very low or absent and, hence, the tumors can be assumed not to be hormonally dependent, may not be as responsive to the above hypothetical approach as are the more differentiated tumors with a significant hormonal profile. Nevertheless, even in non-hormonally associated tumors it may be worthwhile to attempt to alter their hormonal milieu in order to ascertain the value of this therapeutic approach (Table 1).

It should be stressed that the administration of either 5α-reductase suppressors or activators (or those of the oxidative pathway) must be undertaken in conjunction with chemotherapy and/or radiation, since in all probability without these cytotoxic agents, the malignant condition would be greatly aggravated through stimulation of the cells to mitotic activity and, hence, into more aggressive biology. Apparently, such a situation occurs as a result of the "testosterone surge" observed during the early administration of LHRH agonists (48).

Since suppression of the 5α-reductase system usually leads to a much higher activity of the oxidative pathway, the use of such inhibitors, both of steroidal and nonsteroidal nature (25,26,33,45), may offer an opportunity for the utilization of these relatively safe agents in combination with various chemotherapeutic agents or x-ray therapy. Though following orchiectomy or estrogen administration synthesis of testosterone by the testis is almost totally suppressed, the presence of some testosterone in the prostatic gland or cancer is probably related to

TABLE 1. CURRENTLY USED, AVAILABLE OR INVESTIGATED
MODALITIES IN THE TREATMENT OF PROSTATIC CANCER

I. Hormonal
   A. Ablative (Prevention or ablation of androgen, particularly tes-
       tosterone, production)
      1. Orchiectomy
      2. Hypophysectomy
      3. Adrenalectomy
   B. Suppression of LH secretion or effects
      1. Estrogen therapy
      2. LHRH analogs and antagonists
      3. Testosterone or DHT therapy (in conjunction with chemotherapy
        and/or radiation)
   C. Treatment with compounds with high affinity for intracellular
      receptors
      1. Androgen receptors
        a. Steroidal (cyproterone acetate)
        b. Non-steroidal (flutamide, anandron)
      2. Estrogenic receptors (tamoxifen)
      3. Progestin receptors
      4. Prostatein (Emcyt)
   D. Treatment with 5α-reductase inhibitors or activators (various
      substituted steroids)
II. Chemotherapy (including conjugates with steroidal compounds)
III. Radiation and related approaches
IV. Surgical removal

conversion of adrenal steroids to testosterone; thus, the utilization of
agents affecting the 5α-reductase system still has a place even in those
patients who have undergone orchiectomy.

Not only the structural but also the functional heterogeneity of the
human prostatic gland, usually reflected in cancer conditions, which are
additionally characterized by cytogenetic heterogeneity (34,37), make it
difficult to discuss any parameter as being characteristic for the total
gland. As mentioned previously, though the gland undoubtedly depends on
androgens, particularly DHT, for its survival, integrity and function,
the distribution of the enzymatic systems and receptors essential for
these, shows anatomic and cellular variations. Nevertheless, an overview of this androgen effect can be described as follows: testosterone
(T), after entering the prostatic cell (prolactin may possibly play an
effect here (36)), is reduced at position-5 by the 5α-reductase system
yielding the most potent androgen, as far as the prostate is concerned,
dihydrotestosterone (DHT) (Fig. 1). DHT is then bound by a receptor
which subsequently becomes translocated to the nucleus at a possible
specific site on the nuclear matrix (3), leading to transcription of DNA
to yield messenger RNAs, which find their way into the cytoplasm to direct the synthesis of various proteins, including enzymes such as 5α-
reductase, prostatic acid phosphatase and arginase, various receptors,
etc. Some of these are related to the secretory activity of a gland,
but others undoubtedly play an important part in the survival of the
prostatic cells, though such enzymatic systems have not received the
attention of the functionally more specialized ones. The synthesis of

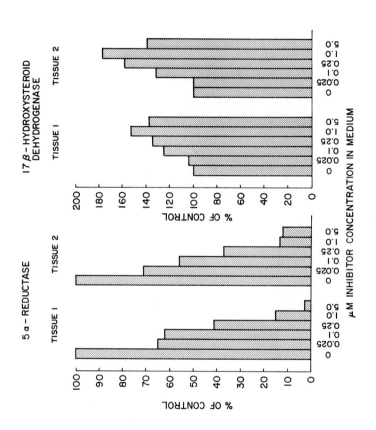

FIG. 1., Effects of various concentrations of 4-methyl-3-oxo-4-aza-5α-pregnane-20(s)-carboxylate (4-MAPC) on the reductive and oxidative metabolism of testosterone in human prostatic carcinoma in culture. The results are from 2 separate explants using different specimens of prostatic tumor. Note severe decrease in 5α-reductase activity and somewhat increased activity of the oxidative pathway (17β-hydroxysteroid dehydrogenase).

TABLE 2. EFFECT OF 6-METHYLENE DERIVATIVES OF PROGESTERONE ON
5α-REDUCTASE ACTIVITY IN HUMAN PROSTATE IN ORGAN CULTURE

Inhibitor	Testosterone	Δ^4A-Dione	DHT	% of Control
None	21.23±2.91	6.94±1.53	19.58±1.84	100
Progesterone	25.37±3.15	7.12±0.45	10.62±1.95*	54
VP-56	24.17±2.99	5.94±0.69	20.73±0.41	105
VP-50	19.07±1.67	3.14±0.26	14.05±0.68**	71
VP-63	21.74±3.04	5.17±0.57	11.45±0.75*	58

Explants were prepared from a specimen of benign prostatic hyperplasia.
Testosterone (0.5 μM) was present in all media; Inhibitor concentrations
were 5.0 μM.
VP-56 = 17α-acetoxy-6-methyl-progesterone (megestrol acetate).
VP-50 = 17α-acetoxy-6-methylene-progesterone
VP-63 = 6-methylene-progesterone
Values are picomoles of metabolite of ^{3}H-testosterone formed per 50 mg
of tissue per 2 hrs; means ± S.E. for 4 determinations.
*p<.025; **p<.05

receptors for androgens, estrogens and progesterone is probably also controlled by the androgen receptor, though the roles played by the estrogen
and progestin receptors are still to be elucidated. Undoubtedly, these
will be found also to play crucial roles, but possibly on a more limited
scale, than that of the androgen receptor. Interfering with these two
systems, i.e., the enzymatic and the receptor, should possibly be given
more attention in designing future approaches for chemotherapy of prostatic cancer. In this, the role played by the oxygenated derivatives of
testosterone, particularly androstenedione, is yet to be settled, particularly in cancerous tissue. Were this and related steroids shown to
be potent compounds in the control of prostatic cell division and survival, inhibition of the oxidative pathway may have to assume an importance akin to that of 5α-reductase, at least in malignant tissue. This
area will be further clarified when specific effects of each endogenous
steroid on cancer cells are clearly delineated in both hormonally dependent and independent prostatic tumors.

Suppression of 5α-reductase activity can be accomplished by a number
of substituted steroids, as well as by a number of chemotherapeutic
agents (35,38). The level of such suppression varies considerably, both
in effectiveness and duration. In vivo, 5α-reductase activity is definitely reduced when patients are orchiectomized or given estrogens
(14,20), both approaches leading to a greatly reduced if not absent levels of testosterone in the circulation, thus leading to reduction of
synthesis of various substances under the control of androgens including
5α-reductase. Generally, when that occurs, the oxidative pathway in the
prostate becomes a major one, including cancerous tissues of that gland
(22). Inhibition or activation of this system will require our further
attention, if the oxygenated steroids are shown to play an important
role in the survival and biology of prostatic cancer.

In Tables 2-5 and Figures 1 and 2 are shown results obtained in our

TABLE 3. EFFECT OF STEROIDAL 4-CHLORO-DERIVATIVES ON 5α-REDUCTASE ACTIVITY IN HUMAN PROSTATE IN ORGAN CULTURE

Inhibitor	Conc. (μM)	Testosterone	Δ^4A-Dione	DHT	% of Control
None	–	28.89±1.89	18.56±2.13	14.08±2.00	100
FB-1	0.5	31.88±2.77	15.89±1.39	13.67±1.31	97
"	1.0	43.16±3.53	19.97±0.72	10.90±0.93	77
"	2.5	36.58±4.25	13.54±1.74	6.71±0.37**	48
"	5.0	42.26±2.10	11.73±1.74	6.00±0.54**	42
FB-7	0.5	31.77±3.08	17.36±0.55	10.08±1.24	71
"	1.0	34.64±1.39	15.89±1.43	9.33±0.47	66
"	2.5	34.28±2.32	18.45±1.52	6.33±0.24**	45
"	5.0	37.45±2.61	17.24±0.67	4.70±0.11*	33

Explants were prepared from benign hyperplastic tissue.
Testosterone was present in all media at a concentration of 0.5 μM.
FB-1 = 4-chloro-testosterone
FB-7 = 4-chloro-17α-hydroxyprogesterone
Values are picomoles of metabolites of ^{3}H-testosterone formed per 50 mg of tissue per 2 hrs; means ± S.E. for 4 determinations. *$p < .005$; **$p < .01$

TABLE 4. EFFECT OF SOME 4-CHLORO-SUBSTITUTED STEROIDS ON 5α-REDUCTASE ACTIVITY IN RAT AND HUMAN PROSTATES IN ORGAN CULTURE

Inhibitor (5μM)	Rat Ventral Prostate 5α-Reduced Products	% Inhibition	Human Prostate (BPH) 5α-Reduced Products	% Inhibition
None	89.60±4.12	–	37.50±7.41[d]	–
4-Chloroandrost-4-ene-17β-ol-3-one	41.23±3.28[a]	54	15.81±2.10[d]	57
23,24-Dinorchol-4-en-22-ol-3-one	51.59±7.52[b]	42	20.15±4.22[e]	46
4-Chloro-23,24-dinorchol-4-en-22-ol-3-one	80.31±3.98[e]	10	30.83±5.04[e]	17
4-Chloropregn-4-ene-3,20-dione	74.13±1.82[d]	17	30.16±4.51[e]	20
4-Chloropreg-4-ene-17α-ol-3,20-dione	11.71±1.45[a]	87	11.33±0.78[c]	70

Values are means of 4 determinations ± S.E.
[a]$p < .0005$ [b]$p < .005$ [c]$p < .01$ [d]$p < .025$ [e]Difference from control not significant
The results are expressed as picomoles/30mg tissue/2 hrs. and picomoles/50mg tissue/2 hrs.

TABLE 5. EFFECT OF A 5α-REDUCTASE INHIBITOR ON THE METABOLIC PATTERN OF TESTOSTERONE
IN EXPLANTS OF HUMAN PROSTATIC CARCINOMA AND ORGAN CULTURE MEDIUM

	Testo-sterone	Polar Metabs.	A-Dione	A-Diol	DHT	A-Diol + DHT
TISSUE						
No Inhibitor	14.38±1.77	0.58±0.40	10.36±1.65	4.66±0.75	19.26±2.80	23.92±3.41
With Inhibitor	22.86±1.15	0.26±0.11	15.94±0.65[b]	1.13±0.22[a]	4.63±0.28[a]	5.76±0.45[a]
MEDIUM						
No Inhibitor	3477±18	19±3	22±5	41±5	38±3	79±6
With Inhibitor	3528±28	12±9	24±3	40±5	33±9	73±13

Values are in picomoles per 50mg of tissue per 2 hrs. or total picomoles recovered from 7.5ml of medium containing 0.5μM testosterone.
Inhibitor was 1.0μM 4-methyl-3-oxo-4-aza-5 -pregnane-20(s)-carboxylate.
All values are means of 4 determinations ± S. E.
[a]p < .005; [b]p < .025

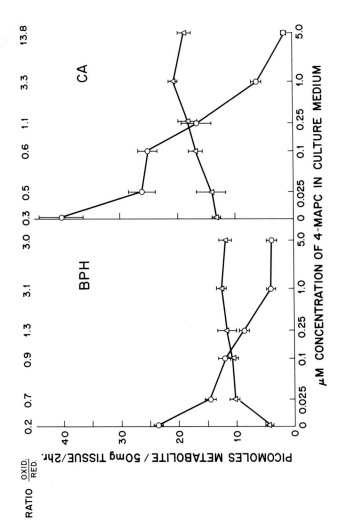

FIG. 2., Products of 5α-reductase and 17β-hydroxysteroid dehydrogenase were measured in explants of human prostate in organ culture. In uninhibited control tissues of both BPH and carcinoma (CA), testosterone was metabolized predominantly via the reductive pathway. The ratio of Δ⁴-androstenedione to DHT was 0.2 for BPH and 0.3 for carcinoma. The addition of increasing amounts of 4-MAPC produced strong inhibition of 5α-reductase, while 17β-hydroxysteroid dehydrogenase activity was progressively enhanced. The alteration in the metabolic pathway was that oxidation to Δ⁴-androstenedione was the predominant metabolic pathway of testosterone. At 1μM inhibitor concentration, the ratio of Δ⁴-androstenedione to DHT was greater than 3.

laboratory with non-cancerous and cancerous rat and human prostatic tissues. These studies utilized explants of prostates in organ culture in which various 5α-reductase inhibitors were used. From the data in Table 2 it can be seen that 6-methylene substitution of progesterone (15-17,29) results in strong inhibitory activity, whereas 6-methyl substitution of megestrol acetate has no effect on 5α-reductase, presumably because of lack of stereochemical specificity for optimal interaction with the target enzyme.

In Tables 3 and 4 are shown results in which the A-ring of the steroid nucleus has been modified to enhance binding to 5α-reductase and render the agent hormonally inactive (4,17). A number of 4-chloro-substituted steroids have been studied by us, with the 4-chloro derivatives of 17α-hydroxyprogesterone being particularly potent inhibitors of 5α-reductase. In Table 5 are shown results with another inhibitor of 5α-reductase (5).

Of interest is the observation that in cases where inhibition of the 5α-reductase system was significant, it was accompanied in some instances by an increase in the oxidative pathway, leading to an increased androstenedione production, but not in other cases. In fact, in some cases a decrease in androstenedione production occurred.

Interference with the receptor-DHT complex activity can be accomplished by various means, including substitution on the receptor for DHT by substances with a much higher affinity for the protein. Included in this group of substances are steroidal (cyproterone acetate) and non-steroidal compounds (flutamide, anandron). The fact that some of the non-steroidal substances are active orally (32), places them in a unique position for their possible use in the treatment of prostatic cancer. It must be again emphasized that the use of substances with a high affinity for the receptor usually does not interfere with 5α-reductase activity and this aspect of prostatic metabolism must be kept in mind when these substances are used as sole treatment agents.

It would appear that the best approach in the treatment of prostatic cancer, once the importance of the reductive and oxidative steroid pathways have been clearly established, is to use both types of agents concomitantly, i.e., 5α-reductase inhibitors and substances with high affinity for the receptor, thus making sure that two hormonally associated systems of crucial importance to prostatic cell survival can be affected, while at the same time chemotherapy or radiation is given. There remains doubt that the use of these hormonally affecting agents per se will be the ultimate approach to the treatment of prostatic cancer; we suggest that they be given in concert with several chemotherapeutic agents and/or ionizing radiation. Combining these various modalities, particularly when dormant cancer cells can be stimulated into mitotic division, as discussed above, should hypothetically yield much better results than afforded by present therapeutic regimens. The recent introduction of LHRH antagonists and agonists (and possibly in the future substances of a similar nature related to prolactin secretion), have added another segment in the treatment of prostatic cancer, for in combination with the other substances mentioned (5α-reductase inhibitors or stimulators and receptor associated substances), this approach may prove to be, in fact, the optimal one available, as based on the present knowledge of prostatic anatomy, physiology, cytogenetics and biochemistry. In the background one must always keep in mind the remarkable heterogeneity, such as cytogenetic, physiologic and anatomic, shown by prostatic cancer, where hormonally sensitive cells would be affected by the regimens outlined above, but cells without such characteristics may require approaches quite different from those delineated herein.

ACKNOWLEDGMENT

Studies emanating from the authors' laboratory and alluded to in this presentation have been supported in part by a grant (CA-15436) from the National Cancer Institute through the National Prostatic Cancer Project.

REFERENCES

1. Altwein, J.E., Orestano, F., and Hohenfellner, R. (1974): Invest. Urol., 12:157-161.
2. Bard, D.R., and Lasnitzki, I. (1977): J. Endocr., 74:1-9.
3. Barrack, E.R. (1982): In: The Nuclear Envelope and the Nuclear Matrix, pp. 247-258. Alan R. Liss, Inc., New York.
4. Batzold, F. (1981): In: The Prostatic Cell: Structure and Function, Part B, edited by G.P. Murphy, A.A. Sandberg and J.P. Karr, pp. 269-282. Alan R. Liss, Inc., New York.
5. Brooks, J.R., Baptista, E.M., Berman, C., Ham, E.A., Hichens, M., Johnston, D.B.R., Primka, R.L., Rasmusson, G.H., Reynolds, G.F., Schmitt, S.M., and Arth, G.E. (1981): Endocrinology, 109:830-836.
6. Brooks, J.R., Berman, D., Glitzer, M.S., Gordon, L.R., Primka, R.L., Reynolds, G.F., and Rasmusson, G.H. (1982): The Prostate, 3:35-44.
7. Bruchovsky, N., McLoughlin, M.G., Rennie, P.S., and To, M.P. (1981): In: The Prostatic Cell: Structure and Function, Part A, pp. 161-175. Alan R. Liss, Inc., New York.
8. Coffey, D.S., and Issacs, J.T. (1979): In: Prostatic Cancer, edited by D.S. Coffey and J.T. Issacs, pp. 233-263. International Union Against Cancer, Geneva, Switzerland.
9. Cowan, R.A., Cowan, S.K., Grant, J.K., and Elder, H.Y. (1977): J. Endocr., 74:111-120.
10. Dupuy, G.M., Roberts, K.D., Bleau, G., and Chapdelaine, A. (1977): J. Steroid Biochem., 8:1145-1151.
11. Farnsworth, W.E. (1969): Invest. Urol., 6:423-427.
12. Ghanadian, R., Masters, J.R.W., and Smith, C.B. (1981): Eur. Urol., 7:169-170.
13. Hammond, G.L. (1978): J. Endocr., 78:7-19.
14. Jenkins, J.S., and McCaffery, V.M. (1974): J. Endocr., 63:517-526.
15. Kadohama, N., Kirdani, R.Y., Murphy, G.P., and Sandberg, A.A. (1977): Oncology, 34:123-128.
16. Kadohama, N., Petrow, V., Lack, L., and Sandberg, A.A. (1983): J. Steroid Biochem., 18:551-558.
17. Kadohama, N., and Sandberg, A.A. (1984): In: In Vitro Models for Cancer Research, edited by M.M. Webber and L. Sekely. CRC Press, Inc., Boca Raton, Florida.
18. Kozák, I., Bartsch, W., Krieg, M., and Voigt, K.-D. (1982): The Prostate, 3:433-438.
19. Krieg, M., Bartsch, W., Janssen, W., and Voigt, K.-D. (1979): J. Steroid Biochem., 11:615-624.
20. Krieg, M., Klötzl, G., Kaufmann, J., and Voigt, K.-D. (1981): Acta Endocrinol., 96:422-432.
21. Lakey, W.H., Bruchovsky, N., Callaway, T., Comeau, T., Lieskovsky, G., Rennie, P., Shnitka, T., and Wilkin, P. (1979): Trans. Am. Assoc. Genitourin. Surg., 71:19-22.

22. Leav, I., Morfin, R.F., Ofner, P., Cavazos, L.F., and Leeds, E.B. (1971): Endocrinology, 89:465-483.
23. Lee, D.K.H., Bird, C.E., and Clark, A.F. (1973): Steroids, 22:677-685.
24. Leinonen, P., Bolton, N.J., Kontturi, M., and Vihko, R. (1982): The Prostate, 3:589-597.
25. Liang, T., and Heiss, C.E. (1981): J. Biol. Chem., 256:7998-8005.
26. Malathi, K., and Gurpide, E. (1977): J. Steroid Biochem., 8:743-746.
27. Moore, R.J., Gazak, J.M., and Wilson, J.D. (1979): J. Clin. Invest., 63:351-257.
28. Morfin, R.F., Leav, I., Charles, J.-F., Cavazos, L.F., Ofner, P., and Floch, H.H. (1977): Cancer, 39:1517-1534.
29. Petrow, V., Wang, Y., Lack, L., and Sandberg, A.A. (1981): Steroids, 38:121-140.
30. Pontes, J.E., Karr, J.P., Kirdani, R.Y., Murphy, G.P., and Sandberg, A.A. (1982): Urology, 19:399-403.
31. Prout, G.R., Jr., Kliman, B., Daly, J.J., Maclaughlin, R.A., and Griffin, P.P. (1976): J. Urol., 116:603-610.
32. Raynaud, J.P., Moguilewsky, M., Lefebvre, F.A., Bélanger, A., and Labrie, F.: The Prostate, (in press).
33. Robaire, B., Covey, D.F., Robinson, C.H., and Ewing, L.L. (1977): J. Steroid Biochem., 8:307-310.
34. Sandberg, A.A. (1980): The Prostate, 1:169-184.
35. Sandberg, A.A. (1981): Urology, 17:34-44.
36. Sandberg, A.A. (1981): In: The Prostatic Cell: Structure and Function, Part B, edited by G.P. Murphy, A.A. Sandberg and J.P. Karr, pp. 55-62. Alan R. Liss, Inc., New York.
37. Sandberg, A.A. (1982): In: Tumor Cell Heterogeneity, edited by A.H. Owens, Jr., D.S. Coffey and S.B. Baylin, pp. 367-397. Academic Press, New York.
38. Sandberg, A.A., and Kadohama, N. (1980): In: Models for Prostate Cancer, edited by G.P. Murphy, pp. 9-29. Alan R. Liss, Inc., New York.
39. Sandberg, A.A., and Karr, J.P. (1983): In: Cancer of the Prostate, edited by G.P. Murphy, pp. 331-343. W.B. Saunders Co., Ltd., London, England.
40. Sandberg, A.A., Müntzing, J., Kadohama, N., Karr, J.P., Sufrin, G., Kirdani, R.Y., and Murphy, G.P. (1977): Cancer Treat. Rep., 61: 289-295.
41. Smith, C.B., Masters, J.R.W., Metacalfe, S.A., and Ghanadian, R.: Eur. J. Cancer, (in press).
42. Sudo, K., Yoshida, K., Akinaga, Y., and Nakayama, R. (1981): Steroids, 38:55-71.
43. Sufrin, G., and Coffey, D.S. (1973): Invest. Urol., 11:45-54.
44. Tokarz, R.R., Harrison, R.W., and Seaver, S.S. (1979): J. Biol. Chem., 254:9178-9184.
45. Verhoeven, G., and Cailleau, J. (1983): J. Steroid Biochem., 18: 365-367.
46. Wada, F., Nishi, N., and Matuo, Y.: The Prostate, (in press).
47. Wenderoth, U.K., George, F.W., and Wilson, J.D. (1983): Endocrinology, 113:569-573.
48. Wenderoth, U.K., Happ, J., Krause, U., Adenauer, H., and Jacobi, G.H. (1982): Eur. Urol., 8:343-347.

Progress in Cancer Research and Therapy,
Vol. 31, edited by F. Bresciani, et al.
Raven Press, New York © 1984.

5α Reductase Deficiency in Man

Julianne Imperato-McGinley

Department of Medicine, Division of Endocrinology and Metabolism, The New York Hospital-Cornell University Medical Center, New York, New York 10021

Significant progress has been made toward defining the role of androgens in sexual differentiation and development. Jost, in pioneer experiments on rabbit fetuses, demonstrated that female organogenesis, i.e., Mullerian stimulation and Wolffian inhibition, will occur in the absence of the gonads (12). Male sexual differentiation is imposed upon the natural tendency of the fetus toward femaleness. Normal male sexual differentiation requires the secretion of testosterone by the Leydig cells and Mullerian inhibiting factor, by the Sertoli cells of the seminiferous tubules (11). More recent studies have shown that testosterone may act as a prehormone in certain androgen dependent target areas. In specific target areas, testosterone can be converted by the microsomal enzyme steroid 5α-reductase to form 5α dihydrotestosterone, a more potent androgen (24). It has been shown that the onset of testosterone production by the fetal testis (rabbit, rat, human) occurs just prior to the onset of male differentiation of the urogenital tract (25). In both urogenital sinus and urogenital tubercle, in rat, rabbit (26) and human (22) fetuses, the capacity to convert testosterone to dihydrotestosterone is present prior to differentiation of these tissues into the prostate and external genitalia. However, synthesis of dihydrotestosterone does not occur in the Wolffian duct until after its differentiation to the epididymis, vas deferens, and seminal vesicles. The data suggest that at least two androgens are involved in sexual differentiation during embryogenesis.

CLINICAL DESCRIPTION

The biochemical and phenotypic evaluation of male pseudohermaphrodites with 5α -reductase deficiency over the years, reveals their significance as unique clinical models, defining major actions for testosterone and dihydrotestosterone in male sexual differentiation and development, and elucidating a role for testosterone in the evolution of male gender identity (3,5,6,8,18). Our major studies have involved a pedigree of 23 families with 38 male pseudohermaphrodites from the Dominican Republic. Other cases have been reported throughout the world (1,2,7,15,20,21,23), including three reports of occurrance in siblings (2,21,23).

Subjects with 5α-reductase deficiency studied to date have perineal hypospadias, and most have separate urethral and vaginal openings within a urogenital sinus. Rarely a blind vaginal pouch opens into the urethra and in one case a blind vaginal pouch was not demonstrated. Wolffian differentiation is normal and the subjects have an epididymis, vas deferens and seminal vesicles. Epididymis and vas deferens were identified at the time of testicular biopsy of 7 affected members of the Domincan kindred. The incidence of cryptorchidism is significantly higher in childhood than adulthood, suggesting that it is not uncommon for the testes to descend during puberty in this condition.

At puberty, there is deepening of the voice, development of a muscular habitus, growth of the phallus (4-6 cm), rugation and hyperpigmentation of the scrotum and testicular descent. The histology of the adult testes in 7 affected Dominican subjects demonstrate Leydig cell hyperplasia. In adult subjects with undescended testes, the seminiferous tubules contain either only Sertoli cells with thickening of the tunica propria, or aberrant spermatogenesis. Some adult subjects with descended testes also exhibit these findings; while others have normal spermatogenesis (9). The prostates are small to absent; and even in a 65 year old subject, it was not palpated or visualized (7). The subjects have erections and there is an ejaculate from the perineal urethra. They have decreased to absent facial hair and decreased body hair.

BIOCHEMICAL EVALUATION

The biochemical abnormalities in this condition have been characterized by the findings of: 1) Normal to elevated levels of plasma testosterone with decreased levels of plasma dihydrotestosterone and an increased plasma testosterone to dihydrotestosterone ratio (3,9,10,18), 2) Decreased conversion of testosterone to dihydrotestosterone in vivo (3,9,10,18), 3) Decreased production of the urinary 5α-reductase metabolites of testosterone, i.e., androsterone and androstanediol with elevated etiocholanolone/androsterone and etiocholanediol/androstanediol ratios (3,9,10,18), 4) Decreased urinary 5α-reduced metabolites of C21 steroids and C19 steroids other than testosterone, i.e., cortisol, corticosterone, 11β-hydroxyandrostenedione and androstenedione (18), 5) Diminished 5α-reductase activity in tissue studies (2,4,13,16,17,19,20,23), 6) Familial differences and genetic heterogeneity in tissue studies of enzyme activity (2,7,13,17), and 7) Autosomal recessive inheritance well-documented in pedigree analysis of the Dominican kindred (3,4,18).

HYPOTHESES

In these subjects, 1) a deficiency of dihydrotestosterone in utero results in a developmental defect which is limited to the external genitalia and prostate, enabling us to conclude that differentiation of these structures appears to be affected through the actions of dihydrotestosterone (Fig. 1).

2) Wolffian differentiation develops normally, suggesting that this is a testosterone, and not a dihydrotestosterone mediated function. This correlates with laboratory studies demonstrating that the genital anlage has high 5α-reductase activity at the time of sexual differentiation; while the Wolffian ductal system does not

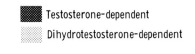

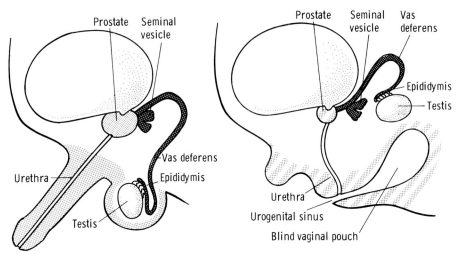

Figure 1.   Schema for the hypothesis for the specific actions of testosterone and dihydrotestosterone in male sexual differentiation <u>in utero</u>.

have the capacity to form dihydrotestosterone until differentiation is completed (22).

3) At puberty, affected males develop rugation and hyperpigmentation of the scrotum, growth of a phallus, an increase in muscle mass and deepening of the voice. Their ultimate height is similar to that of their fathers and normal male siblings. Thus, the aforementioned pubertal events appear to be affected mainly through the actions of testosterone (Fig. 2).

4) Prostatic development and/or enlargement, acne, a normal male distribution of facial and body hair, and temporal recession of the hairline do not occur, and appear to be affected mainly through the actions of dihydrotestosterone. These findings have obvious future clinical implications for the treatment of males with prostatic hypertrophy, acne and baldness, and women with hirsutism and acne through inhibition of 5α-reductase activity (Fig. 2).

5) Affected males have erections, and there is an ejaculate from the perineal urethra. Thus, in the male, the ability to have erections appears to be mediated through the actions of testosterone either directly or via conversion to estradiol. Interestingly, in two subjects, administration of pharmacologic amounts of dihydrotestosterone caused a substantial drop in plasma testosterone with a concomitant loss of libido and the development of impotence (Fig. 2).

6) Plasma LH is frequently elevated with high plasma levels of testosterone, suggesting a role for dihydrotestosterone in the negative feedback control of LH. The elevated plasma LH levels correlate with the light and electron microscopic findings of Leydig cell hyperplasia (9,10,18). Plasma FSH levels are also frequently

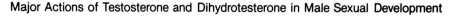

Major Actions of Testosterone and Dihydrotesterone in Male Sexual Development

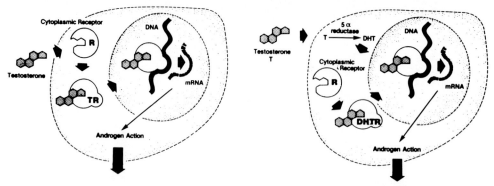

- Muscle Mass Increase
- Penile Enlargement
- Scrotal Enlargement
- Vocal Cord Enlargement
- Skeletal Maturation
- Spermatogenesis
- Pituitary-Gonadal Feedback
- Male Sex Drive, Performance
- Regulation of LH
- Libido Erections

- Increased Facial and Body Hair
- Acne
- Scalp Hair Regression
- Prostrate Enlargement
- Pituitary-Gonadal Feedback
- Regulation of LH

Figure 2.   Schema for the major actions of testosterone and
dihydrotestosterone at puberty.

elevated, which may be a consequence of cryptorchidism with its
resultant effect on spermatogenesis (9,10,18).

ANDROGENS AND GENDER IDENTITY

The psychosexual data demonstrating a gender change from female to
male in 16 of 18 Dominican subjects unambiguously raised as females
in childhood underscores the importance of testosterone exposure of
the brain, in utero, the early postnatal period, and at puberty in
the determination of male gender identity (5,7,8). These subjects
demonstrate that in a nonintervening social environment, when the sex
of rearing is discordant, the testosterone mediated biologic sex will
prevail if the pubertal events are permitted to occur (5,7,8).
Theoretically, under the influence of testosterone "masculinization"
of the brain occurs in utero, and together with the activation of a
testosterone mediated male puberty, a male gender identity develops
despite a female upbringing. This unique experiment of nature
emphasizes the importance of androgens which act as inducers and
activators in the evolution of a male gender identity. Thus, it is
postulated (5,7,8) that in the normal male, the sex of rearing and
testosterone imprinting of the brain act in unison, and together with
the activation of a testosterone mediated male puberty determine the
complete expression of the male gender.

CONCLUSION

Evaluation of the human model of male pseudohermaphrodites with 5α
-reductase deficiency has led us to certin highly significant

hypotheses concerning the actions of T and DHT in male sexual differentiation and development. A natural corollary of this work will be the development and evaluation of a male pseudohermaphroditic animal model with 5α-reductase deficiency (14). The development of an animal model will further elucidate the precise roles of testosterone and dihydrotestosterone in male sexual differentiation and development. Further clarification of the role of dihydrotestosterone in prostatic embryogenesis and development has obvious implications in the treatment of benign prostatic hypertrophy or prostatic carcinoma.

REFERENCES

1. Cantu, M.M., Corona-Rivera, E., Diaz, M., Medina, C., Esquinca, Cortez-Gallegos, V., Vaca, G., and Hernandez, A. (1980): Acta Endocrinol., 94:273-279.
2. Fisher, L.K., Kogut, M.D., Moore, R.J., Goebelsmann, U., Weitzman, J.J., Isaacs, J. Jr., Griffin, J.E., and Wilson, J.D. (1978): J. Clin. Endocrionol. Metab., 47:653-664.
3. Imperato-McGinley, J., Guerrero, L., Gautier, T., and Peterson, R.E. (1974): Science, 186:1213-1215.
4. Imperato-McGinley, J., Guerrero, L., Gautier, T., and Peterson, R.E. (1975): Birth Defects: Original Series, Vol. II, #4, 91-101.
5. Imperato-McGinley, J., Peteron, R.E., Gautier, T., and Sturla, E. (1979): N. Engl. J. Med., 300:1223-1237.
6. Imperato-McGinley, J., Peterson, R.E., Gautier, T., and Sturla, E. (1979): J. Steroid Biochem., 11:637-645.
7. Imperato-McGinley, J., Peterson, R.E., Leshin, M., Griffin, J.E., Cooper, G., Draghi, S., Berenyi, M., and Wilson, J.D. (1980): J. Clin. Endocrinol. Metab., 50:15-22.
8. Imperato-McGinley, J., Peterson, R.E., Gautier, T., and Sturla, E. (1981): In: Clinics in Andrology: Pediatric Andrology Issue, edited by Stanley J. Kogan and E.S.E. Hafez, pp. 99-108. Martinus Nijhoff Publishers B.V., Netherlands.
9. Imperato-McGinley, J., Peterson, R.E., Gautier, T., Cooper, G., Danner, R., Arthur, A., Morris, P.L., Sweeney, W.J., and Shackleton, C. (1982): J. Clin. Endocrinol. Metab., 54:931-941.
10. Imperato-McGinley, J., Peterson, R.E., Gautier, T. (1981): In: Fetal Endocrinology, edited by Miles J. Novy, John A. Resko, pp. 359-382. Academic Press, Inc., New York.
11. Josso, N. (1973): Endocrinology, 93:829-834.
12. Jost, A. (1953): Recent Prog. Hormone Res., 8:379-418.
13. Leshin, M., Griffin, J.E., and Wilson, J.D. (1978): J. Clin. Invest., 62:685-691.
14. Lian, T., Rasmusson, A.H. and Brooks, J.R. (1983): J. Steroid Biochem., 19,1:385-390.
15. Marvais-Jarvis, P., Kuttenn, F., Mowszowicz, I., and Wright, F. (1981): Clin. Endocrinol., 14:459-469.
16. Moore, R.J., Griffin, J.E., and Wilson, J.D. (1975): J. Biol. Chem., 250:7268-7172.
17. Moore, R.J. and Wilson, J.D. (1976): J. Biol. Chem., 251: 5895-5900.
18. Peterson, R.E., Imperato-McGinley, J., Gautier, T., and Sturla, E. (1977): Amer. J. Med., 62:170-191.

19. Pinsky, D.M., Straisfeld, D., Zilahi, B., and St.-G., Hall, C. (1978): Am. J. Med. Genet., 1:407-416.

20. Saenger, P., Goldman, A.S., Levine, L.S., Korth-Schutz, S., Muecke, E.C., Katsumata, M., Doberne, U., and New, M.I. (1978): J. Clin. Endocrinol. Metab., 46:627-634.

21. Savage, M.O., Preece, M.A., Jeffcoate, S.L., Ransley, P.G., Rumsby, G., Mansfield, M.D., and Williams, D.I. (1980: Clin. Endocrinol, 12:397-406.

22. Siiteri,P., and Wilson, J.D. (1974): J. Clin. Endocrinol. Metab., 38:113-125.

23. Walsh, P.C., Madden, J.D., Harrod, M.J., Goldstein, J.L., MacDonald, P.C., and Wilson, J.D. (1974): N. Engl. J. Med., 291:944-949.

24. Wilson, J.D., and Gloyna, R.E. (1970): Recent Prog. Hormone Res., 26:309.

25. Wilson, J.D., and Lasnitzki, I. (1971): Endocrinology, 89:659-668.

26. Wilson, J.D. and Siiteri, P. (1973): Endocrinology, 92: 1182-1191.

27. Wilson, J.D., Harrod, M.J., Goldstein, J.L., Hemsell, D.L. and MacDonald, P.C. (1974): N. Engl. J. Med., 290:1097-1103.

28. Wilson, J.D. (1975): J. Biol. Chem., 250:3498-3504.

Progress in Cancer Research and Therapy,
Vol. 31, edited by F. Bresciani, et al.
Raven Press, New York © 1984.

4-Azasteroids as Inhibitors of 5α-Reductase

Tehming Liang, Jerry R. Brooks, Anne Cheung, Glenn F. Reynolds, and Gary H. Rasmusson

Merck Sharp & Dohme Research Laboratories, Rahway, New Jersey 07065

The hormonal cascade control of the synthesis of androgens by the testes and some steps of androgen action in target cells are shown in Fig. 1. In brief, the hypothalamus releases gonadotropin releasing hormone (GnRH) which stimulates the secretion of luteinizing hormone (LH) by the anterior pituitary (18,20). LH, in turn, stimulates the Leydig cells of the testes to synthesize androgens (4). The major androgen secreted in the adult male is testosterone. After testosterone enters the target cell, probably by diffusion, it is converted to 5α-dihydrotestosterone (DHT) in tissues such as the prostate and the skin. DHT then binds to the cytosol receptor protein to form the DHT-receptor complex. After transformation, the DHT-receptor complex is translocated into the nucleus and eventually activates specific genomes (13). The androgen receptor also binds testosterone, although the affinity is somewhat (2-10 fold) lower than that of DHT (7,10,15,24). In tissues such as skeletal muscle where 5α-reductase activity is low or not present, testosterone binds to the androgen receptor and the testosterone-receptor complex is translocated into the nucleus to exert its effects (13).

Antigonadotropins, which decrease testicular output of androgens via inhibition of gonadotropin secretion, and antiandrogens, which inhibit the binding of androgens to receptor in target tissues, have been shown to be effective for the treatment of androgen dependent diseases. For example, flutamide (16), a nonsteroidal antiandrogen; cyproterone acetate (21), which has both antigonadotropic and antiandrogenic activities; and GnRH agonists (8),

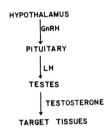

HYPOTHALAMUS
| GnRH
PITUITARY
| LH
TESTES
| TESTOSTERONE
TARGET TISSUES

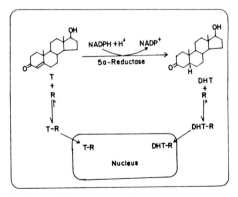

FIG. 1. The hormonal cascade control of testicular synthesis of testosterone and some steps of androgen action in target cells. GnRH, gonadotropin releasing hormone; LH, luteinizing hormone; T, testosterone; R, receptor; DHT, 5α-dihydrotestosterone.

which inhibit gonadotropin secretion when given continuously in large doses, have been shown to be effective for the treatment of prostatic cancer. Cyproterone acetate is also useful for the treatment of acne, hirsutism and alopecia (5). These compounds inhibit the androgen actions mediated by either testosterone or dihydrotestosterone.

We have directed our efforts to the development of inhibitors of 5α-reductase. Such compounds should block those androgen actions requiring DHT, but not those mediated by testosterone. Some potential utilities for 5α-reductase inhibitors include use in the treatment of prostatic cancer, benign prostatic hyperplasia, acne, hirsutism and alopecia. Unlike cyproterone acetate (9) and GnRH agonists (22) which cause impotence in men, 5α-reductase inhibitors should not inhibit libido. This is suggested from the studies of Imperato-McGinley et al (6) on humans with 5α-reductase deficiency. At birth, the males show incomplete differentiation of external genitalia. When they reach puberty, they become muscular and female directed libido develops. They have reduced body and facial hair, no temporal hair line recession, no acne, and the prostate remains small.

4-AZASTEROID AS TRANSITION STATE INHIBITOR OF 5α-REDUCTASE

Our design of 4-azasteroids as inhibitors of 5α-reductase is guided by the hypothesis that enzymatic 5α-reduction of a Δ^4-3-oxo-steroid involves the transfer of a hydrogen from NADPH to the 5α-position of the steroid, which results in a 3-enol transition intermediate (19). The 4-aza substitution of a 3-oxo-5α-steroid would produce a compound with a conformation similar to that of the proposed 3-enol intermediate and as a result would have a high affinity for the enzyme. The effect of 4-aza substitution of a 3-oxo-5α-steroid with a 17β-spiro ether functional group is shown in Fig. 2. The steroid with a $-CH_2-$ at the 4-position does not inhibit the conversion of testosterone to DHT by a rat prostate cell free system. The N-H analog is a good inhibitor of 5α-reductase and the $N-CH_3$ analog is even more active, but the $N-CH_2-CH_3$ derivative is inactive.

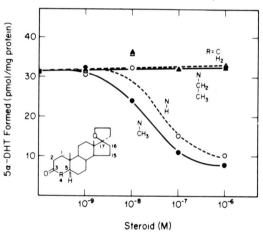

FIG. 2. The effect of substitutions at the 4-position of the steroid on the inhibition of rat prostate 5α-reductase.

INHIBITION OF 5α-REDUCTASE IN VITRO AND IN VIVO BY 4-MA

Synthetic 4-azasteroids were initially tested for their ability to inhibit rat prostate 5α-reductase in vitro and potent inhibitors were then further investigated in animals. 17β-N,N-Diethylcarbamoyl-4-methyl-4-aza-5α-androstan-3-one (4-MA, Fig. 3 R = CH_3) was found to be a potent 5α-reductase inhibitor both in vitro and in vivo. The inhibition of rat prostate 5α-reductase is competitive with testosterone and uncompetitive with NADPH. The apparent Ki is 5.3 ± 0.6 nM (10). The reversible binding of 4-MA to 5α-reductase will be described later. In mature male rats, the concentration of DHT in the ventral prostate is at least 4-fold greater than that of testostrone. The administration of 4-MA to the rats decreased the prostatic concentration of DHT and increased that of testosterone, indicating inhibition of 5α-reductase (1). 4-MA inhibits the growth of the ventral prostate and seminal vesicles of castrated rats given testosterone. The DHT-induced growth of these tissues is less affected by 4-MA (1). Chronic treatment of intact mature male rats with 4-MA reduces the size of the prostate and seminal vesicles (3). 4-MA treatments decreases the size of the prostate in intact dogs (2) and in castrated dogs given testosterone cypionate as shown by Wenderoth et al. (23). 4-MA showed little or no antifertility activity in either male or female rats, and no significant estrogenic, progestational, androgenic or gonadotropin-inhibiting potency (3). A more detailed summary of these earlier in vitro and in vivo studies can be found elsewhere (12,19).

5α-REDUCTASE INHIBITORS WITHOUT AFFINITY FOR ANDROGEN RECEPTOR

4-MA has an affinity for the androgen receptor of rat prostate cytosol, which is approximately 1000-, 120- and 40-fold lower than that of DHT, spironolactone and cyproterone acetate, respectively (8). We, therefore, have directed our efforts to developing 5α-reductase inhibitors which do not have an affinity for the androgen receptor. Fig. 3 compares the abilities of 4-MA

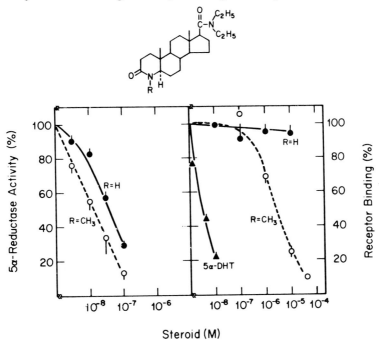

FIG. 3. Inhibition of rat prostate 5α-reductase (left) and the androgen receptor binding of [³H]DHT (right) by 4-MA (R = CH₃) and its des-4-methyl analog (R = H).

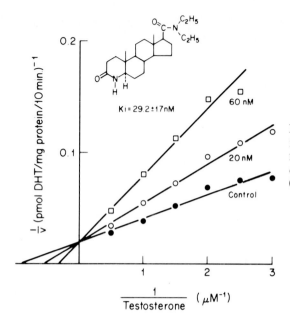

FIG. 4. Lineweaver-Burk plots of inhibition of rat prostate 5α-reductase by 17β-N,N-diethyl-carbamoyl-4-aza-5α-androstan-3-one ([des-4-methyl]4-MA)

(R = CH_3) and its des-4-methyl analog (R = H) to inhibit rat prostate 5α-reductase (Fig. 3, left) and to inhibit ^{3}H-DHT binding to the androgen receptor of rat prostate cytosol (Fig. 3, right). [Des-4-methyl]4-MA is only slightly less potent than 4-MA as an inhibitor of 5α-reductase and it has little affinity for the androgen receptor.   Another 4-N-H steroid, 17β-N,N-diisopropylcarbamoyl-4-aza-androstan-3-one (DIPA) is approximately as potent as 4-MA as an inhibitor of 5α-reductase and it has little affinity for the androgen receptor. Fig. 4 shows that [des-4-methyl]4-MA inhibition

FIG. 5. Lineweaver-Burk plots of inhibition of rat prostate 5α-reductase by 17β-N,N-diisopropyl-carbamoyl-4-aza-5α-androstan-3-one (DIPA).

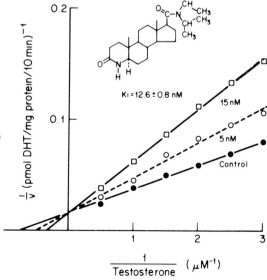

TABLE 1. Effects of DIPA and [des-4-methyl]4-MA on the nuclear uptake of androgens in the rat prostate tissue incubation

Incubation Experiment 1		Radioactivity in nuclei		
			%	
		cpm/mg protein	T	DHT
Control		14771	14	79
[des-4-methyl]4-MA	0.1 μM	13043 ± 441	58 ± 1	36 ± 1
"	1.0 μM	11878	85	9
DIPA	0.1 μM	12086	40	53
"	1.0 μM	11917 ± 501	73 ± 0	19 ± 1
Experiment 2				
Control		12240 ± 1940	13 ± 1	85 ± 1
[des-4-methyl]4-MA	0.1 μM	12053 ± 2066	67 ± 0.4	32 ± 0.7
"	1.0 μM	9645 ± 5	92 ± 0	9 ± 0.1
DIPA	0.1 μM	13658 ± 2028	48 ± 1	51 ± 1
"	1.0 μM	14898 ± 958	77 ± 4	17 ± 1

of rat prostate 5α-reductase is competitive with testosterone, the apparent Ki value being 29.2 ± 1.7 nM. DIPA is also a competitive inhibitor with an apparent Ki value of 12.6 ± 0.8 nM (Fig. 5).

The effect of [des-4-methyl]4-MA and DIPA on nuclear uptake of androgens was investigated in rat prostate tissue incubations. Ventral prostates from castrated rats were minced and incubated with [^{3}H] testosterone in the absence and in the presence of one of these two 4-N-H steroids. The radioactivity in the purified nuclei was extracted and subjected to thin-layer chromatography to separate compounds. As shown in Table 1, in the absence of a 5α-reductase inhibitor, the radioactivity in nuclei was 79-85% DHT and only 13-14% was unmetabolized testosterone. In the presence of [des-4-methyl]4-MA or DIPA, the nuclear concentration of DHT decreased and that of testosterone increased. The total nuclear concentration of testosterone plus DHT (90 to 99% of total) was not significantly affected by either [des-4-methyl]4-MA or DIPA. These results are consistent with the fact that both [des-4-methyl]4-MA and DIPA are inhibitors of 5α-reductase with little affinity for the androgen receptor. [^{3}H]-Testosterone was incubated with minced prostates from castrated rats at 37°C for 40 min. in the absence or presence of a 5α-reductase inhibitor. The radioactivity in purified nuclei is shown.

REVERSIBLE BINDING OF 4-MA TO 5α-REDUCTASE

We have taken advantage of the high affinity of 4-MA for 5α-reductase and developed a binding assay for this enzyme. [^{3}H] 4-MA was incubated with microsomes from rat prostate and liver in the presence and absence of NADPH. The radioactivity bound to microsomes was separated from the free by filtration on a glass fiber filter. Fig. 6 shows that NADPH stimulated the binding of [^{3}H]4-MA to liver and prostate microsomes. The binding stimulated by NADPH was calculated by subtracting the binding in the absence of NADPH from the total. Scatchard analysis of the data shows only a single class of

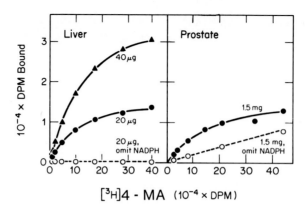

FIG 6. Binding of [^{3}H]4-MA to rat prostate and liver microsomes.
[^{3}H]4-MA was incubated with microsomes in the presence and absence of
NADPH (50 μM) at 0°C for 30 min. [^{3}H]4-MA bound to microsomes was
separated from the free [^{3}H]4-MA by filtration. The amounts of microsomal
protein used are shown in the figure. (Data from reference 11)

binding sites for both liver microsomes (Kd 6.5 ± 0.1 nM, 26.2 ± 1.6 pmol
sites/mg protein) and prostate microsomes (Kd 7 nM, 0.18 pmol sites/mg
protein). Several lines of evidence suggest that the NADPH-dependent binding
is to 5α-reductase. First, the binding capacity of microsomes from the liver
and the prostate is proportional to their levels of 5α-reductase enzymatic
activity. Microsomes from the spleen, the kidney and skeletal muscles showed
no 5α-reductase activity and also had no NADPH-dependent [^{3}H]4-MA binding
activity (Table 2). Second, the relative potency of steroids in inhibiting this
binding correlates with their ability to inhibit the conversion of testosterone
to DHT by the same microsomes (Fig. 7). Third, the binding requires a
cofactor for 5α-reductase. NADPH is 500-fold more effective than NADH.
NADP$^+$ and NAD$^+$ are inactive (Fig. 8). The requirement for NADPH in the
5α-reductase binding of [^{3}H]4-MA suggests that this enzyme binds NADPH
and then [^{3}H]4-MA. Since 4-MA competes with testosterone for the same
binding site, the enzyme may bind NADPH and then testosterone in the
enzymatic reaction.

TABLE 2. Correlation between levels of 5α-reductase activity and NADPH-
dependent [^{3}H]4-MA binding capacity in microsomes of male rat tissues (data
from reference 11)

Microsomes	5α-Reductase activity (pmol DHT formed/mg protein/ 10 min)	NADPH-Dependent binding of ^{3}H 4-MA (dpm (X10^{-2})/ mg protein)
Liver	1520 ± 20	3137 ± 168
Ventral prostate	14.6 ± 3.4	41 ± 2
Spleen	0	0
Kidney	0	0
Skeletal muscle	0	0

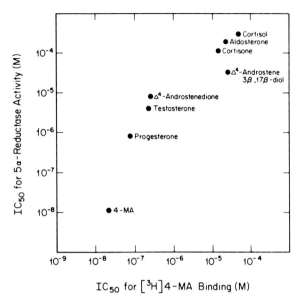

FIG. 7. Correlation between potencies of steroids as inhibitors of 5α-reductase and as inhibitors of [³H]4-MA binding to male rat liver microsomes. The correlation coefficient is 0.92 (data from reference 11).

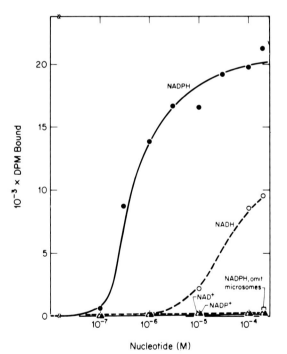

FIG. 8. Nucleotide specificity of [³H]4-MA binding to rat liver microsomes (data from reference 11).

The 5α-reductase binding of [³H] 4-MA is reversible since [³H]4-MA bound to microsomes could be dissociated from the microsomes with an excess of nonradioactive 4-MA. Finally, it was first shown by Yates et al (25) that the liver of female rats has a higher 5α-reductase activity than does that of male rats. Fig. 9 shows that both the 5α-reductase activity and the [³H]4-MA binding capacity of the liver microsomes of female rats are 5-fold higher than those of the liver microsomes of male rats.

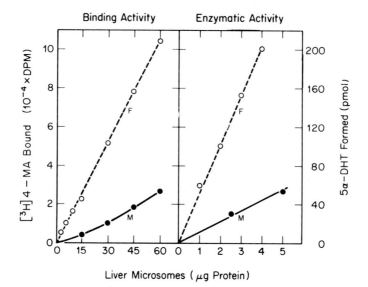

FIG. 9. Comparisons of $[^3H]$4-MA binding capacity and 5α-reductase activity between liver microsomes of male (M) and female rats (F) (data from reference 11).

REFERENCES

1. Brooks, J. S. Baptista, E. M., Berman, C., Ham, E. A., Hichens, M., Johnston, D. B. R., Primka, R. L., Rasmusson, G. H., Reynolds, G. F., Schmitt, S. M., and Arth, G. E. (1981): Endocrinol. 109:830-836.
2. Brooks, J. R., Berman, C., Glitzer, M. S., Gordon, L. R. Primka, R. L., Reynolds, G. F., and Rasmusson, G. H. (1982): The Prostate, 3:35-44.
3. Brooks, J. R., Berman, C., Hichens, M., Primka, R. L., Reynolds, G. F., and Rasmusson, G. H. (1982): Proc. Soc. Exp. Biol. Med., 169:67-73.
4. Hall, P. F. (1970): In: The Androgens of the Testis, edited by K. B. Eik-Nes, pp. 73-115. Marcel Dekker, New York.
5. Hammerstein, J., Meckies, J., Ieo-Rossberg, I., Moltz, and Zielske, F. (1975): J. Steroid Biochem., 6:827-836.
6. Imperato-McGinley, J., Peterson, R. E., Gautier, T., and Sturla, E. (1979): J. Steroid Biochem., 11:637-645.
7. Krieg, M., and Voigt, K. D. (1977): Acta Endocr., 85: supplement 214, 43-89.
8. Labrie, F., Dupont, A., Belanger, A., Lefebvre, F. A., Cusan, L., Reynaud, J. P., Husson, J.M., and Fazekas, A. T. A. (1983): Hormone Res., 18:18-27.
9. Laschet, U., and Laschet, L. (1975): J. Steroid Biochem., 6:821-826.
10. Liang, T., and Heiss, C. E. (1981): J. Biol. Chem., 256:7998-8005.
11. Liang, T., Heiss, C. E., Ostrove, S., Rasmusson, G. H., and Cheung, A. (1983): Endocrinol., 112:1460-1468.
12. Liang, T., Rasmusson, G. H., and Brooks, J. R. (1983): J. Steroid Biochem., 19:385-390.
13. Liao, S. (1977): In: Biochemical Actions of Hormones, edited by G. Litwack, pp. 351-406, Academic Press, New York.
14. Liao, S., Howell, D.K., and Chang, T. M. (1974): Endocrinol., 94:1205-1209.

15. Liao, S., Liang, T., Fang, S., Castaneda, E., and Shao, T.-C. (1973): J. Biol. Chem., 248:6154-6162.
16. Neri, R., and Kassem, N. (1982): In: Hormone Antagonists, edited by M. K. Agarwal, pp. 247-268, Walter de Gruyter, New York.
17. Peets, E. A., Henson, M. F., and Neri, R. (1974): Endocrinol., 94:532-540.
18. Pohl, C. R., and Knobil, E. (1982): Ann. Rev. Physiol., 44:583-593.
19. Rasmusson, G. H., Liang, T., and Brooks, J. R. (1983): In: Gene Regulation by Steroid Hormones II, edited by A. K. Roy and J. H. Clark, pp. 311-334. Springer-Verlag, New York.
20. Schally, A. V. (1978): Science, 202:18-28.
21. Scott, W. W., and Schirmer, K. A. (1966): Trans. Am. Asso. Genito-Urinary Surgeons, 58:54-62.
22. Waxman, J. H., Wass, J. A. H., Hendry, W. F., Whitfield, H. N., Besser, G. M., Malpas, J. S., and Oliver, R. T. D. (1983): British Med. J., 286:1309-1312.
23. Wenderoth, U. K., George, F. W., and Wilson, J. D. (1983): Endocrinol., 113:569-573.
24. Wilson, E. M., and French, F. S. (1976): J. Biol. Chem., 251:5620-5629.
25. Yates, F. E., Herbst, A. L., Urquhart, J. (1958): Endocrinol., 63:887-902.

Progress in Cancer Research and Therapy,
Vol. 31, edited by F. Bresciani, et al.
Raven Press, New York © 1984.

Biological and Clinical Properties of Antiandrogens

Rudolph Neri and Nadim Kassem

Department of Clinical Research, Schering Corporation,
Kenilworth, New Jersey 07033

Interest in antiandrogens arises from the inference that such agents would be therapeutically useful in prostatic hyperplasias and androgen-sensitive dermatologic diseases.

PRECLINICAL STUDIES

I. FLUTAMIDE

Flutamide (propanamide, 2 methyl-N-4-nitro-3-(trifluoromethyl)phenyl is one such agent that was previously reported and was found to be devoid of other hormonal activity.

When orally administered to intact male rats, flutamide significantly reduced prostate and seminal vesicle weights at doses as low as 1 mg/kg (11). Other endocrine structures were not altered. Histological examination of the various tissues revealed marked reductions in the height of the epithelial cells of the seminal vesicles and prostate with no evidence of secretory material within the lumina of the glands. By comparison, cells lining the seminal vesicles of control animals were tall columnar and exhibited secretory granules along with secretory material in the lumen.

In contrast, flutamide, even at high doses up to 50 mg/kg did not affect body or organ weights in female rats treated for three weeks which indicates specificity of this drug for androgen-dependent sex structures.

Flutamide inhibited hypertrophy of the prostate induced by various androgens in orchiectomized rats (11). Flutamide (5-25 mg/kg) significantly inhibited hypertrophy of the ventral prostate induced by testosterone propionate (10 µg/day), testosterone (50 µg/day), dihydrotestosterone (25 µg/day), dehydroepiandrosterone (500 µg/day) and androstenedione (50 µg/day).

II. OTHER ANTIANDROGENS - DNA SYNTHESIS

In addition to flutamide's inhibitory effect on androgen-induced prostatic growth, this agent also inhibits the rate of DNA synthesis in the prostate (18). Orchiectomized rats were given 0.3 mg testosterone propionate subcutaneously together with either flutamide or with other antiandrogenic agents such as cyproterone acetate (1, 2α-methylene 6-chloro Δ^6-17α-hydroxy progesterone, Schering A.G.), MK-316 2'3α' tetrahydrofuran-2'-spiro-17-(6α, 7α difluoromethylene-1α, 2α methylene)-4-androsten-3-one, Merck, R-2956 (17β-hydroxy-2α, 2β, 17α-trimethyl-8α-

estra-4, 9, 11-triene-3-one, Roussel-Uclaf) or medrogestone (6, 17-dimethylpregna-4, 6-diene-3, 20-dione, Ayerst) daily for 3 days. Twenty-four hours after the final injection the prostate was removed, weighed, incubated and processed to measure the rate of DNA synthesis. The results showed that the order of potency in inhibiting the rate in this system was observed to be: flutamide >cyproterone acetate > MK-316 > R-2956 > medrogestone.

III.   STUDIES IN DOGS

Aged dogs with benign prostatic hypertrophy (BPH) - Prostatic hyperplasia occurs spontaneously in a percentage of aged dogs. Thus BPH in dogs was used as a model for the development of chemotherapeutics for the treatment of BPH in man, although the etiological and structural changes of BPH that occur in man are different than those in canines. However, if an antiandrogen can evoke a regression in the glandular epithelia of the human benign hyperplastic prostate (which involves mainly the fibromuscular stroma) the reduction in glandular epithelia may be sufficient to alleviate some of the problems associated with BPH. Consequently flutamide was examined for its ability to reduce the size of the dog hyperplastic prostate.

The compound was orally administered once daily in gelatin capsules at doses of 1, 5, 10, 15, 25 and 50 mg/kg for 6 weeks. In addition, dogs were given flutamide for 1 year. Verification of prostatic hypertrophy was by caliper measurements and biopsy at laparotomy. After 6 weeks treatment, the prostate size was reduced (Table I).

Microscopic examination of the prostate revealed a marked reduction in epithelial cell heights and a loss of acid phosphatase and protein. The minimum effective dose was 5 mg/kg. When flutamide was given daily for 1 year at 5 mg/kg the reduction in prostate size was maintained. Libido and spermatogenesis were not adversely affected since these dogs mated and sired several litters. Eight weeks after flutamide treatment was stopped, the atrophied prostate reverted to its initial hyperplastic state.

TABLE I

Effects of Flutamide on Prostates of Dogs with Benign Prostatic Hyperplasia

6 Wks.[a] Rx mpk	Pre-Treatment				Post-Treatment			
	Body Wt (kg)	Prostate Volume (Cm^3 ± S.E.)	Epith. Cell Ht (μ ± S.E.)	Acid Phos-phatase*	Body Wt (kg)	Prostate Volume (Cm^3 ± S.E.)	Epith. Cell Ht (μ ± S.E.)	Acid Phos.*
0	12.5 ± 1.4	35.2 ± 4.8	33.4 ± 1.8	3	12.0 ± 0.8	36.0 ± 4.2	34.2 ± 1.6	3
1	11.4 ± 1.2	29.6 ± 4.2	31.9 ± 2.1	3	11.7 ± 1.2	23.4 ± 3.2	28.5 ± 1.7	3
5	10.9 ± 1.7	29.3 ± 3.4	30.3 ± 1.9	3	11.7 ± 1.4	6.0 ± 1.2[†]	4.1 ± 0.4[†]	1
10	15.9 ± 2.3	70.5 ± 10.2	41.1 ± 1.3	3	15.6 ± 2.0	13.3 ± 2.4[†]	5.0 ± 0.6[†]	0
15	17.0 ± 1.5	36.5 ± 6.8	31.6 ± 0.9	3	15.3 ± 1.2	10.1 ± 1.8[†]	3.3 ± 0.2[†]	0
25	11.0 ± 1.0	26.1 ± 3.8	27.4 ± 0.8	3	10.5 ± 1.0	3.4 ± 0.8[†]	4.2 ± 0.4[†]	0
50	7.8 ± 0.8	32.1 ± 6.2	29.3 ± 2.4	3	8.0 ± 1.1	5.5 ± 1.2[†]	4.7 ± 0.4	0

[a]6 weeks treatment (mg/kg) 2 animals/group.
*Acid Phosphatase - 3 = strong reaction, 1 = slight reaction and 0 = no reaction.
†Significantly different from pretreatment $p < 0.01$.

TABLE II

Effect of Flutamide on Hair Fat Production, Seminal Vesicle

and Ventral Prostate Weights in Orchiectomized Rats

Compound	Daily Treatment[a]	Initial Body Wt. (g ± S.E.)	Final Body Wt. (g ± S.E.)	Hair Fat Production mg/g of hair/day (mg ± S.E.)	Seminal Vesicles (mg ± S.E.)	Ventral Prostate (mg ± S.E.)
Control	---	194 ± 4	347 ± 15	0.47 ± 0.06*	22.3 ± 3.1*	18.1 ± 1.1*
Testosterone	0.4 mg s.c.	184 ± 2	348 ± 15	1.29 ± 0.04	602.0 ± 22.3	668.0 ± 46.5
Testosterone + Flutamide	0.4 mg s.c. and 20 mg p.o.	186 ± 2	351 ± 14	0.40 ± 0.07*	34.6 ± 4.8*	26.2 ± 1.5*

[a] 6 rats/group, treated daily for 24 days.

* Significantly different from testosterone-treated controls, p ≤ 0.01.

IV. ANTIPROSTATE STUDIES IN THE BABOON

Flutamide, diethylstilbestrol diphosphate and ESTRACYT[R] (Estradiol-nitrogen mustard) were examined for their anti-prostate effects (10). According to the authors, the prostate of this sub-human primate resembles that of man in some respects and was investigated as a possible model for the study of chemotherapeutic agents for cancer of the prostate in humans. Flutamide (5 mg/kg) was injected intramuscularly three times weekly for 4 weeks. Following treatment, all drugs were shown to produce a definite decrease in the weight of the prostate. The mean prostate weight of the three baboons treated with flutamide was 3.44 g, a decrease of 66% from the mean control prostate weight of 10.18 g. ESTRACYT[R] and diethylstilbestrol diphosphate (3 baboons/each) given intravenously in doses of 5 mg/kg reduced the weight of the prostate 32% and 42%, respectively.

V. STUDIES RELATED TO THE SECONDARY THERAPEUTIC ACTIVITIES OF FLUTAMIDE

1. Antisebaceous Gland Activity. Rats - To determine whether flutamide suppresses androgen-sensitive sebaceous glands, flutamide was administered to testosterone-treated orchiectomized rats. The amount of hair fat emanating predominantly from sebaceous glands was measured and expressed as mg/g of hair/day. Seminal vesicle and ventral prostate weights were also recorded.

The results indicated that the rate of hair fat production as well as the weights of the seminal vesicles and ventral prostates were reduced almost to castrate levels (Table II).

Hamsters - Unilateral topical application of flutamide (0.1 - 3.0 mg/kg/14 days) to flank organs (sebaceous glands) of testosterone-treated female hamsters resulted in bilateral reductions in flank organ weight. In addition, inhibition of in vitro incorporation of ^{14}C from radioactive sodium (1-^{14}C) acetate into flank organ lipids occurred (8).

2. Effects of Flutamide on Sexual Behavior and Androgen-Mediated Aggression - Long term studies in rats (11,13,14) and dogs (12) indicated that flutamide, although exerting a marked inhibitory effect on prostate growth, did not alter sexual potency nor libido. To sub-

stantiate these findings a more detailed and sophisticated analysis of
sexual behavior was done in which flutamide was applied to hypothalami
of intact rats. Lesions of the pre-optic nucleus produce a loss of
sexual behavior which is not prevented or reversed by the administration
of androgens. Conversely, the loss of sexual behavior following
castration is reversed by testosterone administered either systemically
or by implanation in the pre-optic nucleus. Therefore, it is
reasonable to assume that direct application of an antiandrogen to such
a site would produce a decrease in sexual behavior. The results
indicated that flutamide (300 μg) implanted* into the preoptic nucleus
of male rats (6/group) did not produce any significant change in the
components of sexual behavior (latency from the time of introduction
of a female to the first intromission; frequency of mounts and intromission to ejaculation; post-ejaculatory interval) when compared to
measures made prior to implantation. Cyproterone acetate,
employed as a standard, was also ineffective in altering sexual
behavior. These studies suggest but do not prove that androgen
receptors in the preoptic nucleus differ quantitatively from those in
peripheral tissues.

Soderstein et al (16) corroborated the ineffectiveness of flutamide
toward inhibiting sexual behavior in male rats. Intact, sexually
experienced males, were given flutamide (50 mg/kg) s.c. daily for 4
weeks and tested for sexual behavior twice weekly during the 4 week
dosing period. No quantitative or qualitative behavioral effects were
noted. Luteinizing and testosterone hormone levels were increased
whereas ventral prostate weights were reduced approximately 50% as
compared to controls.

Flutamide will prevent lordosis in female rats that have been
primed with testosterone. Gladue et al (3) administered testosterone
propionate (250 μg) to ovariectomized rats and observed a lordosis
quotient of over 60% as opposed to a less than 1% in control animals.
The simultaneous administration of testosterone propionate (25 μg) and
flutamide (10 mg/rat) daily for two days reduced the lordosis quotient
to control levels. The simultaneous administration of estradiol benzoate
and progesterone produced a 90% lordosis score. Flutamide had no effect
when given along with estradiol benzoate and progesterone. These
results indicate that flutamide exerts an antiandrogenic effect and is
devoid of anti-estrogenic and anti-progestational activity, substantiating previous findings (11).

Flutamide does not alter sexual behavior in monkeys (5). The sexual
interactions of 10 pairs of rhesus monkeys were observed during a control
and an experimental menstrual cycle of each female. During the experimental cycle the females were treated with flutamide (10 mg/kg, twice
daily throughout menstrual cycle). No alteration in sexual behavior
occurred following flutamide dosing as compared to sexual behavior
during the control cycle.

Many studies have been reported in which testosterone was implicated
as playing a major role in the development and maintenance of
aggressive behavior in mice. Thus, abolishing the main source of
testosterone by orchiectomy will prevent the development of aggressive

---

*Implants prepared by gently melting the materials, dipping the top
 of a pre-weighed length of 27 gauge stainless steel tubing in it
 and allowing a small bead of the material to cool on the tip.

behavior in mice when isolated for 3 weeks. Chronic administration of methyl testosterone returns the incidence of fighting behavior to control values. The simultaneous administration of methyl testosterone (10.7 mg/kg) and flutamide (94.2 mg/kg) did not reduce the incidence of fighting (4). Since in this same study the ventral prostate weights were markedly reduced as compared to methyl-testosterone-treated mice it follows that mechanism for androgen stimulation of secondary sex organ weight differs from that involved in the development and maintenance of aggression resulting from isolation (4).

3. Effect of Flutamide on Spermatogensis - Dhar and Setty (1) administered flutamide (25 mg/kg) orally to rats (150-200 g) (10 rats/ group) once daily for 30 days. No effect on spermatogenesis was observed and Leydig cell morphology was unaltered. The secretory activity of the epididymis either remained unaffected or was stimulated. There was a significant decrease in seminal vesicle and ventral prostate weight and in fructose content of coagulating glands. There was no change in pituitary gland weight. The fertility pattern did not change. These findings are compatible with previous results indicating that flutamide does not inhibit sexual potency in rats.

4. Thrombus Formation in Rats - Uzunova, Ramey and Ramwell (20) studied the role of flutamide in thrombus formation. Insertion of a polyethylene cannula into the abdominal aorta produces occlusive arterial thrombosis in male and female rats. This phenomenon is more manifest in male than in female rats subjected to the same endothelial trauma. The mortality rate is also higher in males that in females. Administration of depo-testosterone cypionate increased thrombus formation resulting in a four-fold increase in the mortality rate in male and female rats. When flutamide (50 mg/kg) was injected subcutaneously once daily for two weeks together with depo-testosterone cypionate (10 mg/kg) subcutaneously twice a week, flutamide decreased thrombus formation and the mortality rate was reduced about 50% as compared to the androgen alone in those rats containing the aortic cannula.

5. Studies on the Mechanism of Action of Flutamide - Flutamide exerts its antiandrogenic effects on male secondary sex structures by an inhibition of androgen uptake and/or inhibition of nuclear binding of the androgens in the target tissues (15). A single 15 mg/kg dose of flutamide or cyproterone acetate, co-administered with i.p. injection of either ^{3}H-testosterone or ^{3}H-dihydrotestosterone inhibited uptake and retention of the labeled androgen by prostate whole tissues and nuclei. Flutamide was demonstrated to inhibit the formation of the nuclear 3-S protein-^{3}H androgen complex in addition to depressing whole tissue uptake and retention of ^{3}H-testosterone. Similar effects were noted with cyproterone acetate. The effects of flutamide on prostate tissue in vitro were shown to be similar, though not as marked, to those observed in vivo. (The in vitro results suggested that flutamide might achieve its results, at least in part, through an active metabolite.)

It was reported that when orally administered flutamide was given to various species including man, the compound was rapidly and extensively metabolized (6). Several metabolites were identified, the major metabolite being Sch 16423 (Hydroxyflutamide). The rapid conversion of flutamide to Sch 16423 and the high plasma levels of Sch 16423 suggest that Sch 16423 may be an active form of flutamide.

Subsequent reports also suggested that this may be correct. Liao et al (7) showed that flutamide suppressed retention of a specific 5-α-dihydrotestosterone in vitro by receptor protein in prostate cytosol and nuclear retention of the androgen-receptor complex during incubation of minced prostate. Cyproterone acetate, employed as a standard, was equipotent to flutamide in vivo, but in vitro, flutamide was found to be 40 times less active than cyproterone acetate. The authors suggested that flutamide's in vivo activity may be attributable to a metabolite.

Mainwaring et al (9) reported similar results. Flutamide, like cyproterone acetate, antagonized testosterone activity in vivo by depressing nuclear binding of 5α-dihydrotestosterone and testosterone-stimulated RNA polymerase activity in rat prostate. Flutamide was less effective in vitro suggesting that the in vivo activity may result from a metabolite of flutamide. Other reports substantiate flutamide's in vivo activity on the cellular events as opposed to flutamide's lessened activity in vitro (21, 2).

Symes et al (19) assessed the potency of several antiandrogens using human benign prostatic tissue in an in vitro system. Slices of tissue were incubated in the presence of ^{3}H-testosterone and the uptake into nuclei was determined. Flutamide competed weakly for uptake, whereas Sch 16423 and cyproterone acetate competed extensively with labeled testosterone.

The conversion of ^{14}C-testosterone (T) to dihydrotestosterone (DHT) and androstanediol (A-diol) was studied in vitro using a crude homogenate of prostates from patients with benign prostatic hypertrophy, (19). Under standard conditions, the mean conversion to DHT was 70% and to A-diol 14%. Addition of various anti-androgens and other substances decreased the T→→DHT conversion to 0-55% and the T→→A-diol to 0-10%. Flutamide was one of the antiandrogens that was an effective inhibitor of T→→DHT.

HUMAN STUDIES

I. INTRODUCTION

For years now, estrogens have been the mainstay of medical therapy for prostatic carcinoma. However, the significant rate of cardiovascular side effects and the subsequent increased risk of death associated with their use, directed the attention of researchers to other modes of anti-androgenic therapy.

Flutamide is a unique antiandrogen that it is devoid of other agonistic or antagonistic activity. It is well absorbed from the GI tract and rapidly and extensively metabolized and excreted in the urine. The plasma half-life of its major metabolite in man is 5-6 hours.

Clinical pharmacological studies in normal male volunteers indicated that flutamide is safe and well-tolerated. The main reported adverse experience was gynecomastia with secretion of colostrum in some volunteers.

In a four week double-blind study, flutamide was compared to placebo or diethylstilbestrol (DES) in forty patients with prostatic cancer refractory to conventional therapy. The short-term efficacy and safety shown by flutamide were encouraging, suggesting a longer-term investigation of its effects on cancer of the prostate.

II. CLINICAL TRIALS

A. Controlled Studies

The clinical efficacy of flutamide in prostatic cancer was studied by 17 investigators who participated in a multicentric randomized double-

TABLE III

Prevalence of Metastases, Elevated Acid Phosphatase and Pain

Number of Patients With	Flutamide 1500 mg (n = 42)	Flutamide 750 mg (n = 39)	DES 1 mg (n = 44)
Metastases	38	36	37
Elevated Acid Phosph.	28	30	35
Pain	20	22	30

blind trial that compared the effects of flutamide and diethylstilbesterol (DES). Eligible for enrollment were patients who had Stage D cancer of the prostate and had received no previous chemotherapy, hormonal treatment or ablative surgery. Surgical intervention to correct urinary retention did not disqualify a patient's admission into the study.

One hundred and twenty five (125) such patients ranging in age from 66 to 85 years were randomly assigned to receive flutamide 1500 mg/day (42 pts.), flutamide 750 mg/day (39 pts.) or DES, 1 mg (44 pts.). The three groups of patients were comparable in respect to the symptoms and signs associated with their disease. The majority of the patients had measurable metastases with elevated serum acid phosphatase and pain as shown in Table III.

EFFICACY CRITERIA

In order to define response to therapy in this multicentric clinical trial, the following acceptable categories of response in cancer patients have been used:

Complete Remission: The disappearance of all objective and subjective signs and symptoms.

Partial Remission: The disappearance or significant improvement of two or more objective and subjective signs and symptoms.

Improvement: The significant improvement of an objective and one or more subjective signs and symptoms.

Stabilization: Refers to arrest of disease progression in both objective and subjective categories.

Failure: None of the above.

RESULTS

The patients were evaluated every two weeks for the first 12 weeks of treatment and every three months thereafter. The overall response of the patients is shown in the following table.

Table IV

Overall Response: Flutamide vs DES
N = 125

Treatment	CR	PR	Imp.	Stab.	Failure	Uneval.*	Total	Time (Wks) to Response + SEM	Duration (Wks.) of Response
Flutamide 1500 mg	0	19	8	4	3	8	42	12.3 + 2.42	24.6 + 8.65
Flutamide 750 mg	0	18	7	7	9	5	39	9.2 + 1.56	36.3 + 7.9
DES 1 mg	1	18	7	4	4	10	44	10.0 + 1.40	39.2 + 5.84

*Unevaluable   (<6 Wks)

These results show that flutamide and DES elicited similar improvement and remissions, and the time to response varied from 10 weeks with
DES to 9.2 weeks with flutamide 750 mg. The duration of response was
calculated from the time the response was first obtained until the time
of disease progression. This is a conservative estimate of the total
benefit time since patients may start to improve prior to actually
obtaining a measured response. The average duration on therapy for the
1500 mg flutamide group (n=42) was 39.02 + 5.5 weeks with a range of
0-192 weeks. For the 750 mg group (n=39) the average duration of therapy
was 41.6 + 7.8 weeks with a range of 1-294 weeks. The DES group (n=44)
had an average duration on therapy of 32.3 + 5.2 weeks with a range of
0-168 weeks. No statistical differences existed between the three groups
in terms of duration on therapy.
    There were 12 deaths during the study: five (5) occurred following
surgery and 7 were non-surgical deaths.
    Survival analyses were obtained on more than 60% of the patients.
The degree of censoring was equally distributed among the three treatment groups. The survival analyses curves were tested for statistical
difference by both the Breslow and the Mantel-Cox tests and were found
to have no statistical difference. The mean survival time for the
flutamide group was about 38.5 months and 32.8 months in the DES group
(Figure 1).

Figure 1:

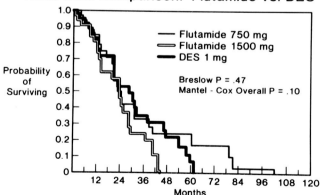

Survival Analysis
Double Blind Comparison: Flutamide vs. DES

In addition, of the 30 DES patients who had pain 19 (i.e., 62%) were relieved of their pain vs 17 of the 22 flutamide 750 mg patients (77%).

SAFETY

Aside from infrequent nausea, diarrhea and dizziness in a small number of patients, the most common adverse experiences were gynecomastia and breast tenderness which occurred in 35% of the patients who were treated with flutamide and 43% of those treated with DES. The most important adverse effects were the thromboembolic/cardiovascular complications. Six (6) of the 44 DES treated patients developed such complications (4 thrombophlebitis, one of whom also had a pulmonary embolus, 1 pulmonary edema, 1 congestive heart failure) and two (2) of the 81 flutamide treated patients developed complications: one patient expired 4 days after enrollment in the study and 13 days following the surgical removal of pelvic lymph node. Death was probably due to a pulmonary embolus secondary to post-operative iliofemoral thrombosis. The patient was included in the safety analysis although it was uncertain whether he actually did receive the drug. The other patient developed a marked granulocytopenia and an inferior myocardial infarction while on flutamide and Bactrim, an antibiotic known to produce agranulocytosis. The myocardial infarct was not attributed to flutamide. For purpose of comparison, the next table shows the incidence of the major side effects of flutamide seen in the controlled study and those reported with estramustine phosphate.

Table V

Comparative Toxicities
Estramustine, DES and Flutamide

| | Estramustine SBA | | Present Study | | |
| | Estramustine | DES | DES | Flutamide | |
	11.5-15.0 mg/kg/day (N-92)	3 mg/day (N-93)	1 mg/day (N-44)	750 mg/day (N-39)	1500 mg/day (N-42)
Cardiovascular Complications	32%	30%	11%	0%	2.4%
Hepatotoxicity	35.8%	38%	2.3%	2.6%	5%
Abdominal Discomfort	12.5%	6.3%	6.8%	2.6%	7%
Gynecomastia	71%	69%	43%	31%	36%

The striking difference between flutamide and the estrogens is very clear, particularly in the most troublesome and hazardous cardiovascular complications where both estramustine and DES 3 mg cause such side effects in approximately a third of the patients. In contrast, flutamide 750 mg did not cause any drug related cardiovascular side effects.

CONCLUSIONS

On the basis of the quality of response seen where flutamide and DES appear to be similar in their effect on Stage D cancer of the prostate, and on the basis of a significantly lower cardiovascular liability of flutamide over DES, it is concluded that flutamide is a safe and efficacious drug in the palliative treatment of cancer of the prostate.

Figure 2:

DISTRIBUTION OF PATIENTS BY PREVIOUS TREATMENT

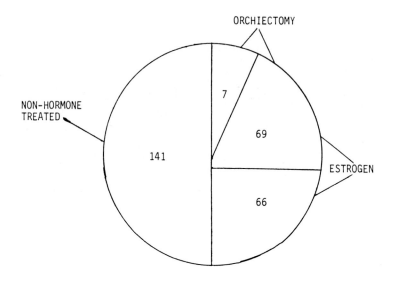

B. OPEN STUDIES

That flutamide is efficacious in prostatic cancer is further supported by the results of an open multicentric study.

In this study, patients with Stage D prostatic cancer, whether previously treated or not were enrolled and treated with flutamide 750 mg a day for as long as they responded to treatment. Two hundred and eighty three (283) patients were studied (Figure 2); 76 were orchiectomized and 207 were not. Of these 207 patients, 66 patients had received estrogens.

In other words, 142 patients were randomly treated with hormonal manipulation medically and/or surgically and 141 patients were not.

Seventy (70) patients were less than 60 years old and the rest were older.

The majority of the patients had measurable metastasis with elevated acid phosphatase and pain.

Table VI

Prevalence of Metastases,
Elevated Acid Phosphatase and Pain
(Flutamide 750 mg)

Patient Status	N	Metastases	Elevated Acid Phosphatase	Pain
Hormone-treated	142	70	84	94
Non-treated	141	91	88	68
Total	283	161	172	162

Flutamide was administered orally at a dose of 750 mg/day for as long as the patients responded to treatment. The criteria for efficacy were similar to those previously described in the flutamide vs. DES study. The results are shown in Table VII.

TABLE VII
OVERALL RESPONSE TO FLUTAMIDE THERAPY N = 283

PR	IMP	STAB	FAILURE	TOTAL	TIME IN WEEKS TO RESPONSE + S.E.	DURATION IN WEEKS OF RESPONSE + S.E.
119	54	67	33	273*	15.1 ± 2.33	25.9 ± 3.52
44%	20%	24%	12%			

*10 patients too early to evaluate.

PR   = Partial Remission
IMP = Improvement
STAB = Stabilization

Sixty-four percent of the patients showed either a partial remission or improvement. Of the 283 patients, 142 were previously treated with estrogens and/or orchiectomy. Twenty-seven percent showed a partial remission and another 22% had an improvement. From this patient population, 76 were refractory to estrogen and/or orchiectomy. Interestingly, a partial remission and improvement occurred in 18% and 20%, respectively, despite the fact that these patients were refractory to prior hormonal or surgical therapy.

The data clearly indicate that flutamide induced remissions not only in previously untreated patients but also in patients who could not tolerate estrogens and in patients whose disease had progressed despite estrogen therapy or orchiectomy.

In addition to its efficacy in untreated and in hormone refractory patients, flutamide's safety is another reason for the particular interest in the drug.

SAFETY

When discussing the safety of flutamide, one has to keep in mind that estrogen therapy for prostatic carcinoma is associated with an increased incidence of cardiovascular complications and deaths.

Estrogens affect several clotting fractors while flutamide does not. The most common adverse experience was breast tenderness and gynecomastia that occurred in about one-third of the patients. Gastrointestinal intolerance occurred in 5% of the patients. No cardiovascular complications were observed that were attributable to flutamide therapy.

In summary, on the basis of the quality of response in orchiectomized as well as nonorchiectomized patients with Stage D cancer of the prostate and on the basis of its low potential for cardiovascular complications, flutamide appears to be a safe and efficacious drug in the treatment of cancer of the prostate.

REFERENCES

1. Dhar, J.D. and Sett, B.S. (1976): Fertil. Steril., 27:566-576.
2. Ghanadian, R., Smith, C.B., Williams, G. and Chisholm, G.D. (1977): Br. J. Urol., 49:695-700.
3. Gladue, B.A., Dohanich, G.P. and Clemens, L.G. (1978): Pharm. Bioch. Behav., 9:827-832.
4. Heilman, R.D., Brugmans, M., Greenslate, F.C. and DaVanzo, J.P. (1976): Psychopharmacology, 47:75-80.
5. Johnson, D.F. and Phoenix, C.H. (1978): Horm. Behav., 11:160-174.
6. Katchen, B. and Buxbaum, S. (1975): J. Clin. Endo. Met., 41: 373-379.
7. Liao, S., Howell, D.K. and Chang, T.M. (1974): Endocrinology, 94:1205-1209.
8. Lutsky, B.N., Budak, M., Koziol, P., Monahan, M. and Neri, R.O. (1975): J. Invest. Dermatol., 64:412-417.
9. Mainwaring, W.I.P., Mangan, F.R., Feherty, P.A. and Freifeld, M. (1974): Molec. Cell. Endocrinol., 1:113-128.
10. Muntzing, J., Varkarakis, M.J., Yamanaka, H., Murphy, G.P. and Sandberg, A.A. (1974): Proc. Soc. Exptl. Biol. Med., 146:849-854.
11. Neri, R.O., Florance, K., Koziol, P. and Vancleave, S. (1972): Endocrinology, 91:427-437.
12. Neri, R.O. and Monahan, M. (1972): Invest. Urol., 10:123-130.
13. Neri, R.O. (1976): In Advances in Sex Hormone Research, edited by S. Singhal and J. Thomas, University Park Press, Baltimore, Vol. 2, pp. 233-262.
14. Neri, R.O. (1977): In Androgens and Antiandrogens, edited by L. Martini and M. Motta, Raven Press, NY pp. 179-189.
15. Peets, E.A., Henson, M.F. and Neri, R.O. (1974): Endocrinology, 94:532-540.
16. Soderstein, P., Gray, G., Damassa, D.A., Smith, E.R. and Davidson, J.J. (1975): Endocrinology, 97:1468-1475.
17. Sogani, P.C. and Whitmore, W.F., Jr. (1979): J. Urol., 122:640-643.
18. Sufrin, G. and Coffey, D.S. (1973): Invest. Urol., 11:45-54.
19. Symes, E.K., Milroy, E.J.G. and Mainwaring, W.I.P. (1978): J. Urol., 120:180-183.
20. Uzunova, A.D., Ramey, E.R. and Ramwel, P.W. (1978): Am. J. Physiol., 234:454-459.
21. Varkarakis, M.J., Kirdani, R.V., Yamanaka, H., Murphy, G.P. and Sandberg, A.A. (1975): Invest. Urol., 12:275-284.

Progress in Cancer Research and Therapy,
Vol. 31, edited by F. Bresciani, et al.
Raven Press, New York © 1984.

Use and Mechanism of Action of the LH-RH Agonist ICI 118630 in the Therapy of Hormone-Sensitive Breast and Prostate Cancer

*R.I. Nicholson, *K.J. Walker, *P. Davies, *A. Turkes,
*A.O. Turkes, *J. Dyas, **R.W. Blamey, **M. Williams,
†M.R.G. Robinson, and *K. Griffiths

*Tenovus Institute for Cancer Research, Welsh National School of Medicine, Heath,
Cardiff, CF4 4XX; **Department of Surgery, City Hospital, Nottingham; and
†Department of Urology, Pontefract General Infirmary, Pontefract,
West Yorkshire, United Kingdom*

In 1977 Dr. Barry Furr and the late Dr. Arthur Walpole from ICI Pharmaceuticals Division (U.K.) approached the Tenovus Institute for Cancer Research to screen a series of luteinising hormone-releasing hormone (LH-RH) agonists which they believed might have interesting endocrinological and antitumour properties. The results obtained at that time clearly showed that in female rats the compounds were able to suppress ovarian activity, reduce circulating levels of oestradiol and cause a decrease in size of oestrogen target tissues (28,30), including an ability to promote extensive regressions in oestrogen receptor positive dimethylbenzanthracene (DMBA)-induced mammary tumours (31,32). Similarly, in male animals the LH-RH agonists decreased circulating levels of testosterone and, at least in young animals, promoted an atrophy of the accessory sex organs (34). Interestingly, the effects observed often resembled those of ovariectomy or orchidectomy, a finding which led to the conclusion that the drugs were eliciting a 'chemical castration-like response' in the gonads (30-32) As a result of these studies and others (17) one of the original compounds, ICI 118630 (D-Ser(Bu^t)^{6}Azaglycine^{10} - LH-RH), was selected for clinical development and is now undergoing phase I trials in both advanced breast (33,35,45,46) and prostate cancer (1,2,33,35,45,46). It is hoped that ICI 118630, together with other LH-RH agonists (7,27,37,47), will prove to be a non-invasive, reversible and non-toxic alternative to the widely used irreversible surgical procedures of oophorectomy in premenopausal women with breast cancer and orchidectomy in men with prostate cancer.

The present communication highlights a number of the endocrinological aspects which have arisen from the early clinical trials of ICI 118630 and relates them to our current knowledge of the mechanism of action of LH-RH agonists in animals and in man.

BREAST CANCER

The patients selected for the study were those with histologically proven carcinoma of the breast who had either recurrent or locally advanced disease and were premenopausal. No patient was entered into the study who had received prior ablative or additive endocrine therapy for either their primary or recurrent disease. ICI 118630 (supplied by ICI Pharmaceuticals Division, Macclesfield, UK in 1ml ampoules containing 500µg of the drug in citrate buffer adjusted to pH 5) was administered (500 or 1000 µg/day) by subcutaneous (s.c.) injection during the morning. Treatment was initiated in the breast clinic of Professor R.W. Blamey. As a consequence of this and the requirement for prompt therapy, an important feature of the study was that ICI 118630 treatment was started at various stages of the menstrual cycle.

Endocrine Effects

The data presented in figure 1 show the hormonal effects of ICI 118630

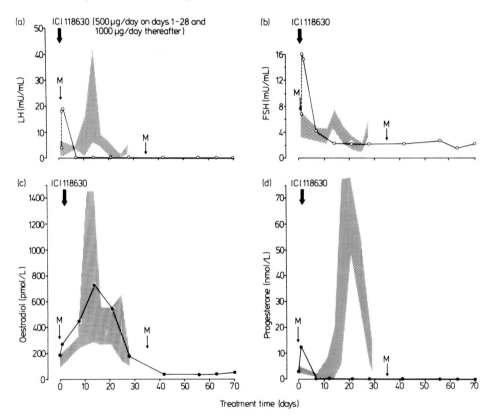

FIG. 1.   Influence of ICI 118630 on plasma hormone levels in a 46 year old premenopausal woman (AH, weight 52 kg) with advanced breast cancer. ICI 118630 was injected (sc) daily during the morning (500 µg/day on days 1-28 and 1000 µg/day thereafter) starting on day 1 of menstruation. Blood samples were withdrawn at time 0, 1h (-----) and 24h (———) and then 24h after the last injection on the days indicated. The samples were assayed for (a) LH, (b) FSH, (c) oestradiol and (d) progesterone. The assays for these hormones have been previously described (35). M = menstruation. Control data from 6 premenopausal postmastectomy or postlumpectomy patients is presented as a range of values for each hormone (see toned area) observed during one complete menstrual cycle.

in a 46 year old female patient (AH) who developed secondary boney
metastases 6 months after mastectomy. Therapy was initiated on day 1
of menstruation. Within 1h of ICI 118630 injection (500µg) there was a
substantial rise in circulating levels of luteinising hormone (LH) and
follicle stimulating hormone (FSH), reaching concentrations in plasma
of 17.7 mu/ml and 16.0 mu/ml respectively. These values were maintained
at 24h. On continued daily administration of ICI 118630 however the
basal plasma levels of the gonadotrophins were reduced to those seen
during the mid-luteal phase of 6 control premenopausal postmastectomy
or postlumpectomy patients. No evidence of a midcycle peak of either
of these hormones was observed. In this patient, plasma oestradiol
values showed a normal progressive follicular rise, followed by a decrease
in concentration during the second half of the cycle (Fig. 1c).
Significantly, however, no evidence for ovulation or formation of an
active corpus luteum was obtained since plasma progesterone, after a
small early rise on day 1, remained low (Fig. 1d). The findings were in
marked contrast to the results obtained in control premenopausal women
with breast cancer where plasma progesterone concentrations of 50 to 80
nmol/L were observed in the second half of the menstrual cycle. A
second menstrual bleeding commenced on day 35 and continued intermittent-
ly during the next 28 days. Plasma concentrations of LH, FSH, oestradiol
and progesterone were low during the remaining 35 day treatment period
and showed no evidence of cyclical activity.

The patterns of LH and FSH release during treatment with the LH-RH
agonist were qualitatively similar in individual patients (not illustrated) and appeared largely independent of whether treatment was
initiated during the follicular (Fig. 2a,b) or luteal (Fig. 3a,b) phases
of the menstrual cycle. Thus, elevated gonadotrophins were observed in
all patients after the first injection of the drug and were followed by
a subsequent reduction in their basal values during the first and second
menstrual cycles. Small rises in circulating oestradiol and progesterone were often associated with the increased plasma concentrations of
the gonadotrophins. This was especially evident when therapy was
initiated during the follicular phase (Fig. 2c,d). On continued treatment, however, while plasma progesterone concentrations fell back to
levels observed during the early follicular phase of control cycles,
oestradiol concentrations continued to increase (Fig. 2c). The levels
obtained, however, were indistinguishable from control late follicular
phase samples. No evidence of ovulation or formation of an active
corpus luteum was seen in these women since plasma progesterone remained
low (Fig. 2d). Plasma oestradiol concentrations decreased towards
menstruation and were low during the remaining 35 day study period.

Initiation of ICI 118630 therapy during the luteal phase of the
menstrual cycle in 3 women did not appreciably affect circulating
oestradiol (Fig. 4) or progesterone (Fig. 3c) in that cycle. Follicular oestradiol production was however evident during the second
recorded cycle although no progesterone production was recorded. Two
of the women subsequently had suppressed oestradiol levels. The remaining patient, however, who showed some persistent follicular activity
throughout treatment also showed small fluctuations in plasma FSH which
appeared to precede the peaks of oestradiol production (Fig. 5).

The decreased plasma concentrations of oestradiol and progesterone
resulting from long-term ICI 118630 treatment were similar to those seen
after oophorectomy or in postmenopausal women, and were substantially
lower than the oestradiol levels observed in control premenopausal

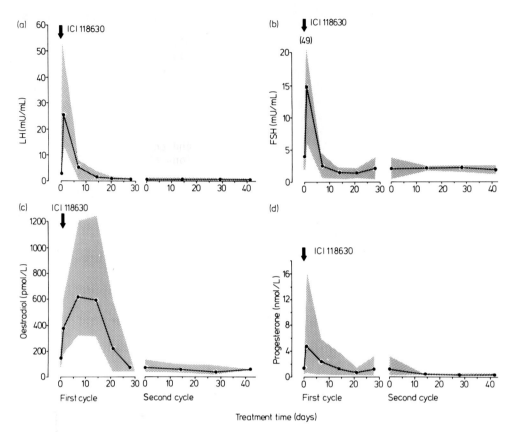

FIG. 2.   Long-term effects of ICI 118630 on plamsa hormone levels in patients with advanced breast cancer. ICI 118630 (500 or 1000 μg) was injected daily for periods up to 70 days in 5 patients. Treatment was initiated during the follicular phase of the menstrual cycle (days 1,3,9, 9 and 15; plasma progesterone (<3nmol/L). Hormonal profiles are divided into the events occurring up to the date of first menstruation and all subsequent events. Blood samples were withdrawn on the days indicated 24h after the last injection of ICI 118630 and assayed for (a) LH, (b) FSH, (c) oestradiol and (d) progesterone. Values are shown as the mean (●——●) ± range.

postmastectomy patients on day 14 of their menstrual cycles (Fig. 6a) or the progesterone values during the mid-luteal phase (Fig. 6b). The alterations in plasma hormones observed during LH-RH agonist therapy were recorded in the absence of side effects.

   The above data in premenopausal women with advanced breast cancer are similar to those reported for the LH-RH agonist buserelin, D-Ser-$(Bu^t)^6 LH-RH^{1-9}$ethylamide (27) and indicate that LH-RH agonists can reduce both follicular and luteal function. Longer term follow-up on increased numbers of patients is now necessary to assess objective tumour responses to ICI 118630.

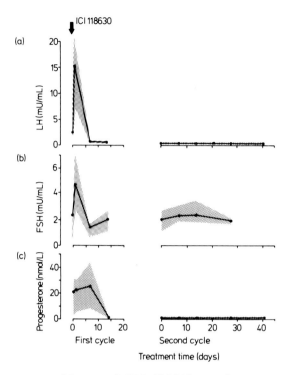

FIG. 3.   Long-term effects of ICI 118630 on plasma hormone levels in
patients with advanced breast cancer.   ICI 118630 was injected daily
for periods upto 45 days in 3 patients.   Treatment was initiated during
the luteal phase of the menstrual cycle (BP, day 18, plasma progesterone
32 nmol/L; S.McG, day 14, progesterone 26 nmol/L and MD, day 36, progesterone 3.7 nmol/L).   The experimental procedure is detailed in the
legend to Fig. 2.   Blood samples were assayed for (a) LH, (b) FSH and
(c) progesterone.

Potential mechanisms of action of ICI 118630 in breast cancer patients

(a) Pituitary desensitization

It is clear from the above studies that the long-term therapy (4-6
weeks) of breast cancer patients with ICI 118630 reduces ovarian activity, producing and maintaining castrate concentrations of both oestradiol and progesterone in plasma (Figs. 4&6).   The most likely explanation for this relatively quiescent state within the ovary relates to the
ability of LH-RH agonists, when administered at high concentrations, to
down-regulate pituitary LH-RH receptors (6) and hence desensitise the
pituitary gland to the releasing hormone properties of the drugs (4,6,
42).   This process eventually results in a fall in circulating levels of
LH and FSH (Figs. 2,3) and thus a withdrawal of support for gonadal
steroidogenic activity (16,39).   It is noteworthy, however, that pituitary desensitization is not an instantaneous event and that the initial
action of these drugs is to promote substantial release of LH and FSH
(Figs. 1-3 and refs. 15,40).   This may lead to two opposing early actions

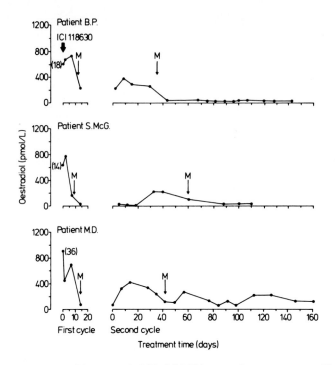

FIG. 4.   Long-term effects of ICI 118630 on plasma oestradiol levels in patients with advanced breast cancer.   Therapy was initiated during the luteal phase.   Experimental procedure is detailed in Figs. 2 and 3.

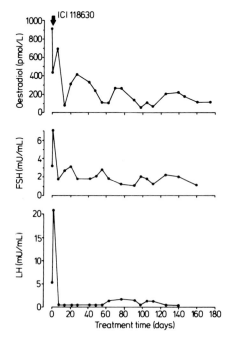

FIG. 5.   Hormonal profile of patient M.D.

on the ovary, an initial stimulation of oestradiol (Fig. lc) and progesterone (Fig. 1d) production, followed by a loss of receptors for LH and
FSH (13,26), the latter phenomenon decreases the sensitivity of the
tissue to gonadotrophins (13,25,26). Unfortunately, it is not possible
from the present data to assess critically the relative contribution of
each of these actions of LH-RH agonists to the rapidity with which ICI
118630 causes ovarian quiescence, although it is evident that a failure
to achieve a full pituitary desensitization may, in some patients, be
associated with persistent follicular activity (Fig. 5 and ref. 27).

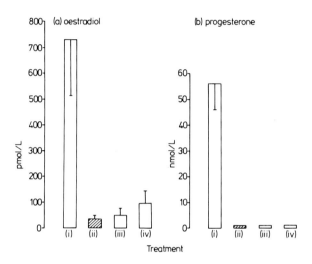

FIG. 6.   Long-term effects of ICI 118630 and oophorectomy on plasma
oestradiol and progesterone levels. (a) Plasma oestradiol levels in
(I) samples removed from control premenopausal postmastectomy patients
on day 14 of their menstrual cycle (n=6), (II) patients with suppressed
ovarian activity resulting from long-term ICI 118630 therapy (n=13) and
(III) 2 month oophorectomised or (IV) postmenopausal postmastectomy
patients (n=16); (b) plasma progesterone levels in (I) samples removed
from control patients on day 25 of their menstrual cycle (n=5), (II),
(III) and (IV) as in (a). Results are presented as the mean ± SEM.

(b) Direct antigonadal actions
     Experiments performed in hypophysectomised female rats have indicated
that LH-RH agonists (41), including ICI 118630 (18,36), are capable of
inhibiting the stimulatory actions of human chorionic gonadotrophin
(hCG) and FSH on ovarian function. These data infer that LH-RH agonists
may have direct inhibitory actions on the ovaries (18,36) and more
specifically on granulosa (23,24) and luteal (5,9,21) cells. The direct
inhibition of ovarian steroidogenesis by LH-RH agonists in the rat
appears to be mediated through ovarian LH-RH binding proteins (9,10,11,
21) which are similar in character to those present in rat anterior
pituitary tissue (10,11,21,38).

No such actions of ICI 118630 were however evident in premenopausal women with advanced breast cancer and both follicular oestradiol production (Figs.1,2&4) and luteal progesterone secretion (Fig. 3), once initiated, appeared to progress normally until menstruation. Similar observations on follicular oestradiol production have been made by Klijn and DeJong in 3 out of 4 patients with advanced breast cancer treated with the LH-RH agonist buserelin (27). Interestingly, two of these women also had elevated progesterone concentrations. These findings are consistent with a failure of LH-RH or an agonistic analogue to effect FSH-stimulated human granulosa synthesis of oestradiol and progesterone in vitro (8). Furthermore, Clayton and Huhtaniemi (12) have been unable to demonstrate LH-RH binding proteins in human corpora lutea using methods which detect rodent ovarian LH-RH receptors. Taken together these data suggest that a direct inhibitory action of LH-RH agonists on human ovarian activity, in the short term, is unlikely.

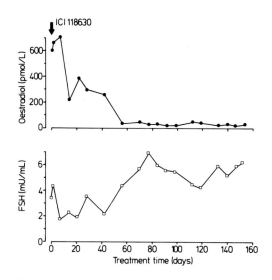

FIG. 7.   Hormonal profile of patient B.P.

On long-term therapy, however, patient B.P. showed a progressive increase in plasma FSH in the presence of castrate values of oestradiol (Fig. 7). This may suggest a direct inhibitory action of ICI 118630 on FSH-induced follicular development in vivo.

PROSTATE CANCER

The patients selected for the study were those with histologically proven carcinoma of the prostate who attended the clinic of M.R.G.R. They had received no previous hormone or cytotoxic therapy. ICI 118630 (100 or 250 μg/day) was administered by injection (s.c.) during the morning.

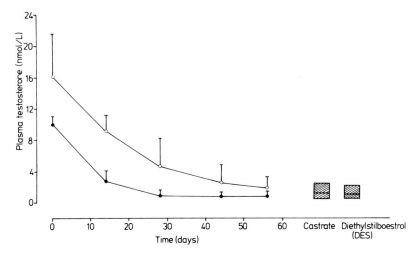

FIG. 8.   Long-term effects of ICI 118630 on plasma testosterone
levels in patients with advanced prostate cancer. ICI 118630 (100 μg,
O or 250 μg,● ; n=4/group) was administered (sc) during the morning.
Blood samples were withdrawn at the times indicated, approximately 24h
after the last injection. The values of testosterone obtained were
compared with those found in either 2-month castrate or diethylstilboestrol (DES, 1 mg td) treated patients.

Endocrine Effects

     The data illustrated in figure 8 show the mean levels of testosterone
in two groups of 4 patients with advanced prostate cancer treated with
either 100μg or 250μg ICI 118630 daily for 58 days. At the highest dose
level plasma testosterone concentrations were suppressed by day 14 and
remained low throughout treatment. The levels obtained were comparable
to those observed in castrate or diethylstilboestrol treated patients.
On the lower dose level (100μg), plasma testosterone concentrations
approximating to those of castrate patients were not achieved until
after 5-6 weeks. A similar suppression in plasma LH and FSH was however
observed in patients with 100μg or 250μg ICI 118630/day (46).

     The hormonal changes were associated with clinical improvements as
assessed by the Criteria of the British Prostate Study Group. These
included a reduction in circulating acid phosphatase levels in 7/8
patients and increased urinary flow. The results were observed in
patients showing minimal side-effects. Similar clinical and hormonal
observations have been made by other groups using ICI 118630 (1,2) and
buserelin (7,37,47).

Potential mechanisms of action of ICI 118630 in prostate cancer patients

     As in premenopausal women the long-term inhibitory action of ICI
118630 on gonadal activity in male patients are most simply explained
by the ability of the drug to cause pituitary desensitation and a withdrawal of gonadotrophin support for testicular function. Thus, de-

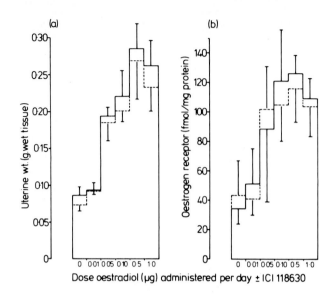

Dose oestradiol (µg) administered per day ± ICI 118630

FIG. 9.   Influence of ICI 118630 on the responsiveness of uteri to
oestradiol in ovariectomised animals (n=5 rats/group). Two week
ovariectomised animals were treated twice daily for 4 days with various
doses of oestradiol (0.005-0.5 µg per injection) in the presence or
absence of ICI 118630 (5 µg bd). On the morning of day 5 (16h after
the last injection) the animals were sacrificed and uteri removed,
weighed and stored at -20°C for subsequent oestrogen-receptor assay
(29). Data are expressed as the mean ± SD. No significant (NS)
differences were observed between the oestradiol and oestradiol plus
ICI 118630 treated groups using either a Student's 't' test or a Mann-
Whitney U-test.

creases in basal plasma LH may be correlated with decreased plasma
testosterone (Fig. 8 (46)). Indeed, in a more detailed study Allen and
her coworkers (2) showed that the sustained rise in plasma LH noted 1,2
and 4h after an initial injection of ICI 118630 (250µg) was obliterated
after 7 days of twice-daily injections of the drug. Interestingly,
however, the testes still retain their sensitivity to the gonadotrophins
in patients with suppressed levels of testosterone resulting from ICI
118630 treatment and show a substantial rise in the level of this
androgen 24, 48 and 72h after the administration of hCG (1). These
data are not consistent with a direct inhibitory action of LH-RH
agonists on gonadal tissue, a concept supported by a failure to detect
LH-RH binding proteins in human leydig cells (11) and an inability of
LH-RH agonists to interfere with short-term testosterone production
in vitro (3,43).

Direct actions of ICI 118630 on oestrogen and androgen target tissues

    Recent reports have shown that treatment of either postmenopausal
women with advanced breast cancer (20) or castrated men with prostate
cancer (2) with LH-RH agonists may be associated with tumour remissions.
Such observations, if verified, may imply direct inhibitory actions of
LH-RH agonists on oestrogen and androgen dependent tumours, a hypothesis

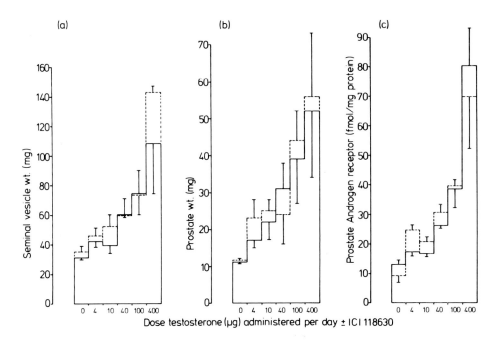

FIG. 10.   Influence of ICI 118630 on the responsiveness of seminal
vesicles and the ventral prostate to testosterone in orchidectomised
rats. Ten day orchidectomised animals (n=5 rats/group, weight approximately 280g) were treated twice daily for 10 days with various doses of
testosterone (2-200 μg/injection) in the presence or absence of ICI 118630
(5 μg bd). On the morning of day 11 (16h after the last injection),
the animals were sacrificed and seminal vesicles and ventral prostate
removed, weighed and the prostate stored at -20°C for androgen receptor
assay. The receptor assay was basically as described by Davies et al,
(14), except that all buffers contained 0.6 KCl.

which has some (44) although not universal (18,36) experimental
support.
    In order to investigate further such actions, the effect of a fixed
concentration of ICI 118630 (5μg bd) on the stimulation of uterine weights
by various concentrations of oestradiol in ovariectomised female rats
or prostate and seminal vesicle weights by testosterone in castrate male
rats has been examined. Fig. 9 shows that ICI 118630, at a dose which
causes pronounced atrophy of oestrogen target tissues in intact animals
(28), has no substantial effect on either uterine weight gain caused by
the daily administration of a wide dose range of oestradiol in castrate
rats (Fig. 9a) or on the oestrogen receptor content of the uteri (Fig.
9b). Similarly, ICI 118630 was without appreciable influence on either
the testosterone-stimulated increase in prostate (Fig. 10b) and seminal
vesicle (Fig. 10a) weights in orchidectomised animals or the prostate
androgen receptor content (Fig. 10c). Moreover, the drug was unable to
prevent the tumour growth-promoting activity of oestradiol in ovariectomised rats bearing DMBA-induced mammary carcinomas (Fig. 11). These data
do not support the concept of direct inhibitory actions of LH-RH agonists
on all oestrogen and androgen target tissues. However, the recent obser-

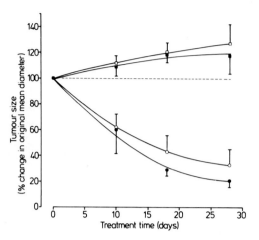

FIG. 11.   Effect of ICI 118630 on the stimulation of DMBA-induced
mammary tumour growth by oestradiol in ovariectomised rats. Tumour-
bearing animals were ovariectomised and injected twice daily with
oestradiol (0.25 µg/injection, □), oestradiol plus ICI 118630 (5 µg/
injection,■), ICI 118630 (●) or saline (O). Tumour size was measured
at the times indicated as the mean of two perpendicular diameters, one
measured across the greatest width. Data are expressed as mean ± SEM.
No significant (NS) differences were observed between oestradiol and
oestradiol plus ICI 118630 treated groups using either a Student's 't'
test or a Mann-Whitney U test.

vation of the presence of LH-RH binding proteins in Dunning rat prostate
tumours, but not in normal rat ventral prostate (22), coupled with the
sensitivity of the model to the inhibitory actions of ICI 118630 (19),
require that the antagonistic properties of LH-RH agonists against test-
tosterone should be examined in this tumour.

CONCLUSIONS AND FUTURE PROSPECTS

   It is evident from the foregoing data that ICI 118630 is able to
promote a decrease in gonadal function in patients with either advanced
breast cancer or prostate cancer. The levels of steroids achieved are
equivalent to those seen in castrate patients. There is every hope
therefore that in the future,the class of drugs to which ICI 118630
belongs, will find a place in the management of these prevalent cancers
and may obviate the need for surgical ablation of the gonads.
   It is considered however, that their true value can only be critically
assessed by controlled trials in which the drug is compared with standard
forms of therapy and which use meaningful criteria of response. Such a
trial is currently underway in South Wales (Co-ordinator, KJW) and will
examine the antitumour efficacy of ICI 118630 with that of subcapsular
orchidectomy in patients with advanced prostate cancer.

ACKNOWLEDGEMENTS

   The authors wish to thank the Tenovus Institute for generous financial
support and ICI Pharmaceuticals Division (UK) for the gift of ICI 118630.

REFERENCES

1. Ahmed, S.R., Shallet, S.M., Brooman, P.J.C., Howell, A., Blacklock, N.J. and Richards, D. (1983): The Lancet, Aug. 20th: 415-418.
2. Allen, J.M., O'Shea, J.P., Mashiter, K., Williams, G. and Bloom, S.R. (1983): Brit. Med. J., 286: 1607-1609.
3. Badger, T.M., Beitins, I.Z., Ostrea, T., Crisafulli, J.M.,Little, R. and Saidel, M.E. (1980): Endocrinology,106: 1149-1153.
4. Berquist, C., Nillius, S.J. and Wade, L. (1979): J. Clin. Endocr. Metab.,49: 472-474.
5. Behrman, H.R., Preston, S.L. and Hall, A.K. (1980): Endocrinology, 107: 656-664.
6. Belchetz, P.E., Plant, T.M., Nakai, Y., Keogh, E.J. and Knobil, E. (1978): Science N.Y. 202: 631-633.
7. Borgmann, V., Hardt, W., Schmidt-Gollwitzer, M., Adenauer, H. and Nagel, R. (1982): The Lancet, May 15th: 1097-1099.
8. Casper, R.F., Erickson, G.F., Rebar, R.W. and Yen, S.S.C. (1982): Fert. and Steril., 37: 406-409.
9. Clayton, R.N., Harwood, J.P. and Catt, K.J. (1979): Nature, 282: 90-93.
10. Clayton, R.N., Katikineni, M., Chan, V., Dufau, M.L. and Catt, K.J. (1980): Proc. Natn. Acad. Sci. U.S.A., 77: 4459-4463.
11. Clayton, R.N. and Catt, K.J. (1981): J. Endocr. Rev., 2:186-209.
12. Clayton, R.N. and Huhtaniemi, I.P. (1982): Nature, 299: 56-59.
13. Conti, M., Harwood, J.P., Hseuh, A.J.W., Dufau, M.L. and Catt, K.J. (1976): J. Biol. Chem., 251: 7729-7731.
14. Davies, P., Thomas, P. and Griffiths, K. (1977): J. Endocrinol., 74: 393-404.
15. de la Cruz, A., de la Cruz, K.G., Arimura, A., Coy, D.H., Vilchez-Martinez, J.A., Coy, E. and Schally, A.V. (1975): Fertil. Steril., 26: 894.
16. Dorrington, J.H. and Armstrong, D.T. (1979): Rec. Prog. Horm. Res., 35: 301-333.
17. Dutta, A.S., Furr, B.J.A., Giles, M.B. and Valcaccia, B. (1978): Biochem. biophys. Res. Commun., 81: 382-390.
18. Furr, B.J.A. and Nicholson, R.I. (1982): J. Reprod. Fert., 64: 529-539.
19. Furr, B.J.A. (1983): AASCR Meeting, San-Diego, Abst. 730.
20. Harvey, H.A., Lipton, A., Santen, R.J. et al. (1981): Proc. Amer. Assoc. Can. Res./Amer. Soc. Clin. Oncol., 22: 444.
21. Harwood, J.P., Clayton, R.N. and Catt,K.J. (1980): Endocrinology, 107: 407-413.
22. Hierowski, M.T., Altamirano, P., Redding, T.W. and Schally, A.V. (1983): Febs Letters, 154: 92-96.
23. Hseuh, A.J.W. and Erickson, G.F. (1979): Science, 204: 854-855.
24. Hseuh, A.J.W., Wang, C. and Erickson, G.F. (1980): Endocrinology, 106: 1697-1705.
25. Hunzicker-Dunn, M. and Birnbaumer, L. (1976): Endocrinol.,99: 211-222.
26. Kledzik, G.S., Cusan, L., Auclair, C., Kelly, P.A. and Labrie, F. (1978): Fert. Steril., 30: 348-353.
27. Klijn, J.G.M. and DeJong, F.H. (1982): The Lancet, May 29: 1213-1216.
28. Maynard, P.V. and Nicholson, R.I. (1979): Brit. J. Cancer, 39: 274-279.

29. Nicholson, R.I., Davies, P.and Griffiths, K.(1978): In: Reviews
        on Endocrine-Related Cancer, ICI Publications, Supplement
        April, pp306-321.
30. Nicholson, R.I., Finney, E. and Maynard, P.V. (1978): J. Endocrinol.,
        79: 51P.
31. Nicholson, R.I. and Maynard, P.V. (1979): Brit. J. Cancer, 39:
        268-273.
32. Nicholson, R.I., Walker, K.J. and Maynard, P.V. (1980): In:
        Breast Cancer: Experimental and Clinical Aspects, edited by
        H.T. Mouridsen and T. Palshof, pp.295-299. Pergamon Press,
        Oxford.
33. Nicholson, R.I., Walker, K.J., Walker, R., Read, G., Blamey, R.W.,
        Campbell, F.C., Plowman, P.N. and Griffiths, K. (1983):
        3rd EORTC Breast Cancer Working Conference, Amsterdam.
        Abst. IX.22.
34. Nicholson, R.I. and Harper, M. (Unpublished).
35. Nicholson, R.I., Walker, K.J., Turkes, A., Turkes, A.O., Dyas, J.,
        Blamey, R.W., Campbell, F.C., Robinson, M.R.G. and Griffiths, K.
        (In Press): J. Steroid Biochem. 18.
36. Nicholson, R.I., Walker, K.J., Harper, M., Phillips, A. and
        Furr, B.J.A. (In Press): In: Reviews on Endocrine-Related Cancer,
        ICI Publications.
37. Trachtenberg, J. (1983): J. Urol.129: 1149-1151.
38. Reeves, J.J., Sequin, C., Lefebvre, F.A., Kelly, P.A. and
        Labrie, F. (1980): Proc. Natn. Acad. Sci. U.S.A., 77:
        5567-5571.
39. Richards, J.S. and Midgley-Rees, A. (1976): Biol. Reprod. 14:
        82-94.
40. Ripple, R.H., Johnson, E.S., White, W.F., Fujino, M., Fukuda, T.
        and Kobayashi, S. (1975): Proc. Soc. Exp. Biol. Med., 148:
        1193-1197.
41. Ripple, R.H. and Johnson, E.S. (1976): Proc. Soc. Exp. Biol.
        Med. 152: 432-436.
42. Sandow, J., Von Rechenberg, W., Jerzabek, G. and Stoll, W.
        (1978): Fert. Steril., 30: 205-209.
43. Sharpe, R.M., Fraser, H.M., Cooper, I. and Rommerts, F.F.G. (1982):
        Ann. N.Y. Acad. Sci.
44. Vilchez-Martinez, J.A. and Pedroza-Garcia, E. (1978): 60th Ann.
        Meeting. End. Soc. U.S.A. Abst. 200: 174.
45. Walker, K.J., Nicholson, R.I., Turkes, A., Turkes, A.O.,
        Blamey, R.W. and Robinson, M. (1983): 2nd Joint Meeting of the
        British Endocrine Societies, York. Abst. 18.
46. Walker, K.J., Nicholson, R.I., Robinson, M., Turkes, A.O., Turkes,
        A. and Griffiths, K. (1983): The Lancet, Aug. 20th: 413-415.
47. Waxman, J.H., Wass, J.A.H., Hendry, W.F., Whitfield, H.N.,
        Besser, G.M., Malpas, J.S. and Oliver, R.T.D. (1983):
        Brit. Med. J., 286: 1309-1312.

Progress in Cancer Research and Therapy,
Vol. 31, edited by F. Bresciani, et al.
Raven Press, New York © 1984.

Combined Antihormonal Treatment in Prostate Cancer: A New Approach Using an LHRH Agonist or Castration and an Antiandrogen

*F. Labrie, *A. Dupont, *A. Bélanger, *C. Labrie,
*Y. Lacourcière, **J.P. Raynaud, **J.M. Husson, † J. Emond,
† J.G. Houle, ‡ J.G. Girard, § G. Monfette, ¶ J.P. Paquet,
#A. Vallières, § § C. Bossé, and ¶ ¶ R. Delisle

*Department of Molecular Endocrinology and Medicine, Le Centre Hospitalier de
L'Université Laval, Québec, G1V 4G2 Canada; **Centre de Recherches
Roussel-UCLAF, Romainville, France; † Hôtel-Dieu Hospital, Lévis, Québec,
Canada; ‡ Asbestos Medical Center, Québec, Canada; § Hôtel-Dieu Hospital,
St. Jérôme, Québec, Canada; ¶ Enfant-Jesus Hospital, Québec, Canada; #Saint
Sacrement Hospital, Québec, Canada; § § Hôtel-Dieu Hospital, Chicoutimi,
Canada; and ¶ ¶ Hôtel-Dieu Hospital, Roberval, Canada

Cancer of the prostate is the second cause of death due to cancer in man and its annual incidence is approximately 40,000 new cases per 100 millions of population in North America. A major advance in the treatment of this disease pertains to the pioneering studies of Huggins and collaborators who have recognized the role of androgens in the evolution of this cancer (26, 27). Following these observations, during the last forty years, neutralization of testicular androgens has been achieved by surgical castration or treatment with high doses of estrogens, two approaches which lead to subjective and/or objective improvement in 60 to 70% of cases for various time intervals (3, 4, 12, 23, 43, 44, 45, 58, 63, 65). However, surgical castration presents psychological limitations for many patients while high doses of estrogens frequently cause lethal cardiovascular complications (12, 63, 64). There was thus the need for a more acceptable way of neutralizing testicular androgens.

The unexpected finding that LHRH (luteinizing hormone-releasing hormone) agonists block testicular testosterone secretion and induce a marked loss in ventral prostate weight in the adult rat (2, 33) opened the possibility of a new approach in the treatment of androgen-dependent diseases, especially cancer of the prostate. Fortunately, among all species studied, man is the most sensitive to the inhibitory effect of LHRH agonist treatment on testicular androgen formation (5, 16, 34, 51) and medical castration can be easily achieved (34-37, 51, 60).

Despite the initial improvement of symptoms after neutralization of androgens of testicular origin in a large proportion of patients, relapse of the disease usually occurs within one or two years (47). Moreover, within 6 months after relapse of the disease, the survival is only approximately 50% (29). Since man is unique among species in having a high secretion of weak adrenal androgens which can be converted into active steroids in the prostate as well as at the periphery, (21, 24, 46), it is quite possible that reactivation of the cancer is due to the androgens of adrenal origin (7, 13, 21, 50). We thus felt important to include neutralization of adrenal androgens in our antihormonal treatment regime.

Knowing that chemical castration can be achieved by LHRH agonists (34), neutralization of the action of adrenal androgens on the cancer was the next problem to be investigated. Following our preliminary studies using an LHRH agonist and a pure antiandrogen in experimental animals (38, 52), we have used the same combined therapy in men with advanced prostatic cancer (35-37). The present report is a continuation of this study in 97 patients at stage D of the disease. The combination therapy was used in 44 previously untreated patients as well as in 24 patients previously treated with DES (diethylstilbestrol). In 9 previously untreated patients, complete androgen neutralization was achieved by surgical castration (instead of LHRH agonist administration) and the antiandrogen. For comparison, in 29 patients showing relapse of the disease after surgical castration, the effect of antiandrogen administration has been studied. In support of our previous suggestion (35-37), the present study clearly indicates that drastic changes in the approach to hormonal therapy in prostatic cancer are appropriate.

PATIENTS, MATERIALS AND METHODS

Ninety-seven patients with histology-proven prostatic adenocarcinoma took part in this study after written informed consent (Table 1). The average age of the patients was 67 (45-85) years. Of the 44 previously untreated patients, complete antihormonal therapy was achieved in 35 patients by combined treatment with the LHRH agonist [D-Ser(TBU)^6, des-Gly-NH$_2$^{10}]LHRH ethylamide (HOE-766, Buserelin), and the pure antiandrogen, 5,5-dimethyl-3[4-nitro-3-(trifluoromethyl)phenyl]-24-imidazolidinedione (RU-23908, Anandron) while 9 were orchiectomized and received the antiandrogen. Buserelin was injected s.c. at the daily dose of 500 µg at 0800 hours while the antiandrogen was given three times daily at 0700, 1500 and 2300 hours at the dose of 100 mg orally. The combined treatment with the LHRH agonist and the antiandrogen was also given to 24 patients previously treated with high doses of DES but showing progression or relapse of the disease. The antiandrogen was started one day before first administration of the LHRH agonist. Twenty-nine previously cas-

TABLE 1. <u>Objective response to the complete removal of androgens</u>

Previous treatment	Months of RX	Current RX	No of pts	% OBJECTIVE RESPONSE				
				Complete	Partial	Stable	Progression	Escape
NIL	9.9 (4-18)	LHRH-A +ANTI-ANDR.	35	9% (3)	71% (25)	20% (7)	0% 0%	2/35
								4.5%
NIL	7.3 (4-11)	CASTR. +ANTI-ANDRO.	9	11% (1)	33% (3)	56% (5)	0% 0	2/44 0/9
DES	8.5 (3-14)	LHRH-A +ANTI-ANDROG.	24	4% (1)	37% (9)	17% (4)	42% (10)	4/14
								25%
CASTR.	8.1 (4-11)	LHRH-A +ANTI-ANDRO.	13	0% 0	8% (1)	31% (4)	61% (8)	6/24 2/5
CASTR. + DES	6.5 (4-10)	ANTI-ANDR.	16	0% 0	19% (3)	12% (2)	69% (11)	0/5

Objective response according to the NPCP criteria to the combined treatment with an LHRH agonist (or surgical castration) and a pure antiandrogen in previously untreated patients with prostate cancer at stage D or previously treated with DES as well as to treatment with the antiandrogen in stage D patients previously castrated.

trated patients, 16 of which had also received high doses of DES, were treated with the antiandrogen alone (Table 1).

Subjective symptoms included prostatism, bone pain and general well-being. Hesitancy to initiate stream, loss of caliber of stream, terminal dribbling, higher frequency of urination, dysuria and urinary incontinence were graded from 0 to +++++, this last symbol representing maximal acceptable signs of urinary obstruction. Pain was graded from 0 to +++++, this last symbol being assigned to patients having bone pain of a degree sufficient for immobilization or requiring intravenous morphine administration. General well-being was assessed in comparison with the general status of the patient and his usual life activities before development of cancer. This included physical activities, appetite, sleep and body weight.

METHODS

Complete clinical, urological, biochemical and radiological evaluation of the patients was performed before starting treatment as described (35-37). Blood samples were taken at days -2, -1 and 0 (time of LHRH administration or surgical castration) as well as at the time intervals indicated in the Legends to Figures for determination of plasma testosterone (T), dihydrotestosterone (DHT), 17-OH-progesterone, androstane-3α,17β-diol, dehydroepiandrosterone (DHEA), dehydroepiandrosterone-sulfate (DHEA-S), 17 β-estradiol (E_2), cortisol, LH, FSH, prolactin and prostatic acid phosphatase by double-antibody radioimmunoassays (6, 34), as well as alkaline phosphatase as part of the SMA-12 performed by Technicon AutoAnalyzer.

Radioimmunoassay data were analyzed using a program based on model II of Rodbard and Lewald (49). Statistical significance was measured according to the multiple-range test of Duncan-Kramer (32). All results are shown as the means ± SEM of duplicate determinations on individual samples.

Prostatic size was assessed by rectal examination as well as by transrectal and transabdominal ultrasonography using a Toshiba probe (model IVA-306A) and scanner (model SAL-20A). Intravenous urography was also performed when indicated. Bone scanning was performed with technetium methylene diphosphonate in all patients using a Dyna camera (series 5, Picker International). Pelvic, thoracic and lumbar spine X-Rays were done routinely. Series of laboratory analyses, including complete blood count, sequential multiple analyzer (SMA-12) and urinalysis, were performed at regular intervals (36, 37). The response criteria developed by the National Prostatic Cancer Project were used (43).

MATERIALS

The nonsteroidal pure antiandrogen Anandron was supplied by Dr. Jacques Gareau, Medical Department, Roussel-Canada Inc., in 50 mg tablets. The LHRH agonist Buserelin was supplied by Dr. A.T.A. Fazekas, Medical Department, Hoechst Canada, Montreal, Quebec, Canada, in the form of an injectable preparation. Material from New England Nuclear was used for measurement of prostatic acid phosphatase by double-antibody radioimmunoassay.

RESULTS

Serum prostatic acid phosphatase

Serum prostatic acid phosphatase (PAP) measured by radioimmunoassay was elevated in 70 out of 97 patients at initiation of treatment. It can be seen in Fig. 1 that serum PAP was rapidly reduced to 45% of pretreatment values as early as 5 days after starting the combined antihormonal therapy using the LHRH agonist and the antiandrogen in previously untreated patients. The serum PAP values progressively decreased and normal values were reached within two months in all except 4 patients who all showed normal serum PAP levels at 4 months. A comparable pattern was seen in the patients previously untreated who were surgically castrated and received the same dose of the antiandrogen (data not shown).

It can be seen in Fig. 2 that a striking difference is observed when the same treatment is applied to patients previously treated with DES and showing relapse of the disease. In fact, although serum PAP levels decreased to normal values in some patients, the levels of serum PAP

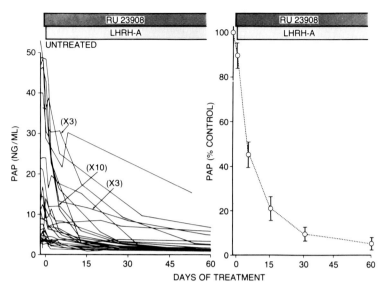

Fig. 1. Effect of combined treatment with an LHRH agonist
(HOE-766) and a pure antiandrogen (RU23908) on serum PAP
levels in previously untreated patients with advanced (stage
D2) prostatic cancer. Individual values are shown on the
left panel while means ± SEM are illustrated on the right
panel (25 patients).

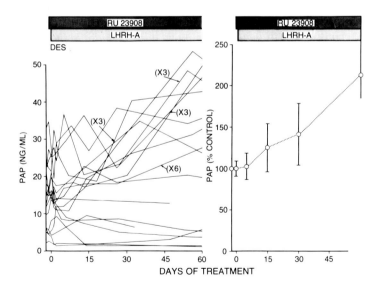

Fig. 2. Effect of combined treatment with an LHRH agonist
(HOE-766) and a pure antiandrogen (RU23908) on serum PAP
levels in patients with advanced (stage D2) prostatic cancer
previously treated with diethylstilbestrol. Individual
values are shown on the left panel while means ± SEM are
illustrated on the right panel (9 patients).

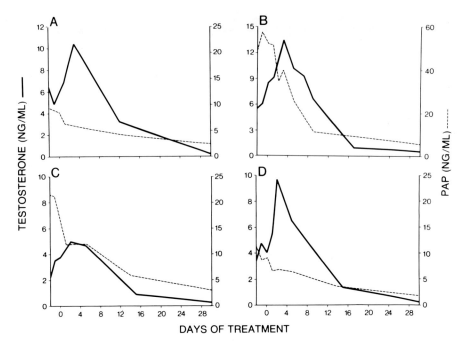

Fig. 3. Changes in serum PAP and testosterone levels during the first month of treatment in four previously untreated patients having advanced prostatic cancer and receiving the combined administration of the LHRH agonist HOE-766 and the pure antiandrogen RU23908. Note the rapid and marked decrease in serum PAP concentration in the presence of elevated serum T levels, thus indicating the efficiency of the antiandrogen at the dose used.

continued to increase in 11 out of 24 patients. Similarly, in patients previously castrated, stabilization or an increase of serum PAP levels was seen in 75% of patients (data not shown).

As already seen in the first adult man treated with a high dose of an LHRH agonist (34), treatment with LHRH agonists alone is always accompanied by a rise in serum T and DHT concentration which lasts for 5 to 15 days (22, 35-37, 51, 61) and is accompanied in a significant proportion of cases by a flare of the cancer (22, 51, 61). It is thus of great interest to see in Fig. 1 and 3 that a 55% decrease in serum PAP is already observed during the first 5 days of treatment with the LHRH agonist at a time when serum androgens are increased by 100 to 200% (p $<$ 0.01, Fig. 3).

Hormonal

Before treatment, except in patients treated with high doses of DES, or castrated, serum steroid values were within

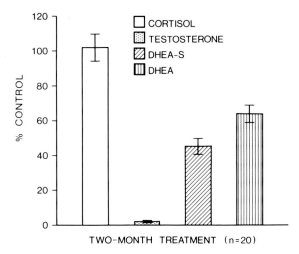

Fig. 4. Effect of 2-month combined treatment with the LHRH agonist (HOE-766) and the antiandrogen RU23908 on serum levels of cortisol (F), testosterone (T), dehydroepiandrosterone (DHEA) and dehydroepiandrosterone sulfate (DHEA-S) in 20 previously untreated patients having prostatic cancer. Control levels of F, T, DHEA-S and DHEA were respectively 156 ± 6, 5.44 ± 0.44, 834 ± 147 and 1.9 ± 0.3 ng/ml.

the normal range. As expected, chronic administration of the LHRH agonist in combination with RU23908 led to a marked inhibition of serum T levels to 2.50 ± 0.03% of control. It was also found, somewhat surprisingly, that serum levels of DHEAS and DHEA were also decreased to 45.0 ± 4.7 and 64 ± 5.0% of control, respectively, while serum cortisol levels remained unchanged (Fig. 4).

Bone scanning

In 32 previously untreated patients having metastatic disease, the combined therapy led to at least a 50% decrease in uptake accompanied by a normalization of serum PAP and no appearance of new lesions. A complete disappearance of bone lesions was seen within 5 months in 4 patients, thus indicating complete objective response. In the other 12 patients classified as stable, serum PAP levels are decreasing but have not yet reached normal values. A most important finding is that none of the 44 previously untreated patients receiving the combination therapy showed progression of the disease (Table 1).

Clinical signs and symptoms

In the previously untreated patients, a rapid and complete relief of pain was observed in all patients presenting this symptom before treatment. Disappearance of bone pain was seen within a few days. In patients previously treated with DES, complete removal of androgens also led to a disap-

pearance of pain in all patients while in patients previously castrated, disappearance of pain was seen in 12 out of 16
patients. A partial relief of pain was obtained in the 4
others. Although more difficult to evaluate due to the frequent concomitant presence of benign prostatic hyperplasia,
signs of prostatism were improved in 80 to 100% of patients.
The improvement in signs of prostatism was confirmed by
rectal examination as well as by transrectal and transabdominal echography in all cases. Improvement in performance
and well-being (appetite, sleep, general activity and body
weight) was seen in 100% of previously untreated patients
while an approximately 60% improvement was seen in the
patients previously treated with DES or castrated.

As shown earlier (35-37), approximately 50% of patients
receiving the combined therapy developed, to various
degrees, climateric-like vasomotor phenomena consisting of
perspiration and hot flushes. These symptoms decreased or
disappeared after a few months of treatment. Most patients
complained of a decrease in libido and erectile potency
after two to three weeks of treatment. However, in a few
cases, libido and erectile potency were maintained despite
complete androgen neutralization. No serious side-effects
were observed.

As revealed by a series of standard biochemical and hema-
tological tests, treatment with the LHRH agonist and the
antiandrogen has no detectable effect on any of the following parameters: complete (WBC, RBC, hemoglobin, hematocrit
and platelets) and differential blood count, γ-glutamyl
transaminase, glutamic oxaloacetic transaminase, glutamic
pyruvic transferase, lactic dehydrogenase, creatinine, total
biliburin and other parameters of blood biochemistry (SMA-
12).

DISCUSSION

As the duration of treatment and the number of patients
included in this study increases, a most consequent conclusion which clearly appears is that prostate cancer in man is
extremely sensitive to androgens. In fact, when complete
androgen neutralization is achieved in patients previously
untreated, a positive objective response assessed according
to the criteria of the National Prostatic Cancer Project is
observed in more than 95% of patients. In fact, in 44
patients who received the combined therapy with the LHRH
agonist or surgical castration, and the antiandrogen, no
progression of the disease was observed in any patient.

It is important to provide further information on the
only two patients who have shown relapse after 6 and 9
months, respectively. In one patient, although complete
disappearance of bone metastases had occurred, one tumor
developed after 9 months of treatment at the level of the
prostate but local radiotherapy could apparently control the
disease. The second patient was admitted bedridden at the
emergency room with complete urinary obstruction and hydro-
nephrosis as well as with an important oedema of the left
leg due to large lymp nodes of the left iliac chain. Two

PROSTATE CANCER

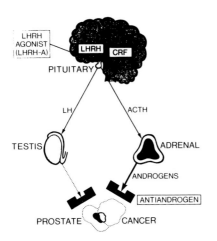

COMPLETE ANDROGEN WITHDRAWAL
LHRH-A + ANTIANDROGEN

a) LHRH-A BLOCKS THE FORMATION OF MALE
HORMONES (ANDROGENS) BY THE TESTIS

b) ANTIANDROGEN PREVENTS THE ACTION
OF ANDROGENS OF ADRENAL AND
TESTICULAR ORIGIN

c) COMBINATION OF BOTH DRUGS SHOULD
EXERT MAXIMAL INHIBITORY EFFECTS ON
CANCER GROWTH BY ELIMINATING ALL
ANDROGENIC STIMULATION

ADVANTAGES

— ELIMINATES THE ACTION OF ALL ANDROGENS

— NO SECONDARY EFFECTS

— CAN BE ADMINISTERED EARLY IN ORDER
TO PREVENT DISSEMINATION OF CANCER
TO OTHER TISSUES AND DEVELOPMENT
OF ANDROGEN-INSENSITIVE CELL CLONES

Fig. 5. Schematic representation of the combined treatment
with an LHRH agonist and a pure antiandrogen in prostate
cancer.

months after the beginning of treatment, 95% of the oedema
of the left leg had disappeared and the patient became
ambulatory. By the third month of treatment, the catheter
could be removed and the general status of the patient was
excellent. However, 6 months later, the patient started
complaining of abdominal pain and the signs of urinary
obstruction as well as the oedema of the left leg reappear-
ed. It should be mentioned that these two patients had a
life expentancy of less than four weeks at the beginning of
treatment. In the 42 other patients, remission is still
continuing.

Since patients at stage D2 have an average of at least
ten metastases each, for a total of at least 460 metastases,
and only two tumors were apparently hormone-insensitive (or
become insensitive), the present data indicate that even at
the late metastatic stage, more than 99% of prostatic tumors
are androgen-sensitive. This finding has major implications
for therapy. In a large study, including 600 patients who
could be followed up to five years, Nesbit and Baum (45)
concluded that 30% of patients with metastases showed no
response whatever to castration and/or estrogen therapy, an
indication, according to the authors, of a high incidence of
androgen independence. The same percentage of patients with
advanced prostatic cancer who responded to androgen therapy
has been reported by Menon and Walsh (41) and Whitmore (65).
The most likely explanation for this major difference between our results and those of previous studies is that previous hormonal therapy was limited to the neutralization of
androgens of testicular origin by surgical castration and/or
high doses of estrogens while the present approach achieves
complete neutralization of all androgens of both testicular
and adrenal origin (Fig. 5).

In fact, the standard hormonal therapy leaves 5 to 10% of circulating androgens of adrenal origin (7, 13, 50). It is most likely that prostatic carcinoma is composed of heterogenous populations of cells which differ in their requirement for androgens to perform vital cellular processes. Thus, after partial removal of androgens by castration, high doses of estrogens or LHRH agonist treatment alone, the most androgen-dependent cells regress, thus accounting for the 60 to 70% positive response previously reported (3, 4, 12, 26, 27, 43-45, 51, 58, 64). When complete neutralization of all androgens is achieved by the present approach, more than 99% of the tumors regress, thus indicating their extremely high degree of androgen sensitivity.

After neutralization of testicular androgens by surgical castration, high doses of estrogens or LHRH agonists alone, the adrenals continue to secrete a large amount of weak androgens and also low amounts of testosterone. These weak adrenal androgens may be converted into strong androgens in prostatic tissue (1, 21) as well as the peripheral level. The skin does in fact convert DHEAS and DHEA into androstenedione and DHT (20, 53, 57). Even blood cells can transform androstenedione into T (10, 62) while the brain can transform DHEA into T and DHT (31).

That androgens of adrenal origin play a role in prostatic cancer after removal of testicular androgens is clearly demonstrated by the finding that relatively high levels of DHT have been found to accumulate in prostatic cancer tissue in patients after surgical castration (21). That cancer cells which are androgen-sensitive remain active after surgical castration or high doses of estrogens is also clearly illustrated by the finding that 33 to 39% of patients already castrated or treated with estrogens showed a positive response to the antiandrogen Flutamide (56, 59). Moreover, following adrenal androgen suppression with aminoglutethimide in patients who had become refractory to orchiectomy and exogenous estrogens, a favorable response was observed in 3 out 7 patients (50). In a similar study, Robinson et al. (48) found a 50% significant palliation. Side-effects do however limit the acceptability of such treatment. In agreement with the above-mentioned data and our study, bilateral adrenalectomy has been found to be associated with palliation in 20 to 70% of patients with advanced prostatic carcinoma who had become refractory to castration or estrogen therapy (7, 39-42). Surgical hypophysectomy has also been found to transiently improve the disease in approximately 50% of patients (17).

That low levels of circulating androgens are important in prostatic cancer is further indicated by the close correlation observed between plasma testosterone levels and the evolution of prostatic cancer (15). Thus, in cases with serum T levels between 0.34 and 0.57 ng/ml, partial response was observed in only 37% of cases while, when T values were between 0.1 and 0.24 ng/ml, a positive response was seen in 60% of cases. This is further supported by the data of Sciarra et al. (55) who showed that remission after bilateral castration occurred in a group where serum T decreased to 0.3 ± 0.2 ng/ml while no remission occurred in 10 out of 27 patients where T levels were 1.4 ± 0.2 ng/ml. That the adrenal androgens were responsible for these high levels of androgens was confirmed by the marked inhibitory effect of dexamethasone on serum androgen levels in these patients. Thus, although serum androgen levels are markedly reduced after surgical or medical castration by estrogens or LHRH agonist treatment, basal circulating levels of testosterone are not negligible while stress due to many causes can further increase serum androgen levels.

Another most important conclusion which can be drawn from the present study is that a large proportion of prostatic cancer cells which continue to grow under the influence of androgens of adrenal origin become insensitive to androgens in this "androgen-poor" milieu. This is clearly demonstrated by the finding that complete androgen neutralization in patients previously treated with estrogens or castrated leads to only 30 to 40% positive/objective responses as compared to more than 95% in previously untreated patients. The much lower rate of response observed in previously treated patients indicates a marked increase in the proportion of androgen-insensitive cancer cells in these patients. The relatively low rate of response observed after removal of adrenal androgens in previously treated patients in our study is in agreement with the data obtained in the same category of patients following surgical or medical adrenalectomy (7, 25, 28, 39, 42).

It is thus clear that in these patients, neutralization of testicular androgens left an important proportion of cells growing in an "androgen-poor" milieu. This transformation of androgen-sensitive into androgen-insensitive cells in the "androgen-poor" environment is similar to the finding in pregnancy-dependent spontaneous mammary tumors in mice which normally regress after parturition but fail to regress after repeated pregnancies (18) as well as androgen-sensitive mouse mammary tumors which become insensitive after prolonged exposure to low androgens (30).

These two predominant findings, namely extremely high androgen sensitivity of prostatic cancer not previously treated and the transformation into androgen-insensitive cells in the presence of androgens of adrenal origin have major implications for the choice of early vs late hormonal therapy in prostatic cancer as well as complete versus partial neutralization of androgens.

Supporting arguments for prompt initiation of therapy upon diagnosis of advanced prostatic cancer are the following:

1) untreated stage C or D prostatic carcinoma is usually progressive (12, 63).

2) reduction of tumor load should increase the effectiveness of intrinsic antitumor defenses and antitumor therapies (54) and

3) progressive disease is more likely to affect quality of life than treatment (12, 23, 43).

Late treatment of prostatic cancer until symptoms of metastases developed was based on the supposition that a cancer can be controlled only for a fixed and limited period of time and that treatment should be at best used when palliation is needed. This has led some authors to recommend late endocrine therapy (4, 8, 9, 63). Much of these conclusions are however influenced by the serious cardiovascular side-effects related to the use of estrogens. In addition, the suggestion of late endocrine therapy is based on the supposition that hormone-insensitive cells are present early in the tumors and are those responsible for the ultimate failure of hormonal therapy (40, 43). However, complete removal of androgens of both testicular and adrenal origins shows that more than 99% of prostatic tumors, even at the stage of metastases, are still androgen-sensitive. Instead of being present at the beginning of treatment, our data clearly indicate that the androgen-insensitive cells appear when the tumor cells are exposed to the "low androgen" milieu provided by the adrenal androgens.

Hormone dependence of prostatic cancer cells is a characteristic of the tissue of origin. This property of cancer cells can be progressively lost during cell division (14, 53). It is logical that as the disease advances, a greater chance of appearance of androgen-resistant cell clones develops. In animal models, survival is related to the size of the tumor at the time treatment is administered (19). Our present data strongly support the suggestion (4, 11, 23, 43) that antihormonal therapy should be started as early as possible after diagnosis, at least in advanced prostatic cancer.

Another important finding in the present study is that concomitant treatment with the pure antiandrogen completely prevents flare-up of the disease, a complication unfortunately observed in a significant proportion of patients treated with LHRH agonists alone (22, 51, 61). With the present knowledge, there remains no rationale for the use of LHRH agonists alone since the effect of the initial rise in serum androgens can be so easily prevented, thus eliminating any unnecessary risk to the patient.

Due to its excellent tolerance and lack of secondary effects other than those related to hypoandrogenecity, the present findings strongly suggest that complete androgen neutralization achieved by the present approach should be initiated as early as possible after diagnosis (at least at stage C and D) in order to obtain remission in a greater proportion of patients and to minimize the appearance of androgen-insensitive cell clones, thus improving the quality of life and faciliting the possible application of other treatments such as radiotherapy and/or chemotherapy in the cases developing androgen-independent tumors.

REFERENCES

1. Acevedo, H.F., and Goldziecker, J.W. (1965): Biochim. Biophys. Acta., 97:564-570.
2. Auclair, C., Kelly, P.A., Coy, D.H., Schally, A.V., and Labrie, F. (1977): Endocrinology, 101:1890-1893.

3. Bailar, J.C., Byar, D.P., and Vet. Adm. Coop. Urol. Res. Group (1970): Cancer, 26: 257-259.
4. Barnes, R.W., and Ninan, C.A. (1972): J. Urol., 108:897-900.
5. Bélanger, A., Auclair, C., Ferland, L., and Labrie, F. (1980a): J. Steroid Biochem., 13: 191-196.
6. Bélanger, A., Caron, S., and Picard, V. (1980b): J. Steroid Biochem., 13:185-190.
7. Bhanalaph, T., Varkarakis, M.J., and Murphy, G.P. (1974): Ann. Surg. 179:17-23.
8. Blackard, C.E., The Veteran's Administration Cooperative Urology Research Group (1975a): Cancer Chemother. Rep., 59:225-227.
9. Blackard, C.E., Byar, D.P., Seal, U.S., Doe, R.P. and VACURG (1975b): New Engl. J. Med., 291:751-755.
10. Blaquier, J., Forchielli, E. and Dorfman, R.I. (1967): Acta Endocrinol., 55:697-699.
11. Bracci, U., and Di Silverio, F. (1973): Proc. XLVI Congr. Soc. Ital. Urol., 2:207-210.
12. Byar, D.P. (1973): Cancer, 32:1126-1130.
13. Cowley, T.H., Brownsey, B.G., Harper, M.E., Peeling, W.B., and Griffiths, K. (1976): Acta Endocrinol., 81:310-320.
14. De Grouchy, J. (1973): Biomedicine, 18: 6-8.
15. Di Silverio, F. (1975): In: Hormone therapy of prostatic cancer, edited by U. Bracci and F. Di Silverio, pp. 47-58. Rome, Cofese, Palerno.
16. Faure, N., Labrie, F., Lemay, A., Bélanger, A., Gourdeau, Y., Laroche, B., and Robert, G. (1982): Fertil. Steril., 37:416-424.
17. Fergusson, J.D. (1975): In: Hormonal Therapy of Prostatic Cancer, edited by U. Bracci and F. Di Silverio, pp. 201-207. Cofese Edizioni, Palerno.
18. Foulds, L. (1949): Brit. J. Cancer, 3: 345-375.
19. Fowler, J.E. Jr., and Whitmore, W.F. Jr. (1980): J. Urol., 126:372-375.
20. Gallegos, A.J., and Berliner, D.L. (1967): J. Clin. Endocrinol. Metab., 27:1214-1218.
21. Geller, J., Albert, J., Loza, D., Geller, S., Stoeltzing, W., and De La Vega, D. (1978): J. Clin. Endocrinol. Metab., 46: 440-444.
22. Glode, L.M. (Abbott Prostatic Cancer Study) (1982): LASCO Proc., Abst., p. 110.
23. Grayhack, J.T. and Kozlowski, J.M. (1980): Urol. Clin. North Amer., 7: 639-643.
24. Harper, M.E., Peeling, W.B., Cowley, T., Bronsey, B.G., Phillips, M.E.Z., Groom, G., Fahmy, D.R., and Griffiths, K. (1974): Acta Endocrinol., 81: 409-426.
25. Harrisson, J.H., Thorn, G.W., and Jenkins, D. (1953): N. Engl. J. Med., 248: 86-92.
26. Huggins, C., and Hodges, C.V. (1941): Cancer Res., 1: 293-297.
27. Huggins, C., Stevens, R.E., and Hodges, C.W. (1941): Arch. Surg., 43: 209-223.
28. Huggins, C., and Scott, W.W. (1945): Ann. Surg., 122:1031-1032.

29. Johnson, D.E., Kaesler, K.E., and Ayala, A.G. (1975): J. Surg. Oncol. 7:9-15.
30. King, R.J.B., Cambray, G.J., Jagus-Smith, R., Robinson, J.H., and Smith, J.A. (1977): In: Receptors and Mechanism of action of Steroid Hormones, edited by J.R. Pasqualini, p. 215, Marcel Dekker, New York.
31. Knapstein, P., David, A., Wu, C.H., Archer, D.F., Flickinger, G.L., and Touchstone, J.C. (1968): Steroids 11: 885-886.
32. Kramer, C.Y. (1956): Biometrics, 12:307-310.
33. Labrie, F., Auclair, C., Cusan, L., Kelly, P.A., Pelletier, G., and Ferland, L. (1978): In: Endocrine approach to male contraception, Int. J. Andrology, suppl.2, pp. 303-308.
34. Labrie, F., Bélanger, A., Cusan, L., Séguin, C., Pelletier, G., Kelly, P.A., Lefebvre, F.A., Lemay, A., and Raynaud, J.P. (1980): J. Androl., 1:209-228.
35. Labrie, F., Dupont, A., Bélanger, A., Cusan, L., Lacourcière, Y., Monfette, G., Laberge, J.G., Emond, J.P., Fazekas, A.T.A., Raynaud, J.P. and Husson, J.M. (1982) J. Clin. Invest. Med., 5: 267-275.
36. Labrie, F., Dupont, A., Bélanger, A., Lacoursière, Y., Raynaud, J.P., Husson, J.M., Gareau, J., Fazekas, A.T.A., Sandow, J., Monfette, G., Girard, J.G., Emond, J. and Houle, J.G. (1983a): The Prostate, in press.
37. Labrie, J., Dupont, A., Bélanger, A., Lefebvre, F.A., Cusan, L., Raynaud, J.P., Husson, J.M. and Fazekas, A.T.A. (1983b) Hormone Res., 18:18-27.
38. Lefebvre, F.A., Séguin, C., Bélanger, A., Caron, S., Sairam, M.R., Raynaud, J.P., and Labrie, F. (1982): The Prostate, 3:569-578.
39. MacFarlane, D.A., Thomas, L.P., and Harrison, J.H. (1960): Amer. J. Surg. 99:562-572.
40. Markland, F.S., Chiopp, R.T., Cosgrove, M.D., and Howard, E.B. (1978: Cancer Res., 38:2818-2826.
41. Menon, M. and Walsh, P.C. (1979): In: Prostatic Cancer, edited by G.P. Murphy, Littleton, Massachusetts, PSG Publishing Co., pp. 175-200.
42. Morales, P.A., Brendler, H. and Hotchkiss, R.S. (1955): J. Urol., 73: 399-409.
43. Murphy, G.P. and Slack, N.H. (1980): Urol. Clin. North Amer., 7:631-638.
44. Nesbit, R.M. and Plumb, R.T. (1946): Surgery, 20:263-266.
45. Nesbit, R.M. and Baum, W.C. (1950): JAMA, 143:1317-1320.
46. Pike, A., Peeling, W.B., Haerper, M.E., Pierrepoint, C.G., and Griffiths, K. (1970): Biochem. J., 120: 443-449.
47. Resnick, M.I., and Grayhack, J.T. (1975): Urol. Clin. North Amer., 2:141-161.
48. Robinson, M.R.G., Shearer, R.J., and Fergusson, J.D. (1974): Brit. J. Urol., 46: 555-559.
49. Rodbard, D., and Lewald, J.E. (1970): In: Second Karolinska Symposium on Research Methods in Reproductive Endocrinology, edited by E. Diczfalusy, Copenhagen, Bogtrykleriet Forum, pp. 79-103.

50. Sanford, E.J., Paulson, D.F., Rohner, T.J., Drago, J.R., Santen, R.J. and Bardin, C.W. (1977): J. Urol., 118:1019-1021.

51. Santen, R.J., Warner, B., Demers, L.M., Dufau, M., and Smith, J. (1983): In: LHRH and its analogs - a new class of contraceptive and therapeutic agents, edited by B. Vickery, J.J. Nestor, Jr. and E.S.E. Hafez, MTP Press, Lancaster-Boston, in press.

52. Séguin, C., Cusan, L., Bélanger, A., Kelly, P.A., Labrie, F., and Raynaud, J.P. (1981): Mol. Cell. Endocrinol., 21:37-41.

53. Schubert, G.E. (1975): In: Hormone Therapy of Prostate Cancer, edited by U. Bracci and F. Di Silverio, Rome, cofese, Palerno, pp. 43-45.

54. Silver, R., Young, R., and Holland, J. (1977): Am. J. Med., 63: 772-787.

55. Sciarra, F., Piro, C., Concolino, G., and Conti, C. (1968): Folia Endocrinol., 4: 423-430.

56. Sogani, P.C., Ray, B., and Whitmore, W.F. Jr. (1975): Urology, 6:164-166.

57. Sommerville, I.F., Flamigni, C., Collins, W.P., Koullapis, E.N., and Dewhurst, C.J. (1971): Proc. Roy Soc. Med., 64:845-847.

58. Staubiz, W.J., Oberlkircher, O.J. and Lent, M.H. (1954): J. Urol., 72: 939-945.

59. Stoliar, B., and Albert, D.J. (1974): J. Urol., 111: 803-807.

60. Tolis, G., Ackman, D., Stellos, A., Mehta, A., Labrie, F., Fazekas, A.T.A., Comaru-Schally, A.M. & Schally, A.V. (1982): Proc. Natl. Acad. Sci. USA, 79:1658-1662.

61. Trachtenberg, J. (1983): J. Urol., 129:1149-1152.

62. Van der Molen, H.J., and Groen, D. (1968): Acta Endocrinol., 58:419-444.

63. Veterans Administration Cooperative Urological Research Group (1967a) J. Urol., 100: 59-65.

64. Veterans Administration Cooperative Urological Research Group (1967b) J. Urol., 98:516-522.

65. Whitmore, W.F. Jr. (1956) Amer. J. Med., 21:697-713.

Progress in Cancer Research and Therapy,
Vol. 31, edited by F. Bresciani, et al.
Raven Press, New York © 1984.

Studies of Steroid Hormone Receptors in Brain

*Jan-Åke Gustafsson, *,† Zhao-Ying Yu, *Örjan Wrange, and † Lars Granholm

Department of Medical Nutrition, Huddinge University Hospital, S-141 86 Huddinge; and † Department of Neurosurgery, Karolinska Hospital, S-104 01 Stockholm, Sweden

Various steroid hormones are used in clinical practice for several disorders. A prerequisite for the steroidal effect is the presence of specific receptor proteins for the steroid hormones in the respective target tissues. A correlation between tissue content of steroid receptors and response to hormone therapy in advanced breast cancer was first described by Jensen and co-workers (31). These authors used quantitation of the estrogen receptor (ER) as the basis for the predictive test. Numerous investigators (51,52) have subsequently confirmed the correlation between presence of ER in breast cancer tissue and response to endocrine therapy and, furthermore, similar correlations seem to exist also with respect to other endocrine-related malignancies. Measurement of glucocorticoid receptors (GR) has been suggested as a predictive instrument when individualizing the therapy in certain forms of leukemia (38,41). ER and progestin receptor (PR) levels in endometrial cancer tissue may offer some guidance when treating patients with breast disease (3). The concentration of androgen receptor (AR) in prostatic carcinoma seemed to be correlated to the response of these patients to endocrine therapy (27,58). Finally steroid hormone receptors have been identified in several other types of neoplasia, e.g. malignant melanoma (15) and colonic carcinoma (45,47), etc. and it has been suggested that the presence of steroid receptors in these tissues is indicative of a certain hormonal responsiveness.

Many years ago glucocorticoid steroids were found to affect cerebral edema in cases of neurological disease (18,37,70). Glucocorticoid hormones are now widely used in neurological and neurosurgical practice (5,46,55,56,60,61). The effect of glucocorticoid hormones on the water and electrolyte content of the brain has been examined in cases of brain edema caused by intracranial tumors (25,75). The clinical use of glucocorticoid steroids in brain edema of various origin, however, is based on clinical experience from direct observations of the condition of the patients. Thus, the treatment of various forms of brain edema is to a large extent based on clinical impressions and the literature contains numerous, frequently contradictory reports on the beneficial effects of steroid hormone treatment in such conditions (1,5,18,23,46,66,79). Treatment with glucocorticoid hormones is expensive and may also give rise to a number of unwanted secondary effects and complications.

The mechanism of action of glucocorticoids on brain edema is unknown. During recent years several investigators have found that glucocorticoid hormones act by binding to specific soluble intracellular receptor proteins in the target cells. The formation of a steroid-receptor complex is the first step in a series of events leading to the biological effects induced by these hormones (for a review, see ref. 4,64). The first report on the presence of ER in intracranial meningiomas was from Donnell et al (13). In view of the limited knowledge concerning mechanisms of steroid action in human brain it was considered of interest to investigate this tissue somewhat further.

PREVIOUS INVESTIGATIONS

Brain edema

Brain edema remains a very great problem in the field of neurology and neurosurgery in spite of the intense investigations and numerous therapeutic attempts which have been performed during the last twenty years (for review, see ref. 16,29,35,73,76,78). An accepted classification of brain edema has been given by Klatzo (35,36). A few modifications have been made to include various clinical situations in patients with intracranial hypertension. Experimentally, cerebral edema has been divided into two distinct types, vasogenic and cytotoxic edema. The vasogenic edema is characterized mainly by a transudation of plasma proteins into the extracellular space due to increased permeability (35,36). In cytotoxic brain edema the blood-brain barrier is intact and the condition is characterized by cellular swelling, especially of the astrocytes (35). Fishman (16) has described a third type of brain edema - interstitial edema (hydrocephalic edema), due to the transependymal movement of cerebrospinal fluid from the ventricle and infiltrating adjacent brain tissue. Ischemic edema associated with cerebral ischemia begins as a cytotoxic edema and subsequently becomes vasogenic (16,78). Experimental models indicate that edema around brain tumors and in connection with head injuries most closely resembles the vasogenic type (16,29,73). It has been shown, experimentally and clinically, that vasogenic brain edema in certain conditions may be reduced by the use of glucocorticoids (73,76).

The use of glucocorticoids in the treatment of brain edema related to brain tumors, cerebral infarctions and head injuries, has been extensively discussed in the literature (5,9,46,60,79,80). As stated above, the mechanisms of steroid hormone action in the treatment of brain edema is still unknown.

Steroid hormone treatment of brain edema

A large number of publications exists on various aspects of steroidal treatment of brain edema. The results are not infrequently contradictory. There seems to be an agreement with regard to the beneficial effect of steroid treatment in case of the (vasogenic) edema caused by intracranial metastases and particularly malignant gliomas, whereas there is much less conviction concerning the effect of treatment in edema of traumatic or ischemic origin (1,9,23,62,79).

Steroid hormone receptors

Available data indicate that various steroid hormones act in a similar way in their respective target organs (30,40,64,91). Common to all steroids is that they interact with a receptor molecule, an intracellular protein which binds the hormone with a high affinity and a low capacity. The receptor protein is specific for one class of steroid hormones. The current concept of steroid hormone action is that the steroid diffuses passively from the blood over the cell membrane of the target cell and binds to the receptor to form a steroid-receptor complex which is subsequently translocated to the cell nucleus where it binds to DNA. This is followed by the appearance of specific mRNA sequences in the cytoplasm, coding for proteins which are responsible for the biological effects of the hormone.

GR in brain tissue

Several investigations have reported on the presence of GR in rat brain (48-50,85). Most of these studies were designed to characterize the properties of GR and to localize GR in different anatomical areas of the rat brain (11,12,48,72,81-83,87). In 1979 a first report appeared on the distribution of GR in human brain specimens obtained at autopsy (83).

ER and PR in meningioma

Meningioma is an intracranial tumor which does not occur infrequently and which accounts for about 13-18% of all intracranial neoplasms (22,96). 2/3 of all intracranial meningiomas and 80% of all spinal meningiomas occur in women (42,54,71). Furthermore, these tumors are known to progress rapidly during pregnancy (21,33,69) and a statistically significant association has been demonstrated between meningioma and breast cancer (77). In 1979, Donnell et al (13) first reported on the presence of ER in six cases of intracranial meningioma. Two other publications describe the presence of ER and PR in meningioma (67) and ER in acoustic neuroma (32). The presence of sex steroid receptors in meningioma and the clinical observations described above indicate that hormonal factors may participate in the control of the growth of meningioma.

Computerized tomography in brain edema

Computerized tomography can often give an exact location and suggest a more specific histological diagnosis of an intracranial lesion than previously used techniques (2,26). The simple, painless, and hazardless nature of computerized tomography makes it an ideal diagnostic tool for neurological disorders. Intracranial lesions, otherwise poorly defined, can frequently be much better visualized by means of intravenous administration of iodinated contrast media immediately prior to the examination (17). In order to determine accurately the effect on the extent of edema on different occasions, a head fixation system such as that described by Bergström et al (6) can be used. In modern CT-scanners, the attenuation numbers of the brain tumor and the edema zone and surrounding brain tissue can be very accurately determined as well as the geographic distribution of the edema (14,39).

THE SCOPE OF THE PRESENT STUDY

The aim of the present work has been to study various aspects on steroid hormone receptors in brain tissue from rat and man. Special interest has been devoted to the presence of steroid hormone receptors in intracranial tumors. The existence of a possible correlation between the levels of these receptors and the presence of brain edema has been studied using computerized tomography. Furthermore, the effect of glucocorticoid treatment of brain edema has been followed during repeated examinations with computerized tomography. Based on these studies, attempts are made to answer the following questions:

1) Does the GR in human brain have the same chemical characteristics as that present in rat brain?

2) Is it possible to use measurement of GR in brain tissue as a basis for a predictive test on individual responsiveness to dexamethasone treatment in a variety of intracranial disorders?

3) Is there a correlation between the content of GR in intracranial disorders and the tumor attenuation, the amount of edema and the effect of steroid treatment as studied by CT?

4) Can determination of the steroid hormone receptor pattern in specific brain tumors give an indication with regard to the particular hormonal sensitivity of that tumor?

MATERIALS AND METHODS

Ligands

^{3}H-Dexamethasone was used as a ligand in GR measurements (92-94). ER and PR receptors were assayed using ^{3}H-estradiol and ^{3}H-R 5020 respectively, as ligands (95).

Animals and cytosol preparation

Male Sprague-Dawley rats were adrenalectomized at 8 weeks of age 2-6 days prior to the experiment (92). The animals were given a standard pellet diet supplemented with 9 g NaCl/l solution to drink.

Animals were killed by perfusion via the heart with ice-cold buffer A (20 mM Tris-HCl, pH 7.4, 1 mM disodium-EDTA, 10% (w/v) glycerol and 2 mM 2-hydroxyethylmercaptan) under ether anaesthesia. The brain was taken out and placed in ice-cold buffer A for 1 min. The tissue was minced and homogenized in an all glass Potter-Elvehjem homogenizer. The brain homogenate was centrifuged at 175,000 x g for 40 min. The supernatant following centrifugation was used as cytosol.

Normal and neoplastic human brain tissue

Human cerebral or cerebellar tissue and intracranial tumor tissue were obtained from patients subjected to surgery at the Department of Neurosurgery, Karolinska Hospital. Cerebellar resections are used at this department as a routine to facilitate the access to pontine angle tumors. Also in other cases brain tissue was used for analysis only when a resection was necessary to give access to the tumor. Sampling of tumor or brain tissue for receptor analysis was only performed on patients where glucocorticoid therapy was withheld before and during surgery. Human brain tissue and tumor samples were stored at -70°C immediately following resection. The procedures for homogenization and cytosol preparation were the same as those described above for obtaining rat brain cytosol (92-95). On each occasion of tumor sampling, tumor material was also sent to the Department of Pathology at the Karolinska Hospital to obtain a histological diagnosis. The various specimens have been seen by a number of pathologists but all specimens were also reviewed by a neuropathologist (93-95).

Incubation

For receptor measurement incubations were carried out with tritium-labelled ligand in the presence or absence of a 100-fold excess of unlabelled ligand dissolved in ethanol (92-95). Binding in the presence of excess of unlabelled ligand represented nonspecific (nonsaturable) binding.

Protein determination

A preliminary estimation of the cytosolic protein concentration was obtained by expressing the difference in optical density at 280 and 310nm ($A_{280-310 \ nm}$). The cytosolic protein was also measured according to Lowry et al (44) using bovine serum albumin as standard.

Limited proteolysis

Cytosol preparations previously incubated with tritium-labelled steroids in the presence or absence of competing unlabelled steroids were routinely incubated with 0.5 μg trypsin/$A_{280-310 \ nm}$ for 30 min at 10°C when measuring GR receptors (92,93). In case of ER assays, 5 μg of trypsin/$A_{280-310 \ nm}$ was used (95).

Dextran-coated charcoal treatment

In order to remove unbound steroid from the incubation mixture, dextran-coated charcoal suspension corresponding to one-third of the incubation volume and yielding a final concentration of 1% (w/v) charcoal and 0.1% (w/v) dextran, was added. After mixing, the sample tubes were kept on ice for 10 min and centrifuged at 3,000 x g for 10 min at 0°C. The supernatant obtained after DCC treatment was taken for isoelectric focusing analysis.

Isoelectric focusing in polyacrylamide gel

Two hundred µl of supernatant was assayed using isoelectric focusing in polyacrylamide gel, containing 2.4% (w/v) Ampholine, pH range 3.5-9.5 (92-95).

Sucrose gradient centrifugation

The cytosolic progestin receptor concentration was measured essentially as described previously (68) using sucrose gradient centrifugation (95).

Other techniques used

CT studies were performed at the Department of Neuroradiology, Karolinska Hospital, with a GE CT/8800 scanner (94). The contrast material was Isopacque Cerebral (280 mg/ml) given intravenously as a bolus of 1 ml per kg of body weight of the patient. The slice thickness was 10 mm for the large lesions and 5 mm for the smaller ones. Attenuation values, contrast enhancement, volume of the tumor and edema and other parameters were evaluated by CT. The techniques used to estimate tumor and edema volumes and the fixation technique facilitating repeated examinations of identical intracranial regions are described in Hatam et al (24).

RESULTS AND DISCUSSION

GR in brain

Qualitative comparison of GR in cytosol from human and rat brain
The characteristics of the GR in cytosol from human brain were investigated using isoelectric focusing in polyacrylamide gel. The ^{3}H-dexamethasone-GR complexes from both rat and human brain had very similar isoelectric points (6.15 + 0.04 and 6.10 + 0.06 for the human and rat receptor, respectively) (92).

Since limited trypsin digestion has previously been used to compare the GR in various tissues in the rat (8,87-89), the same method was used in the present investigation to compare the human and rat brain cytosolic GR. The trypsin-induced fragmentation patterns of the GR from human and rat brain were very similar when analyzed using isoelectric focusing.

Comparative studies with regard to ligand specificity of the human and rat brain GR were also performed using unlabelled dexamethasone, betamethasone, cortisol and corticosterone as receptors. No differences in ligand specificity were observed between the human and rat brain GR.

In conclusion, the hormone specificity and the protein structure of the glucocorticoid receptors in human and rat brain are similar.

GR in intracranial tumors

Tissue samples from twenty patients with various intracranial tumors and one case of cerebral contusion were analyzed with regard to the concentration of cytosolic GR. The highest receptor concentration was noted in a metastatic tumor and the lowest receptor value was found in a case of cerebral contusion. The concentration of receptor was higher in the periphery than in the central part of the partially necrotic tumors. Cerebral metastases contained a higher GR concentration than meningiomas. The receptor levels in neuromas were lower than in meningiomas but higher than in gliomas. Most of the tumors had a higher receptor concentration than the surrounding cerebral or cerebellar tissue(93).

The GR concentrations in the various tumor types were compared to the clinical response to dexamethasone as described by Reulen et al (74). A correlation was observed between the receptor concentration and the clinical response when treating the tumor-associated brain edema with synthetic glucocorticoid steroids. However, one exception to this general trend was observed, namely in case of meningiomas, which despite a high GR concentration do not respond particularly well to steroid treatment. This discrepancy prompted an examination regarding the effect of dexamethasone treatment on peritumoral brain edema as evaluated by computerized tomography. The lack of correlation between GR content and steroid effects on brain edema in cases of meningioma is further discussed in the section on CT-findings.

As stated above the lowest GR concentration recorded was in a case of cerebral contusion. Although it is premature to draw any conclusions on the basis of one single observation it is interesting to note that edema formation may be different in traumatic cases, involving cytotoxic or ischemic mechanisms. Further work on receptor concentrations in traumatically contused brain tissue may help to verify why ischemic edema is generally relatively insensitive to glucocorticoid treatment.

CT-findings and glucocorticoid steroids

Malignant brain tumors, e.g. cerebral metastases and glioblastomas, are frequently associated with extensive peritumoral vasogenic edema. This condition has a relatively typical appearance in CT-examinations (14,86). Vasogenic edema is at least partially caused by increased permeability of tumor vessels. The abnormal permeability results in a leakage of plasma constituents outside the tumor, accumulating in the extravascular space as peritumoral edema (7,16,20,43,65). CT-scans of various intracranial tumors frequently display an appearance typical for a particular type of tumor with respect to attenuation values, contrast enhancement, volume of the tumor and volume of the surrounding edema.

No definite correlation was found between tumor concentration of GR and edema volume or tumor size as estimated by CT (94). However, some correlation existed between GR concentration and attenuation as well as contrast enhancement of the tumor. The positive correlation between GR level and contrast enhancement, reinforced by reports in the literature that contrast enhancement is affected by glucocorticoids (10,19), support the contention that contrast enhancement is mainly due to extravasation of contrast material and that steroid-receptor interaction is important in the regulation of the vascular permeability of tumors.

In a prospective study (24), the effect of dexamethasone on brain edema was evaluated by CT in 14 patients with brain tumors. A CT-study was performed immediately prior to the initiation of the treatment and at regular intervals during 18-19 days thereafter. The volume and attenuation of the edema were measured and related both to time following the beginning of the treatment and to the relative levels of GR in the various tumor types. In 5 cases of meningioma only minor changes were recorded with respect to the volume of the edema. A substantial decrease in edema volume was noted in 2 out of 4 cases of glioma whereas the remaining 2 cases showed a small decrease in edema volume following dexamethasone treatment. For 3 metastatic tumors a decrease in edema volume which was linear with time was noted during the entire follow-up period. In one case of acoustic neuroma a marked decrease in edema volume was also noted after dexamethasone treatment. These CT-findings are in agreement with the previously made statement that there is a parallelism between the response to steroid treatment and the amount of GR except in meningioma.

The lack of sensitivity of meningiomas to steroid treatment in spite of the relatively large amounts of GR present in these tumors remains to be explained. It is poosible that the extensive amount of peritumoral edema found at CT-examinations of meningiomas may be of more cytotoxic than vasogenic origin. Finally it may be mentioned that it has been reported that steroid treatment effectively reduces edema in tumors with pronounced contrast enhancement but without increased vascularity as documented by angiography (63). Meningiomas most often show a pronounced enhancement and also usually display an increased vascularity.

Mineralocorticoid receptor (MR) in rat kidney and hippocampus

Even if receptors for estrogens, androgens, progestins and glucocorticoids have been described in the CNS, it has been difficult to demonstrate with certainty the existence of a specific MR in this tissue. Recently, a reproducible and simple technique for the detection and measurement of MR in brain tissue has been developed (59). This method is based on selective saturation of the GR binding sites with the synthetic "pure" glucocorticoid RU 26988 followed by a labelling of MR with ^{3}H-aldosterone; the radioactive steroid-MR complex is measured by isoelectric focusing in slabs of polyacrylamide gel.

The characterization and quantitation of MR in rat kidney and hippocampus have been carried out in our laboratory and have been described by Wrange & Yu (90). The apparent dissociation constant for aldosterone was 5.1×10^{-10} M and the competition experiments with various steroids showed that progesterone, corticosterone, cortisol and dexamethasone were potent competitors with ^{3}H-aldosterone for binding to the receptor. When limited proteolytic digestion of GR and MR was performed followed by analysis with isoelectric focusing in polyacrylamide gel it was found that the two receptor proteins fragmented in distinctly different ways. On the other hand, MR from rat kidney and rat hippocampus, respectively, had identical proteolytic fragmentation patterns. An anti-GR antibody did not show any cross-reactivity to MR. Taken together, these findings indicate that rat kidney and rat hippocampus contain an MR with similar properties in the two tissues but distinctly different from the GR.

MR in intracranial tumors

The same method as described by Wrange & Yu (90) was also used for quantitating MR in various intracranial tumors. The order of tumor types with respect to average concentration of MR was gliomas >

metastases > neuromas > meningiomas. The corresponding order with respect to average concentration of GR was metastases > meningiomas > acoustic neuromas > gliomas.

The biological significance of the presence of MR in intracranial tumors is uncertain. Since a derangement of the intracellular sodium equilibrium causing excessive uptake of water and astrocyte swelling was suggested to be involved in the pathogenesis of cytotoxic brain edema (29,34), mineralocorticoids may play a role in the cause and process of cytotoxic edema.

Estrogen and progestin receptors in meningiomas

Tissue samples from 16 meningioma patients were analyzed with respect to cytosolic estrogen receptor concentration using isoelectric focusing and eleven of the sixteen cases were also analysed for cytosolic progestin receptor concentration using sucrose gradient centrifugation. Fifteen of the sixteen (94%) and nine of the eleven (82%) meningiomas had detectable estrogen and progestin receptors, respectively(95). The mean estrogen receptor concentration in female subjects was 8.9 fmol/mg protein and in males 3.0 fmol/mg protein. In addition to the meningiomas, four samples each of acoustic neuroma, astrocytoma and glioblastoma were also examined for the content of estrogen receptor. Except for one case of acoustic neuroma these intracranial tumors contained no detectable estrogen receptors. Furthermore, five samples of peritumoral brain tissue did not contain detectable estrogen receptors. However, a sample of amygdala tissue from a patient with a low grade glioma in the temporal lobe contained 4.6 fmol estrogen receptor per mg protein. Taken together these results indicate that both estrogen and progestin receptors are usually present in meningiomas of both male and female origin and that estrogen receptors do not frequently occur in other intracranial neoplasms.

A positive correlation (r = 0.87) was found between estrogen and progestin receptor levels in the same tumor tissue in female patients. This is in agreement with previous findings on the sex steroid receptor profile in human breast cancer specimens (52). Several studies have demonstrated that estrogens may induce progestin receptors in estrogen target tissues, such as the uterus (57) and rat brain (53). The presence of progestin receptors in a tissue may therefore be taken as an indication that the tissue is responsive to estrogens.

The demonstration and measurement of estrogen and progestin receptors in meningiomas in the human confirm and extend previous reports of Donnell et al (13) and Poisson et al (67) on the presence of sex steroid receptors in meningiomas. The results give further support to the contention that selective endocrine therapy may be worth trying in meningiomas, especially in poor-risk patients or in inoperable tumors.

Acknowledgements

This work was supported by grants from the Swedish Medical Research Council (13x-2819), the Royal Swedish Academy of Science and LEO Research Foundation.

REFERENCES

1. Alexander E Jr (1972): Clin. Neurosurg. 19:240
2. Ambrose J (1973): Br. J. Radiol. 46:1023.
3. Andersson DG (1965): Am. J. Obstet. Gynecol. 92:87.
4. Baxter JD, Rousseau GG (1979): Berlin, Springer-Verlag, p. 638.
5. Beks JWF, Doorenbos H, Walstra GJM (1972): In Reulen HJ, Schürmann K (eds): Steroids and Brain Edema, Springer-Verlag, Berlin/Heidelberg/New York, p. 233.
6. Bergström M, Boethius J, Eriksson L, Greitz T, Ribbe T, Widén L (1981): J. Compt. Assist. Tomogr. 5:136.
7. Brightman MW, Klatzo I, Olsson Y, Reese JS (1970): J. Neurol. Sci. 10:215.
8. Carlstedt-Duke J, Gustafsson J-Å, Wrange Ö (1977): Biochim. Biophys. Acta 497:507.
9. Cooper PR, Moody S, Clark WK, Kirkpatrick J, Maravilla K, Gould AL, Drane W (1979): J. Neurosurg. 51:307.
10. Crocker EF, Zimmerman RA, Phelps ME, Kuhl DE (1976): Radiology 119:471.
11. De Kloet ER, McEwen BS (1976): Biochim. Biophys. Acta (Amst.) 421:115.
12. De Kloet ER, Wallach G, McEwen BS (1975): Endocrinology 96:598.
13. Donnell MS, Meyer GA, Donegan WL (1979): J. Neurosurg. 50:499.
14. Drayer BP, Rosenbaum AE (1979): J. Comput. Assist. Tomogr. 3:317.
15. Fischer RJ, Niefeld JP, Lippman ME (1976): Lancet 2:337.
16. Fishman RA (1975): New Eng. J. Med. 293:706.
17. Gado MH, Phelps ME, Coleman RE (1975): Radiology 117:589.
18. Galicich JH, French LA, (1961): Amer. Practit. 12:169.
19. Gerber AM, Salvolaine ER (1980): Neurosurgery 6:282.
20. Go KG, Gazendam J, van der Meulen-Woldendrop DA, Teelken AW (1980): In Cervos-Navarro J, Ferszt R (eds): Advances in Neurology, Vol. 28, Brain Edema, Raven Press, New York p. 9.
21. Goldstein PI, Rosenberg S, Smith RW (1972): Am. J. Obstet. Gynecol. 112:297.
22. Green JR, Waggener JD, Kriegsfeld BA (1976): In Thomson RA, Greene JR (eds): Advances in Neurology, Vol. 15, Neoplasia in the Central Nervous System. Raven Press, New York, p. 51.
23. Gutterman P, Schenkin HA (1970): J. Neurosurg. 32:330.
24. Hatam A, Yu Z-Y, Bergström M, Berggren B-M, Greitz T (1982): J. Comput. Assist. Tomogr. 6:586.
25. Herrman H-D, Neuenfeldt D, Dittman J, Palleske H (1972): In Reulen HJ, Schürmann K (eds): Steroid and Brain Edema. Springer-Verlag, Berlin/Heidelberg/New York, p. 77.
26. Hounsfield G (1973): Br. J. Radiol. 46:1016.
27. Huggins C, Hodges CV (1941): Cancer Res. 1:293.
28. Ignelzi RJ (1979): Neurosurgery 4:338.
29. Ignelzi RJ (1980): In Cervos-Navarro J, Ferszt R (eds): Advances in Neurology, Vol. 28, Brain Edema, Raven Press, New York, p. 281.
30. Jensen EV, De Sombre ER (1973): Science 182:126.
31. Jensen EV, Jacobson HJ (1962): Rec. Progr. Horm. Res. 18:414.
32. Kasantikul V, Brown WJ (1981): Surg. Neurol. 15:105.
33. Kempers RD, Miller RH (1963): Am. J. Obstet. Gynecol. 87:858.
34. Kirsch WM, Ignelzi RJ (1976): In Morley TP (ed): Current Controversies in Neurosurgery. Saunders Co., Philadelphia, p. 595.
35. Klatzo I (1967): J. Neuropathol. Exp. Neurol. 24:1.

36. Klatzo I, Wisniewski H, Steinwall O, Streicher E (1967): In Klatzo I, Seitelberger F (eds): Symposium on Brain Edema. Springer-Verlag, New York, p. 554.
37. Kofman S, Garvin JS, Nagamani D, Taylor SG (1957): J. Amer. Med. Ass. 163:1473.
38. Konior Yarbro GS, Lippman ME, Johnson GE, Leventhal BG (1977): Cancer Res. 37:2688.
39. Lanksch W, Oettinger W, Baethmann A et al (1976): In Pappius HM, Feindel W (eds): Dynamics of Brain Edema. Springer-Verlag, New York, p. 283.
40. Liao S (1975): Int. Rev. Cytol. 41:87.
41. Lippman ME, Perry S, Thompson EB (1975): Am. J. Med. 59:224.
42. Lombardi G, Passerini A (1961): Radiology 76:381.
43. Long DM, Hartman JF, French LA (1966): Neurology (Minneap.) 16:521.
44. Lowry OH, Rosebrough NJ, Farr AL, Randall RJ (1951): J. Biol. Chem. 193:265.
45. Maillot KV, Hermanek P, Gentsch HH, Ober KG (1980): In Wittliff JL, Dapunt O (eds): Steroid Receptors and Hormone-Dependent Neoplasia. Ch. 32. Masson Publishing USA, Inc., New York, p. 215.
46. Maxwell RE, Long DM, French LA (1972): In Reulen HJ, Schürmann K (eds): Steroids and Brain Edema. Springer-Verlag, Berlin/-Heidelberg/New York.
47. McClendon JE, Appleby D, Claudon DB, Donegan WL, De Cosse JJ (1977): Arch. Surg. 112:240.
48. McEwen BS, Davis PG, Parsons B, Pfaff DW (1979): In Cowan WM, Hall ZW, Kandel ER (eds): Annual Review of Neuroscience. Ann. Rev. Inc., Palo Alto, Calif. 2:65.
49. McEwen BS, de Kloet R, Wallach G (1976): Brain Res. 105:129.
50. McEwen BS, Gerlach JL, Micco DJ Jr (1975): In Issacson R, Pribam K (eds): The hippocampus: A comprehensive Treatise. Plenum, New York, p. 285.
51. McGuire WL, Carbone PP, Vollmer EP (1975): Raven Press, New York.
52. McGuire WL, Horwitz KB, Pearson OH, Segaloff A (1977): Cancer 39:2934.
53. McLusky NJ, McEwen BW (1980): Brain Res. 189:262.
54. Mealey I Jr, Carter IE (1968): Obstet. Gynecol. 32:204.
55. Meinig G, Aulich A, Wende S, Reulen HJ (1976): In Pappius HM, Feindel W (eds): Dynamics of Brain Edema. Springer-Verlag, Berlin/Heidelberg/New York.
56. Meinig G, Reulen HJ, Simon RS, Schürman K (1980): In Cervos-Navarro J, Ferszt R (eds): Advances in Neurology, Vol. 28, Brain Edema. Raven Press, New York, p. 471.
57. Milgrom E, Luu Thi M, Atger M, Baulieu E-E (1973): J. Biol. Chem. 248:6366.
58. Mobbs BG, Johnson JE, Conolly JG (1980): In Wittliff JL, Dapunt O (eds):Steroid Receptors and Hormone-Dependent Neoplasia. Ch. 16. Masson Publishing USA, Ubc., New York, p. 139.
59. Moguilewsky M, Raynaud JP (1980): J. Steroid Biochem. 12:309.
60. Mulley G, Wilcox RG, Mitchell JR (1978): Brit. Med. J. 2:994.
61. O´Brien MD (1979): A review. Stroke 10:623.
62. Norris JW (1976): Arch. Neurol. 33:69.
63. Oi S, Galicich JH (1977): Neurol. Med. Chir. 17 (Part II):63.
64. O´Malley BW, Birnbaumer L (1978): Academic Press, New York.
65. Patberg WR, Go KG, Teelken AW (1977): Exp. Neurol. 54:141.

66. Plum F, Posner JB, Alvard EC (1963): Arch. Neurol. 9:571.
67. Poisson M, Magdelenat H, Fencin JF, Blubel JM, Philippon J,
    Pertuiset B, Buge A (1980): Rev. Neurol. (Paris) 139:193.
68. Powell B, Carola RE, Chamness GC, McGuire WE (1979): Cancer Res.
    39:1678.
69. Rand CW, Andler M (1950): Arch. Neurol. Psdychiat. 63:1.
70. Rasmussen T, Gulati DR (1962): J. Neurosurg. 19:535.
71. Rausing A, Ybo W, Stenflo I (1970): Acta Neurol. Scand. 46:102.
72. Rees HD, Stumpf WE, Sar M (1975): In Stumpf WE, Grant LD (eds):
    Anatomical Neuroendocrinology. Karger, Basel, p. 262.
73. Reulen HJ (1976): Brit. J. Anaesth. 48:741.
74. Reulen HJ, Hadjidimos A, Hase U (1973): In Schürman K, Brock M,
    Reulen HJ, Voth D (eds): Advances in Neurosurgery I. Brain
    edema. Cerebello-Pontine Angle Tumours. Springer-Verlag,
    Berlin/Heidelberg/New York, p. 92.
75. Reulen HJ, Hadjidimos A, Schürmann K (1972): In Reulen HJ,
    Schürmann K (eds): Steroids and Brain Edema. Springer-Verlag,
    Berlin/Heidelberg/New York,, p. 239.
76. Reulen HJ, Schürmann K (1972): Steroids and Brain Edema.
    Springer-Verlag, Berlin/Heidelberg/New York.
77. Schoenberg BS, Christine BW, Whisnant JP (1975): Neurology
    25:705.
78. Sherman DG, Easton JD (1980): Postgrad. Med. 68:107.
79. Siegel BA, Studer RK, Potchen EJ (1972): Arch. Neurol. 27:209.
80. Sparacio RR, Lin T-H, Cook AW (1965): Surg. Gynecol. Obstet.
    121:513.
81. Stumpf WE (1971): Am. Zoologist. 11:725.
82. Stumpf WE, Sar M (1975): In Stumpf WE, Grant LD (eds): Anatomical
    Neuroendocrinology. Karger, Basel, p.254.
83. Tsuboi S (1978): Folia Endocrin. (Jap.) 54:966.
84. Tsuboi S, Kawashima R, Tomioka O, Nakata M, Sakamoto N, Fujita T
    (1979): Brain Res. 179:181.
85. Warembourg M (1975): Brain Res. 89:61.
86. Wende S, Aulich A, Kretschmar K, Lang S, Grumme T, Meese W,
    Lanksch W, Kazner E, Steinhoff H (1977): In DuBolay GH (ed):
    First European Seminar on Computer Axial Tomography in Clinical
    Practice. Springer-Verlag, New York, p. 118.
87. Wrange Ö (1979): Biochim. Biophys. Acta 582:346.
88. Wrange Ö, Carlstedt-Duke J, Gustafsson J-Å (1979): J. Biol. Chem.
    254:9284.
89. Wrange Ö, Gustafsson J-Å (1978): J. Biol. Chem. 253:856.
90. Wrange Ö, Yu Z-Y (1983): Endocrinology 113:243.
91. Yamamoto KR, Alberts BM (1976): Rev. Biochem. 45:721.
92. Yu Z-Y, Wrange Ö, Boethius J, Gustafsson J-Å, Granholm L (1981a):
    Brain Res. 223:325.
93. Yu Z-Y, Wrange Ö, Boethius J, Hatam A, Granholm L, Gustafsson J-Å
    (1981b): J. Neurosurg. 55:757.
94. Yu Z-Y, Hatam A, Bergström M, Greitz T (1981c): J. Comput. Assist.
    Tomogr. 5:619.
95. Yu Z-Y, Wrange Ö, Haglund B, Granholm L, Gustafsson J-Å (1982): J.
    Steroid Biochem.16:451.
96. Zulch KI, Mennel HD (1974): In Vinken PI, Bruyn GW (eds): Handbook
    of Clinical Neurology, Vol. 16. Tumors of the Brain and Skull.
    Part 1. North-Holland Publishers, Amsterdam, p. 1.

*Progress in Cancer Research and Therapy,
Vol. 31*, edited by F. Bresciani, et al.
Raven Press, New York © 1984.

Sex Steroid Receptors in Human Meningioma and Glioma

*B.F. Pertuiset, **M. Moguilewsky, † H. Magdelenat,
‡ P.M. Martin, **D. Philibert, and *M. Poisson

*Clinique Neurologique (Pr. A. Buge), Pitié-Salpétrière, 75651 Paris; **Centre de
Recherche Roussel-UCLAF, 93230 Romainville; † Laboratoire de Radiopathologie,
Institut Curie, 75231 Paris; and ‡ Cancérologie Expérimentale, Nord,
13326 Marseille, France*

In recent years, growing interest has been focused on estrogen (E), progestin (P) and androgen (A) receptors (R) in human meningioma and glioma, i.e., in benign and malignant intracranial (or spinal) tumors (3,6,8,11,13,14-16,19,20-23,30-33). Although these tumors arise in the leptomeningeal and glial tissues respectively which for long were not considered to be hormone-sensitive (10,34), the presence of sex-steroid receptors has been investigated because epidemiological and clinical data point to sex-hormone sensitivity in some patients (1,2,5,17,28,29).

This chapter contains a brief review of the data on which our present research is based and also an overview of our joint experience on the detection of ER, PR, and AR in 110 meningioma and 20 glioma in adult patients (13,20,22,23).

MENINGIOMA

Rationale for Sex Steroid Studies

Meningioma are diagnosed most frequently between 35 and 55 years, very rarely in childhood and rarely after 75 years (5,34). They are more frequent in females (F) than in males (M), the F/M ratio being about 2.5:1 for intracranial tumors and 9:1 for spinal canal tumors (10). In 101 meningioma assayed for steroid hormone receptors over the last 3 years (13,20,22,23), we recorded a F/M ratio of 2.2:1 for intracranial tumors in agreement with published data. For patients in their thirties and forties (n=38) (Fig. 1), the F/M ratio was 3.75:1 suggesting that estradiol and/or progesterone may act on tumor growth in premenopausal women.

In the large series of Cushing and Eisenhardt (5), the mean age was 42.5 years in females and many of the patients had a long clinical history before diagnosis. The slow growth pattern of most meningioma is also illustrated by the 5 years mean recurrence delay reported by Crampton and Gautier-Smith (4). These data suggest that many meningioma, at least in females, start to grow during the period of maximum gonadal activity. Moreover, the relapsing course of meningioma during pregnancy (usually during the last four months) (2,17) further supports a role of sex hormones as does the more than chance association of these tumors with breast cancer (28) and obesity (1).

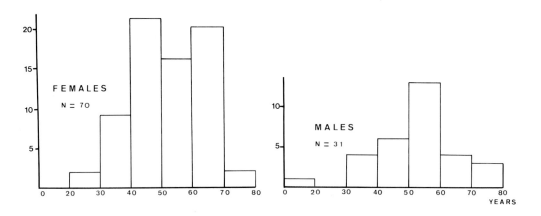

FIG. 1. Distribution of patients with intracranial meningioma (n=101)
according to age.

Biochemical Assay Methodology

All surgical specimens were immediately frozen, stored at -80°C and
assayed within two months (13,20,22,23). In two series of meningioma
(13,22), the tissue was homogenized in high strength buffer (0.4 M KCl)
for the measurement of both cytosolic and nuclear receptors (Rcn). ERcn
and PRcn were evaluated with a 2-point assay (5 nM of labelled ligand
with and without cold ligand) using respectively (^{3}H) RU 2858 (Moxestrol) and (^{3}H) R 5020 (Promegestone) as tags, since neither of these
ligands, unlike the natural hormones, binds to any great extent to contaminating plasma proteins (25,26). In a third series of tumors (23), cytosolic receptors (Rc) were assayed with these same tags for ER and PR, and
with (^{3}H) RU 1881 (Methyltrienolone) for AR (27). An excess of triamcinolone acetonide was added to prevent RU 1881 binding to PR and to glucocorticoid (G) and mineralocorticoid receptors. By using increasing ligand
concentrations, the dissociation constant (Kd) could be determined in
each case. In a fourth series of tumors (20), nuclear ER (ERn) and PR
(PRn) were assayed with (^{3}H) RU 2858 and (^{3}H) RU 27987 (21S-hydroxy-
metabolite of R 5020) respectively. RU 27987 has the considerable advantage over R 5020 of lower non-specific binding in the detection of nuclear binding to PR (19).
The specificity of (^{3}H) R 5020 (13,23) and (^{3}H) RU 1881 (23)
binding sites was assessed by incubating the cytosols with 5 nM of
radioligand in the presence of increasing concentrations of competing
steroids.
Bound steroids were measured by the dextran-coated charcoal (DCC)
adsorption technique (13,22,23) except in the last series (20) where ERn
and PRn were evaluated by measuring directly the radioactivity in the
washed 800xg pellet (unpurified nuclei). A cut-off value of 100 femtomoles per gram of tissue (fmol/gT) and/or a Kd value in the nM range were
chosen as criteria of receptor positivity. The protein (prot.) and DNA
(7) contents of all samples were calculated.
Finally, five meningioma were analyzed by sucrose density gradient
(SDG) centrifugation (13).

Assay Results

Estrogen receptor.
In a first series of meningioma, low levels of cytosolic and/or nuclear (^{3}H) RU 2858 binding sites were recorded in 70% (43/60) of tumors (mean : 300 fmol/gT, range : 110-2100) (13-22). In two further series (20,23), similar levels of high affinity (mean Kd : 3.10^{-9} M) cytosolic binding sites were detected in only 30% (14/46) of tumors (mean : 360 fmol/gT ; range : 150-1000) in agreement with the 33% (40/118) overall positivity rate recorded by teams using radiolabelled estradiol to assay ER. These teams however only detected minute amounts of binding sites (3,6,11,14,16,31-33) whereas Blankenstein et al. (3) using stricter criteria found no estradiol binding sites in any of their samples.

Since we found a higher ERcn than ERc incidence and also high PR values (Table 1), we hypothesized that ERc might be translocated into the nuclei by elevated plasma estradiol levels even though ERcn levels did not seem to be related to age or gynecological status (13,22). We were able to detect low levels (mean : 300 fmol/gT) of (^{3}H) RU 2858 nuclear binding sites in 8/20 samples (20) but these results are subject to caution since the highest levels (up to 1500 fmol/gT) were recorded in 2-point assays. Furthermore, they do not corroborate a previous report on 4 cases (13) nor data by Markwalder et al. (14) who found no evidence for nuclear estradiol binding sites in 12 meningioma.

Progestin receptor.
Since the first report by Poisson et al. in 1980 (22), many other teams have recorded the presence of PR, i.e., (^{3}H) R 5020 binding sites, in a high proportion of meningioma, usually in moderate to high levels (3,13,14-16,20-23,30-33). We detected cytosolic and/or nuclear PR in 97% (62/64) of tumors in two series (13,22) and cytosolic PR in 93% (43/46) of tumors in two other series (20,23). These values are in agreement with the overall 73% (71/97) positivity rate calculated from the literature (3,14,16,30-33). The mean levels reported by Magdelenat et al. (13) (PRc and/or PRn), Markwalder et al. (14) and Blankenstein et al. (3) (high affinity PRc) are 5000 fmol/gT, 1500 fmol/gT and 200 fmol/mg prot. respectively.

TABLE 1. Positivity rate of (^{3}H)RU 2858, (^{3}H)R 5020 and (^{3}H)RU 1881 binding sites in a joint experience on 110 meningioma[a]

Binding sites	(^{3}H) RU 2858 (ER)	(^{3}H) R 5020 (PR)	(^{3}H) RU 1881 (AR)
cytosolic and/ or nuclear	70% (43/60)	97% (62/64)	ND[c]
cytosolic	30% (14/46)	93% (43/46)	92% (23/25)
nuclear	33% (8/24)[b]	71% (15/21)	ND

[a] References 13,20,22,23   [b] 4 cases from ref.13 plus 20 from ref.20
[c] not determined

Cytosolic (^{3}H) R 5020 binding sites have been well characterized with regard to affinity (Kd in the nM order), sedimentation coefficient in a SDG (unique 8-9 S peak under low salt conditions) and specificity (only progestins, i.e.,norgestrel and progesterone, compete significantly). These results suggest that a classic PR is present in meningioma tissue (3,13,14,20,23,31,33). The detection of nuclear (^{3}H) RU 27987 binding sites in 15/21 samples (20) (range : 150 - 6500 fmol/gT) furthermore supports the concept of a functional PR in meningioma.

Previous indications (13) that PRcn levels were higher in females than in males were not confirmed by further results on PRc (20,23) nor by a report by Markwalder et al. (14).

The influence of preoperative dexamethasone therapy on PR levels was also considered (13), particularly because (^{3}H) R 5020 binding to GR can be excluded in these samples. We found no difference between PR concentrations in samples from treated and untreated patients (23).

In our series (13,20-23) and those of others (14,31,32), PR levels were higher in tumors of the meningotheliomatous and transitional subtypes than of the fibroblastic subtype. There was no relationship between PR levels and mitotic figure rate or tumor vascularization (21,23).

Androgen receptor.
We have found high affinity (mean Kd : 3.10^{-9} M) cytosolic (^{3}H)-RU 1881 binding sites in 23 out of 25 meningioma samples (Table 1) obtained from 23 patients (23). The mean level was 2265 fmol/gT (range : 120-8300 fmol/gT) in cases with detectable binding sites. The androgen specificity of the cytosolic (^{3}H) RU1881 binding sites was determined in a single case (23) and is now illustrated by a second case in Fig. 2. The sample was obtained from a 68 years old female with an intracranial meningioma and no glucocorticoid therapy prior to surgery. The concentration of high affinity cytosolic (^{3}H) RU 1881 binding sites was 1400 fmol/gT. In the presence of a 100-fold excess of triamcinolone acetonide, specific androgen binding was observed since only compounds with known androgenic

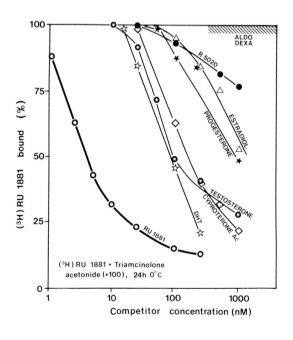

FIG. 2. Specificity of cytosolic androgen binding sites in a meningioma from a female patient with no glucocorticoid therapy prior to surgery.

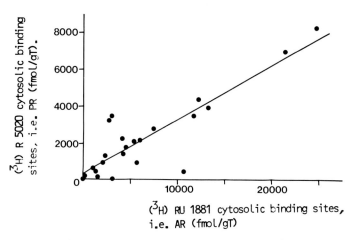

FIG. 3. Correlation between PR and AR concentrations in meningioma from 23 patients (r = 0.88).

activity (e.g. dihydrotestosterone and testosterone) competed for (^{3}H) RU 1881 binding whereas compounds belonging to other hormone classes had little or no effect.

Interestingly, we found a marked correlation (r = 0.88) between (^{3}H) R 5020 and (^{3}H) RU 1881 high affinity cytosolic binding sites, i.e., between PR and AR concentrations respectively, in a recent series of meningioma obtained from 23 patients (23) (Fig. 3). The figure contains 23 points for a series of 25 meningioma (23) since the 3 samples obtained from the same patient (cases n° 19,20 and 21) were recorded as a single point (mean PR and AR concentrations were calculated from the 3 samples). Using radiolabelled dihydrotestosterone, Schnegg et al. (30) detected cytosolic AR in two tumors (2/9) from female patients. The AR concentration and Kd were respectively 20 fmol/mg prot. and 1.42 10^{-9}M in fibroplastic meningioma and 13 fmol/mg prot. and 0.29 10^{-9}M in a "syncitial" meningioma. In contrast to our data, Schnegg et al. did not detect PR in their tumors with AR.

GLIOMA

Glioma are devastating brain tumors of various degrees of malignancy. They are more frequent in male patients, the male : female being about 3 : 2 in adults (29,34). Since animal data have suggested some sex-hormone sensitivity of chemically-induced glioma in rats (9), we have (22,23), like other teams (30,32,33), investigated the presence of sex-steroid receptors in human intracranial glioma using methods similar to those reported above for meningioma (13,22,23).
We detected small amounts of cytosolic (^{3}H) RU 2858 binding sites in 2 glioma (2/9) obtained from female patients (concentrations : 1370 and 500 fmol/gT), whereas we found only minute concentrations of cyto-solic (^{3}H) R 5020 binding sites in 2 other cases (2/9) (23). Vaquero et al. (32) detected very low levels of so-called estrogen receptors in the glioblastoma they studied (concentration : 1.65 fmol/mg prot.). Overall, estrogen and progestin binding sites have been detected (biochemical assays) in respectively 3/21 and 2/13 of the cases published so far (22,23,30,32,33).

TABLE 2. (^{3}H) RU 1881 cytosolic and nuclear binding sites in 11 human intracranial glioma

Case N°	Sex/age (in yr)	Histological type	Binding site level[a]	
			cytosol	nucleus
1	F/54	Astrocytoma	190[b]	0
2	F/67	Anaplastic astrocytoma	240	110
3	F/61	Glioblastoma	350[b]	0
4	M/26	Astrocytoma	0	270
5	M/39	Astrocytoma	280	0
6	M/50	Astrocytoma	100	0
7	M/26	Anaplastic astrocytoma	300[b]	0
8	M/52	Glioblastoma	240[b]	0
9	M/60	Glioblastoma	100	0
10	M/60	Glioblastoma	790[b]	150
11	M/71	Glioblastoma	220	500

[a] in fmol/gT   [b] Kd value in the range : 1-2 nM

We were able to detect small amounts of cytosolic (^{3}H) RU 1881 binding sites in 8/9 glioma (23). The mean concentration was 440 fmol/gT in cases with detectable binding sites (range : 115-1100 fmol/gT). This led us to investigate 11 more surgical samples for cytosolic and nuclear androgen binding sites (Table 2). Cytosolic (^{3}H) RU 1881 binding sites were present in 8/11 tumors with a mean concentration of 330 fmol/gT (range : 190-790 fmol/gT) and a Kd in the nM order (range : $1-2.10^{-9}$M). Nuclear binding sites were detectable in only 4 glioma (4/11) in very low concentrations (range : 110-500 fmol/gT). No obvious relationship was noted between (^{3}H) RU 1881 binding site levels and patient sex and age, or tumor histological type.

DISCUSSION

A general consensus seems to exist regarding the presence of a true PR in meningioma (3,13,14-16,20-23,30-33). Using a histochemical technique, Hinton et al. (8) showed that the binding sites are present in tumor cells and this has been confirmed by the lack of a correlation between PR levels and the degree of tumor vascularization (13,21,23). Our present data strongly support the additional presence of a true AR in meningioma tissue, whereas the presence of ER remains a moot point (3,6,13,14,23, 33).

It would seem that in meningioma high PR levels can be associated with low or undetectable cytosolic ER and inconclusive nuclear ER, in contrast to the known regulation of PR through ER in, for instance, normal and pathological breast tissues (3,13,14,20,22,23,32,33). It is noteworthy that this apparently non-estrogenic modulation of PR has already been demonstrated in rat cerebral cortex (12,18). On the other hand, we found a good correlation between PRc and ARc which raises several hypotheses including a possible androgenic modulation of PR.

The presence of high levels of PR in well-differentiated meningotheliomatous and transitional meningioma, i.e., tumors which share many ultrastructural features with normal arachnoid cells (10), and the apparent absence of PR in other intracranial tumors such as glioma (23, 30, 32) and acoustic neurinoma (22,32) suggest that PR may be a marker of leptomeningeal cells. This concept is supported by the recent discovery by our team of high affinity (^{3}H) R 5020 binding sites in normal leptomeninges of adult patients (13,24).

It is not yet known whether PR and AR have any biological function in meningioma tissue. The study of the metabolism of sex-hormones in tumors (15), in vitro experiments on cells cultured in conditions enabling their differentiation and finally clinical trials with hormone agonists and antagonists (anti-progestins ?) should help to establish their significance and the relevance of sex-hormone (or anti-hormone) treatment of patients with inoperable and/or recurrent meningioma.

The demonstration of cytosolic and/or nuclear androgen binding sites, i.e., high affinity (^{3}H) RU 1881 binding sites, in intracranial glioma deserves attention, especially since these tumors are more frequent in males and have a very bad prognosis. At this point, it is not clear, however, whether these androgen binding sites are true AR and are capable of mediating any adjuvant endocrine therapy by, for instance, anti-androgens. As for meningioma, further in vivo and in vitro studies, as well as clinical trials, should help to clarify their role and that of androgens (and estrogens) in the biology of these tumors.

REFERENCES

1. Bellur, S.N., Chandra, V., and Anderson, R.J. (1983) : Ann. Neurol., 13 : 346–347.
2. Bickerstaff, E.R., Small, J.M. and Guest, I.A. (1958) : J. Neurol. Neurosurg. Psychiatry, 21 : 89–91.
3. Blankestein, M.A., Blaauw, G., Lamberts, W.J., and Mulder, E. (1983) : Eur. J. Cancer Clin. Oncol., 19 : 365–370.
4. Crompton, M.R. and Gautier-Smith, P.C. (1970) : J. Neurol. Neurosurg. Psychiatry, 33 : 80–87.
5. Cushing, H. and Eisenhardt, L. (1938) : Meningiomas. Their Classification, Regional Behavior, Life History, and Surgical End Results. Charles C. Thomas, Sprinfield.
6. Donnell, M.S., Meyer, G.A., and Donegan, W.L. (1979) : J. Neurosurg., 50 : 499–502.
7. Fiszer-Szafarz, B., Szafarz, D., and Guevara de Murillo, A. (1981) : Anal. Biochem., 110 : 165–170.
8. Hinton, D., Mobbs, B.G., Sima, A., and Hanna, W. (1982) : Biochemical Assay of Estrogen and Progesterone Receptors and their Cellular Localization in Human Intracranial Meningiomas. In : Abstracts of IX Intl. Congress of Neuropathology, n° 138, P. 179, Vienna.
9. Hopewell, J.W. (1975) : Neuropath. Appl. Neurobiol., 1. : 141–148.
10. Kepes, J.J. (1982) : Meningiomas. Biology, Pathology and Differential Diagnosis. Masson Publishing USA, New York.
11. Kobayashi, S., Mizuno, T., Tobioka, N., Ichimura, H., Samoto, T., Tanaka, H., Masaoka, A., Wakabayashi, S., Umemura, S., Fukuoka, H., and Nagai, H., (1982) : Gann, 73 : 439–445.
12. MacLusky, N.J. and McEwen, B.S. (1978) : Nature, 274 : 276–278.
13. Magdelenat, H., Pertuiset, B.F., Poisson, M., Martin, P.M., Philippon, J., Pertuiset, B., and Buge, A. (1982) : Acta Neurochir., 64 : 199–213.

14. Markwalder, T.M., Zava, D.T., Goldhirsch, A., and Markwalder, R. (1983) : Surg. Neurol., 20 : 42–47.
15. Martin, P.M., Fournier, S., Rieg, A.M., Magdelenat, H., Hassoun, J., Pertuiset, B.F., Poisson, M., Vigouroux, R.P., and Toga, M. (1983) : J. steroid Biochem., suppl. 19 : 166 S.
16. Martuza, R.L., MacLauglin, D.T., and Ojemann, R.G. (1981) : Neurosurg., 9 : 665–671.
17. Michelsen, J.J. and New, P.F.J. (1969) : J. Neurol. Neurosurg. Psychiatry, 32 : 305–307.
18. Moguilewsky, M. and Raynaud, J.P. (1979) : Brain Res., 164 : 165–175.
19. Moguilewsky, M., Philibert, D., Bouton, M.M., and Raynaud, J.P. (1983) : J. steroid Biochem., suppl. 19 : 126 S.
20. Moguilewsky, M., Pertuiset, B.F., Verzat, C., Philibert, D. Philippon, J., and Poisson, M. (1983) : J. steroid Biochem., suppl. 19 : 165 S.
21. Pertuiset, B.F., Magdelenat, H., Boutry, J.M., Hauw J.J., Foncin, J.F., Kujas, M., Poisson, M., and Escourolle, R. (1982) : Progestin Receptors in Meningiomas : Relation to Histological Type and in vitro Cell Kinetic Study. In : Abstracts of IX Intl. Congress of Neuropathology, n° D2 10, p. 64, Vienna.
22. Poisson, M., Magdelenat, H., Foncin, J.F., Bleibel, J.M., Philippon, J., Pertuiset, B., and Buge A. (1980) : Rev. Neurol. (Paris), 136 : 193–203.
23. Poisson, M., Pertuiset, B.F., Hauw, J.J., Philippon, J., Buge, A., Moguilewsky, M., and Philibert, D. (1983) : J. Neuro-Oncol., 1 : 179–189.
24. Poisson, M., Magdelenat, H., Martin, P.M., Pertuiset, B.F., Hauw, J.J., Fohanno, D., Sichez, J.P., Vigouroux, R.P., and Buge A. : Rev. Neurol. (Paris) (in press).
25. Raynaud J.P. (1977) : In : Progesterone Receptors in Normal and Neoplastic Tissues : R5020, a Tag for the Progestin Receptor, edited by W.L. McGuire, J.P. Raynaud and E.E. Baulieu, pp. 9–21. Raven Press, New York.
26. Raynaud, J.P., Martin P.M., Bouton, M.M., and Ojasoo, T. (1978) : Cancer Res., 38 : 3044–3050.
27. Raynaud, J.P., Bouton M.M., and Martin, P.M. (1980) : In : Steroid Receptors, Metabolism and Prostatic Cancer : Human Prostate, Hyperplasia and Adenocarcinoma : Steroid Hormone Receptor Assays and Therapy, edited by F.H. Schroeder and H.H. de Voogt, pp. 165–181. Excerpta Medica, Amsterdam.
28. Schoenberg, B.S., Christine, B.W., and Whisnant, J.P. (1975) : Cancer, 25: 705–712.
29. Schoenberg, B.S. (1978) : In : Advances in Neurology vol 19 : Epidemiology of Primary Nervous System Neoplasms, edited by B.S. Schoenberg. Raven Press, New York.
30. Schnegg, J.F., Gomez, F., Lemarchand-Beraud, T., and de Tribolet, N. (1981): Surg. Neurol., 15 : 415–418.
31. Tilzer, L.L., Plapp, F.V., Evans, J.P., Stone, D., and Alward, K. (1982) : Cancer, 49 : 633–636.
32. Vaquero, J., Marcos, M.L., Martinez, R., and Bravo, G. (1983) : Surg. Neurol., 19 : 11–13.
33. Yu, Z.Y., Wrange, Ö., Haglund, B., Granholm, L. and Gustafsson, J.Å., (1982) : J. steroid Biochem., 16 : 451–456.
34. Zülch, K.J. (1965) : Brain Tumors : Their Biology and Pathology. Springer Publishing Company, New York.

Progress in Cancer Research and Therapy,
Vol. 31, edited by F. Bresciani, et al.
Raven Press, New York © 1984.

Clinical and Biochemical Features of Ectopic Hormone-Producing Tumors: Possible Mechanism of Hormone Production

H. Imura, S. Matsukura, Y. Nakai, K. Nakao, S. Oki, I. Tanaka, T. Tsukada, and T. Yoshimasa

Second Division, Department of Internal Medicine, and Department of Clinical Nutrition, Kyoto University Faculty of Medicine, Shogoin, Sakyo-ku, Kyoto 606, Japan

It is well-known that a variety of endocrine manifestations associated with non-endocrine tumors are caused by ectopic production of hormones by tumors. The ectopic hormone production has been defined to be a phenomenon that certain neoplasms produce hormones not usually produced by tissues from which the neoplasms have arisen. For example, ACTH production by tumors other than those of the pituitary, such as oat-cell carcinoma of the lung, has been considered to be ectopic ACTH production. However, recent advances in detecting small amounts of hormones in tissues have thrown doubts upon the classical definition of ectopic hormone production. It is now well established that small amounts of ACTH are produced in a variety of extrapituitary tissues, such as the brain, gastrointestinal tract, adrenal medulla, pancreatic islets and thyroid (Imura et al, 1982). Therefore, islet-cell tumors or gastrointestinal carcinoids producing ACTH cannot be defined as ectopic ACTH producing tumors. More perplexing was the observation by Iwasa et al (1983) that immunologically active ACTH precursor was detected in almost all human non-neoplastic tissues. If this is true, then all ectopic ACTH-producing tumors are no longer "ectopic" in the strict sense. Similar problems exist in other ectopic hormone producing tumors. Ectopic human chorionic gonadotropin (hCG) production has been reported in patients with carcinomas of the lung, stomach, liver, kidney and adrenal, considering that hCG is normally produced only in trophoblastic tissues (Imura, 1980). However, immunoreactive hCG has been reported to exist in a variety of normal non-trophoblastic tissues of adults and fetuses (Yoshimoto et al, 1977; Huhtaniemi et al, 1978). If this immunoreactive hCG is really hCG and not cross-reacting materials, hCG-producing tumors of the liver and colon cannot be defined to be "ectopic". Accumulating evidence in recent years suggests that many other hormones are also produced in various tissues other than the major site of production. Therefore, the differentiation of "ectopic" from "eutopic" hormone production has become very difficult. In this paper, however, I would like to define tentatively the "ectopic" hormone production as production of a hormone by a neoplasm arising from an organ which is not accepted as the major site of production of the hormone in question.

Although many studies have been described on various ectopic hormone producing tumors, ectopic ACTH-producing tumors have been most extensively studied. In this article, we would like to discuss clinical and biochemical features of ectopic ACTH-producing tumors and possible mechanisms responsible for that production in tumors, based on studies performed in our laboratory.

CLINICAL FEATURES OF ECTOPIC
ACTH-PRODUCING TUMORS

Ectopic ACTH production was originally considered to be an uncommon manifestation of tumors. However, increased awareness of such a syndrome and increased availability of sensitive assay procedures have shown that ectopic ACTH-production is a universal concomitant of certain neoplasms, although associations of clinical and biochemical abnormalities are uncommon. Previously, ectopic ACTH producing tumor and ectopic ACTH syndrome were used as synonyms. We should differentiate, however, ectopic ACTH syndrome (clinical and/or biochemical abnormalities) from ectopic ACTH production that includes silent ACTH production. In our series, we have had 37 patients with ectopic ACTH-producing tumors, who showed laboratory data of hyperadrenocorticism. As shown in Table 1, 15 of 37 patients had signs of Cushing's syndrome, such as moon face and truncal obesity. As compared with Cushing's syndrome of other etiologies, truncal obesity tended to be less prominent in ectopic ACTH syndrome. All patients with Cushing's syndrome had extrapulmonary tumors, and none of the patients with bronchogenic carcinoma showed signs of Cushing's syndrome in our series. The reason for such discrepancy is unknown, but may be explained by the rapid clinical course and/or cachexia in patients with bronchogenic carcinoma.

The existence of hyperadrenocorticism was demonstrated by increased urinary 17-OHCS excretion, elevated plasma cortisol, absence of diurnal

TABLE 1. Ectopic ACTH syndrome studied in this series

Histology of Tumors		No of Patients
Lung		14
Oat-cell ca.	7	
Adenocarcinoma	4	
Large-cell undifferentiated ca.	2	
Squamous cell ca.	1	
Thymic tumor		8
Carcinoid		5
Bronchus	3	
Stomach	1	
Duodenum	1	
Medullary ca. of the thyroid		3
Islet cell ca.		3
Miscellaneous		4
Clinical and laboratory findings		
Cushing's syndrome	present	15
	absent	22
Hyperadrenocorticism	present at first exam.	29
	appeared at later period	8

rhythmicity and lack of the suppression by a small dose dexamethasone. Such laboratory findings were noted at the first examination in 29 of our series of patients. In the remaining 8 patients, adrenocortical function was within normal limits on the first examination, but definitely elevated in the later period of the disease. This indicates that repeated endocrine examinations are required to diagnose tumor-associated hyperadrenocorticism.

One of the difficult problems in the diagnosis of ectopic ACTH syndrome is the differentiation from Cushing's disease. Even though patients have definite signs or X-ray findings of extrapituitary tumors, still the possibility of the co-existence of ACTH-producing pituitary microadenoma cannot be ruled out. When tumors are occult, the differential diagnosis becomes much more difficult. In our series, 95 % of patients with ectopic ACTH syndrome did not suppress by a large dose of dexamethasone. It is well-known, however, that some patients with Cushing's disease do not suppress by a large dose dexamethasone. In addition, some patients with ectopic ACTH syndrome show apparent suppression of urinary 17-OHCS due to periodic secretion of the hormone by tumors. One of the promising procedures at present for the differential diagnosis is the response to corticotropin-releasing factor (CRF). We have performed CRF tests in 6 patients with Cushing's disease and a patient with ectopic ACTH syndrome. All patients with Cushing's disease showed normal or rather exaggerated response of plasma ACTH to the intravenous injection of 100 μg of ovine CRF, whereas a patient with ectopic ACTH syndrome due to medullary carcinoma of the thyroid did not. Interestingly, the latter patient responded remarkably to lysine vasopressin (Shimatsu et al, 1983). This suggests that the CRF test may be applicable to the differential diagnosis of Cushing's disease and ectopic ACTH syndrome. It is possible, however, that some patients with Cushing's disease may not respond to CRF and that some patients with ectopic ACTH syndrome may respond to CRF, because we have found that rat median eminence extract, containing CRF, stimulated ACTH release from ectopic ACTH-producing tumors in vitro (Hirata et al, 1979). Further studies are required to evaluate the diagnostic value of the CRF test.

Histological diagnosis of ectopic ACTH-producing tumors associated with hyperadrenocorticism are shown in Table 1. As already well-known, bronchogenic carcinomas are the most common, followed by thymic tumors (possibly carcinoid), carcinoids of various organs, islet-cell tumors and medullary thyroid carcinoma. Among bronchogenic carcinomas, small-cell or oat-cell carcinomas are the most common. All these tumors are considered to have arisen from APUD cells (Pearse, 1968) or paraneurons (Fujita, 1976), which have characteristics of neuroendocrine cells. As distinct from silent ACTH production, as will be discussed later, tumors associated with hyperadrenocorticism derived from non-APUD cells are relatively uncommon, being 21 % in our series.

During the same period that we studied these patients, we could detect ACTH in an other 17 tumors. In 11, adrenocortical function test before death was within normal limits. In the remaining 6, the test was not performed. Ectopic ACTH production was suspected, because of tumor histologies, presence of hypokalemia or other reasons. These results suggested that silent ACTH production is common in some tumors and prompted us to study the incidence of ACTH production in patients with primary lung cancer as will be discussed later.

Another characteristic feature of ectopic ACTH production is the simultaneous production of multiple hormones. In our series of 37 patients, there were two patients with a syndrome of inappropriate

TABLE 2. <u>Two cases of multiple hormone-producing tumor</u>

Age & Sex	Case 1 63 M		Case 2 39 F	
Histology	Bronchogenic ca. Polymorphocellular type		Thymic carcinoid	
Cardinal Manifestation	Gynecomostia		Hypercalcemia	
Tissue Hormones	hCG	3.9	PTH	38.2*
	hCG–α	3.3	Calcitonin	12.7
	hCG–β	3.0	ACTH	0.5
	hPL	270	β–MSH[+]	2.9
	ACTH	2.9	α–MSH	0.5
	β–MSH[+]	8.2	Gastrin	0.7
	Calcitonin	14.7		
	Gastrin	0.8		

expressed as ng/g tissue except for * ng/mg dry weight
+ β– or τ–LPH measured as β–MSH–like immunoreactivity

secretion of antidiuretic hormone (ADH), whose tumors contained not only ADH, but ACTH and β–MSH–like immunoreactivity (Hirata et al, 1976a). In two patients listed in Table 2, we could detect a variety of hormones in tumors suggesting the production of multiple hormones. Both patients had laboratory data of hyperadrenocorticism but lacked signs of Cushing's syndrome. If we measure many hormones in tumors, we may be able to detect multiple hormones. Recent studies have shown that ACTH, β–LPH (β–MSH–like immunoreactivity) and β–endorphin are derived from a common precursor. Therefore, simultaneous production of these hormones in a tumor could always occur. However, ectopic ACTH–producing tumors often produce calcitonin, ADH and other hormones which are not derived from the common precursor molecule. Production of multiple hormones by tumors are usually asymptomatic, and the association of clinical syndromes of excess of more than two hormones seems very uncommon.

INCIDENCE OF ECTOPIC ACTH SYNDROME AND ECTOPIC ACTH PRODUCTION

In order to clarify the incidence of ectopic ACTH syndrome (hyperadrenocorticism), we performed adrenal function tests in 78 unselected patients with primary lung cancer (Imura et al, 1978) and found hyperadrenocorticism, especially the absence of diurnal rhythm of plasma cortisol and lack of suppression by a small dose of dexamethasone, in 8 patients (Table 3). Four had oat-cell carcinoma or small-cell undifferentiated carcinoma. Thus, the incidence of hyperadrenocorticism in primary lung cancer seems to be approximately 10 %. Although we did not measure plasma ACTH in these patients, other investigators reported increased plasma ACTH levels in 72 - 88 % of such patients (Ayvazian et al, 1975; Wolfsen and Odell, 1979).

In order to determine the incidence of ectopic ACTH production, we measured immunoreactive ACTH, calcitonin and human chorionic gonadotropin (hCG) in 47 unselected bronchogenic carcinomas of various histologies (Imura et al, 1978). As shown in Table 3, immunoreactive ACTH was detected in 64 % of all tumors and oat-cell carcinoma gave the highest percentage. Immunoreactive calcitonin was detected in 65 % and hCG in 34 %. Many tumors contained more than two hormones, again showing that production of multiple hormones is common, especially in bronchogenic carcinomas. Similar results were obtained by Abe et al

TABLE 3. Incidence of ectopic ACTH syndrome and ectopic hormone production in bronchogenic carcinoma

Histology	Hyperadreno-corticism (%)	Tomur Hormones (%)		
		ACTH	Calcitonin	hCG
No. of Patients	80	47	29	31
Oat-cell ca.*	50	71	85	25
Large-cell undifferentiated ca.	9	60	83	67
Adenocarcinoma	5	100	67	0
Squamous cell ca.	4	29	22	30
Carcinoid	50	–	–	–
Not firmly determined	11	–	–	–
Total	10	64	65	34

* includes small-cell undifferentiated ca.

(1983). However, Gewirtz and Yalow (1974) and Odell et al (1977) reported that 92 to 100 % of bronchogenic carcinomas contained ACTH. Moreover, Odell et al (1977) found ACTH at similarly high percentage in tumors other than bronchogenic carcinomas, although Gewirtz and Yalow (1974) reported lower values. Thus, there are still some disagreements in the percentage of unselected tumors in which ACTH can be detected. It is evident, however, that ectopic ACTH production is a common concomitant of neoplasms, although the association of clinical and/or biochemical abnormalities is rather uncommon.

BIOCHEMICAL CHARACTERISTICS OF ACTH AND RELATED PEPTIDES IN TUMORS

The nature of ACTH produced by tumors has been a matter of interest for a long time. If ACTH is produced in tumors by abnormalities in the regulation of gene expression, one would expect ACTH in tumor to be similar in structure to its counterpart in the pituitary. Since antigenic determinants and biologically active sites are usually different in hormone molecules, we thought that comparison of biological and immunological activities of tumor ACTH might give some information regarding its nature. In our previous studies, we found a remarkable dissociation between biologic and immunologic activities of ACTH in some tumor tissues studied (Imura et al, 1973). This suggested to us the presence of a biologically less active form of ACTH.

We then studied size heterogeneity of tumor ACTH by gel filtration. As reported by Gewirtz and Yalow (1974), we also found that both the pituitary and tumors have different molecular forms of ACTH; big, intermediate and little forms. Little ACTH was eluted at the position of authentic ACTH, whereas big ACTH appeared a little behind the elution position of human albumin (Imura et al, 1974, 1978). The proportion of big ACTH in total ACTH-like immunoreactivity tended to be higher in tumors than in the pituitary and some tumors contained almost exclusively big ACTH. Since big ACTH has, if any, little biologic activity, a marked dissociation between biologic and immunologic activity of tumor ACTH can be explained by the predominance of big ACTH.

Using an in vitro system, we demonstrated that labeled amino acid was first incorporated into big ACTH fraction of tumors (Hirata et al, 1975). This suggested to us that big ACTH would be a biosynthetic precursor. Nakanishi et al (1979) have determined the amino acid sequence of the precursor of ACTH by studying the nucleotide sequence of DNA complementary to messenger RNA (mRNA) coding for the precursor. This

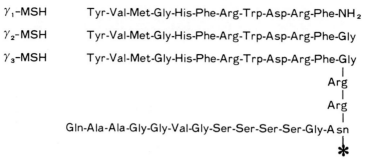

γ_1-MSH   Tyr-Val-Met-Gly-His-Phe-Arg-Trp-Asp-Arg-Phe-NH$_2$

γ_2-MSH   Tyr-Val-Met-Gly-His-Phe-Arg-Trp-Asp-Arg-Phe-Gly

γ_3-MSH   Tyr-Val-Met-Gly-His-Phe-Arg-Trp-Asp-Arg-Phe-Gly
                                                                          |
                                                                         Arg
                                                                          |
                                                                         Arg
                                                                          |
            Gln-Ala-Ala-Gly-Gly-Val-Gly-Ser-Ser-Ser-Ser-Gly-Asn
                                                                          *

FIG. 1.   Amino acid sequences of γ_1-, γ_2- and γ_3-MSH. Asterisk shows
           possible site of N-glycosylation.

precursor molecule, named preproACTH/β-LPH or preproopiomelanocortin,
contained β-lipotropin (β-LPH) in the C-terminus. Next to β-LPH, there
exists ACTH. In the previously unknown N-terminal portion, there is
another melanotropin (MSH)-like structure, named γ-MSH. The structure
of preproACTH/γ-LPH gave an explanation for the previous observations

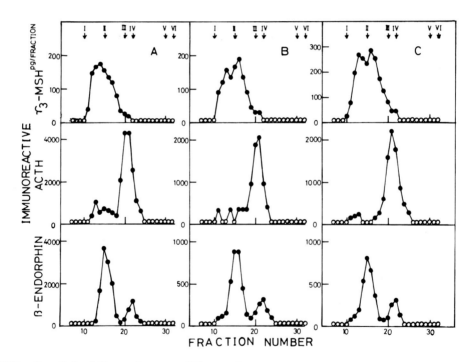

FIG. 2.   Gel filtration profiles of γ-MSH-LI, ACTH-LI and β-EP-LI in
           human pituitary extracts on a column of Bio-Gel P-60, 0.7 x 52
           cm. Each fraction obtained from the column was subjected to
           radioimmunoassays for γ_3-MSH, ACTH and β-endorphin. Markers
           used were blue dextran (I), mouse 16 K fragment (II), β-LPH
           (III), ACTH (IV), γ_3-MSH (V) and iodine (VI).

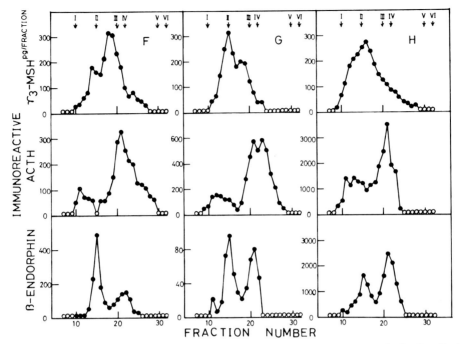

FIG. 3. Gel filtration profiles of γ-MSH-LI, ACTH-LI and β-EP-LI in
three ectopic ACTH-producing tumors. See legend for Fig. 2.

that ectopic ACTH producing tumors contained also β-LPH, γ-LPH (β-LPH 1-58) and β-endorphin (β-LPH 61-91) (Hirata et al, 1976b; Orth et al, 1978).

In order to study molecular forms of ACTH and related peptides in tumor tissues, we set up radioimmunoassays for ACTH, β-endorphin and $γ_3$-MSH (27 amino acid peptide having γ-MSH at the N-terminus) (Fig. 1). Fig. 2 and 3 show gel filtration profiles of extracts of human pituitaries and ectopic ACTH producing tumors. In pituitaries, the proportion of big ACTH to total immunoreactive ACTH was below 20 %, whereas it tended to be higher in tumors. Although not shown in this figure, we had a case who showed almost exclusively big ACTH (Hirata et al, 1976c). Immunoreactive β-endorphin was composed of two peaks: one eluted at the position of β-LPH and was considered to be β-LPH which cross-reacted equally to β-endorphin with β-endorphin antisera; the other eluted at the position of authentic β-endorphin and was considered to be β-endorphin itself. In human pituitaries, β-LPH was predominant with a minor peak of β-endorphin (Fig. 2). On the other hand, the ratio of β-LPH to β-endorphin was variable in tumors (Fig. 3), suggesting different processing of β-LPH to β-endorphin between the pituitary and tumors. Immunoreactive γ-MSH consisted of a single broad peak in the pituitary, eluted near the position of β-LPH (Fig. 2). This was named big γ-MSH. In ectopic ACTH-producing tumors, gel filtration patterns varied in different tumors. There were an intermediate form and even a trace of little form of γ-MSH-like immunoreactivity eluted behind big γ-MSH, but earlier than $γ_3$-MSH (Tanaka et al, 1981). To further characterize big, intermediate and little γ-MSH, we studied their binding to concanavalin A (Con-A)-agarose. Although data are not shown, big γ-MSH was adsorbed to the lectin column and eluted by α-methyl-D-mannopyranoside. This suggests that big γ-MSH is a glycoprotein. Since the elution position of big γ-MSH coincides with that of mouse 16 K fragment and, since only γ_3-MSH has a N-glycosylation site in the proACTH/β-LPH molecule, big γ-MSH is considered to be a large N-terminal peptide having γ_3-MSH at the C-terminus. When tumor extracts were subjected to Con-A-agarose column, less γ-MSH-like immunoreactivity was adsorbed to the column as with pituitary γ-MSH. In particular, a tumor γ-MSH of predominantly intermediate form was less adsorbed to the column. This suggests that there exist some abnormalities in glycosylation of big γ-MSH in tumors (Tanaka et al, 1981). Similar abnormalities were observed in hCG produced by tumors (Yoshimoto et al, 1979).

Although normal human pituitaries contain only big γ-MSH, we have observed that human extrapituitary tissues and bovine neurointermediate pituitary contain little γ-MSH eluted near the position of β-endorphin (Imura et al, 1982). This little γ-MSH seems to be a glycosylated form of γ_3-MSH, since it is adsorbed to Con-A-agarose and since γ_3-MSH has a glycosylation site, Asn-X-Ser. Although not clear in Fig. 3, some tumors seemed to contain little γ-MSH. This suggests that the processing of big γ-MSH is different between the pituitary and tumors. Furthermore, we were able to detect γ_1-MSH-like immunoreactivity in one of 6 ectopic ACTH producing tumors (Tanaka et al, 1983). Gel filtration studies revealed that γ_1-MSH-like peptide is not γ_1-MSH itself but a large peptide having γ_1-MSH at the C-terminus. γ_1-MSH consists of the N-terminal amino acids of γ_3-MSH (Fig. 1) and there exists Arg-Arg next to the C-terminus of γ_1-MSH. This pair of basic amino acids does not seem to be cleaved in the pituitary, since the glycosylated C-terminal portion hinders the enzymatic cleavage. In fact, we failed to detect γ_1-MSH in normal pituitaries. In some tumors, however, the glycosylation of γ_3-MSH is lacking or abnormal and γ_1-MSH-like peptide can be produced from big γ-MSH.

Fig 4 schematically shows the processing of proACTH/β-LPH in human pituitary and extra-pituitary tissues. In the pituitary, major final products are big γ-MSH (N-terminal fragment), ACTH and β-LPH, with a minor amount of β-endorphin. On the other hand, the processing of β-LPH to β-endorphin is almost complete in extrapituitary tissues. ACTH is further split into α-MSH and corticotropin-like intermediate lobe peptide (CLIP). Big γ-MSH is processed to little γ-MSH to some extent. Further processing of β-endorphin to small molecular forms and γ-LPH to β-MSH may occur in some tissues. Our studies demonstrate that there are several abnormalities in the processing of proACTH/β-LPH in tumors.

(1) Abnormalities in glycosylation of prohormones: The translation product directed by mRNA for the precursor has a signal peptide, which is cleaved when the translation product crosses the membranes of the endoplasmic reticulum. The remaining portion is glycosylated at the Asn residue in the γ_3-MSH portion and possibly at the Thr residue of the N-terminal portion. In some tumors, the glycosylation is either lacking or abnormal and big γ-MSH has less affinity to Con-A. Since the glycosylation is considered to be prerequisite for appropriate processing, abnormalities in glycosylation may cause abnormal processing of the precursor protein.

(2) Limited processing of prohormone: Processing of proACTH/β-LPH to β-LPH and ACTH in tumors is limited to variable extents as compared with that in the pituitary. In some tumors, only big ACTH, possibly proACTH/β-LPH, could be detected.

(3) Accelerated processing of peptides derived from proACTH/β-LPH: In the pituitary, β-LPH, ACTH and big γ-MSH are the major final pro-

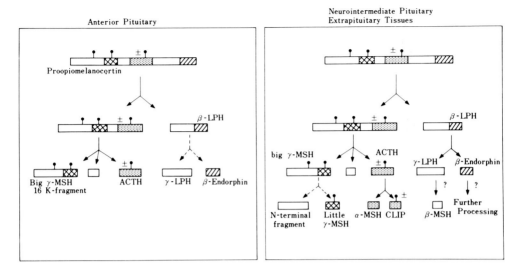

FIG. 4. Processing of proACTH/β-LPH in the anterior pituitary (left) and the neurointermediate pituitary or extrapituitary tissues (right).

ducts, although β-endorphin is produced to some extent. In tumors, the conversion of β-LPH to β-endorphin is accelerated to variable extents. β-Endorphin is not further processed in the pituitary, but may be processed to smaller peptides in tumors (Suda et al, 1982). It is possible that β-MSH is produced from β- and γ-LPH in tumors (Ueda et al, 1980), although artifactual production could not be ruled out. ACTH is not further processed in the human pituitary but split into α-MSH and CLIP in some tumors. We were able to detect α-MSH in 4 of 33 tumors studied. In the pituitary, big γ-MSH is the final product, whereas little γ-MSH may be produced in some tumors. In addition, γ₁-MSH like peptide is also produced in certain tumors. Although such accelerated processings in tumors resemble those in non-neoplastic extrapituitary tissues to some extent, they varies in different tumors and are abnormal in some tumors compared with extrapituitary tissues.

MESSENGER RNA (mRNA) AND DNA CODING FOR PROACTH/β-LPH
IN ECTOPIC ACTH-PRODUCING TUMORS

Ectopic ACTH-producing tumors elaborate ACTH, β-LPH, β-endorphin and γ-MSH, all of which are derived from the common precursor, proACTH/β-LPH. This suggests that proACTH/β-LPH is produced in ectopic ACTH producing tumors as it is in the pituitary. To demonstrate whether mRNA and its translation product in tumors are the same as those in the pituitary, we first studied mRNA from a thymic carcinoid and a human pituitary by the RNA blot hybridization analysis (Tsukada et al, 1981). RNA was extracted from these tissues and electrophoresed on an agarose gel. ^{32}P-labeled cDNA for bovine proACTH/β-LPH was used as a hybridization probe. As shown in Fig. 5, RNA from the tumor showed two bands, the major one co-migrated with RNA from the pituitary and the minor one moved more slowly. The former had an apparent molecular weight of 3.7 x

10^5 (1,100 nucleotides). The nature of the larger RNA is not known, because it was too small in amount to clone.

We next studied cell-free translation product directed by mRNA. Reticulocyte lysate cell-free protein synthesizing system was used and the products formed were immunoprecipitated and electrophoresed on SDS-polyacrylamide gel. RNAs from the human pituitary and a thymic carcinoid yielded a single radioactive product with an identical mobility corresponding to an apparent molecular weight of 38,000. An excess of ACTH 1-24 or β-endorphin competed with the binding of the translation

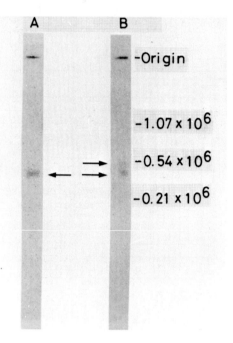

FIG. 5. Hybridization analysis of RNA from the human pituitary (A) and an ectopic ACTH-producing tumor (B) with ^{32}P-labeled cDNA. The RNA markers used were Escherichia coli 23 S rRNA ($\underline{Mr}$ 10.7 x 10^5), 16 S rRNA ($\underline{Mr}$ 5.4 x 10^5) and rabbit α- and β-globulin mRNA ($\underline{Ms}$ 2.1 x 10^5). (Reproduced from 29)

product with respective antibodies. Further studies have suggested that the products directed by pituitary and tumor mRNA are identical. It appears, therefore, that a large mRNA detected by the RNA blot hybridization analysis might give the same translation product as that by mRNA of regular size or not been translated. These results suggest that the major mRNA species produced by tumors is indistinguishable from the mRNA of the human pituitary. Very recently, DeBold et al (1983) succeeded in partially sequencing DNA complementary to mRNA for proACTH/β-LPH in an tumor and observed that the sequence of the β-MSH-β-endorphin portion is the same as that of cDNA for pituitary mRNA. Interestingly, they observed also two species of mRNA coding for proACTH/β-LPH from a tumor as we did in a thymic carcinoid, although the difference of these two mRNAs was not known.

The next question was whether genomic DNA in tumors is identical to that in normal tissue. DNA was extracted from normal human tissue, ectopic ACTH-producing tumors and non-ACTH-producing human tumors and digested with the restriction endonuclease, Hind III, Eco R1 or Bam H1. Then the products were electrophoresed, transferred onto DBM-paper and hybridized with ^{32}P-labeled cDNA encoding bovine proACTH/β-LPH. As shown in Fig. 6, human placenta, ACTH-producing thymic carcinoid and lung cancer, and 5 apparently non-ACTH-producing human tumors gave

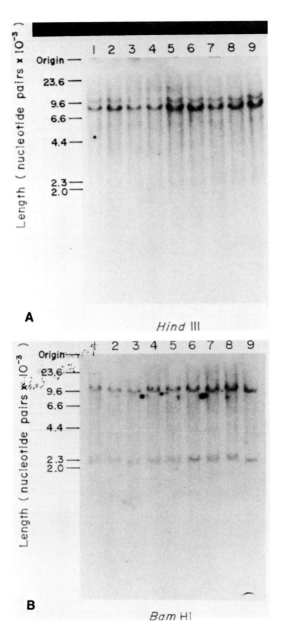

FIG. 6. Hybridization analysis of DNA from human placenta (1), ACTH-producing thymic carcinoid (2) and lung cancer (3), non-ACTH-producing stomach cancer (4), medullary thyroid carcinomas (5,6), pheochromocytoma (7), bronchial carcinoid (8) and thymoma (9). ^{32}P-cDNA for proACTH/β-LPH was used. As restriction enzymes, Hind III (A) and Bam Hl (B) were used.

TABLE 4. Contents of immunoreactive ACTH, β-endorphin,
          Met-enkephalin and Leu-enkephalin
          in ectopic ACTH-producing tumors

Tumor	ACTH	β-EP	Met-enk	Leu-enk
Medullary thyroid ca.	756	588	112	61
Thymic carcinoid	434	502	432	243
Oat-cell ca.	28	36	3.7	1.4

ng/g tissue

identical DNA fragments after Hind III digestion. Similar results were
obtained with other restriction enzymes.

These results indicate that there exists no detectable length poly-
morphism in and near proACTH/β-LPH gene in most of clones of ectopic
ACTH-producing tumors. Since it is still unknown whether or not the DNA
structure is identical in all cells of a tumor, we cannot conclude that
genomic DNA and its adjacent area in ectopic ACTH-producing cells are
identical to those in normal pituitary. Immunoperoxidase staining
revealed that tumors used for DNA analysis contained cells stained with
anti-ACTH, anti-β-endorphin and anti-γ-MSH antisera, although only a
limited number of tumor cells could be stained (unpublished observation). Further studies are required before concluding that there are no
abnormalities in and near the proACTH/β-LPH gene in tumor cells producing ACTH, although we have failed thus far to find abnormalities.

PRODUCTION OF PEPTIDES EVOLUTIONARY RELATED TO
ACTH IN ECTOPIC ACTH PRODUCING TUMORS

Recent studies by Numa and his associates (Noda et al, 1982; Kakidani
et al, 1982) have shown that proenkephalin A, the precursor of Met-
enkephalin and Leu-enkephalin, and proenkephalin B, the precursor of
dynorphin and α-neo-endorphin, have structures very similar to proACTH/
β-LPH. Moreover, the organization of genes of proenkephalin A and B is
very similar to that of proACTH/β-LPH, having three exons divided by two
intervening sequences and having most of the protein-coding region in
exon III. These results suggest that the genes of three opioid peptide
precursors have evolved from a single precursor, possibly by gene
duplication. Another related peptide is corticotropin-releasing factor
(CRF) which stimulates release of ACTH from the pituitary. The precursor of CRF has a region with sequence homology to ACTH (Furutani et
al, 1983). Interestingly, it has also a sequence resembling neurophysin
II, a peptide sharing the precursor with vasopressin. It is of interest, therefore, to study whether genes for these peptides are expressed
simultaneously in ectopic ACTH-producing tumors.

We measured immunoreactive ACTH, β-endorphin, Met-enkephalin and
Leu-enkephalin in three ectopic ACTH-producing tumors. All tumors
contained immunoreactive Met-enkephalin and Leu-enkephalin. Further
studies with high performance, reverse phase liquid chromatography
showed that tumors contained Met-enkephalin and Leu-enkephalin (unpublished observation). Although more extensive studies are required,
it is likely that many ectopic ACTH-producing tumors produce Met-
enkephalin and Leu-enkephalin simultaneously.

Since sensitive radioimmunoassay for human CRF was not available, we measured biologic activity of CRF in ectopic ACTH-producing tumors (Yamamoto et al, 1976). The pituitary incubation method was used, combined with in vivo steroidogenic assay for ACTH. Of 7 ectopic ACTH-producing tumors, 6 had significant amount of biologic CRF activity. On the other hand, only one of 5 non-ACTH-producing tumors showed CRF-like activity. The contribution of vasopressin to CRF-like activity seemed, if any, minimal, because the dose-response relationship of tumor extract was clearly different from that of vasopressin. Although studies are required using radioimmunoassay for human CRF, it appears that many ectopic ACTH-producing tumors simultaneously elaborate CRF.

These results suggest that Met-enkephalin, Leu-enkephalin and CRF are produced in many but not all ectopic ectopic ACTH-producing tumors. It is still premature to draw conclusion, but it is possible that some genes with special relationship to proACTH/β-LPH gene are expressed in ectopic ACTH-producing tumors.

MECHANISMS FOR ECTOPIC ACTH PRODUCTION

The mechanism by which tumors elaborate ACTH and other hormones is not yet understood. The possibility that mutation of genes fortuitously encodes the ACTH precursor is unlikely, because the precursor in tumors seems identical to that in the pituitary. As mentioned above, a variety of tissues are considered to have neuroendocrine cells that produce ACTH, since not only ACTH and β-LPH but also mRNA for ACTH/β-LPH precursor are detected in these tissues. If tumors arise from such neuroendocrine cells, they produce ACTH or other hormones. Carcinoids are examples of such tumors and produce relatively large amounts of ACTH. However, tumors which are considered to have arisen from cells other than neuroendocrine cells, such as adenocarcinoma, also produce ACTH though usually less in amount. This can not be explained by the neuroendocrine cell hypothesis. Simple derepression of once repressed gene during the process of development seems unlikely, since direct measurements using nucleic acid hybridization techniques have failed to detect significant gene derepression in transformed cells (Williams et al, 1977).

There seem to be two possibilities to explain ACTH production in adenocarcinoma or other tumors. One is that some tumor cells differentiate towards neuroendocrine cells, thus gaining the ability to produce hormones. An alternate explanation is that tumor cells produce hormones due to abnormalities in regulation of gene expression. Such abnormalities can account for the following observations on ectopic ACTH syndrome. (1) The precursor of ACTH in tumors seems identical to that in the pituitary, although post-translational processing of the precursor is often different in tumors. (2) No gross abnormalities in genomic DNA and mRNA encoding proACTH/β-LPH could be detected in tumor tissues. (3) Production of multiple hormones is common in ectopic ACTH-producing tumors. (4) Ectopic ACTH production is a universal concomitant of neoplasms.

ACKNOWLEDGEMENT

A part of these studies was supported by cancer research grants from the Ministry of Education, Science and Culture, the Ministry of Health and Welfare, Japan, and the Princess Takamatsu Cancer Research Foundation. Thanks are also due to Drs. S. Numa and S. Nakanishi, Department of Medical Chemistry, Kyoto University, for help and advice to the RNA and DNA studies.

REFERENCES

1. Abe, K., Kameya, T., Yamaguchi, K., Kikuchi, K., Adachi, I., Tanaka, M., Kimura, S., Kodama, T., Shimosato, Y., and Ishikawa, S. (1983): In: Endocrine Lung in Health and Disease, edited by K.L. Becker and A.F. Gazdar, W.B. Saunders, in press.

2. Ayvazian, L.F., Schneider, B., Gewirtz, G., and Yalow, S. (1975): Am. Rev. Resp. Dis., 111: 279-287.

3. DeBold, C.R., Schworer, M.E., Connor, T.B., Bird, R.E., and Orth, D.N. (1983): Science, 220: 721-723.

4. Fujita, T. (1976): In: Chromaffin, Enterochromaffine and Related Cells, edited by R.E. Coupland and T. Fujita, pp. 204-208, Elsevier, Amsterdam.

5. Furutani, Y., Morimoto, Y., Shibahara, S., Noda, M., Takahashi, H., Hirose, T., Asai, M., Inayama, S., Hayashida, H., Miyata, T., and Numa, S. (1983): Nature, 301: 537-540.

6. Gewirtz, G., and Yalow, R.S. (1974): J. Clin. Invest., 53: 1022-1032.

7. Hirata, Y., Yamamoto, H., Matsukura, S., and Imura, H. (1975): J. Clin. Endocrinol. Metab., 41: 106-114.

8. Hirata, Y., Matsukura, S., Imura, H., Yakura, T., Iijima, S., Nagase, C., and Itoh, M. (1976a): Cancer, 38: 2575-2582.

9. Hirata, Y., Matsukura, H., Imura, H., Nakamura, M., and Tanaka, A. (1976b): J. Clin. Endocrinol. Metab., 42: 33-40.

10. Hirata, Y., Sakamoto, N., Yamamoto, H., Matsukura, S., Imura, H., and Okada, S. (1976c): Cancer, 37: 317-321.

11. Hirata, Y., Yoshimi, H., Matsukura, S., and Imura, H. (1979): J. Clin. Endocrinol. Metab., 49: 317-321.

12. Huhtaniemi, I.F., Koreabrot, C.C., and Jaffe, R.B. (1978): J. Clin. Endocrinol. Metab., 46: 894-997.

13. Imura, H. (1980): Clin. Endocrinol. Metab., 9: 235-260.

14. Imura, H., Matsukura, S., Yamamoto, H., Hirata, Y., Nakai, Y., and Matsuyama, H. (1973): Jap. J. Clin. Oncol., 6: 7-12.

15. Imura, H., Matsukura, S., Yamamoto, H., Hirata, Y., and Nakai, Y. (1974): Saishin-Igaku (Modern Medicine), 29: 1745-1750.

16. Imura, H., Nakai, Y., Nakao, K., Oki, S., Matsukura, S., Hirata, Y., Fukase, M., Hattori, M., Yoshimi, H., and Sueoka, S. (1978): Protein Nucl. Acid Enzyme, 23: 641-656.

17. Imura, H., Nakai, Y., Nakao, K., Oki, S., Fukata, J., Tanaka, I., Kinoshita, F., Tsukada, T., and Yoshimasa, T. (1982): In: Pituitary Hormones and Related Peptides, edited by M. Motta, M. Zanisi and F. Piva, pp. 243-269, Academic Press, London, New York.

18. Iwasa, S., Laborde, N.P., and Odell, W.P. (1983): Program and Abstract, 65th Annual Meeting, Endocrine Society, p.321.

19. Kakidani, H., Furutani, Y., Takahashi, H., Noda, M., Morimoto, Y., Hirose, T., Asai, M., Inayama, S., Nakanishi, S., and Numa, S. (1982): Nature, 298: 245-249.

20. Nakanishi, S., Inoue, A., Kita, T., Nakamura, M., Chang, A.C.Y., Cohen, S.N., and Numa, S. (1979): Nature, 278: 423-427.

21. Noda, M., Furutani, Y., Takahashi, H., Toyosato, M., Hirose, T., Inoyama, S., Nakatani, S., and Numa, S. (1982): Nature, 295: 202-206.

22. Odell, W.D., Wolfsen, A., Yoshimoto, Y., Weitzman, R., Fisher, D., and Hirose, K. (1977): Trans. Assoc. Am. Physicians, 90: 204-227.

23. Orth, D.N., Guillemin, R., Ling, N., and Nicholson, W.E. (1978): J. Clin. Endocrinol. Metab., 46: 849-852.

24. Pearse, A.G.E. (1968): Proc. R. Soc. Ser. B., 170: 71-80.
25. Shimatsu, A., Kato, Y., Tanaka, I., Nakai, Y., Fukunaga, M., and Imura, H. (1983): Clin. Endocrinol., 18: 119-125.
26. Suda, T., Tozawa, F., Yamaguchi, H., Shibasaki, T., Demura, H., and Shizume, K. (1982): J. Clin. Endocrinol. Metab., 54: 167-171.
27. Tanaka, I., Nakai, Y., Nakao, K., Oki, S., Fukata, J., and Imura, H. (1981): Clin. Endocrinol., 15: 353-361.
28. Tanaka, I., Nakai, Y., Nakao, K., Oki, S., Yoshimasa, Y., and Imura, H. (1983): J. Clin. Endocrinol. Metab., 56: 1080-1083.
29. Tsukada, T., Nakai, Y., Jingami, H., Imura, H., Taii, S., Nakanishi, S., and Numa, S. (1981): Biochem. Biophys. Res. Commun., 98: 535-540.
30. Ueda, M., Takeuchi, T., Abe, K., Miyakawa, S., Ohnami, S., and Yanaihara, N. (1980): J. Clin. Endocrinol. Metab., 50: 550-556.
31. Williams, J.G., Hoffman, R., and Penman, S. (1977): Cell, 11: 901-907.
32. Wolfsen, A.R., and Odell, W.D. (1979): Am. J. Med., 66: 765-772.
33. Yamamoto, H., Hirata, Y., Matsukura, S., Imura, H., Nakamura, M., and Tanaka, A. (1976): Acta endocr., 82: 183-192.
34. Yoshimoto, Y., Wolfsen, A.R., and Odell, W.D. (1977): Science, 197: 575-579.
35. Yoshimoto, Y., Wolfsen, A.R., and Odell, W.D. (1979): Am. J. Med., 67: 414-420.

Progress in Cancer Research and Therapy,
Vol. 31, edited by F. Bresciani, et al.
Raven Press, New York © 1984.

GH-Secreting Adenomas: Pathophysiology and Pharmacological Treatment

A. Liuzzi, P.G. Chiodini, G. Verde, G. Oppizzi, and D. Dallabonzana

Division of Endocrinology, Ospedale Niguarda, 20162 Milan, Italy

It is well established that in normal humans the release of GH from the pituitary is under the control of somatostatin and of growth hormone releasing factor (GRF) which respectively inhibit and stimulate the release of GH by the somatotrophic cells. The secretion of these two neurohormones is in turn regulated at the hypothalamic level by neurotransmitters and, in particular, by the cerebral monoamines. This scheme of functional organization is present but qualitatively, and probably quantitatively, deranged in acromegaly.

The aim of this work is to summarize the present status of the pathophysiology of acromegaly with particular emphasis on those aspects of practical relevance for understanding the problems related to the neuropharmacological treatment of this disease.

PATHOPHYSIOLOGY

The studies on the pathophysiology of GH release from GH secreting adenomas have evidenced a number of derangements from the normal subjects both at hypothalamic and at pituitary levels. In fact, an abnormal hypothalamic control of GH release is documented by the lack of the sleep related GH increase in acromegaly (8) as well as by the frequent failure in releasing GH in response to stimuli such as arginine infusion (31) or insulin hypoglycemia (21) which act at the hypothalamic level: in addition, a peculiar finding of GH secretion in acromegaly is impaired suppression or paradoxical response to glucose load (2).

Of major relevance is however the behavior of GH release following neuroactive agents acting at the level of the tumoral somatotrops.Saito et al(51)showed that thyrotrophic hormone releasing hormone (TRH) which is ineffective in stimulating GH release in normal subjects, is a powerful releaser of the hormone in a consistent proportion of acromegalics and a similar effect,but of lower incidence has been reported for LHRH (49).

In 1972 Liuzzi et al (30) demonstrated that L-dopa,which increases GH levels in normal subjects,is followed by an inhibition of GH release in acromegalic patients.The same group showed that more specific dopamine agonists (DA) such as apomorphine (9)and in particular bromocriptine(Br),a long lasting dopaminergic drug(32),could lower GH levels in about 50% of the patients.

A meaningful step in the study of the pathophysiology of GH releasing adenomas was the finding of a homogeneity between the presence or absence of the GH releasing effect of TRH and of the GH lowering activity of DA(33).It was thus possible to separate the acromegalic population into responsive and non-responsive patients.Since in responsive patients the behavior of GH strictly resembles that of prolactin (PRL), the existence of a mammosomatotropic cell capable of releasing GH and PRL or,at least of a tumoral somatotrop with receptorial properties of the normal lactotrop was hypothesized (34). This view was strengthened by the demonstration that the inhibitory effect of DA on GH release is due to the activation of dopaminergic receptors on the tumoral somatotrops (7).It has been recently shown however,that dopamine receptors inhibiting GH release are also present on the normal GH secreting cells (57);thus,the GH-lowering effect of dopamine agonists in acromegaly may be viewed not as paradoxical but rather as an amplification of a normal phenomenon.The GH releasing effect of TRH,present in several pathological conditions, might be explained by the hypothesis of Muller et al (38) that,in acromegaly, pituitary and hypothalamus are functionally disconnected. The cells of the GH nonresponders lacking dopamine receptors would bear a higher degree of dedifferentiation.

Recently,Spada et al(54)have reported that,depending on the dose added in vitro,dopamine can either stimulate or inhibit GH release from human GH secreting adenomas.According to these data,the tumoral somatotrops would possess either stimulatory or inhibitory dopaminergic receptors and the responsiveness to DA would depend on the balance between these two receptor types.

The identification of a neuropeptide capable of inhibiting GH release,somatostatin (6),led to the hypothesis that a deficiency of this neurohormone might be responsible for the GH hypersecretion in acromegaly (4).This view was supported by the possibility of reverting the paradoxical increase of GH to glucose load by somatostatin infusion (23),and by the finding of normal and not elevated somato- statin levels in the cerebrospinal fluid of acromegalics (42);however the infusion of maximally inhibitory doses of somatostatin in a large series of patients evidenced a wide range of sensitivity to this peptide,several patients being fully desensitized.This finding suggests individual changes in somatotrop sensitivity rather than a hypothalamic de- ficiency of somatostatin in acromegaly (41).

An excess of GRF has been hypothesized as an etiologic factor in acromegaly since 1969 (14) and in 1971 (22) an in- creased GRF activity in the serum of some acromegalic pa- tients was shown.A 44 aminoacid peptide capable of selec- tively stimulating GH release both in vitro (48) and in vivo (60),has been recently isolated from a human pancreatic cell tumor. So far,a limited number of acromegalic patients has been tested with synthetic GRF (67)so that any conclusion on the effects of GRF on GH release in acromegaly would be inconsistent.From the preliminary data however,there appears to be a marked degree of individual variability to the GH releasing effect of GRF.

Collectively the present knowledge on the pathophysiology of GH secretion in acromegaly points to the pituitary as the site of most of the abnormalities of the secretory dynamic of GH in this disease.This conclusion,however,does not ex- clude a primitive derangement in the hypothalamic control of GH secretion and,in particular,an excessive secretion of GRF may be hypothesized.

It has been shown in fact that when GRF is hypersecreted by a pancreatic tumor,an acromegalic disease develops in Which both a positive response to TRH and GH inhibition during dopamine infusion is present (59).

Thus,it is possible that long-lasting changes in the hypothalamic tone of some neurohormones or neurotransmitters may alter the receptorial properties of the GH secreting cells that become sensitive to stimulatory or inhibitory inputs ineffective in normal conditions.

MEDICAL TREATMENT

Effects on GH levels

The ability of dopamine agonists to inhibit GH secretion

in acromegaly has provided an effective basis for the medical treatment of acromegaly. Although all DA capable of directly stimulating dopamine receptors inhibit GH release in acromegaly (Tab.1) only a few of these,namely Br (10), lisuride (62),methergoline (11),pergolide (25), CU-32085 (3) have been used in the medical treatment of this disease due to their prolonged activity.

As far as the data with Br are concerned, most studies in the literature (35) agree that,by the chronic administration of this drug,GH levels can be consistently suppressed in acromegaly.The percentage of responsive patients shows a wide variability in the different series ranging from 100% (1) to 0% (29).These discrepancies are most probably due to the lack of common criteria in assessing the treatment effectiveness.

In our opinion, treatment may be considered as effective when a reduction of at least 50% below the pretreatment GH values is obtained. In our series of 72 patients collected since 1974,a 50% reduction of GH levels has been achieved during Br treatment in 52.6% of the patients and a normalisation of hormone levels in 26% of these (i.e. GH levels below 5 ng/ml).This figure fits with the data of most of the studies of the literature.In particular,Quabbe (46) has reported that 27% of his patients had their GH levels normalized by Br.

There is general agreement that treatment has to be started with low drug doses in order to avoid the side effects of dopamine agonists such as nausea,vomiting,and postural hypotension, but the problem of the maintenance dose has been largely discussed.

It has been reported (63) that,by increasing the dose of Br to 60 mg/day,the percentage of responsive patients may be increased;other studies have demonstrated that the maximal dose of Br to be used is 20 mg/day (50).In accordance with the latter study,in our series , doses higher than 20 mg/day neither determined a more marked decrease of GH levels in patients responsive to lower doses,nor a GH lowering effect in unresponsive patients.

The GH inhibition by DA can be maintained even for seven years in those patients in whom the side effects do not prevent the administration of effective doses of the drug.In our experience no changes in hematopoietic,hepatic and renal function or adverse effects on the cardiovascular apparatus derive from these prolonged treatments.

Although it has been reported that after treament,withdrawal GH levels may be lower than those measured in pretreatment conditions (58),we have constantly found that drug withdrawal,even after years of treatment,is followed by a sharp increase (within 24-48 hours) of GH levels to the basal values.In addition,the TRH induced GH release is not impaired by the chronic administration of DA (3).These data suggest that DA only impair the release and not the synthesis of GH in acromegaly.

Since only some acromegalics are responsive to DA in terms of GH secretion,the problem of selecting these patients in order to avoid a useless prolonged treatment has been raised. In our experience,an acute test is a very useful tool for this purpose.Oral administration of 2.5 mg of Br or 0.3mg of lisuride allows one to distinguish responders or nonresponders on the the basis of a percent GH inhibition below the basal levels of at least 50%.This is an arbitrary limit and provides only a rough distinction between the two groups. It should be noted however that when the percent maximal GH decrease observed during the acute test is compared to that obtained during the chronic treatment a significant correlation is found.

The use of the acute test as predictive of the treatment effectiveness is not generally accepted (63) ;this is mainly due to the criteria on which evaluation of the results of the treatment relies. We stress that the acute test is a reliable index only when the percent inhibitions of GH levels between acute and chronic DA administration are compared.

Although DA are the most effective agents in controlling GH hypersecretion in acromegaly,since 1970,when Lawrence et al(28)reported that medroxyprogesterone-acetate could lower GH levels in a group of patients,several neuropharmacological attempts to treat this disease have been made.

Since the serotoninergic system is stimulatory on GH release in normal humans (53),drugs with antiserotoninergic properties have been used.Previous reports(20)have failed to evidence an inhibitory effect on GH secretion in acromegaly by cyproheptadine,but recently Kato et al (24) have obtained a consistent reduction of GH levels in 3 out 4 acromegalics chronically treated with 16-24 mg/day of the drug.Other drugs with antiserotoninergic properties such as methergoline or methysergide can lower GH levels in acromegaly,however this effect is most probably due to a dopaminergic activity of these compounds (11,40).

In 1974 Cryer et al (15) showed that an infusion of the alfa-adrenergic blocking drug,phentolamine,could lower GH levels in acromegalic patients.In our studies however (36), the chronic treatment with phenoxybenzamine up to the maximal tolerate dose of 60 mg/day,in patients responsive to phentolamine infusion,did not modify GH levels.

Tamoxifen,an antiestrogen compound,potentiates the inhibitory effect of dopamine on PRL release in vitro [16]. However,in accordance with the report of Lamberts et al (27) we found that the administration of 20 mg/day of tamoxifen to patients under bromocriptine treatment did not show any addittive effect in lowering GH levels.

Lastly,the attempt to achieve a stable suppression of GH levels by retarded forms of somatostatin was unsuccessul(36)

Clinical and metabolic effects of DA

The pharmacological treatment with DA is accompanied by improvement of clinical features and of some metabolic parameters deranged by GH hypersecretion such as glucose tolerance or hyperhydroxyprolinuria.A widely discussed problem is whether these changes are linked with the GH lowering effect of DA.Although these clinical and metabolic parameters generally improve only in GH responsive patients, there is indisputable evidence that they can also be observed independently of a lowering of GH levels (3,58).

It has been recently (17) shown that Br can alter the proportion between the "little" biologically active GH and the "big",less active form of the hormone,in favor of the latter. In addition,Wass et al(65) have demonstrated that in some patients Br can lower somatomedin-C levels without altering GH concentrations.

It has also been shown that separate plasma samples may not be representative of the actual daily GH secretion since clinical and metabolic changes appears to be correlated with the behavior of urinary but not of plasma GH (19).

Effects of DA on tumor size

The problem of an antitumor effect of DA on GH secreting adenomas has been raised by the studies of Wass et al (63) showing improvements of visual field defects in acromegalic patients under Br treatment and of Wass et al (64) who demonstrated indirect signs of tumor shrinkage (i.e remineralization of sella walls) in similar patients. They also showed by computed tomography (CT) evidence of tumor shrinkage after 11 months of Br treatment in one patient.

Unlike macroprolactinomas,however,the number of acromegalics studied is low.McGregor et al (37) did not evidence signs of tumor shrinkage in 4 patients treated for 3 months with 20 mg/day of Br;on the contrary,clear cut signs of tumor size reduction were evidenced by Spark et al(55) in 3 out of 3 patients,by Wollesen et al (66) in 2 out 3 patients and by Wass et al (65) in 2 out 2 patients.

In the recent years,we have studied 23 patients selected
out of a series of 41 acromegalics,due to the presence of
large(more than 10 mm) adenomas.Fourteen patients have been
treated with Br (5-20 mg/day) and 9 patients with lisuride
(0.6 -2.0 mg/day) for periods ranging from 8 to 30 months
(mean 12.6 + 1.8). Serial CT performed throughout treatment
allowed to evidence a reduction of tumor size only in two
patients(-30% and -40% of the pretreatment tumor area);in
the remaining patients the size of the tumor was unchanged.
    In the two patients,shrinkage of the tumor was observed
in the CT performed after 6 and 7 months of treatment with
Br and no further shrinkage was observed in the other CTs
performed after up to 19 months of treatment.
    If the data on GH levels and tumor size are compared,it
is evident that in none of the GH nonresponsive patients was
any tumor shrinkage obtained and that the two patients whose
tumor shrank were both GH responders.However,in 7 out of 9
9 GH responsive patients the tumor size was not affected by
the treatment.

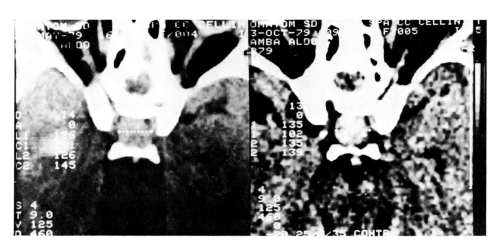

FIG. 1,Computed tomographies before(left) and after(right)
8 months of treatment with 20 mg/day of bromocriptine in a
GH nonresponsive patient.The size of the tumor is unchanged.

    It is interesting to note that all 8 GH secreting aden-
omas reported to shrink were GH responders with a possible
exception of one patient (65);moreover,in accordance with
our data,two of the patients of McGregor et al (37) whose
tumor did not shrink,were GH responders.
    Although the data so far collected give evidence that DA
can determine a size reduction of GH secreting tumors,it is
still unknown by which mechanisms this effect is brought
about.Ergot alkaloids possess a vasoconstrictive activity

that may reduce blood supply to the tumor thus determining necrotic phenomena and ultimately tumor shrinkage; however neither Br (13) nor lisuride (44) have a strong vaso-constrictive activity; moreover should this effect be re-sponsible for tumor shrinkage, it would have occurred also in GH nonresponsive patients.

Br exerts an antimitotic effect on human fibroblasts (43) and normal rat lactotropes (56); however evidence for such an effect has not been collected on rat (26) and human (45) PRL secreting tumors in vitro. As far as Br effects on GH secreting adenomas are concerned, Reganchary et al(47) failed to evidence any change by electron microscopy suggestive of an antimitotic activity; this patient however was GH non-responsive. Although some of the patients whose tumor shrank during DA administration were hyperprolactinemic, (55,65) we feel it unlikely that the reduction in size of the tumor of our two patients was due to a drug effect on the lactotropic portion of the tumor, since they had normal or only slightly elevated PRL levels.

Lastly, it is possible, but still unproven, that similarly to what has been shown for macroprolactinomas, DA may reduce the cellular volume (39,61).

Whatever the mechanisms of action may be, the incidence of tumor shrinkage of GH secreting adenomas is, in our ex-perience, far lower than that reported for macroprolactinomas (12).

We cannot exclude the possibility that the use of higher drug doses might have increased the percentage of tumor shrinkage in our series; however, the two patients who showed tumor shrinkage were treated with doses of Br as low as 5 or 7.5 mg/day that are superimposable on those adopted by Spark et al (55) in their two responsive patients. In addition, doses of Br of 20 and even 30 mg/day were ineffective in the 4 patients of McGregor et al(37) and in 1 of the 3 patients re-ported by Wollesen et al (66).

CONCLUSIONS

The conclusions that can be drawn after almost ten years since the introduction of the DA treatment of acromegaly may be summarized as follows: long lasting dopamine agonists are effective in controlling, even for years, the GH hyper-secretion in a consistent proportion of patients.

In the GH responsive patients, and even in some GH non-responders, an amelioration of the clinical symptoms of the disease can be observed together with an improvement of metabolic parameters deranged by GH hypersecretion. However,

even in these favourably treated patients,interruption of
treatment is followed by an almost immediate rise of GH
levels.

As far as tumor growth is concerned,enlargement of the
tumor is a very infrequent event during DA treatment (52).
However,on the basis of our data, tumor shrinkage can be
obtained only in a minority of GH responsive patients.Thus,
DA treatment of acromegaly is a very useful tool when reduction of GH levels is the aim of the therapy when surgery
or X-ray have either failed or are contraindicated.However,
DA treatment is only of limited value when the therapeutic
goal is to achieve shrinkage of the adenoma.

ACKNOWLEDGMENT

This work was supported by CNR,Special Project "Control of
Neoplastic Growth",grant no 820033496.

REFERENCES

1. Althoff,P.H.,Bottger,B.,Harz,C.,Rosak,C.,and Schoffling,
   K.(1981):Acta Endocrinol.(Suppl.),243:Abst.231.
2. Beck,P.,Parker,M.L.,and Daughaday,W.H.(1966):J.Clin.
   Endocrinol.Metab.,26,463-9.
3. Belforte,L.,Camanni,F.,Chiodini,P.G.,Liuzzi,A.,Massara,
   F.,Molinatti,G.M.,Muller,E.E.,and Silvestrini,F.(1977):
   Acta Endocrinol.,85,235-40.
4. Besser,G.M.,Mortimer,C.H.,Carr,D.,Schally,A.V.,Coy,D.H.,
   Evered,D.,Kastin,A.J.,Tunbridge,W.M.G.,Thorner,M.D.,and
   Hall,R.(1974):Br.Med.J.,1:352-5.
5. Besser,G.M.,Wass,J.A.,Grossman,A.,Moult,P.J.A.and
   Bouloux,P.(1983):In Lisuride and Other Dopamine
   Agonists edited by D.B.Calne,pp239-47.Raven Press,NY
6. Brazeau,P.,Vale,W.,Burgus,R.,Ling,N.,Butcher,M.,Rivier,
   J.,and Guillemin,R. (1973):Science,179:77-9.
7. Bression,D.,Brandi,A.M.,Nousbaum,A.,and Pellion,F.(1981)
   Acta Endocrinol.(Suppl.),243:Abst.241.
8. Chihara,K.,Kato,Y.,Abe,H.,Furomoto,M.,Maeda,K.,and Imura
   H.(1977):J.Clin.Endocrinol.Metab.,44:78-84.
9. Chiodini,P.G.,Liuzzi,A.,Botalla,L.,Cremascoli,G.,and
   Silvestrini,F.(1974):J.Clin.Endocrinol.Metab.,38:200-6.
10. Chiodini,P.G.,Liuzzi,A.,Botalla,L.,Cremascoli,G.Muller,
    E.E.,and Silvestrini,F.(1975):J.Clin.Endocrinol.Metab.,
    40:705-8.
11. Chiodini,P.G.,Liuzzi,A.,Muller,E.E.,Botalla,L.,Cremasco-
    li,G.,Oppizzi,G.,Verde,G.,,and Silvestrini F.(1976):J.
    Clin.Endocrinol.Metab.,43:356-63.

12. Chiodini,P.G.,Liuzzi,A.,Cozzi,R.,Oppizzi,G.,Dallabonza-
    na,D.Spelta,B.,Silvestrini,F.,Borghi,G.,Luccarelli,G.,
    Rainer,E.,and Horowski,R.(1981):J.Clin.Endocrinol.
    Metab.,40:705-8.

13. Clark,B.J.,Fluckiger,E.,Loew,D.M.,and Vigouret,J.M.
    (1978):Triangle,17:21-29.

14. Cryer,P.E.,Daughaday,W.H.(1969):J.Clin.Endocrinol.Metab.
    29:386-93.

15. Cryer,P.E.,and Daughaday,W.H.(1974):J.Clin.Endocrinol.
    Metab.,39:658-63.

16. de Quiada,M.,Timmermans,H.A.T.,Lamberts,S.W.J.,and
    MacLeod, R.M.(1980):Endocrinology,106:702-9.

17. Dietz,A.,Schopol,J.,Eversmann,T.,and von Werder,K.(1981)
    Acta Endocrinol.(Suppl.),240:70.

18. Dunn,P.,Donald,R.,and Espiner,A.(1977):Clin.Endocrinol.,
    7:273-9.

19. Eskildsen,P.C.,Svenden,P.A.,Vang,L.,and Nerup,J.(1978):
    Acta Endocrinol.,87:687-94.

20. Feldman,J.,Plonk,J.W.,and Bivens,C.H.(1976):Clin.
    Endocrinol.,5:71-8.

21. Glick,S.M.,Roth,J.,Yalow,R.S.,and Berson,S.A.(1965):Rec.
    Progr.Horm.Res.,21:241-83.

22. Hagen,T.C.,Lawrence,A.M.,and Kirsteins,L.(1971):J.Clin.
    Endocrinol.Metab.,33:448-51.

23. Hall,R.,Besser,G.M.,Schally,A.V.,Coy,D.H.,Evered,D,
    Goldie,D.J.,Kastin,A.J.,McNeilly,A.J.,Mortimer,C.H.
    Phenekos,C.,Tunbridge,W.M.G.,and Weightman,D.(1973)
    :Lancet,2:581-6.

24. Kato,Y.,Kabayama,Y.,and Ohta,H.(1983):65th Meeting
    Endocr.Soc.,Abst.197.

25. Kendall-Taylor,P.,and Upstill-Goddard,G.(1983):64th
    Meet.Endocr.Soc.,Abst.98.

26. Lamberts,S.W.,MacLeod,R.M.,and Robet,M.(1979):
    Endocrinology,104:65-70.

27. Lamberts,S.W.J.,de Quiada,M.,and Klin,J.G.M.(1980):J.
    Endocrinol.Invest.,4:43-50.

28. Lawrence,A.M.,and Kirsteins,L.(1970):J.Clin.Endocrinol.
    Metab.,30:646-51.

29. Lindholm,J.,Riishede,J.,Vestergaard,S.,Hummer,L.,Faber,
    O.,and Hagen,C.(1981):N.Engl.J.Med.,304:1450-3.

30. Liuzzi,A.,Chiodini,P.G.,Botalla,L.,Cremascoli,G.,and
    Silvestrini,F.(1972):J.Clin.Endocrinol.Metab.,35:
    941-3.

31. Liuzzi,A.,Chiodini,P.G.,Botalla,L.,Cremascoli,G.,and
    Tosi,M.(1973):Folia Endocrinol.,26:503-10.

32. Liuzzi,A.,Chiodini,P.G.,Botalla,L.,Cremascoli,G.,Muller,

E.E.,and Silvestrini,F.(1974):J.Clin.Endocrinol.Metab.,
38:910-2.

33. Liuzzi,A.,Chiodini,P.G.,Botalla,L.,Silvestrini,F.,and
Muller,E.E.(1974):J.Clin.Endocrinol.Metab.,39:871-6.

34. Liuzzi,A.,Panerai,A.E.,Chiodini,P.G.,Secchi,C.,Cocchi,
D.,Botalla,L.,Silvestrini,F.,and Muller,E.E(1976):
In:Growth Hormone and Related Peptides,edited by
A.Pecile,and E.E.Muller,pp.236-51.Excerpta Medica,
Amsterdam.

35. Chiodini,P.G.,and Liuzzi,A.(1979):The Regulation of
Growth Hormone Secretion.Eden Press,Montreal.

36. Liuzzi,A.,Chiodini,P.G.,Verde,G.,Cozzi,R.,Botalla,L.,
and Silvestrini,F.(1981):In:Endocrinology 1980,
edited by Cumming,J.A.,Funder,J.W.,and Mendelson,
F.A.O.,pp719-24.Elsevier,Amsterdam.

37. McGregor,A.M.,Scanlon,M.F.,Hall,R.,and Hall,K.(1979):Br.
Med.J.,2:700-3.

38. Muller,E.E.,Liuzzi,A.,Cocchi,D.,Panerai,A.E.,Oppizzi,G.,
Locatelli,V.,Mantegazza,P.,Silvestrini,F.,and
Chiodini,P.G.(1977):In:Nonstriatal Dopaminergic
Neurons,edited by E.Costa,and G.L.Gessa,pp127-38.
Raven Press,New York.

39. Nissim,M.,Ambrosi,B.,Bernasconi,V.,Giannattasio,G.,
Giovannelli,M.A.,Bassetti,M.,Vaccari,V.,Moriondo,
P.,Spada,A.,Travaglini,P.,and Faglia,G.(1982):J.
Endocrinol.Invest.,5:409-15.

40. Oppizzi,G.,Verde,G.,De Stefano,L.,Cozzi,R.,Botalla,L.,
Liuzzi,A.,and Chiodini,P.G.(1977):Clin.Endocrinol.,
7:267-72.

41. Oppizzi,G.,Botalla,L.,Verde,G.,Cozzi,R.,Liuzzi,A.,and
Chiodini,P.G.(1981):J.Clin.Endocrinol.Metab.,51:
616-9.

42. Patel,Y.C.,Krishna,R.,and Reichlin,S.(1977):N.Engl.J.
Med.,296:529-33.

43. Petrini,M.,Giampietro,O.,and Ambrogi,F.(1981):Drugs
Exptl.Clin.Res.,5:649-52.

44. Podvalova,I.,and Dlabac,A.(1972):Res.Clin.Stud.Headache,
3:325-8.

45. Prysor-Jones,R.A.,Kennedy,S.J.,O'Sullivan,J.P.,and
Jenkins,J.S.(1981):Acta Endocrinol.,98:14-23.

46. Quabbe,H.J.(1981):Acta Endocrinol.(Suppl.),240:Abst.66.

47. Reganchary,S.S.,Tomita,T,Jefferies,B.K,and Watanabe,I.
(1982):Neurosurgery,10:242-9.

48. Rivier,J.,Spiess,J.,Thorner,M.,and Vale,W.(1983):Nature,
300:276-8.

49. Rubin,A.L.,Levin,S.R.,Bernstein,R.G.,Tyrrell,J.B.,Noacco
C.,and Forsham,P.H.(1973):J.Clin.Endocrinol.Metab.,
37:160-2.

50. Sachdev,J.,Tunbridge,W.G.M.,Weightman,D.R.,Gomez-Pan,A., and Hall,R.(1975):Lancet,2:1164-8.

51. Saito,S.,Abe,K.,Yoshida,H.,Kaneko,T.,Nakamura,E.,Shiruzu N.,and Yanaihara,N.(1971):Endocrinol.Jpn.,17:101-8.

52. Salti,I.S.,and Istfan,N.(1979):N.Engl.J.Med.,301:386-91.

53. Smythe,G.A.,and Lazarus,L.(1974):J.Clin.Invest.,54:116-21.

54. Spada,A.,and Sartorio,A.,Bassetti,M.,Pezzo,G.and Giannattasio,G.(1982):J.Clin.Endocrinol.Metab.,55:734-9.

55. Spark,R.F.,Baker,R.,Bienford,C.,and Borgland,R.(1982): J.A.M.A.,247:312-7.

56. Stepien,H.,Wolamink,A.,and Pawlikowski,M.(1978):J.Neur. Transm.,42:239-44.

57. Tallo,D.,and Malarkey,W.B.(1981):J.Clin.Endocrinol. Metab.,53:1278-81.

58. Thorner,M.O.,Chail,A.,Aitken,M.,Benker,G.,Bloom,S.R., Mortimer,C.H.,Sanders,P.,Stuart Mason,A.,and Besser,G.M.,(1975):Br.Med.J.,1:299-303.

59. Thorner,M.O.,Perryman,R.L.,Cronin,M.J.,Rogol,A.D., Draznin,M.,Johanson,A.,Vale,W.,Horvath,E.,and Kovacs,K.(1982):J.Clin.Invest.,70:965-977.

60. Thorner,M.O.,Spiess,J.,Vance,M.L.,Rogol,A.D.,Kaiser, D.L.,Webster,J.D.,Rivier,J.Borges,J.L.,Bloom,S.R., Cronin,M.J.,Evans,W.S.,and MacLeod,R.M.(1983):Lancet, 2:24-8.

61. Tindall,G.T.,Kovacs,K.,Horvath,E.,and Thorner,M.O.(1982) J.Clin.Endocrinol.Metab.,55:1178-83.

62. Verde,G.,Chiodini,P.G.,Liuzzi,A.,Cozzi,R.,Spelta,B., Dallabonzana,D.,Rainer,E.,and Horowski,R.(1979): J.Endocrinol.Invest.,4:405-9.

63. Wass,J.A.H.,Thorner,M.O.,Morris,D.V.,Rees,L.H.,Stuart Mason,A.,Jones,A.E.,and Besser,G.M.(1977):Br.Med. J.,1:875-8.

64. Wass,J.A.H.,Moult,P.J.,Thorner,M.O,Dacie,J.E., Charlsworth,M.,Jones,M.E.,and Besser,G.M.(1979): Lancet,2:66-9.

65. Wass,J.A.H.,Williams,J.,Charlsworth,M.,Kinosley,D.P.E., Halliday,A.M.,Doniack,I.Rees,L.H.,MacDonald,V.I., and Besser,G.M.(1982):Br.Med.J.,284:1908-11.

66. Wollesen,F.,Andersen,T.,and Kerle,A.(1982):Ann.Int. Med.,96:281-6.

67. Wood,S.M.,Ch'Ng,J.L.C.,Adams,E.F.,Webster,J.D.,Joplin, G.F.,Mashiter,K.,and Bloom,S.R.(1983):Br.Med.J., 286:1687-91.

Progress in Cancer Research and Therapy,
Vol. 31, edited by F. Bresciani, et al.
Raven Press, New York © 1984.

Peptide Hormones in Various Types of Gastro-Entero-Pancreatic Tumors: Immunohistochemical Patterns and Evolutionary Background

*S. Falkmer, **H. Mårtensson, **A. Nobin, and † F. Sundler

*Department of Pathology, University of Lund, Malmö General Hospital, S-214 01 Malmö; **Department of Surgery, University of Lund, University Hospital, S-221 85 Lund; and † Department of Histology, University of Lund, S-223 62 Lund, Sweden*

For several reasons, tumors of the gastro-entero-pancreatic (GEP) neuroendocrine system are of particular interest in cancer research. They offer unique possibilities to follow tumor cell differentiation because their autonomous growth is usually accompanied by likewise autonomous synthesis and release of well-known neurohormonal peptides and/or biogenic amines. This hormone production and secretion may also evoke characteristic clinical syndromes; they can often be cured by extirpation of the GEP endocrine tumor or by drug-induced suppression of its hormone production. The hormonal peptides and amines can also be used as tumor markers to facilitate the clinical diagnosis and to monitor the course of the disease. The two facts that the tumors most often are multihormonal and that a whole spectrum of nodular hyperplasias, genuine adenomas and outspoken carcinomas can occur in several endocrine organs more or less concomitantly - the so-called multiple endocrine adenopathy (MEA) - have initiated an intense scientific research about the onto- and phylogenetic evolution of the neuroendocrine system and its neurohormonal peptides (4,5,8,9).

Despite the fact that the GEP endocrine neoplasms at present fascinate a broad spectrum of scientists in biomedical cancer research, a correct clinical-pathological diagnosis can be difficult to make in the individual case; the same statement applies to the prognosis, *i.e.* our efforts to predict the subsequent course of the disease. This implies that there is a need for a better definition and classification of these tumors.

The aim of the present report is to summarize the "state of the art" as regards the immunohistochemical (IHC) pattern of GEP neurohormonal peptides and its evolutionary background in the tumor pathology of the large neuroendocrine system. In addition, we suggest on the basis of our recent findings, a "flow chart" scheme for an optimal and complete investigation of GEP neuroendocrine tumors.

BRIEF CLINICO-PATHOLOGICAL BACKGROUND

In a clinical retrospective analysis of 156 patients with gastrointestinal carcinoid tumors (20), and in correlated, clinical, histopathological, and IHC studies of GEP endocrine neoplasms of man (1,2,19, 21), we have recently been able to show that most GEP endocrine tumors are asymptomatic and have no, or rather few, specific symptoms. For the ileal carcinoids this results in a high incidence of metastases at the time of operation. The greatest prevalence of clinical symptoms of endocrine disorder occurs in the endocrine neoplasms of the stomach/duodenum and the pancreatic islet parenchyma; here the tumors can give rise to specific symptoms in about half the number of patients. These poor possibilities to detect GEP neuroendocrine tumors pre-operatively also imply that the correct diagnosis is often not made until at the histopathological examination, not seldom as a surprise.

As to the survival rate, it was found that, for the classical ileal carcinoid, this was correlated to the size of the primary tumor and, of course, to the extent of the metastases (19,20); moreover, it is well known that carcinoids in the appendix and in the rectum usually are small and only exceptionally give rise to metastases; consequently, they are essentially of rather benign character. Efforts to use the microscopic growth pattern of the tumor parenchyma for classification and prognostic purposes have, so far, not been particularly successful (14,19).

IHC PATTERN OF NEUROHORMONAL PEPTIDES AND CLINICAL PICTURE OF GEP

ENDOCRINE NEOPLASMS

In our studies of patients with neuroendocrine tumors of the GEP organs we have evaluated our IHC observations against the background of not only the clinical picture but also the results of a conventional histopathological classification of carcinoid tumors by means of their location (32) growth pattern (14,27), tinctorial features (10), and serotonin content. So far, supplementary ultrastructural examinations and radioimmunoassays (RIA) of neurohormones in the blood and the tumors have only been performed to a limited extent.

"Foregut Carcinoids".
As described in detail in a more comprehensive report (2), based on a retrospective study of 27 patients with endocrine tumors of the stomach, duodenum, upper jejunum, and pancreas - 6,5,2, and 14 patients, respectively, - the majority of these neoplasms were found to be multihormonal with a pattern of neurohormone immunoreactive tumor cells well in conformity with that of their cells of origin. Thus, some of the carcinoids of the stomach, duodenum and upper jejunum were found to contain gastrin, somatostatin, and PP (pancreatic polypeptide) immunoreactive cells, whereas the islet-cell tumors of the pancreas often showed a great variety of insulin, somatostatin, glucagon, PP, VIP (vasoactive intestinal polypeptide), substance P, neurotensin, enkephalin, calcitonin, and ACTH (adrenocorticotropic hormone) immunoreactive tumor cells. In 13 of the 27 patients overt signs of endocrine disorder were observed clinically, in most cases associated with elevated peptide hormone levels in the blood. The most common and distinct syndromes observed were the hypoglycemic ("insulinoma") (with hyperinsulinemia), the hyperglycemic, cutaneous ("glucagonoma") (with hyperglucagonemia), the ulcerogenic

("Zollinger-Ellison") ("with hypergastrinemia), the diarrheogenic ("VIP-oma" or "Verner-Morrison") (with high VIP levels in the blood) and the Cushing syndrome (with high blood levels of cortisol). Of these 13 patients, 10 had their tumors in the pancreas, 2 in the stomach, and 1 in the duodenum.

The most common immunoreactive GEP neurohormonal peptide in the islet-cell tumors was PP, followed in incidence by somatostatin, insulin, glucagon, gastrin and VIP. The prevalence of PP immunoreactive tumor cells is in conformity with the recent report that PP can be used as a specific marker for GEP endocrine tumors (22). No clear-cut association could be found between the peptide hormone content of these multihormonal endocrine neoplasms and their size or growth pattern, their tinctorial reactions and contents of serotonin cells, and the sex and age of the patients, as well as the subsequent course of the disease. Not only argyrophil but also argentaffin tumors were observed. Members of families with MEA, type 1, occurred; they often had multiple tumor nodules in their pancreas.

These observations agree with those recently made by others as summarized in some recent overviews (5,12,13); here it is stressed how necessary an IHC analysis of the tumor parenchyma is for a precise classification. Pancreatic endocrine neoplasms are obvious models of tumor cell heterogeneity (13) and all authors of reports of recent investigations with modern IHC techniques of gastroduodenal carcinoids seem to agree that these tumors also produce a variety of neurohormonal peptides and, in addition, biogenic amines (5). Additional secretory products of the foregut carcinoids obviously exist and remain to be isolated and identified; a typical example is the ECL tumors of the stomach; they have been claimed to be part of a recently described clinical syndrome, consisting of achylia, pernicious anemia, and hypergastrinemia (28). Other clinical syndromes remain to be better characterized and defined before they can be generally recognized; two typical examples are those due to overproduction of somatostatin and PP. For the first one of these two examples some constellations of signs and clinical symptoms have already been suggested; for the second one any clinical syndrome associated with the elevated PP-levels in blood have not yet been described. The "somatostatinoma" syndrome comprises, in addition to hypersomatostatinemia, steatorrhea, mild diabetes mellitus, and cholelithiasis (5, 15).

Of evolutionary interest is the fact that some GEP peptide hormone immunoreactive cells seem to be less prone to become neoplastically transformed than the others (8, 9). A typical example is the GIP ("gastric inhibitory peptide" or "glucose-dependent insulinotropic peptide") cells; no clear-cut GIP-producing tumor has, so far, been described. GIP has been claimed to be the most recent addition to the secretin/glucagon family, assuming that most GEP neurohormonal peptides have developed from a hypothetical ancestral peptide molecule by gene duplications and independent evolution of the mutated products (9). Phylogenetical studies indicate that GIP is mainly a vertebrate hormone involved in the enteroinsular axis (7). Could it be that neuroendocrine cells of low evolutionary age are more resistant to neoplastic transformation?

"Midgut Carcinoids".

In comparison with the variegated pattern of neurohormonal peptide immunoreactive tumor cells shown by the GEP endocrine tumors of foregut origin, that of the classical ileal and appendiceal carcinoids displays an astonishingly narrow spectrum of such cells; at least this statement applies to retrospective studies where IHC investigations have been made of sections of paraffin-embedded specimens, fixed in conventional 10% formalin (19). Apart from the rather ubiquitous presence of serotonin in these usually argentaffin tumor cells, it is – among the neurohormonal peptides – practically only substance P immunoreactivity that is more regularly displayed by the tumor cells (Fig. 1). The classical carcinoid syndrome, essentially evoked by serotonin overproduction by metastatic nodules in the liver, is the only clinical syndrome associated with midgut carcinoids (19); they are often discovered as an incidental finding at appendectomy or at autopsy (19). It has been claimed that many patients die with their carcinoids instead of from them (3).

This allegedly occurring relative monotony in the IHC and clinical-pathological features of the midgut carcinoids is at present being questioned. By recent correlated ultrastructural (EM) and light-micro-scopical examinations it has been shown that small-gut carcinoids usually consist of at least two kinds of tumor cells, *viz.* argentaffin cells with pleomorphic secretion granules of EC (entero-chromaffin) cell type and argyrophil cells with more uncharacteristic spherical granules (18). Moreover, already in retrospective studies of conventional type, it could be found that also somatostatin, glicentin, PP, gastrin, neurotensin, and motilin immunoreactive tumor cells could exceptionally occur in small-gut carcinoids although always as minority cell populations (17,29,30,33).

In order to see whether these somewhat diverging opinions about the IHC pattern of midgut carcinoids of small-gut origin could be due to differences in the techniques used for tissue precessing, we made an IHC study of 14 ileal carcinoids with liver and/or lymph node metastases, where we compared the results after conventional histopathological routines and after optimal tissue processing (2). Some clinical-pathological data about the patients are given in Table 1.

The primary tumors and some of the metastatic nodules were investigated on sections from paraffin-embedded specimens fixed according to conventional histopathological routines in 10% formalin. After the diagnosis had been established histopathologically, new biopsy specimens were taken from one or two of the metastatic nodules in the liver and/or lymph nodes; this time they were fixed by techniques designed to preserve optimally the neurohormone peptide immunoreactivity of the tumor cells.

Two different histochemical procedures were used, both gave the same results. Specimens of the tumor parenchyma were, immediately after excision, frozen in a mixture of propane and propylene, cooled to the temperature of liquid nitrogen, and freeze-dried. Then, they were fixed for 3 hours at 55°C in diethylpyrocarbonate (DEPC) (24) and embedded in paraffin *in vacuo*. Sections, 5-6 μm thick, were cut and used for the IHC analysis. Alternatively, the tumor specimens were immersed for 24 hours in ice-cold, 0.1 M phosphate buffered, 10% formalin, pH 7.2. After thorough rinsing for several days in the same buffer with 5-10% of sucrose added, the specimens were frozen on dry CO_2-ice and cut on a cryostat microtome at -20°C; the sections were about 15 μm thick.

TABLE 1. Some clinico-pathological data of 14 patients with ileal carcinoid tumors, used for studies of the role of different techniques for tissue processing in the IHC analysis of the pattern
of neurohormonal peptides in the tumor cells (cf. TABLE 2).

Patient		Primary Tumor		Clinical Picture			
Ini-ti-als	Age/Sex	Num-ber	Approx. Size (cm)	High Blood Levels of		Car-cinoid Syn-drome?	Follow Up (Years after operation)
				5-HT	Subst. P		
K.B.	70/M	Mult.	1-2	+	nt	No	Alive; 4
M.A.	63/M	Solit.	1-2	(+)	+	No	Alive; 4
G.R.	53/F	Mult.	1-2	+	nt	No	Dead; 1½
A.S.	67/F	Mult.	>2	+	−	Yes	Alive; 2
G.B.	70/F	Mult.	>2	+	+	Yes	Alive; 2½
I.N.	55/M	Solit.	>2	(+)	−	No	Alive; 2½
S.P.	71/M	Mult.	1-2	+	+	Yes	Dead; 2
S.M.	47/F	Solit.	1-2	+	nt	Yes	Dead; 1
M.G.	32/M	Solit.	1-2	+	+	Yes	Alive; 7
A.R.	49/M	Solit.	>2	+	+	Yes	Alive; 2
I.A.	55/F	Solit.	>2	+	+	Yes	Alive; 2
M.T.	64/F	Solit.	1-2	+	+	No	Alive; 1
R.B.	40/M	Mult.	>2	+	nt	Yes	Dead; 1
K.E.P.	53/M	Solit.	<1	+	+	Yes	Dead; 2

a) Increased blood levels of serotonin were assessed both via assays of
5-hydroxytryptamine in blood and/or in platelet-poor plasma and/or via
assays of 5-hydroxy-indole-acetic-acid in the urine. The actual numerical
values are given in a separate report (21)

b) + = At least two of the three techniques used to test the presence of
hyperserotoninemia gave increased values.
(+) = Only one of the three techniques used to test the presence of
hyperserotoninemia gave increased values.

c) + = Significantly increased concentrations of substance P. The actual
numerical values are given in a separate report (21)
  − = Normal concentrations of substance P
 nt = Not tested

Additional tumor specimens were, after initial freeze-drying, fixed by
exposure to formaldehyde vapor for detection of serotonin by the
Falck-Hillarp procedure (19, 21).
    The paraffin and cryostat microtome sections were incubated with
16 different antisera, raised against the following mammalian neurohormonal peptides: Somatostatin, glucagon, glicentin, PP, (both human and
bovine), secretin, VIP, GIP, gastrin, CCK (cholecystokinin), substance P,
neurotensin, ACTH, enkephalin (both "leu"- and "met"-forms), and motilin.
Both the immunofluorescence and the peroxidase-anti-peroxidase (PAP)
procedures were used. Additional methodological details are given in a
separate report (21). A selection of the same antisera was used to test
the presence of the neurohormone peptide immunoreactive tumor cells in
the primary tumors.

Not even by means of these two improved histotechniques were we able
to detect any regularly occurring neurohormone immunoreactive tumor cells
other than substance P cells in these metastases of primary ileal
carcinoids. All the tumors also showed serotonin containing cells. Both
the substance P and serotonin tumor cells were majority cell populations
(Fig. 1). With the exception of one of the primary tumors that harboured
a few enkephalin cells, no other neurohormone immunoreactive tumor cells
were found.

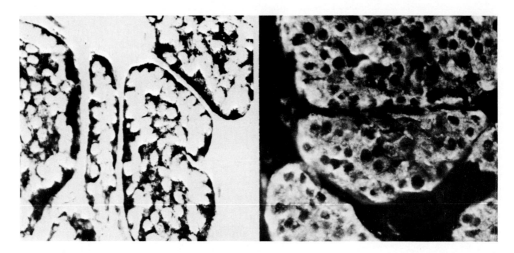

Fig. 1. Medium-power photomicrographs of sections of a liver metastasis
of a primary ileal carcinoid (Case "I.A." in Tables 1 and 2), processed
by histotechniques optimal for demonstration of neurohormonal peptide
immunoreactivity and serotonin in the tumor cells. The tumor nodule shows
the typical insular growth pattern. The PAP procedure for the detection
of substance P immunoreactive tumor cells (left) reveals that they (black
cells with white nuclei) occur as a majority cell population. Likewise,
the Falck-Hillarp technique for histochemical demonstration of serotonin
tumor cells (cf. 9,21) (right) shows that practically all the tumor cells
contain this biogenic amine (bright cells with dark nuclei).

x 500 (left and right)

A striking contrast was obtained when the same antisera were applied
in IHC analyses of the sections from the primary tumors fixed and
embedded for routine histopathological examination; here, only a few of
the sections showed any substance P immunoreactive tumor cells and none
exhibited any other kind of immunoreactivity with the antisera used
(Table 2). The presence of serotonin in the tumor cells could be
visualized in all tumor nodules of all the cases, irrespective of the
technique used for tissue processing.

We have, consequently, shown that substance P - or other members of
its large tachykinin family, like eledoisin, physalaemin (26) - is
almost as common a constituent of the tumor cells of ileal carcinoids
as serotonin, and that both hormones, to some extent, can be used as

TABLE 2. Differences between conventional and optimal histotechniques in IHC analyses of the occurrence of GEP neurohormone immunoreactive tumor cells in primary tumors and in metastatic nodules in the liver and/or the lymph nodes of ileal carcinoids from the same patients as in TABLE 1.

Patient Initials	Histotechnical Procedure for Tissue Processing							
	Conventional Methods[a]				Optimal Histotechniques[b]			
	Primary Tumor		Metastatic Nodules		Primary Tumor		Metastatic Nodules	
	Subst P	Other N.h.p.	Subst P	Other N.h.p.	Subst P	Other N.h.p.	Subst P	Other N.h.p.
K.B.	+	0	+	0	nt	nt	+	0
M.A.	–	0	–	0	nt	nt	+	0
G.R.	–	0	–	0	nt	nt	0	0
A.S.	–	0	–	0	++	0	+	0
G.B.	–	0	–	0	++	Enk	+	0
I.N.	–	0	–	0	nt	nt	+	0
S.P.	–	0	–	0	nt	nt	+	0
S.M.	–	0	–	0	nt	nt	+	0
M.G.	–	0	–	0	nt	nt	+	0
A.R.	–	0	–	0	nt	nt	+	0
I.A.	–	0	–	0	nr	nt	++	0
M.T.	–	0	–	0	+	0	+	0
R.B.	–	0	–	0	+	0	+	0
K.E.P.	–	0	–	0	+	0	+	0

[a] Fixation in 10% formalin, followed by routine paraffin embedding.

[b] Immediate freezing, followed by freeze-drying, fixation in DEPC and paraffin embedding *in vacuo*. Alternatively: Fixation in 10% buffered formalin, followed by thorough rinsing in sucrose buffer and cryostat microtome sectioning (Same results with both procedures).

Enk = Enkephalin
nt = not tested
0 = no immunoreactive cells
+ = moderate numbers of immunoreactive cells
++ = numerous immunoreactive cells
N.h.p. = Neurohormonal peptides

markers for these tumors. The possibilities to demonstrate substance P by means of an IHC analysis of biopsy specimens, or of material obtained at gut resection, or even at autopsy, depend, however, to a great extent on the techniques used for tissue processing; the results shown in Table 2 drastically illustrate how vulnerable substance P is to the rather poor histotechniques used for conventional histopathological assessments.

On the other hand, our inability to demonstrate any regularly occurring additional kinds of GEP neurohormone immunoreactive tumor cells in these 14 midgut tumors can obviously not be explained as a result of poor IHC analysis procedures. Explanations for the discrepancy between our results

and those of others must be sought elsewhere, for instance in differences
in the composition of the tumor material and in the specificity
of the antisera used (21). Consequently, we still think that it is
justified to characterize the midgut carcinoids, particularly those from
the ileum, as serotonin-producing endocrine tumors with a distinctly
narrow spectrum of GEP neurohormonal peptides, essentially consisting
of substance P.

"Hindgut Carcinoids".

It surprised most investigators when it recently was realized that
the clinically silent classical rectal carcinoid often shows such a broad
spectrum of GEP neurohormone immunoreactive tumor cells as has, by now,
been reported independently from a rather great number of pathology laboratories (1,5,23). In our own series of 25 cases, studied "retrospec-
tively" without any optimal tissue processing techniques, no less than
21 were found to contain tumor cells displaying GEP neurohormone peptide
immunoreactivity (1). Of these 21 cases, 11 harboured more than one kind
of hormone. In contrast, only 4 of the tumors were found to contain serotonin. Majority cell populations could be made up by PP and/or glucagon/
/glicentin immunoreactive tumor cells. Other more or less commonly found
GEP neurohormonal peptides were insulin, somatostatin, substance P,
enkephalin, and β-endorphin. Our results have been confirmed by others
(5,23). Antisera raised against other GEP neurohormonal peptides, such
as secretin, VIP, GIP, gastrin, CCK, neurotensin, motilin, calcitonin,
and ACTH, have, so far, failed to demonstrate any immunoreactive tumor
cells (5). Both non-argyrophil, argyrophil, and even argentaffin rectal
carcinoids occur. The growth pattern showed wide variations. The tumors
were clinically benign and evoked no signs or symptoms of endocrine
disorder.

Quite recently, it has been shown by means of an IHC analysis, using
a region-specific PP antiserum and an antiserum raised against a newly
discovered member of the PP family, *viz.*, PYY, (the polypeptide YY), that
the tumor cells of the rectal carcinoids contain a PP-like molecule
rather than genuine PP, and that PYY immunoreactive tumor cells are rare
(31) despite the fact that PYY cells are rather common in normal human
colon and rectum (6).

Except for the presence of insulin and enkephalin/endorphin immunoreactive tumor cells (1), the kinds of GEP neurohormonal peptides discovered by IHC in our rectal carcinoids can be said to reflect the GEP
hormone production of their cells of origin (5). The appearance of insulin cells in these tumors is of great phylogenetical interest; in deuterostomian invertebrates, including amphioxus, there is no islet parenchyma, and the insulin cells occur as open types in the mucosa of the
alimentary tract (9). In the rectal carcinoids the tumor cells have,
thus, regressed to a prevertebrate evolutionary stage (see below).
Whether this statement applies also to the enkephalin/endorphin immunoreactive cells remains to be investigated; the phylogeny of the epithelial opioid immunoreactive cells in the mucosa of the alimentary tract
is still incompletely known.

Classification, Based on Neurohormone Peptide Contents.

From the accounts given above of the pattern of neurohormone peptide
contents in foregut, midgut, and hindgut carcinoid tumor cells, and of
their associated clinical signs and symptoms of endocrine disorders, it
is obvious that marked differences exist between these three main groups
of endocrine tumors of the GEP organs. The differences can be used for a

combined anatomical and functional classification of these neoplasms.
The main features of such a classification have been summarized in
Table 3.

In the individual case, particularly when only a biopsy specimen
from a metastatic nodule is available for examination, all additional
facts about the details of the IHC pattern of the tumor cells must be
taken into account, as well as their ultrastructure (2,5,19). Additional
basic data about the size and multiplicity of the tumor, the extent of
its metastatic nodules, its serotonin content, and its growth pattern
should, of course, also be included in the ultimate diagnosis in order
to try to adequately predict the subsequent course of the disease
(see below).

TABLE 3. Classification scheme for GEP neuroendocrine tumors, based on
their anatomical localization and on their spectrum of neurohormonal immunoreactive tumor cells and associated clinical
signs and symptoms of endocrine disorder

Tumor Origin	Organ	Immunohisto-chemical Pattern	Clinical Symptoms	Prognosis
Foregut	Stomach Duodenum Pancreas Jejunum	Multihormonal	Several Kinds of Syndromes	Variable
Midgut	Ileum	Few Neuro-hormones	Carcinoid Syndrome	Variable
	Appendix		No	Good
Hindgut	Colon Rectum	Multihormonal	No	Good

SUGGESTED MODE OF APPROACH FOR AN OPTIMAL HISTOPATHOLOGIC

CLASSIFICATION OF GEP ENDOCRINE TUMORS

In Fig. 2 an oversimplified "flow chart" scheme is given, illustrating the mode of approach used in our laboratories for a histopathological assessment and classification of a tumor that, from its gross aspects
and its microscopic growth pattern can be suspected to be a GEP neuroendocrine neoplasm.

Diagnostic Principles.
The endocrine character of a tumor is usually recognized from its
microscopic growth pattern; the provisional diagnosis can then be confirmed by means of the Grimelius silver nitrate procedure; it is a well-
-known and technically simple method (10,33). Alternatively, neuron-
-specific enolase (12,13,25) can be used; it is a more expensive and
complicated technique, sometimes difficult to evaluate, but has the
advantage that it also detects those GEP endocrine cells that are non-
-argyrophil or only faintly argyrophil with the Grimelius technique,
viz. the insulin, somatostatin, PP, and CCK cells (10,25). In practice,

identification of these four endocrine cell types is, however, not a diagnostic problem; they are easily identified in the next step in our diagnostic "flow chart", *viz*. the IHC analyses, usually be means of the PAP method (Fig. 2). Additional diagnostic accuracy can then be obtained via a supplementary ultrastructural analysis. A typical example is when a biopsy specimen of a metastatic nodule from an unknown primary tumor should be further analyzed after the findings of argyrophil tumor cells with immunoreactivity against substance P; the presence of pleomorphic secretion granules (and serotonin fluorescence) in the tumor cells will then confirm the preliminary diagnosis of a metastasis from a primary carcinoid in the ileum. Another example is the ECL tumor of the stomach, where the parenchymal cells can be only faintly argyrophilic or even non--argyrophilic (usually falsely so, due to poor fixation) and completely devoid of any kind of GEP neurohormone immunoreactivity; here, an electron micro-scopical examination (even on conventionally fixed and paraffin embedded specimens, can establish the correct diagnosis, as described in one of our actual cases (2).

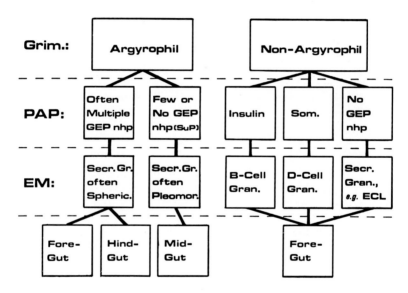

FIG. 2. "Flow chart" scheme for a histopathological-IHC-ultrastructural analysis of GEP endocrine tumors.
Grim = Grimelius' silver nitrate procedure
PAP = The Peroxidase-Anti-Peroxidase IHC method
EM   = Electron Microscopy
nhp   = Neuro-hormonal peptides
Su P = Substance P
Sect.Gr = Secretion Granules

Finally, with all the morphologic and IHC data at hand, together with the results of a thorough clinical investigation of the patient (Table 3), it should be possible, in the individual case to arrive at a correct diagnosis, even pre-operatively when only a biopsy specimen is

available for examination, and to give at least a fair prediction of the
subsequent course of the disease. The ultimate clinico-pathological
diagnosis of a GEP neuroendocrine neoplasm should then contain at least
the following information:
1. Its site of origin;
2. Its histopathological features, as regards;
    A) Growth pattern and differentiation;
    B) Presence of argyrophil/argentaffin cells;
    C) Occurrence of metastatic nodules;
3. Its IHC spectrum of GEP neurohormones;
4. Signs or symptoms of endocrine disorder.

    A practical example of such an ultimate diagnosis would then be
(case "A.R." in Tables 1 and 2): "Endocrine tumor - argentaffin carcinoma
(carcinoid) - of the ileum; high differentiation ("insular" type),
invading the whole gut wall; lymph node and liver metastases; serotonin
and substance P production; carcinoid syndrome".

    Ideal Preservation of Tumor Specimens.
    When a pre-operative diagnosis of an endocrine GEP tumor seems
justified, for instance from a histopathologic and IHC analysis of the
kind outlined above of a biopsy specimen of a metastasis, and a complete
analysis of the tumor parenchyma for scientific purposes is aimed at,
we would - on the basis of our experience, so far - suggest that the
following procedure for tissue preservation is followed at the main subsequent surgical intervention for extirpation of the primary tumor and/or
(additional) metastatic nodules:
    As soon as specimens from the tumor parenchyma can be taken, already
early at laparotomy, small thin pieces should immediately be excised for
the following purposes.
1. For optimal tissue processing for IHC investigations of the presence
    of GEP neurohormonal peptides: Immersion fixation in phosphate
    buffered 4% formaldehyde (=10% formalin), pH 7.2, at 0-4°C.
2. For ultrastructural examination: Immersion fixation in a mixture of
    1% glutaraldehyde and 3% formaldehyde, followed by postfixation in
    OsO_4.
3. For RIA of the presence of GEP neurohormonal peptides: Deep freezing,
    for instance on dry CO_2-ice, and subsequent preservation at -20°C
    (or lower).
4. For routine histopathological diagnosis: Immersion fixation in Bouin's
    fluid at room temperature. Conventional immersion fixation in 10%
    formalin can be made of the rest of the tissue specimens obtained at
    the surgical intervention.
    If this protocol is followed, adequate material can be secured, not
only for a complete histopathological and IHC diagnosis, but also for
supplementary ultrastructural examinations and a correlated biochemical
analysis of the tumor parenchyma with possibilities to isolate and
identify the neurohormonal peptides produced by the tumor cells.

EVOLUTIONARY ASPECTS

    Some phylogenetic   explanations and speculations have already been
given above; one example is the absence of GIP cells in foregut carcinoids; another is the appearance of insulin cells in hindgut carcinoids.
The neurohormonal pattern displayed by the tumor cells is generally in
good conformity with the spectrum of neuroendocrine cells present in the
different parts of the GEP organs (1,2,5,6,13,31). Exceptions can usual-

ly be well explained with some knowledge of the phylogeny and ontogeny of the neurohormonal peptides and their cells of origin.

As accounted for in a recent review of the ontogeny and phylogeny of the neuroendocrine system (9), the GEP endocrine cells have evolved from neurally programmed progenitor cells. Although it has been claimed that some of the well-known GEP neurohormonal peptides occur already in unicellular eukaryote - and even prokaryote - organisms as messenger substances for intercellular communication (16), it is not until the level of the coelenterates that their presence is well established by means of correlated IHC examination and RIA (8,11). Here, they occur only in the nervous system, among the peptides isolated are substance P, neurotensin, CCK, and bombesin (11). Analogous investigations of the central nervous system of larval and adult stages of protostomian invertebrates (annelids; insects) confirm that apparently all the GEP neurohormonal peptides are present in neurosecretory cells before they appear in the alimentary tract mucosa and its associated glands. In deuterostomian invertebrates and in vertebrates, practically all the GEP neurohormonal peptides show a dual distribution in the central nervous system and the digestive tract, recently referred to as the brain-gut axis (7). With the advent of the first vertebrates some 600 million years ago, the neuroendocrine system underwent further specialization, with the appearance of such compact endocrine glands as the pituitary, the thyroid, and the adrenal glands, as well as the islet parenchyma, first occurring as a separate islet organ, later on included in the pancreas as the islets of Langerhans(7,9). In the normal gut of adult vertebrates no insulin cells have ever been found (9).

Ontogenetically, the neuroendocrine system essentially follows the famous Haeckel principle, *i.e.* " the ontogeny recapitulates phylogeny" (9). Consequently, when the GEP endocrine tumors show IHC features different from those of their cells of origin, their neoplastically transformed cells show a regression towards both a phylogenetically and ontogenetically earlier evolutionary stage. A typical example is the appearance of gastrin immunoreactive cells in islet-cell tumors. Although gastrin cells are not found in the mammalian pancreatic islet parenchyma after birth, they are well known to be transiently present during fetal life, for instance in rats (7).

SUMMARY

GEP endocrine tumors are of great importance in cancer research, mainly due to their autonomous production of neurohormonal peptides and biogenic amines. Because of rather uncharacteristic clinical symptoms, they are often not detected until histopathologic examination. Diagnosis is usually based on their gross features and their rather typical microscopic growth patterns. By means of a comprehensive IHC analysis of the tumor cells, supplemented by ultrastructural examination and RIA, a more precise diagnosis and functional classification can, however, be attained. The IHC pattern of neurohormonal peptides is to a great extent rather characteristic for GEP endocrine tumors of different anatomical sites and reflects that of their cells of origin.

Thus, GEP endocrine tumors of foregut type, *i.e.* carcinoids in the stomach, duodenum, and upper jejunum, and pancreatic islet-cell tumors, show a variegated pattern of neurohormonal peptides; most of them are multihormonal; they are known to be combined with several clinical endocrine syndromes. In contrast, endocrine tumors of midgut origin, *i.e.* the classical ileal and appendiceal carcinoids, show a surprisingly narrow spectrum of GEP neurohormonal peptides, essentially containing only substance P. In addition, the tumor cells regularly harbour serotonin. Whereas metastasizing ileal carcinoids can evoke the carcinoid syndrome, appendiceal ones usually run a benign course and give no symptoms of endocrine disorder. Hindgut endocrine tumors, notably the rectal carcinoid, are often multihormonal, displaying a broad spectrum of GEP hormone immunoreactive tumor cells, as a rule characteristic for their cells of origin. Like the appendiceal carcinoids they only rarely metastasize and do not give rise to any endocrine syndromes.

In an investigation of the role of the technique used for tissue processing in the IHC analysis of the hormonal pattern of ileal carcinoids, it was found that substance P is particularly vulnerable to poor histotechniques, and that optimal tissue preservation did not markedly increase the number of neurohormonal peptides that could be detected in these tumor cells.

A "flow-chart" is given for a routine histopathological and IHC analysis of GEP endocrine tumors, including suggestions for optimal tissue processing in the operation theater, and some classification principles. Lastly, the fundamental features in the onto- and phylogenetical background of the neurohormonal peptide production of these tumor cells are outlined.

ACKNOWLEDGMENT

This work was supported by grants from the Swedish Medical Research Council (Projects No. 12X-718 and 12X-4499), the Swedish Diabetes Association, the Cancer Research Foundation at Malmo General Hospital, the Albert Pahlsson Foundation, and the Medical Faculty at the University of Lund.

REFERENCES

1. Alumets, J., Alm, P., Falkmer, S., Håkanson, R., Ljungberg, O., Mårtensson, H., Sundler, F., and Tibblin, S. (1981): *Cancer,* 48:2409-2415.
2. Alumets, J., Sundler, F., Falkmer, S., Ljungberg, O., Håkanson, R., Mårtensson, H., Nobin, A., and Lasson, Å.(1983): *Ultrastruct. Pathol.,* 5:469-486.
3. Berge, T., and Linell, F. (1976): *Acta Path.Microbiol.Scand.Sect.A,* 84:322-330.
4. Creutzfeldt, W. (1984): In: *Evolution and Tumour Pathology of the Neuroendocrine System,* edited by S.Falkmer, R. Håkanson, and F. Sundler (in press). Elsevier, Amsterdam.
5. Dayal, Y., and Wolfe, H.J. (1984): In: *Evolution and Tumour Pathology of the Neuroendocrine System,* edited by S. Falkmer, R. Håkanson,. and F. Sundler (in press). Elsevier, Amsterdam.
6. El-Salhy, M., Grimelius, L., Wilander, E., Ryberg, B., Terenius, L., Lundberg, J.M. and Tatemoto, K. (1983): *Histochemistry,* 77:15-23.
7. Falkmer, S., El-Salhy, M., and Titlbach, M. (1984): In: *Evolution and Tumour Pathology of the Neuroendocrine System,* edited by S. Falkmer, R. Håkanson, and F. Sundler (in press). Elsevier, Amsterdam.

8. Falkmer, S., and Grimmelikhuijzen, C.J.P. (1981): In: *Phyletic App-roaches to Cancer*, edited by C.J. Dawe, J.C. Harshbarger, S. Kondo, T. Sugimura and S. Takayama, pp. 333-346. Japan Sci. Soc. Press, Tokyo

9. Falkmer, S., and Van Noorden, S. (1983): Handb.Exp. Pharmacol. 66/I:81-119.

10. Grimelius, L., and Wilander, E. (1980): *Invest. Cell. Path.*, 3:3-12.

11. Grimmelikhuijzen, C.J.P. (1984): In: *Evolution and Tumour Pathology of the Neuroendocrine System*, edited by S. Falkmer, R. Håkanson, and F. Sundler (in press). Elsevier, Amsterdam.

12. Heitz, P.U., Kasper, M., Polak, J.M., and Klöppel, G. (1982): *Hum. Pathol.*, 13:263-271.

13. Heitz, P.U., and Klöppel, G. (1984): In: *Evolution and Tumour Patho-logy of the Neuroendocrine System*, edited by S. Falkmer, R. Håkanson, and F. Sundler (in press). Elsevier, Amsterdam.

14. Johnson, L.A., Lavin, P., Moertel, C.G., Weiland, L., Dayal, Y., Doos, W.G., Geller, S.A., Cooper, H.S., Nime, F., Masse, S., Simson, I.W., Sumner, H., Fölsch, E., and Engström, P. (1983): *Cancer*, 51:882-889.

15. Larsson, L.-I., Holst, J.J., Kuhl, C., Lundqvist, G., Hirsch, M.A., Ingemansson, S., Lindkaer-Jensen, S., Rehfeld, J.F. and Schwartz, T.W. (1977): *Lancet*, 1:666-668.

16. LeRoith, D., and Roth, J. (1984): In: *Evolution and Tumour Pathology of the Neuroendocrine System*, edited by S. Falkmer, R. Håkanson, and F. Sundler (in press). Elsevier, Amsterdam.

17. Lundqvist, M., and Wilander, E. (1981): *Acta Path.Microbiol.Scand. Sect.A.* 89:335-337.

18. Lundqvist, M., and Wilander, E. (1982): *Acta Path.Microbiol.Immunol. Scand. Sect.A*, 90:317-321.

19. Mårtensson, H. (1983): *Gut Endocrine Tumors; On the Classification, Diagnosis, and Treatment with Special Reference to Midgut Tumors*. Bull. Dept. Surg., Univ. Lund, 43:1-49.

20. Mårtensson, H., Nobin, A,, and Sundler, F. (1983): *Acta Chir.Scand.*, 149:607-616.

21. Mårtensson, H., Nobin, A., Sundler, F., and Falkmer, S. (1984) Ann. Surg. (Submitted)

22. Öberg, K., Grimelius, L., Lundqvist, G., and Lörelius, L.-E. (1981): *Acta Med. Scand.* 210:145-152.

23. O'Brian, D.S., Dayal, Y., De Lellis, R.A., Tischler, A.S., Bendon, R., and Wolfe, H.J. (1982): *Am.J.Surg.Pathol.*, 6:131-142.

24. Pearse, A.G.E., and Polak, J.M. (1975): *Histochem.J.*, 7:179-186.

25. Polak, J.M., Bloom, S.R., and Marangos, P.J. (1984): In: *Evolution and Tumour Pathology of the Neuroendocrine System*, edited by S. Falkmer, R. Håkanson, and F. Sundler (in press). Elsevier, Amsterdam.

26. Skrabanek, P., and Powell, D. (1983): *Substance P.* Annual Res.Rev., 3:1-184.

27. Soga, J., and Tazawa, K. (1971): *Cancer*, 28:990-998.

28. Wilander, E. (1980): *Virch.Arch. (Pathol.Anat.)*, 387:371-373.

29. Wilander, E., and El-Salhy, M. (1981): *Acta Path.Microbiol.Scand. Sect.A*, 89:247-250.

30. Wilander, E., Grimelius, L., Portela-Gomes, G., Lundquist, G., Skoog, V., and Westermark, P. (1979): *Scand.J.Gastroent* 14: Suppl. 53:19-25.

31. Wilander, E., El-Salhy, M., Lundqvist, M., Grimelius, L., Terenius,

L., Lundberg, J.M., Tatemoto, K., and Schwartz, T.W. (1983): *Virch.Arch. (Pathol.Anat.)*, 401:67-72.

32. Williams, E.D., and Sandler, M. (1963): *Lancet* 1:238-239.

33. Yang, K., Ulich, T., Cheng, L., and Lewin, K.J. (1983): *Cancer*, 51:1918-1926.

Progress in Cancer Research and Therapy,
Vol. 31, edited by F. Bresciani, et al.
Raven Press, New York © 1984.

Hypercalcemia of Malignancy: Pathogenesis and Treatment

A. Valentin-Opran and P.J. Meunier

*U. 234 INSERM "Pathologie des Tissus Calcifiés," Faculté A. Carrel,
69008 Lyon, France*

Malignancy is one of the most frequent etiologies of hypercalcemia (HCa), second only to hyperparathyroidism (HPT) (19).
Actually, HCa is a common complication in cancer patients,
estimates of its incidence varying from 10 to 20% (28). HCa
is not only responsible for gastrointestinal, renal and neu-
rologic symptoms, but it is also potentially lethal. Thus,
numerous studies have tried to explain its pathogenesis and
to establish its best treatment.

PATHOGENESIS

The main cause of HCa is increased bone resorption, associated with decreased bone formation. In addition, as kidneys
are major regulatory organs of calcium homeostasis, any alteration in renal function, especially dehydration, might precipitate acute HCa. Because it is a disturbance of the bone re-
modelling system, the condition is prone to abrupt shifts
from normal to very high levels of serum calcium, jeopardi-
zing the patient's life much more than other etiologies of
HCa (22).
    No single pathogenetic hypothesis can apply to all forms
of malignant states. Three types of HCa of malignancy must
therefore be considered :
1 - Hematologic malignancies,
2 - Humoral hypercalcemia of malignancy (HHM)
3 - Solid tumors with bone metastases.

Hypercalcemia and hematologic malignancies

Multiple myeloma is the most common example in this group.
HCa is found in about 30% of patients at the time of presentation, and myelomatous patients represent about 20% of all patients with the HCa of malignancy (21).
    In order to understand the mechanisms of the HCa and bone
destruction in multiple myeloma, we have done an histomorphometric study on undecalcified iliac bone biopsies in 118 such
patients. We observed that the main mechanism of bone destruction is osteoclastic. The total trabecular resorption surfaces

were increased by 85%, as compared to healthy controls. The number of osteoclasts was higher in bone areas massively infiltrated by malignant plasma cells, compared to areas that appeared not to be infiltrated. In addition, although more osteoblasts were present, their individual activities were significantly reduced as demonstrated by decreased thickness of osteoid seams and decreased calcification rates (38).

The osteoclastic activation and osteoblastic depression are probably related to the secretion by myeloma cells of a soluble factor, similar to, or the same as, the lymphokine Osteoclast Activating Factor (OAF) (12). This macromolecular protein (13) is secreted by activated B and T lymphocytes (5). The secretion is dependent on monocyte prostaglandin production (40) and requires c.AMP accumulation in lymphocytes (41). In vitro, OAF causes release of calcium by stimulating osteoclastic resorption, while inhibiting collagen synthesis (24). OAF has been found to be produced by established myeloma cell lines, cultures of marrow aspirates and bone explants from myelomatous patients (18, 8). It is also released by lymphoid cell lines, including Burkitt's lymphoma (17).

Humoral Hypercalcemia of malignancy (HHM)

HHM represents about 10% of all patients with the HCa of malignancy. It is associated mainly with cancers of lung, kidney and squamous cell carcinoma of head and neck.

Bone histomorphometric studies in patients having HHM showed increased osteoclastic surfaces contrasting with markedly decreased osteoblastic surfaces (30). This skeletal imbalance in calcium metabolism is due to ectopic secretion of a humoral factor by the tumor cells. However, the nature of the tumoral mediator is still unclear and has been the subject of many speculations. Among these factors, parathyroid hormone (PTH) and prostaglandins (PgS) have been the most extensively studied.

a) Role of ectopic PTH secretion.
Since the clinical picture of the HHM resembled hyperparathyroidism in many respects, it was thought that PTH was responsible for the syndrome. Against this hypothesis is the fact that no such hymoral HCa has ever been found to fulfil all the criteria of ectopic secretion of PTH. Very recently, Simpson et al. (27) have produced new arguments against PTH involvement, using a specific DNA-mRNA hybridization assay. It is based on the principle of base pair hybridization of cloned PTH-DNA with PTH-mRNA. The authors examined 13 human tumors and 3 animal tumors. Five of the human tumors were obtained from hypercalcemic patients. In none of these tumors could they detect the presence of PTH-mRNA.

b) Role of prostaglandins.
There is evidence in vitro and in vivo that tumor cells can produce and secrete excessive amounts of PgE_2 which then act on the skeleton to induce HCa. These results derive mainly from studies in two animal models : the $HSDM_1$ fibrosarcoma in the mouse and the VX_2 carcinoma in the rabbit (34). Evidence

is lacking however that PgS are the humoral factors responsible for HCa in patients. For example, PgE_2, the most potent bone resorbing Pg., is rapidly metabolized in lung, and, for this reason, plasma levels are too low for a metabolic effect in hypercalcemic patients. Furthermore, while treatment of animals with inhibitors of Pg synthesis, such as indomethacin or hydrocortisone, can prevent or reverse HCa (32), it has generally failed to do so in patients with HHM (6).

c) Role of other factors.

It now appears likely that the factor(s) responsible in most cases of HHM are neither PTH, nor PgS, but a family of polypeptides, related to Transforming Growth Factors (TGF). TGF share some of the features observed in "Epidermal Growth Factor" (EGF) or in "Platelet derived Growth Factor" (PDGF), both of which are able to enhance local PgE_2 production by bone (33, 11).

TGFs are identified by the following properties (29) :
They confer a transformed phenotype on untransformed target cells. The transformed phenotype is characterized by changes in cellular shape, loss of density-dependent inhibition of growth in monolayer culture and acquisition of anchorage-independent growth of untransformed cells in soft agar.
They promote cell growth and replication.
Some of them compete with EGF for receptor binding, although they are structurally and antigenically different from EGF (35).

TGF have been detected in conditioned media of cultured tumor cells (25) in tumor cell extracts (25), and recently in the urine of patients with cancer (36) and thereby named Tumor derived Transforming Growth Factors.

Tumor derived TGFs have been demonstrated to produce HHM in two animal models and in one patient with cancer and HCa. These models have been studied especially by Mundy et al. (20).

Leydig Cell-tumors occur spontaneously in aged inbred Fisher rats, which then become hypercalcemic, hypercalciuric and hypophosphatemic. HCa is due to increased bone resorption. When the tumor is removed, the serum calcium falls to the normal range. Leydig cell tumors, from hypercalcemic animals, have been established in culture and have been shown to produce a bone resorbing factor, present in conditioned media and in tumor extracts. After extraction, lyophilization and chromatography, bone resorbing activity was eluted with proteins of a molecular weight of aproximately 30 000 d. A factor found to have TGF characteristics and activity, coeluted with the peak of bone resorbing activity.

The Walker rat breast tumor model is a spontaneous Fisher rat breast tumor which has at least two distinct variants : one normocalcemic, the other inducing HHM. This second variant also induces hypophosphatemia, hyperphosphaturia, increased nephrogenous cAMP and increased urinary excretion of PgE. All these features resemble those observed in patients with HHM. Using the same approach as for Leydig cell tumors, Mundy et al have demonstrated that the hypercalcemic variant, but not the normocalcemic, released a TGF of approwimately 25 000 d. Fractions containing this factor also stimulated-bone resorption in vitro. However, unlike the factor released by

Leydig cell tumors, this TGF does not compete with EGF for receptor binding, indicating that it may have different properties.

Finaly, a patient with renal cancer, a single osteolytic bone lesion, lung metastases and HCa, has been also studied and found to present in his urine a TGF of approximately 10 000 d. Column-purified fractions also stimulated bone resorbing activity in vitro. Tumor extracts from the same patient also contained a 17 000 d. TGF.

It is sure however that not all tumor derived TGFs stimulate bone resorption, and more studies are needed to identify those responsible for HHM.

Solid tumors with bone metastases

Seventy per cent of all patients with HCa of malignancy belong to this group (21). Clinical observation suggests that HCa is related in this condition to the extent of metastatic bone disease and bone destruction. In such patients resorption surfaces are greater than formation surfaces (16), generating more calcium than the normal homeostatic mechanisms can handle. Several different cell types may be involved in the destruction of bone at metastatic sites. Osteoclasts are the major resorbing cells. Lymphocytes and monocytes develop complex interactions with each other and with osteoclasts. Tumor cells may also play a direct role in bone destruction, especially at the final stages of metastasis (9, 7).

The capacity to destroy bone might be related to the production by tumor cells of collagenolytic enzymes. Such activity has been demonstrated in breast cancer, one of the tumors most frequently metastasizing to bone. Collagenolytic enzyme secretion in these cells seems to be under hormonal control, beeing stimulated by estrogens (10).

The presence of tumor cells in a metastatic site also provokes a cell-mediated immune response which leads to the accumulation of activated lymphocytes and monocytes in and around the tumor deposit (37). Activated lymphocytes release the lymphokine osteoclast activating factor. In addition, monocytes can resorb bone directly (15) and also release prostaglandins which could be responsible for activating osteoclasts.

Nevertheless, the major cellular mechanism of bone resorption in metastatic cancer is osteoclastic. Osteoclasts can be activated by the presence of a tumor metastasis in bone. Tumor cells in vitro produce local factors which could be responsible for osteoclast activation, such as prostaglandins (1). Using the Estradiol Receptor-positive (ER+) MCF-7 breast cancer cell line (39), we have observed that Pg production by tumor cells is followed by increased osteoclastic bone resorption in vitro. Both Pg production and bone resorption were stimulated by exposure of tumor cells to estradiol. Thus, the presence of estradiol receptors in breast cancer cells might explain HCa in those patients treated with estrogens. The osteolytic response potentiated by estradiol might also explain the early osteotropism of some breast cancers. There have been many clinical reports indicating that ER+ breast

tumors metastasize to viscera (3, 26, 31). Indeed, under estradiol stimulation, ER+ breast tumors may secrete more PgE_2
which would permit the tumor cells to implant in bone.

TREATMENT

HCa of malignancy is a complex disturbance. The review of
all the general and specific therapeutic agents that have
been used is too long to be developped in this paper.

However, beside the usual treatments, the usefulness of the
diphosphonates as a new treatment for HCa must be stressed.
These are synthetic analogues of pyrophosphate that inhibit
osteoclastic bone resorption as well as retard or inhibit the
deposition of hydroxyapatite crystals on bone collagen. The
most currently tested diphosphonates are : sodium etidronate
(EHDP), amino hydroxypropane diphosphonate (APD) and dichlo-
romethilene diphosphonate (Cl_2MDP). APD and Cl_2MDP have the
advantage of inhibiting bone resorption at doses that do not
affect mineralization of newly formed osteoid. Studies published by different authors (14, 23) as well as those done
in our Clinic show the effectiveness of diphosphonates to
treat HCa. In a double-blind cross-over study conducted by
Chapuy et al (4), we assessed the effects of Cl_2MDP against
placebo on : serum calcium level and urinary excretion of
calcium and hydroxyproline in 5 hypercalcemic patients with
breast or renal cancer. Cl_2MDP was given orally for 4 weeks.
Four patients experienced a rapid and significant decrease in
serum calcium and urinary calcium excretion. There was also
an increase in alkaline phosphatase. However, Cl_2MDP failed
to decrease the urinary hydroxyproline excretion.

In order to obtain a more rapid fall in calcium plasma levels, Charhon et al in our group (unpublished data) have conducted an open study using parenteral diphosphonates to treat
HCa in multiple myeloma. Four hypercalcemic patients have received daily intravenous EHDP at a dose of 4.3 mg/kg-day.
Three to eight days of EHDP infusion were sufficient to nor
malise serum calcium in all patients. Urinary excretion of
calcium and hydroxyproline decreased in the same time. One
patient who relapsed one week after the end of EHDP treatment,
has been successfully treated thereafter with IV Cl_2MDP at
5 mg/kg-day for 3 days. No adverse effects have been observed
during this study. Serum alkaline phosphatase and creatinine
levels remained in the normal range. Although there is a recent report of renal failure associated with IV diphosphonates.
(2) EHDP was administered in that study at much higher doses
than in our patients.

Diphosphonates appear to hold promise in the treatment of
HCa of malignancy and may also be useful in the prevention of
osteolytic metastases. However, more studies are needed to
assess the tolerance and the duration of their effects.

Acknowledgements : We acknowledge Pr G.R Mundy for providing
part of the scientific material presented in this paper. This
work has been also done in "Laboratoire de Biologie Médicale"
Dr Saez, Centre Anticancéreux L. Bérard.
We acknowledge Mrs Navarro for technical assistance.

REFERENCES

1. Benett, A., Mc Donald, A.M., Stamford, I.F., Charlier, E.
   M., Simson, J.S., and Zebro, O. (1977) Lancet, ii : 624-
   626.
2. Bounameaux, H.M., Schifferli, J., Montani, J.P., Jung, A.
   and Chatelanat, F. (1983) Lancet, i : 471.
3. Campbell, F.C., Blamey, R.W., Elston, C.W., Nicholson, R.
   I., Griffiths, K., and Haybittle, J.L. (1981) Br. J. Cancer, 44 : 456-459.
4. Chapuy, M.C., Meunier, P.J., Alexandre, C.M. and Vignon,
   E.P. (1980) J. Clin. Invest., 65 : 1243-1247.
5. Chen, P., Trummel, C., Horton, J., Baker, J.J., and Oppenheim, J.J. (1976) Eur. J. Immunol., 6 : 732-736.
6. Combes, R.C., Neville, A.M., Bondy, P.J. (1976) Prostaglandins, 12 : 1027-1035.
7. Eilon, G., and Mundy, G.R. (1978) Nature, 276 : 726-728
8. Cailani, S., Mc Limans, W.F., Mundy, G.R., Nussbaum, A.,
   Roholt, O., and Ziegel, R. (1976) Cancer Res., 26 : 1299-
   1304.
9. Galasko, C.S.B., and Benett, A. (1976) Nature, 263 : 508-
   510.
10. Heuson, J.C., Pasteels, J.L., Legros, N., Heuson-Stiennon
    J., and Leclerq, G. (1975) Cancer Res., 35 : 2039-2048.
11. Hohmann, E., Levine, L., Antoniades, H.N., and Tashjian,
    A.H. Jr. (1981) In 63[d] Ann. Meeting of the Endocrine So-
    ciety. p. 237 Abstr. 619.
12. Horton, J.E., Raisz, L.G., Simmons, H.A., Oppenheim, J.J.
    and Mergenhagen, S.E. (1972) Science, 177 : 793-795.
13. Horton, J.E., Koopman, W.J., Farrar, J.J., Fuller-Bonnar,
    J., and Mergenhagen, S.E. (1979) Cell. Immunol., 43 : 1-
    10.
14. Jung, A., Van Ouwenaller, C., Chantraine, A., and Cour-
    voisier, B. (1981) Cancer, 48 : 1922-1925.
15. Kahn, A.J., Stewart, C.L., and Teitelbaum, S.L. (1978) :
    Science, 199 : 988-990
16. McDonnel, G.D., Dunstan, C.R., Evans, R.A., Carter, J.N.,
    Hills, E., Wong, S.U.P., and McNeil, D.R. (1982) J. Clin.
    Endocrinol. Metab., 55 : 1066-1072.
17. Mundy, G.R., Luben, R.A., Raisz, L.G., Oppenheim, J.J.,
    and Buell, D.R. (1974) N. Eng. J. Med., 290 : 867-871.
18. Mundy, G.R., Raisz, L.G., Cooper, R.A., Schehter, G.P.,
    and Salmon, S.E. (1974) N. Eng. J. Med., 291 : 1041-1046.
19. Mundy, G.R., Cove, D.H., and Fisken, R. (1980) Lancet, i:
    1317-1320.
20. Mundy, G.R., Ibbotson, K.J., D'Souza, S.M., Simpson, E.L.
    Jacobs, J.W., and Martin, T.J. Submitted to N. Eng. J.
    Med. in 1983.
21. Myers, W.P.L. (1960) Arch. Surg., 80 : 308-318.
22. Parfitt, A.M. (1979) Metab. Bone Dis. and Rel. Res., 1 :
    279-283, 1979.
23. Paterson, A.D., Kanis, J.A., Cameron, E.C., Douglas, D.L.
    Beard, D.J., Preston, F.E., and Russell, R.G.G. (1983) :
    Br. J. Haematol., 54 : 121-132.

24. Raisz, L.G., Luben, R.A., Mundy, G.R., Dietrich, J.W., Horton, J.E. and Trummel, C.L. (1975) J. Clin. Invest., 56, : 408-419.
25. Roberts, A.B., Anzano, M.A., Lamb, L.C., Smith, J.M., Frolik, C.A., Marquardt, H., Todaro, G.J., and Sporn, M. B. (1982) Nature (London), 795 : 417-419.
26. Samaan, N.A., Buzdar, A.V., Aldinger, K.A., Schultz, P.N. Yang, K.P., Romsdahl, M.M. and Martin, R. (1981) Cancer, 47 : 554-560.
27. Simpson, E.L., Mundy, G.R., D"Souza, S.M., Ibbotson, K.J. Bockman, R., and Jacobs, J.W. (1983) N. Eng. J. Med., 309 : 325-330.
28. Singer, F.R., Sharp, C.F. and Rude R.K. (1979) Mineral Electrolyte Metabolism, 2 : 161-178.
29. Sporn, M.B. and Todaro, G.J. (1980) N. Eng. J. Med., 303 878-880.
30. Stewart, A.F., Vignery, A., Silverglate, A., Ravin, N.D., Livols, V., Broadus, A.E., and Baron, R. (1982) J. Clin. Endocrinol. & Metab., 55 : 219-227.
31. Stewart, J.F., King, R.J.B., Sexton, S.A., Millis, R.R., Rubens, R.D., and Hayward, J.L. (1981) Europ. J. Cancer, 17 : 449-453.
32. Tashjian, A.H. Jr., Voelkel, E.F., Goldhaber P., and Levine, L. (1973) Prostaglandins, 3, 515.
33. Tashjian, A.H. Jr. and Levine, L. (1978) Biochem. Biophys. Res. Commun., 85 : 966-975.
34. Tashjian, A.J. Jr., Voelkel, E.F., and Levine, L. (1982): In : Prostaglandins and Cancer : First International Conference, edited by A.R. Liss, pp. 513-523, A.R. Liss Inc., New York.
35. Todaro, G.J., Fryling, C. and de Larco, J.E. (1980) : Proc. Natl. Acad. Sci. (USA), 77 : 5258-5262.
36. Twardzik, D.R., Sherwin, S.A., Ranchalis, J., and Todaro G.J. (1982) J. Natl. Cancer Inst., 69 : 793-798.
37. Underwood, J.C.E. (1974) A review. Br. J. Cancer, 30 : 538-548.
38. Valentin-Opran, A., Charhon, S.A., Meunier, P.J., Edouard C.M., and Arlot, M.E. (1982) Br. J. Haematol., 52 : 601-610.
39. Valentin-Opran, A., Eilon, G., Saez, S., Mundy, B.R. : Submitted to J. Clin. Invest. in 1983.
40. Yoneda, T., and Mundy, G.R. (1979)J. Exp. Med., 150 : 338-350.
41. Yoneda, T., and Mundy, G.R. (1982) Calcif. Tissue Int., 34 : 204-208.

Progress in Cancer Research and Therapy,
Vol. 31, edited by F. Bresciani, et al.
Raven Press, New York © 1984.

Tumor-Associated Hypercalcemia

C. Gennari, G. Francini, R. Nami, S. Gonnelli, and M. Montagnani

Institute of Medical Semeiotics, University of Siena, 53100 Siena, Italy

Hypercalcemia in malignancy represents approximately one-third of all cases of hypercalcemia (18).

In 262 consecutive patients with malignant disease, we found 71 cases of hypercalcemia (27%) and 55 normocalcemic cases with evident bone metastases (21%) as demonstrated by bone scanning and X-rays. Of the 71 cases with hypercalcemia, 55 presented evidence of bone metastases, whereas in 16 hypercalcemic patients the skeleton appeared not to have been invaded by neoplastic cells.

In patients presenting neoplasms, hypercalcemia is more often encountered in some types of tumor. The most frequent tumors causing hypercalcemia, as observed in our patients, were in order of importance: lung and breast followed by myeloma, thyroid, kidney, head and neck, gut and female genital tract.

MECHANISMS OF HYPERCALCEMIA IN MALIGNANCY

Two primary mechanisms for hypercalcemia are involved in patients with the forementioned neoplasms: the first being bone resorption directly by tumor cells metastasized to bone, the second being bone resorption by humoral factors tied to the neoplasm in the absence of bone metastasis.

The nature of these humoral factors, involved in malignant hypercalcemia, has yet to be fully defined. On the basis of clinical similarities between primitive hyperparathyroidism and malignant hypercalcemia, the first humoral factor isolated was a substance similar to parathormone (PTH) - the hormone physiologically involved in stimulating osteoclastic activity - produced by ectopic tumor secretion, especially by some lung neoplasms (1,2). The second factor identified was a prostaglandin, and in particular the PGE type (21,22,25), which exerts a potent stimulatory effect on bone resorption (15); high circulating levels of PGE have been observed in patients with neoplastic hypercalcemia (21) and in some cases the treatment with indomethacin - an inhibitor in prostaglandin synthesis - corrected the hypercalcemia (4). Another identified factor was the "Osteoclast Activating Factor" (OAF) (16), a lymphokine produced by the lympho-monocyte system in neoplastic patients, particularly in patients with myeloma, probably by prostaglandin stimulation (28); OAF, like other bone resorbing hormones, increases the number and activity of osteoclasts. Evidence has been recently given on another factor, yet to be identified, presenting some renal effects similar to those of PTH such as increasing the production of nephrogenous cAMP and reducing the tubular phosphorus threshold (24).

Hypercalcemia is maintained by humoral factors in approximately one-third of the cases; in the remaining two-thirds, hypercalcemia is associated with widespread osteolytic bone metastases. The mechanism of bone destruction in metastases is still unclear. Some studies have suggested that tumor cells may directly resorb bone, probably by the release of proteolytic enzymes (9). In recent studies evidence has been given that tumor cells migrate chemotactically in response to a factor released by resorbing bones (19): this factor, which has been isolated, is also chemotactic for monocytes. This could imply the presence of a local humoral mechanism tied to direct bone destruction by tumor cells.

SIGNS AND SYMPTOMS

Bone metastases cause severe pain and occasionally pathologic fractures.

The clinical presentation of hypercalcemia involves three systems; the neuromuscular, gastrointestinal and renal. The neuromuscular features of hypercalcemia include confusion and lethargy, lapsing rapidly into stupor and coma when serum calcium concentration exceeds 13 mg/dl. The main symptoms of muscular system are weakness and fatigue; the cardiac signs are primarily a shortening of QT in the electrocardiogram and have a potential risk fo syncope and death. The gastrointestinal features of hyper calcemia are nausea, vomiting, constipation and abdominal pain. The renal features are polyuria and polydipsia, and less frequently recurrent renal stones and nephrocalcinosis. There are also less frequent signs such as pruritus, hypertension and band keratopathy.The high serum calcium levels increases the sensitivity to pain by reducing the pain threshold of opiate receptors.

The clinical manifestations of hypercalcemia in malignancy often develop very rapidly: this characteristic facilitates the precocious presence of clinical manifestations when the serum calcium level is only marginally increased. This differentiates the hypercalcemia of malignancy from that of primary hyperparathyroidism, in which the increase in serum calcium is less rapid and symptoms appear when calcium levels reach clear pathologic values.

DIAGNOSIS

In order to define the clinical characteristics of tumoral hypercalcemia, a series of diagnostic tests must be performed.

The first diagnostic point is to establish the degree and extention of bone destruction caused by neoplastic cells. This can be accomplished by skeletal X-rays and bone scan. For evidencing bone metastases, radio-nuclide bone scanning seems to be more sensitive than X-rays. In addition, by using labeled diphosphonates, particularly ^{99}Tc-dichloromethylene diphosphonate (MClDP), the skeletal uptake of the tracer, reflecting the metabolic activity, can be accurately quantified by measuring its 24-hour whole body retention (WBR) (10). The number of hot spots on the bone scan and the WBR of the tracer provide a sensitive measure of increased bone turnover in areas of metastatic involvement. However, the retention of ^{99}Tc-MClDP is related more to the osteoblastic than to the osteoclastic activity (11), both being variably present in metastatic cancer. The osteoclastic component can be better analyzed by urinary hydroxyproline measurement which mainly reflects the breakdown of bone collagen. Increased excretion of hydroxyproline is at least as sensitive an indicator of precocious bone metastases as is bone-scanning (18).

In our cases of malignant hypercalcemia, there was a significant correlation between urinary hydroxyproline excretion and the number of metastases as assessed by skeletal X-rays and bone scan (Figure 1). On the contrary, no significant correlation was found between the number of metastases and the WBR of tracer (Figure 2) and between the urinary hydroxyproline excretion and WBR of labeled diphosphonate (Figure 3).

The second diagnostic point is to ascertain the presence of presumed humoral factors stimulating osteoclastic bone resorption, particularly in the differential diagnosis between primary hyperparathyroidism and malignant disease, which are the two most common causes of hypercalcemia. Considering that primary hyperparathyroidism is associated with hypercalcemia, hypophosphatemia, lowering of the renal phosphate threshold, elevated levels of immunoreactive PTH (iPTH) and enhanced urinary excretion of nephrogenous cyclic AMP (NcAMP), the diagnostic tests to be used in the diagnosis of patients with hypercalcemia are serum calcium, serum phosphorus, serum PTH radioimmunoassay, tubular reabsorption of phosphate and urinary NcAMP.

The quantity of cAMP produced by the kidney under the stimulus of PTH, is considered to be the best index of parathyroid activity (5). In recent studies it has been observed that some patients with tumoral hypercalcemia present high values of NcAMP, suggesting a condition of ectopic hyperparathyroidism due to the secretion of PTH-like substances by the tumor (24). The ectopic secretion of PTH can also be demonstrated by determining the circulating levels of iPTH (20,23). The radioimmunoassay determination of the PGE is also useful for classing those patients with tumoral hypercalcemia, showing an increased plasma PGE concentration (8, 12). In some cases the elevated production of PGE by the neoplastic cells can be documented before the skeleton is involved. In 4 cases of carcinoma of the breast, the determination of the PGE in the venous blood, performed before the mastectomy, demonstrated clearly pathologic levels of PGE in the axillary vein homolateral to the tumor, and superior to those found in the controlateral cubital vein. These data are compatible with the hypothesis that the originating tumor often produces high quantities of PGE early in its development (25).

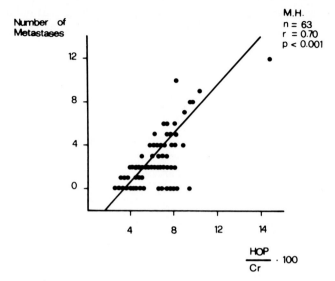

FIG. 1: Correlation between the number of metastases and the urinary
excretion of hydroxyproline in 63 cases of malignant hypercalcemia.

In 62 patients with tumoral hypercalcemia we employed the forementioned tests, comparing the results with those obtained from a group of 63
normocalcemic cancer patients without evident bone metastasis who were
matched as to age, sex and type of tumor. The hypercalcemic patients
were subdivided into two groups; those with high levels of NcAMP (n=15)
and those with low or low-normal values of NcAMP (n=47). The determina-

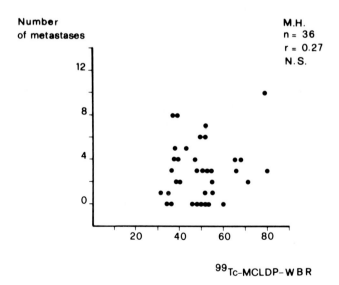

FIG. 2: Correlation between the number of metastases and the 24-hour
whole body retention (WBR) of ^{99}Tc-dichloromethylene diphosphonate
(MCLDP) in 36 cases of malignant hypercalcemia.

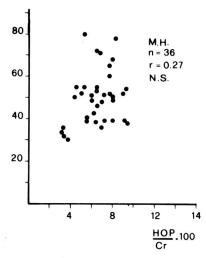

FIG. 3: Correlation between the 24-hour whole body retention of ^{99}Tc-MCLDP and the urinary hydroxyproline excretion corrected for creatinine in 36 cases of malignant hypercalcemia.

tion of the serum levels of iPTH (C-terminal antibody) gave elevated values in 5 of 15 patients with high NcAMP. In these 5 patients, all presenting with a squamous cell tumor of the lung, such a finding suggested a syndrome of ectopic secretion of PTH. In the other 47 patients with low or low-normal NcAMP the circulating levels of iPTH were found to be within normal limits. The measurement of the serum levels of PGE demonstrated elevated values in 4 out of 15 cases with high NcAMP (3 cases of breast cancer, 1 case of renal cancer) and in 24 cases out of 47 with low or low-normal levels of NcAMP. The measurement of the serum phosphate level showed a hypophosphatemia in 11 cases with high NcAMP and only in 3 cases with low NcAMP levels. In all hypophosphatemic cases the tubular reabsorption of phosphate (P_R) resulted lower than normal, confirming a condition of hyperphosphaturia.

On the basis of these determinations the 62 hypercalcemic patients can be divided into 5 groups according to the levels of PTH, NcAMP, P_R and PGE found in each (Table 1).

TABLE 1. Malignant hypercalcemia n=62

iPTH	NcAMP	P_R	PGE	n
High	High	Low	Normal	5
Normal	High	Low	Normal	6
Normal	High	Low	High	4
Normal	Normal	Normal	High	26
Normal	Normal	Normal	Normal	21

In the 21 patients with normal values of all parameters considered the mechanism of hypercalcemia is probably of a direct type due to neoplastic cells metastasized to the skeleton.In fact, in 19 of these patients the X-rays and the bone scan documented the presence of bone metastases. In the 26 cases with high levels of PGE and normal levels of the other parameters, one can hypothesize a humoral mechanism of stimulation of the osteoclasts based on the local or distant production of PGE.In fact in approximately one-third of these patients no bone metastases were observed. Only 5 patients had the humoral signs of hyperparathyroidism, compatible with the hypothesis of an ectopic secretion of PTH. In 10 other cases the circulating levels of iPTH were found to be normal but the renal effects of the hormone were evident with high values of NcAMP and low values of P_R. These data support the hypothesis of the presence of a renotropic factor which resembles native PTH in its ability to stimulate tubular adenylate cyclase and to inhibit tubular phosphate reabsorption (24).

The subdivision of neoplastic hypercalcemia, according to these criteria, is certainly debatable in that we still don't completely known how many or which may be the factors and mechanisms that induce osteolysis in malignancy. However, the possibility of identifying the presence of some of the known factors can be important, not so much on the pathophysiologic level as on the level of clinical treatment of hypercalcemia. In fact, from these determinations we can draw indications for the use of drugs that interfere with the mechanism of osteolysis.

TREATMENT

The management of patients with malignant hypercalcemia is determined by the degree and the stability of the condition and by the presence of symptoms. This approach tends to divide the hypercalcemic patients with malignancy into two groups, the first in which serum calcium exceeds 13 mg/dl, tends rapidly to rise with patients being fully symptomatic. These cases presenting with a hypercalcemic crisis require prompt treatment. The second group includes patients with serum calcium levels between 10.5-13.0 mg/dl and with a latent clinical stage of the syndrome. These cases, in which the condition presents a relative stability require a chronic treatment of hypercalcemia.

Emergency Treatment of Hypercalcemia (Table 2)

The emergency treatment of hypercalcemia should begin with intravenous saline to re-expand the extracellular fluid and restore the glomerular filtration rate. Besides the classical treatment with fluids, loop diuretics as furosemide, intravenous phosphate or EDTA, the calcium chelating agent, we have now at our disposal different drugs: glucocorticoids, mithramycin and calcitonin.

Glucocorticoids act too slowly and their effects are unpredictable (26). Mithramycin presents high hepatic and renal toxicity, its side ef-

TABLE 2. Emergency treatment of hypercalcemia

Drug	Dose
Saline	4-6 L/day
Furosemide	100 mg i.v.
Phosphates	50 mM i.v.
EDTA	50 mg/Kg i.v.
Glucocorticoids	400 mg/day i.v.(hydrocortisone)
Mithramycin	25 mcg/Kg i.v.
Calcitonin	200-800 MRC units/day i.m.

fects are cumulative and the onset of its action is too slow (7).

At present the emergency treatment of choice seems to be calcitonin, the naturally occurring inhibitor of bone resorption. The hormone is immediately acting without toxicity. The only disadvantage is that sometimes the calcium lowering activity of calcitonin is only transient; this loss of activity may be due to down-regulation of calcitonin receptors on bone cells which occurs in the continued presence of the hormone (24). This phenomenon can be prevented by the use of glucocorticoids in combination with calcitonin (24).

Chronic Treatment of Hypercalcemia (Table 3)

Long-term treatment of malignant hypercalcemia is indicated in cases in which the increase in serum calcium levels is moderate and relatively stable.

Many of these patients are currently treated by chemoterapy. Even though in some cases chemotherapy is capable of transiently reducing serum calcium levels into the normal range, it does not however improve bone involvement in the majority of patients. In fact, in 23 cases of malignant hypercalcemia that we treated with chemotherapeutic regimens for

TABLE 3. Chronic treatment of hypercalcemia

Drug	Dose
Phosphate	1-3 g/day orally
Mithramycin	15-25 mcg/Kg i.v.
Glucocorticoids	40-60 mg/day orally (Prednisone)
Indomethacin	150 mg/day orally
Diphosphonates	EHDP 10-20 mg/Kg/day orally
	APD 10-15 mg/Kg/day orally
	Cl_2MDP 20-25 mg/Kg/day orally
Calcitonin	100 MRC Units/day i.m.

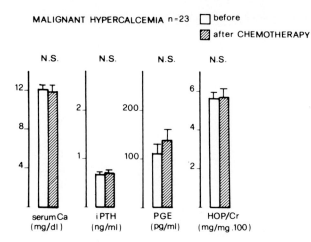

FIG. 4: Effects of a 3-month period of treatment
with chemotherapeutic agents on serum calcium,
iPTH and PGE levels, and on the urinary excretion
of hydroxyproline corrected for creatinine in 23
cases of malignant hypercalcemia. Values are
expressed as mean±standard error of the mean.

three months, the serum calcium level and urinary hydroxyproline excretion were not modified (Figure 4). The drugs that can be actually combined with chemotherapy are indomethacin, diphosphonates and calcitonin
besides phosphates, mithramycin and glucocorticoids. Indomethacin,which
could be indicated in cases of hypercalcemia in which PGE may play a pathogenetic role, has proven to be disappointing in the treatment of hy-

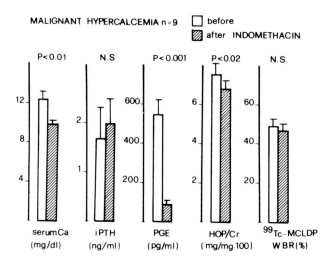

FIG. 5: Effects of indomethacin (150 mg/day for one month) in the treatment of 9 cases of malignant hypercalcemia.

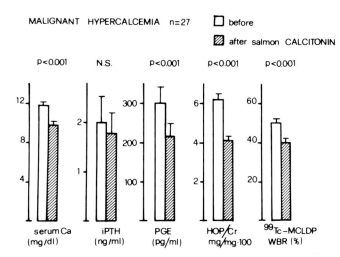

FIG. 6: Effects of salmon calcitonin (100 MRC Units/day by i.m. injection for three months) in the treatment of 27 cases of malignant hypercalcemia.

percalcemic crisis, in which the drug acts much to slowly. This is well evident when indomethacin is compared to calcitonin treatment. We have treated 9 patients presenting with moderate malignant hypercalcemia and high levels of serum PGE for one month with indomethacin in combination with chemotherapy (Figure 5). At the end of treatment, the serum calcium was found to be within normal limits and serum PGE levels were extremely low; nevertheless the two indexes of bone involvement, urinary excretion of hydroxyproline and WBR of labeled diphosphonate, were poorly affected. The failure of indomethacin to reduce hydroxyproline excretion in patients with malignant hypercalcemia has also been described in other studies (6).

Diphosphonates are new pharmacologic agents, characterized by a P-C-P bond in their structure, which exert an inhibitory activity on osteoclastic bone resorption. Until now three different diphosphonates have been employed by the oral route in the treatment of malignant hypercalcemia: disodium etidronate (EHDP) (14), dichloromethylene diphosphonate (Cl_2MDP) (13) and aminohydroxypropylidene bisphosphonate (APD) (27). EHDP and Cl_2MDP have proven to be very effective in the treatment of hypercalcemic crisis if administered intravenously (14). The major limitation of diphosphonate therapy is that they impair not only the dissolution but also the growth of crystals of mineralized bone. In this sense EHDP has proven to cause osteomalacia with an increase in unmineralized osteoid tissue. In addition, APD has demonstrated a particular toxicity, with the appearance of an unexplained fever occurring within the first few days of treatment.

At present, calcitonin seems to be the treatment of choice even in long-term management of malignant hypercalcemia. The hormone, employed for three months in combination with chemotherapy in 27 patients, had significantly reduced not only serum calcium and PGE levels but also the indexes of bone involvement, urinary excretion of hydroxyproline and the 24-hour WBR retention of labeled diphosphonate (Figure 6). The only disadvantage being that it has to be administered by injection.

In conclusion we can now say that the treatment of patients with malignant hypercalcemia, largely determined by its clinical presentation, can utilize many different drugs which even if they aren't the most ideal agents, they do succeed in correcting this severe complication of the neoplastic patient.

REFERENCES

1. Bender, R.A. and Hansen, H. (1974): Ann. Intern. Med., 80:205-208.
2. Berson, S.A. and Yalow, R.S. (1966): Science, 154:907-909
3. Binstock, M.L. and Mundy, G.R. (1980): Ann. Intern. Med., 93:269-272.
4. Brereton, H.D., Haluska, P.V., Alexander, R.W., Mason, D.M., Keiser, H.R. and De Vita, V.T. Jr. (1974): N. Engl. J. Med. 291:83-85.
5. Broadus, A.E. (1979): Nephron, 23:136-141.
6. Coombes, R.C., Neville, A.M., Bondy P.K. and Powles, T.J. (1976): Prostaglandins, 12:1027-1035.
7. Coombes, R.C., Dady, P. and Parsons, C. (1980): Metab. Bone Dis. Rel. Res., 2:199-202.
8. Demers, L.M., Allegra, J.C., Harvey, H.A., Lipton, A., Luderer, J.R., Mortel, R. and Brenner, D.E. (1977): Cancer, 39:1559-1562.
9. Eilon, G. and Mundy, G.R. (1978): Nature, 276:726-728.
10. Fogelman, I., Bessent, R.G., Turner, J.G., Citrin, D.L., Boyle, I.T. and Greig, W.R. (1978): J. Nucl. Med., 19:270-275.
11. Fogelman, I., Bessent, R.G., Beastall, G. and Boyle, I.T. (1980): Ann. Intern. Med., 92:65-67.
12. Gennari C.(1980): In: Calcitonin 1980, Chemistry, Physiology, Pharmacology and Clinical Aspects, edited by A. Pecile, pp.277-287. Excerpta Medica, Amsterdam.
13. Jacobs, T.P., Siris, E.S., Bilezikian, J.P., Baquiran, D.C., Shane, E. and Canfield, R.E. (1981): Ann. Intern. Med., 94:312-316.
14. Jung, A. (1982): Am. J. Med., 72:221-226.
15. Klein, D.C. and Raisz, L.G. (1970): Endocrinol., 85:657-661.
16. Mundy, G.R., Cooper, L.G., Schecter, R.A. and Salmon, S.E. (1974): N. Engl. J. Med., 291:1041-1046.
17. Mundy, G.R. and Martin, T.J. (1982): Metabolism, 31:1247-1277.
18. Niell, H.B., Palmieri, G., Neely, C.L. and Mc Donald, M.W. (1981): Arch. Intern. Med., 141:1471-1473.
19. Orr, F.W., Varani, J., Gondek, M.D., Ward, P.A. and Mundy, G.R. (1980): Am. J. Path., 99:43-52.
20. Raisz, L.G., Chaitanya, H.Y., Bockman, R.S. and Bower, B.F. (1979): Ann. Int. Med., 91:739-740.
21. Robertson, R.P., Baylink, D.J., Metz, S.A. and Cummings, K.B. (1976): J. Clin. Endocrinol. Metab., 43:1330-1335.

22. Seyberth, H.W., Segre, G.V., Morgan, J.L., Sweetman, B.J., Potts, J. T. Jr and Oates, J.A. (1975):N. Engl. J. Med., 293:1278-1283.
23. Skrabanek, P., McPartlin, J. and Powell, D. (1980): Medicine, 59: 262-282.
24. Stewart, A.F., Horst, R., Deftos, L.J., Cadman, E.C., Lang, R. and Broadus, A.E. (1980): N. Engl. J. Med., 303:1377-1383.
25. Tashjian, A.H.Jr (1978): Cancer Res., 38:4138-4141.
26. Thalassinos, N.C. and Joplin, G. (1970): Lancet, 2:537-538.
27. Van Breukelen, F.J.M., Bijvoet, O.L.M. and Van Oosterom, A.T. (1979): Lancet, 1:803-805.
28. Yoneda, T. and Mundy, G.R. (1979): J. Exp. Med., 149:279-283.

Progress in Cancer Research and Therapy,
Vol. 31, edited by F. Bresciani, et al.
Raven Press, New York © 1984.

Estrogen-Responsive Creatine Kinase in Normal and Neoplastic Human Breast

*D. Amroch, **S. Cox, † A. Shaer, † S. Malnick, † S. Chatsubi,
**R. Hallowes, and † A.M. Kaye

†*Department of Hormone Research, The Weizmann Institute of Science, Rehovot,
76100 Israel; *Department of Surgery A, Kaplan Hospital, Rehovot, Israel; and
**Tissue Cell Relationship Laboratory, Imperial Cancer Research Fund,
London, WC2A 3PX United Kingdom*

An easily detectable and quantifiable protein induced by estrogen in human breast tumors could potentially be a better predictor of a tumor response to endocrine therapy than the exclusive use of the concentrations of estrogen and/or progesterone receptors currently employed (10,11). If the response were capable of being detected in vitro in biopsy samples and if the response were rapid, these characteristics would favor its use as a response indicator. Our recent identification (14) of the estrogen induced protein of rat uterus as the brain type isozyme of creatine kinase (CKBB) adds ease of quantitation to the known rapidity of its induction both in vivo (1) and in vitro (6). An increase in its rate of synthesis within 1 h of estrogen administration has been found throughout the reproductive system of the female rat (7,13), including the estrogen rich regions of the pre-optic area and the hypothalamus in the brain (13), as well as in DMBA induced mammary tumors (8,12).

METHODS

Preparation and culture of epithelial "organoids"

Tissue dissociation. Normal tissue from reduction mammoplasties was dissociated as previosuly described by Stampfer et al. (15). The breast tissue was cut into pieces of approximately 1 cm^3 and suspended in an enzyme digestion mixture, containing Type I collagenase (250 U/ml), hyaluronidase (100 U/ml) and bovine serum albumin (BSA, 0.25%) dissolved in RPMI 1640, for 16 to 24 h at 37°C. The suspension obtained was centrifuged at 600xg (10 min) and the supernatant discarded. These steps remove the fat.

The pellet obtained in the previous step was resuspended in fresh digestion mixture in plastic centrifuge tubes. The tubes were then placed on a tube rotator for 5-6 h at 37°C. After this incubation, the tubes were left to stand (10-15 min) which allowed the organoids (lobular and ductal epithelial structures devoid of stroma) to settle. Approximately half the supernatant suspension was removed and replaced with RPMI 1640 at 37°C. The above procedure was repeated three times. The tubes were

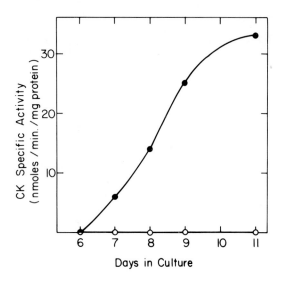

FIG. 1. Creatine kinase (CK) activity in epithelial organoids from normal human breast after exposure to estrogen. Organoids from 6 day-old
to 11 day-old cultures were incubated for 16 h before harvesting in either 0.001% ethanol vehicle (o) or in 10^{-9}M estradiol-17β (●).

then centrifuged at 60xg (3 min) and the supernatant suspension removed.
This procedure removes the fibroblasts from the suspension.
     The resulting pellet was resuspended in fresh digestion mixture and
replaced on the tube rotator at 37°C. After 1 h, the tubes were removed, placed on a tube rotator at room temperature and left overnight.
The suspension was passed through a series of polyester filters ranging
from 1,000 μm to 95 μm pore size. At each stage, the filter was invert-
ed after the suspension was passed through it and the collected organoids washed in RPMI 1640 plus BSA (0.25%) for 3-4 h to remove the enzymes. The organoids were then refiltered and suspended in RPMI 1640
plus BSA (0.25%). The fraction used in the following experiments was
the 200 μm fraction which contains both ductal and lobular structures.

     Culture. The organoids were plated, in 40 mm culture dishes contain-
ing 1.5 ml of rat tail collagen gel (4), in a small volume (200 μl) of
medium to ensure maximal contact with the substrate. The dishes were
placed in a humidified incubator (5% CO_2) overnight to allow maximum attachment. The following morning, 2 ml of medium (RPMI 1640) containing
insulin (1 μg/ml), hydrocortisone (10 ng/ml), epidermal growth factor (5
ng/ml) and transferrin (5 μg/ml) was added to the dishes.

Preparation of Enzyme Extracts

     Tissues were homogenized in 3-6 volumes of homogenization buffer con-
sisting of: 50 mM Tris HCl pH 6.8, 5 mM magnesium acetate, 2.5 mM dithiothreitol (DTT), 0.4 mM disodium EDTA and 250 mM sucrose, using a
glass-glass homogenizer. Cytosols were obtained by ultra-centrifugation
at 4°C at a minimum of 1.5×10^{6}g x min for each cm of liquid height in
the centrifugation tube.

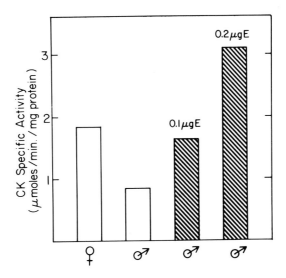

FIG. 2. Creatine kinase activity in the MX-1 transplantable human mammary carcinoma grown in athymic mice. Mice were either untreated (open bars) or given injections of 20 or 40 ng of estradiol-17β/day for 5 days (lined bars).

Assay of Creatine Kinase

Samples of cytosols were assayed in an automatic recording spectrophotometer at a wavelength of 340 nM and a temperature of 30°C, in a volume of 0.5 or 1 ml total assay mixture.

The creatine kinase assay, adjusted to a pH of 6.7, contained in 1.0 ml volume: 50 mM imidazole acetate buffer, 25 mM creatine phosphate, 20 mM D-glucose, 20 mM N-acetyl cysteine, 10 mM magnesium acetate 5 mM disodium EDTA, 2 mM ADP, 2 mM DTT, 2 mM NAD, 50 μM diadenosine pentaphosphate (myokinase inhibitor), 2.4 units of glucose-6-phosphate dehydrogenase (from Leuconostoc), 1.6 units of hexokinase and 10 μg bovine serum albumin.

Separation of Creatine Kinase Enzymes by Step Gradient Chromatography

Column chromatography was performed as described previously for enolase isozyme separation (8) with slight modifications. Cytosol fractions were adjusted to pH 7.9 and NaCl added to reach a concentration of 20 mM. Aggregates were removed by centrifugation and samples were applied to a 1 ml volume DEAE cellulose column in a 5 ml plastic syringe. The MM isozyme passed through the column without absorbtion; the MB isozyme was eluted with 40 mM NaCl, 100 mM Tris HCl (pH 6.4), and 0.4 mM EDTA; the BB isozyme was eluted with 250 mM NaCl in the same buffer.

Protein was assayed by the Bradford method (2), using bovine serum albumin (Sigma) as the protein standard.

RESULTS AND DISCUSSION

We have reported (9) that fragments of normal human breast show an increase in creatine kinase BB activity after being incubated in 3 x

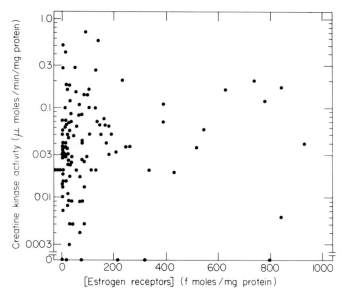

FIG. 3. Lack of correlation between the concentration of estrogen receptors and total creatine kinase activity in human mammary tumors.
Note that creatine kinase activity is plotted on a logarithmic scale.

10^{-8}M estradiol for 2 h. Both fat and non-fat portions of normal breast
were responsive.

In order to have a system which was exclusively epithelial, we cultured the lobular and ductal fragments of human epithelial tissue derived by enzyme digestion and filtration from reduction mammoplasties.
These morphologically intact structures termed "organoids", show responsiveness to estrogen (FIG. 1.), after their first week in culture, by an
increase in growth accompanied by an increasing responsiveness in terms
of the stimulation of creatine kinase activity after 16 h incubation in
10^{-9}M estradiol-17β, but no response to the same concentration of estra-
diol-17α.

A convenient system for investigation of responsiveness of human
breast tumor is the MX1 human tumor grown in athymic mice (FIG. 2).
This tumor shows presumptive estrogen responsiveness in that the specific activity of creatine kinase in the tumor is twice as high when grown
in female as compared to male mice. This assumption is confirmed by the
administration of estrogen to male mice bearing the tumor which causes
the specific activity of CK to increase to the same level as when grown
in females. Doubling the dose of estrogen can produce tumors growing in
male mice having twice the CK specific activity of those growing in untreated females (FIG. 2).

To begin to analyze the possible usefulness of CK for predicting
clinical response to endocrine therapy, we examined the possible relationship between K activity in human breast carcinomas and their concentration of estrogen receptors. Paradoxically, a perfect correlation
in this case would mean that CK activity in the tumors would not add any
further information to that given by the concentrations of receptors.

As shown in FIGS. 3 and 4, there is no correlation between endogenous
CK activity and estrogen or progesterone receptor concentration, a situ-

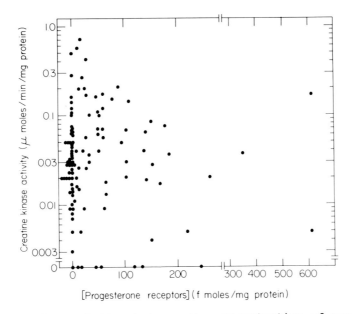

FIG. 4. Lack of correlation between the concentration of progesterone receptors and total creatine kinase activity in human mammary tumors. Note that creatine kinase activity is plotted on a logarithmic scale.

ation paralleled by several parameters which have been tested for estrogen responsiveness (3,5). Since the specific activity of CK in breast tumors shows no correlation with steroid hormone receptor concentration, the best, albeit imperfect, predictor of responsiveness, we must consider the other 2 parameters which a priori seem more promising as indicators, that is, responsiveness in vitro and CK isozyme distribution.

The responsiveness of normal breast fragments mentioned previously is shown (FIG. 5) in comparison with benign breast tumors and secondary carcinomas. This graph shows the change in creatine kinase activity of normal breast tissue fragments incubated for 2 h in 3×10^{-8} M estradiol. Eight out of 10 normal breast samples showed responses. Combining the data in FIGS. 5 and 6 we have found that 4 out of 19 benign and 22 out of 43 malignant tumors show in vitro CK responses to estradiol. Among this group were 10 secondary carcinomas (FIG. 5) of which 4 showed a response – close to the 50% proportion shown by the primary tumors. The distribution of these cases of breast cancer according to receptor status is shown in TABLE 1. Within the group which is positive for both estrogen and progesterone receptors approximately two thirds show estrogen stimulated creatine kinase. In addition, 40% of breast cancer cases which show estrogen but not progesterone receptors are responsive by the creatine kinase test. These data are therefore roughly consistent with the proportion of clinical responses, and will be the starting point for a long term clinical follow up to see whether or not CK responsiveness can add to the predictive usefulness of receptor assays.

The third parameter of CK which can be determined easily is the ratio of the CKBB-isozyme (which is estrogen responsive) to the MM or muscle type isozyme and the MB or cardiac characteristic isozyme. While the bulk of human breast tumors show preponderantly or exclusively the BB isozyme of CK, tumors with preponderantly the MM isozyme in their cyto-

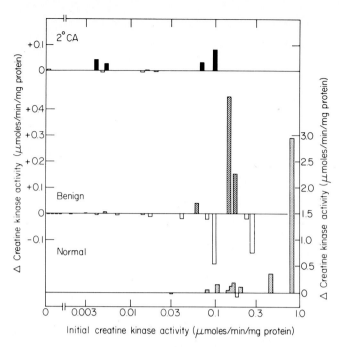

FIG. 5. Change in creatine kinase activity due to *in vitro* estrogen treatment of secondary mammary carcinomas, benign tumors and normal human breast. Fragments of normal breast were incubated for 2 h in 3×10^{-8}M estradiol 17β, secondary mammary carcinomas for 16 h in 10^{-9}M estradiol 17β and benign tumors in either of these two conditions. Note that initial creatine kinase activity is plotted on a logarithmic scale.

sol do appear, and some MB form is found in some tumors (FIG. 7). Whether the additional parameter of distribution of CK isozymes will add anything to the predictive power of receptor analysis, or of combined receptor analysis and CK responsiveness tests, will also be determined in the long-term follow up which is now underway.

SUMMARY

The identification of the "estrogen-induced protein" of rat uterus as the BB isozyme of creatine kinase (CK) and its stimulation by estrogen in other organs of the female rat reproductive system led to a survey of human breast tissue for similar estrogen responsiveness. Epithelial "organoids" cultured from normal human breast showed increasing responsiveness to a 16 h exposure to 1 nM estradiol-17β measured as an increase in creatine kinase specific activity, during the period between 7 and 11 days in culture. The MX-1 human breast cancer, transplanted into athymic mice, showed two times the CK specific activity when grown in ♀ as compared to ♂ mice. The specific activity of CK from tumors in ♂ mice was doubled and quadrupled by daily administration of 0.1 and 0.2 ug of estradiol-17β, respectively. When CK specific activity was meas-

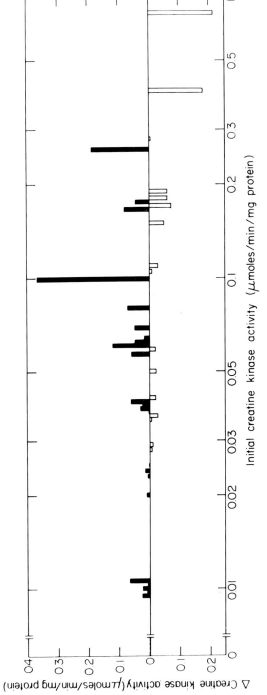

FIG. 6. Change in creatine kinase activity due to estradiol treatment in primary mammary carcinomas. Fragments or slices of tumors were incubated for 2 h in 3 x 10^{-9}M estradiol-17β or overnight (usually 16 h) in 10^{-9}M estradiol-17β. Note that initial activity is plotted on a logarithmic scale.

TABLE 1.   Responsiveness of human breast carcinomas as related to their
estrogen (E) and progesterone (P) receptor status.

Receptor state	Creatine kinase responsive	
$E^- P^-$	1/4	(25%)
$E^- P^+$	0/2	(0)
$E^+ P^-$	4/10	(40%)
$E^+ P^+$	13/19	(68%)

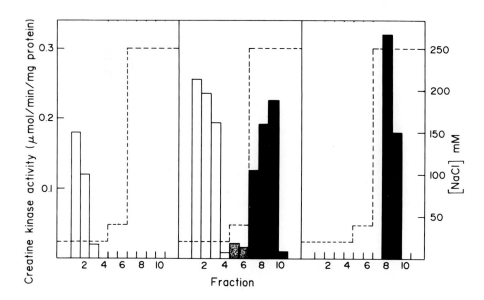

FIG. 7.   Examples of the variation of creatine kinase isozyme composition of human mammary tumors. Open bars, MM isozyme; stippled bars, MB
isozyme; black bars BB isozyme.

ured in fragments of human breast tumors, obtained at biopsy, following
incubation in estradiol-17β, 4 out of 19 benign tumors and 26 out of 53
malignant tumors demonstrated an increase in CK specific activity, in
contrast to fragments of normal breast which showed an increase in 8 out
of 10 cases. These data are the first results in a long-term study to
examine the possible correlation between in vitro responsiveness of tumors to estrogen and clinical response to endocrine therapy.

Acknowledgements

    This work was initiated during the tenure by A.M.K. of an EMBO short
term fellowship at the I.C.R.F. and was supported in part by grants from
the Ford Foundation, The Population Council and the Rockefeller Foundation, New York to the late Prof. H.R. Lindner. A.M.K. is the incumbent
of the Joseph Moss Professorial Chair in Molecular Endocrinology.

REFERENCES

1. Barnea, A. and Gorski, J. (1970): Biochemistry, 9:1899-1904.
2. Bradford, M.M. (1976): Anal. Biochem., 72:248-254.
3. Duffy, M.J. and O'Connell, M. (1981): Europ. J. Cancer, 17:711-714.
4. Hallowes, R.C., Bone, E.J., and Jones, W. (1980): In: Tissue Culture in Medical Research (II), edited by R.J. Richards and K.T. Rajan.
5. Ip, M., Milholland, R.J., Rosen, F. and Untae, K. (1979): Science, 203:361-363.
6. Katzenellenbogen, B.S. and Gorski, J. (1972): J. Biol. Chem., 247:1299-1305.
7. Katzman, P.A., Larson, D.L., and Podratz, K.C. (1971): In: The Sex Steroids: Molecular Mechanisms, edited by K.W. McKerns, pp. 107-147, Appleton-Century-Crofts, New York.
8. Kaye, A.M., Reiss, N., Iacobelli, S., Bartoccioni, E., and Marchetti, P. (1980): In: Hormones and Cancer, edited by S. Iacobelli, R.J.B. King, H.R. Lindner and M.E. Lippman, pp. 41-52, Raven Press, N.Y.
9. Kaye, A.M., Reiss, N., Shaer, A., Sluyser, M., Iacobelli, S., Amroch, D., and Soffer, Y. (1981): J. Steroid Biochem., 15:69-75.
10. King, R.J.B., Stewart, J.F., Millis, R.R., Rubens, R.D., and Hayward, J.L. (1982): Breast Cancer Res. and Treatment., 2:339-346.
11. McGuire, W.L. (1980): In: Hormones and Cancer, edited by S. Iacobelli, R.J.B. King, H.R. Lindner and M.E. Lippman, pp. 337-343, Raven Press, N.Y.
12. Mairesse, N., Galand, P., Henson, J.C. and LeClercq, G. (1976): Arch I. Phys., 84:1089-1090.
13. Malnick, S.D.H., Shaer, A., Soreq, H., and Kaye, A.M. (1983): Endocrinology, 113:1907-1909.
14. Reiss, N.A. and Kaye, A.M. (1981): J. Biol. Chem. 256:5741-5749.
15. Stampfer, M., Hallowes, R.C., and Hackett, A.J. (1980): In Vitro, 16:415-425.

Progress in Cancer Research and Therapy,
Vol. 31, edited by F. Bresciani, et al.
Raven Press, New York © 1984.

Hormone-Dependent Creatine Kinase in Human Endometrium

*G. Scambia, *V. Natoli, *P. Marchetti, **A.M. Kaye,
*S. Iacobelli, and N. Gentiloni

*Laboratorio di Endocrinologia Molecolare, Università Cattolica, 00168 Rome; and
**Department of Hormone Research, The Weizmann Institute of Science,
Rehovot, Israel

Endocrine therapy is of importance in the management of patients with inoperable advanced or recurrent endometrial cancer. It is now widely accepted that only one in three of these patients respond in some way to progestin therapy (3,12,14). Hence the need for prognostic indicators which may help in the selection of patients sensitive to therapy. The encouraging results obtained in breast cancer (13) have prompted some investigators to look for steroid hormone receptors in endometrial cancer (6,21). While it is still too soon to draw definite conclusions, the information available seems to indicate that the knowledge of steroid hormone receptor status in the tumor tissue may prove to be an accurate, although not perfect indicator of the patient's response to progestin therapy (2,5,18). Therefore great interest is now being focused on the search for new markers of steroid hormone action which could serve as better indicators of hormone-dependency in endometrial cancer.

Previous work from this and other laboratories has shown that the so called estrogen "Induced Protein" (IP) of rat uterus may prove to be a very sensitive and specific marker of estrogen action (8-10,19,28). Recently, the major component of IP has been identified as the BB isoenzyme of Creatine Kinase (CK-BB) (22).

As regards human endometrium, previous reports have demonstrated that CK-BB accounts for about 75-95% of total Creatine Kinase activity in this tissue (15). It has also been demonstrated that CK-BB is preferentially located in the luminal as well as glandular epithelial cells (27).

The aim of the present study was to investigate whether CK-BB could serve as an indicator of hormone responsiveness in endometrial cancer.

METHODS

Endometrial samples were obtained by curettage or hysterectomy, washed with saline and frozen at -80°C. Tissues were histologically dated as described by Noyes et al. (20).

For in vitro steroid treatment, fragments of endometrium were incubated in Hancks balanced salt solution containing 10 nM of the hormone to be tested at 37°C under an atmosphere of 95% O_2 and 5% CO_2. The final concentration of ethanol (contributed by the hormone solution) in the incubation medium was 0.5%. This same ethanol concentration was present in control incubations. After incubation samples were frozen at -80°C.

For in vivo steroid treatment, ten postmenopausal women with advanced endometrial cancer were administered 400 mg/day oral medroxyprogesterone acetate for seven days. Endometrial samples were taken before and after the period of treatment.

For steroid hormone receptor assay tissues were homogenized in 10 mM Tris HCl, 1.5 mM EDTA, 0.02% NaN_3, 10% glycerol, 12 mM monothyoglycerol (TENMG). The estrogen and progesterone receptor concentrations were measured by incubating 100 μl of cytosol with 10 nM ^{3}H-estradiol (100 μl) or 40 nM ^{3}H R5020 (100 μl) in TENMG respectively, for 18 h at 4°C. Non specific binding was estimated from parallel sets of tubes containing a 200-fold molar excess of non radioactive diethylstilbestrol or R5020 respectively. After incubation the tubes were placed in an icewater bath and dextran charcoal was added. After 15 minutes tubes were centrifuged at 4° C and radioactivity in the supernatant counted.

Preparation of enzyme extracts, separation of Creatine Kinase isoenzymes and enzyme assay were performed as previously described (11).

Protein was determined by the Bradford method (4), using bovine serum albumin as the standard.

RESULTS

CK-BB in Normal Endometrium

Initially we measured CK-BB in specimens of normal endometrium. As shown in Fig.1, significantly higher CK-BB levels were found in secretory (1.34±0.8 U/mg protein) than in proliferative endometrium (0.5±0.26 U/mg protein), extending our previous findings (11).

In the subsequent experiments the effect of endogenously added steroid hormones on CK-BB activity was investigated. Endometrial explants collected at surgery were incubated for five hours in the presence of 10 nM of either estradiol or progesterone. As shown in Fig.2, estradiol failed to show a consistent stimulatory effect on CK-BB activity. On the contrary there was a decrease of enzyme activity in eleven out of sixteen samples examined. The inhibitory effect was more evident in tissues showing a secretory histology than in those in the proliferative stage. Pro-

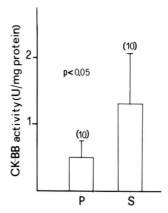

FIG. 1. CK-BB activity in normal proliferative (P) and secretory (S) endometrium. Results are expressed as mean values±S.D.; p<0.05 by Student's t test.
     The number of cases assayed is shown in brackets.

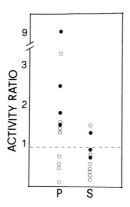

FIG. 2. In vitro effect of estradiol (○) and progesterone (●) on CK-BB
       activity in normal proliferative (P) and secretory (S) endometrium.
       Results are expressed as activity ratio hormone treated/control.

gesterone, however, increased CK-BB activity in five out of seven specimens tested. The samples showing no inductive effect had a late secretory
histology. It is possible that in these particular samples, CK-BB was already maximally stimulated by endogenous progesterone.

Taken togheter these results indicate that, unlike in rat uterus, the
activity of CK-BB in human endometrium is primarily progesterone- rather
than estrogen-dependent. This is not, however, the only example, since
other enzyme activities such as 17β-hydroxysteroid dehydrogenase, peroxidase, glucose-6-phosphate dehydrogenase and the enzymes involved in gly-
cogen metabolism which are estrogen-responsive in rat uterus are proge-
sterone-responsive in human endometrium (7,16,17,23,25,26).

CK-BB in Endometrial Cancer

Fig.3 shows the activities of CK-BB in hyperplastic and neoplastic

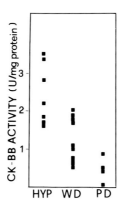

FIG. 3. CK-BB activity in specimens from hyperplastic (HYP) and neoplas-
       tic endometrial tissues (WD, well differentiated and PD, poorly
       differentiated carcinoma).

TABLE 1. <u>Effect of MPA° on CK-BB activity in human endometrial</u>
<u>cancer</u>

| Case | ER | PR | CK-BB activity |
	(fmoles/mg protein)		increase
Well differentiated			
1	444	1058	+++
2	54	94	+++
3	–	2261	+++
4	35	190	+++
Moderately differentiated			
5	28	–	–
6	63	81	++
Poorly differentiated			
7	–	–	–
8	17	57	–
9	–	20	++
10	–	19	+++

°400 mg/day orally, 7 days
+++ CK-BB activity increase   100%
++ CK-BB activity increase   50%
– No increase

endometrium. High activities of CK-BB were found in all 8 hyperplastic tissues examined. In the 14 endometrial cancer specimens examined, the activity was found to be comparable to that seen in normal endometrium (cf. Fig. 1). The more differentiated tumors tended to have CK-BB activities (1.19±0.57 U/mg protein) resembling those seen in the normal secretory tissue, whereas the less differentiated tumors tended to have lower activities (0.48±0.38 U/mg protein) similar to proliferative tissue. In this respect CK-BB is similar to progesterone receptor (24).

Table 1 shows the in vivo effect of medroxyprogesterone acetate on CK-BB activity in postmenopausal women with endometrial cancer. In this test the progesterone was administered orally at a dose of 400 mg per day for seven days. In seven out of ten patients examined progestin treatment increased CK-BB in the tumor tissue. It is interesting to note that the increase of the enzyme activity was present in all well differentiated tumors. As regards the relationship to receptor status, all tumors responding to the progestin contained progesterone receptors. Two of the three samples showing no inductive effect had no progesterone receptors, whereas the other had measurable levels of progesterone receptors. This could indicate the presence of non-functional receptor sites.

DISCUSSION

In this paper we have shown that CK-BB is present and steroid inducible in normal and neoplastic human endometrium. On the basis of the results obtained, we suggest that in humans the activity of CK-BB is proge-
sterone- rather than estrogen-dependent, as it is in rodents. Amroch and
coworkers (1) recently reported that CK-BB is estrogen-inducible in normal and neoplastic human breast tissue. This supports the hypothesis that
the steroid dependence of this isoenzyme is not only species-specific but
also organ-specific. Further studies involving human breast and endometrial cancer cell lines are necessary to clarify the hormonal modulation
of this isoenzyme in humans.

Our study is a first survey of the possible application of CK-BB as a
marker of hormone sensitivity in human endometrial cancer. The results
of the dynamic test using medroxyprogesterone acetate seem to indicate
that the induction of CK-BB may constitute a sensitive marker of responsiveness to endocrine therapy better than the presence or concentration
of hormone receptors.

REFERENCES

1. Amroch, D., Shaer, A., Malnick, S., Cox, S., Chatsubi, I., Hallowes,
   R. and Kaye, A.M. (1983): J. Steroid Biochem., 19: 114 S.
2. Benraad, T.H.J., Friberg, L.G., Koenders, A.J.M. and Kullander, S.
   (1980): Acta Obstet. Gynecol. Scand. 59:155-159.
3. Bonte, J. (1983): In: Role of Medroxyprogesterone in Endocrine Related
   Tumors, edited by L. Campio, G. Robustelli Della Cuna and R.W. Taylor,
   pp. 141-156, Raven Press, New York.
4. Bradford, M.M. (1976): Analyt. Biochem., 72:248-254.
5. Creasman,W.T., McCarty, K.S., Barton, T.K. and McCarty, K.S. Jr.
   (1980): Obstet. Gynecol., 55:363-370.
6. Ehrlich, C.E., Cleary, R.E. and Young, P.C.M. (1978): In: Endometrial
   Cancer, edited by M.G. Brush, R.J.B. King and R.W. Taylor, pp. 258-
   264, Balliere Tyndall, London.
7. Holinka, C.F. and Gurpide, E. (1981): J. Steroid Biochem., 15:183-192.
8. Iacobelli, S. (1973): Nature New Biol., 245, 144:154-155.
9. Iacobelli, S., King, R.J.B. and Vokaer, A. (1977): Biochem. Biophys.
   Res. Commun., 76, 4: 1230-1237.
10. Kaye, A.M., Reiss, N., Iacobelli, S., Bartoccioni, E. and Marchetti, P.
    (1980): In: Hormones and Cancer, edited by S. Iacobelli, R.J.B. King,
    H.R. Lindner, M.E. Lippman, pp. 41-52, Raven Press, New York.
11. Kaye, A.M., Reiss, N., Shaer, A., Sluyser, M., Iacobelli, S., Amroch,
    D. and Soffer, Y. (1981): J. Steroid Biochem., 15: 69-75.
12. Kelley, R.M. and Baker, W.H. (1961): N. Engl. J. Med., 264: 216-222.
13. Knight, W.A., Osborne, C.K., Yochmowitz, M.G., McGuire, W.L. (1980):
    Ann. Clin. Res. 12: 202-207.
14. Kohorn, E.I. (1978): In: Endometrial Cancer, edited by M.G. Brush, R.
    J.B. King, R.W. Taylor, pp. 179-187, Balliere Tindall, London.
15. Lang, H. (1981): In: Creatine-Kinase Isoenzymes, edited by H. Lang,
    pp. 242-269, Springer-Verlag, Berlin.
16. Lyttle, C.R. and De Sombre, E.R. (1977): Proc. Natl. Acad. Sci. 74:
    3162-3166.
17. Lucas, F.V., Carnes, V.M., Schmidt, H.J., Siyes, D.R. and Hall, D.G.
    (1964): Am. J. Obstet. Gynecol. 88: 965-970.

18. Martin, P.M., Rolland, P.H., Gammerre, M., Serment, H. and Toga, M. (1979): Int. J. Cancer, 23: 321–329.
19. Notides, A. and Gorski, J. (1966): Proc. Natl. Acad. Sci. USA, 56: 230–235.
20. Noyes, R.H., Hertig, A.T. and Rock, J. (1950): Fertil. Steril.,1::32–35.
21. Pollow, K., Schmidt-Goll Witzer, M. and Pollow, B. (1978): In: Endometrial Cancer, edited by M.G. Brush, R.J.B. King and R.W. Taylor, pp. 265–274, Balliere Tindall, London.
22. Reiss, N.A. and Kaye, A.M. (1981): J. Biol. Chem. 256: 5741–5749.
23. Richardson, G.S. and McLaughlin, D.T. (1978): UICC Technical Report, Geneva vol. 42, 63.
24. Satyaswaroop, P.G. and Mortel, R. (1981): Am. J. Obstet. Gynecol., 15, 140: 620–623.
25. Tseng, L. and Gurpide, E. (1975): Endocrinology 97: 825–833.
26. Wahawison, R. and Gorell, T.A. (1980): Steroids, 36: 115–129.
27. Wald, L.E., Li, C.Y. and Hamburger, M.A. (1981): Am. J. Clin. Pathol. 75: 327–332.
28. Walker, M.D., Negreanu, V., Gozes, I. and Kaye, A.M. (1979): FEBS lett., 98: 187–191.

Progress in Cancer Research and Therapy,
Vol. 31, edited by F. Bresciani, et al.
Raven Press, New York © 1984.

Elevated Serum Tissue Polypeptide Antigen Concentration in Medullary Thyroid Carcinoma

*E. Martino, *G. Bambini, *F. Aghini-Lombardi, *E. Motz,
*R. Lari, *F. Pacini, *L. Baschieri, and **A. Pinchera

*Patologia Medica 2 and **Endocrinologia e Medicina Costituzionale,
University of Pisa, 56100 Pisa, Italy*

Medullary thyroid carcinoma (MTC)is a differentiated metastasizing tumor arising from parafollicular C cells, secreting large amounts of calcitonin (CT).Serum CT concentration is considered the most reliable humoral index for the diagnosis and the follow-up of this type of thyroid tumor (1,9),although in the past years elevated values of other substances have been found in the serum of the patients with MTC, such as carcino-embryonic antigen, ACTH,MSH,beta-lipotropin,prostaglandins, serotonin, corticotropin releasing factor and substance P (2,7,8,9,10, 11,21).

Tissue polypeptide antigen (TPA) is a substance identified and characterized by Bjorklund and Bjorklund (4) in human neoplastic cell membranes as well as in fetal tissues and placenta (5,6). Recently several studies using a specific and sensitive radioimmunoassay reported detectable amounts of TPA in serum of normal subjects and elevated serum concentrations in patients with different malignant neoplasia (3,13,15,16,20). No data are available, at our knowledge, on circulating TPA in patients with MTC. In the present study we report the results of serum TPA assay in a group of 21 patients with MTC, compared with CT,carcino-embryonic antigen (CEA) and thyroglobulin (Tg) determinations.

Materials and Methods

Patients.

The study group included 21 patients (7 males and 14 females,aging between 26 and 75 yr) with histologically documented MTC. Total thyroidectomy had been previously performed in 20 patients and subtotal thyroidectomy in the remaining one; local or distant metastases were present in 19 cases.All patients were euthyroid on L-thyroxine replacement theraphy. At the time of the study no inflammatory or infectious diseases were pre

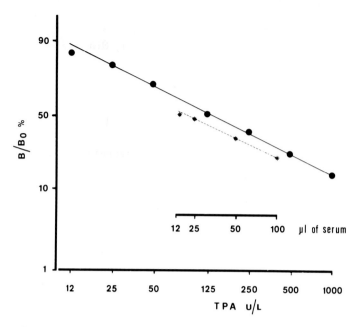

Fig.1.Parallelism between TPA standard (●——●) and
immunoreactive material (*----*) detected in
serum of a patient with MTC.Values in abscissa
are in log scale.

sent. Fourthy-five healthy subjects (23 males and 22 females,aging betwe
en 21 and 64 yr) were investigated as controls.

Tumor Markers Determination

  Blood samples were collected at 8-10 a.m. from overnight fasted subje
cts. Sera were immediately separated in cold centrifuge and stored at
-20°C until assayed. In order to avoid the interassay variations all
samples were measured in duplicate in the same run.

  TPA Determination.Serum TPA was assayed by specific radioimmunoassay
using a commercial kit (TPA-RIA kit Prolifigen,Sangtec Medical, Bromma,
Sweden) kindly supplied by Byk-Gulden Italia S.p.A., Milan. The assay was
performed as described by the manifacturer; the sensitivity of the assay
was 12 U/L. The intraassay coefficient of variation was less than 7%.No
cross reactivity was found with CEA,CT and Tg.The analysis of immunoreactivity of circulating TPA in patients with MTC showed that serial dilution curves of serum were virtually parallel to the standard curve (Fig 1).

  CEA Determination.The assay for CEA determination was performed using
a commercial kit (CEAK-PR,Sorin Biomedica,Saluggia,Italy). The intraassay
coefficient of variation was less than 5%.

  CT Determination.The RIA-MAT Calcitonin II kit (Byk-Mallinkrodt Radio-
pharmaceutica,Dietzenbach,W.Germany) was used for serum CT measurement.
The intraassay coefficient of variation was less than 5%.

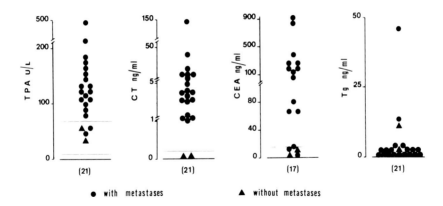

Fig. 2 Individual values of TPA,CT,CEA and Tg in patients
with MTC.The horizontal lines represent the normal
range.

Tg Determination.Serum thyroglobulin was assayed by an immunoradiome-
tric method previously described (14) using HTGK kit,Sorin Biomedica,Sa-
luggia,Italy.The minimun detectable value was 3 ng/ml.Circulating anti-
thyroglobulin autoantibodies.determined by passive haemoagglutination
with commercial kit (Fujizoki Pharmaceutical Co.,Tokyo,Japan), were undetectable in all sera.

Results

Serum TPA concentration in normal controls was 38.0+3.2 U/L (mean±SE),
ranging between 12.0 and 69.0 U/L. Elevated serum TPA values were observed in MTC patients, with a mean value of 135.0+21.0 U/L (p< 0.0005 vs
control). As illustrated in Figure 2 elevated values of serum TPA were
found in 17 out of 21 patients (80%) and were comprised in the normal
range in 4 patients,two of whom had no evidence of metastases and were
apparently free of disease. The incidence of elevated serum TPA leves was
even higher (89%) when only patients with metastases were considered.Se--
rum CT values were elevated in all patients with metastatic MTC with a
mean value of 17.8+7.9 ng/ml,while normal concentrations were found in
the two patients without metastases. Serum CEA was measured in 17 patien
ts and elevated concentrations were observed in 12 (70%), with a mean va
lue of 153.2+50.2 ng/ml;normal values were found in 3 patients with metastases and in the two patients apparently free of disease.Excluding the
patients with no evidence of metastases, the incidence of elevated serum
CEA was 80%. Serum Tg was undetectable in 18 patients, detectable in two
patients with small thyroid residual tissue, with values within the range of normal subjects (< 3-39 ng/ml),and slightly elevated in the patient
submitted to subtotal thyroidectomy.
The comparative statistical analysis of serum TPA and the other tumor
markers showed no significant correlation between TPA and CEA (Fig.3),
CT and Tg.

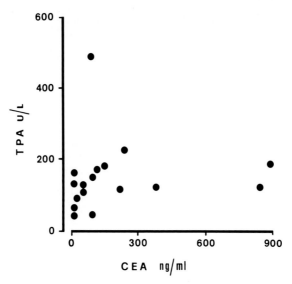

Fig.3 Linear regression analysis between serum TPA and CEA
     in MTC. p was not significant by Pearson correlation
     coefficient.

Discussion

   Elevated serum TPA concentrations are known to be associated with lar
ge number of human tumors with an incidence as high as 70-85% in cancer
of breast, lung,gastro-intestinal tract,pancreas,cervix-uterus, leukemia,
and with lower incidence (50-60%) in prostatic cancer and malignant
melanoma (3,13,15,16,17,20). In our series of medullary thyroid
carcinoma we have found elevated TPA values in 89% of patients with
documented metastases, suggesting that TPA may be considered a marker
although not specific, of MTC.
Bjorklund et al. (5,6) reported that TPA is released from highly
growing multiplying human cancer cells "in vitro". This findings
is corroborated by various clinical studies (3,13,15,16,17,20,23)
indicating that TPA is present in serum of patients with progressive
malignant diseases. These observations are in keeping with our results
on metastatic MTC, since this tumor is the most aggressive differentiated
thyroid cancer. Elevated TPA values have been observed in patients
with inflammatory or infectious disease in absence of malignancies
(12,19,23). On this regard the presence of such noneoplastic diseases
was excluded in our patients.
The analysis of the immunoreactivity of circulating TPA in the serum
of one MTC patients with high TPA value clearly showed the specificity
of the assay.
In agreement with other reports (2,7,8,9,10) in the present study
elevated values of CEA have been observed in 12 of 15 (80%) patients
with metastatic MTC. Although this incidence is slightly lower than

that of TPA, more extensive studies are needed in order to prove whether TPA is a marker more sensitive than CEA. In addition, the lack of correlation between serum TPA and CEA values suggests that different factors may be involved in the serum elevation of these two markers. Undetectable values of serum Tg were found in all patients previously submitted to total thyroidectomy, while detectable values were observed only in patients with residual thyroid tissue. This data are in agreement with other studies (18,22) and are in keeping with the notion that medullary thyroid cancer arises from parafollicular C cells which are unable to synthetize Tg.

In conclusion, this study indicates that serum TPA is an additional humoral marker of metastatic MTC, which can be employed in addition to CT, which remains the most specific marker.

References

1.   Aurbach, G.D., Marx, S.J., and Spiegel, A.M. (1981): In: Textbook of Endocrinology, edited by R.H. Williams, pp. 1017-1019. Saunders Co., Philadelphia.

2.   Baschieri, L., Giani, C., Mariotti, S., Busnardo, B., Girelli, M.E., and Pinchera, A. (1982): In: Markers for diagnosis and and monitoring od human cancer, edited by M.I. Colnaghi, G.L. Buraggi and M. Ghione, pp. 258-265. Academic Press, New York.

3.   Bjorklund, B., (1978): Antibiotics Chemoter., 22: 16-31.

4.   Bjorklund, B., and Bjorklund, V. (1957): Int. Arch. Allergy Appl. Immun., 10: 153-159.

5.   Bjorklund, B., Bjorklund, V., Lundstrom, R., and Eklund, G., (1976): In: Advances in Experimental Medicine and Biology, vol. 73B, Edited by Friedman, Escobar and Reichard, p. 357. Plenum Press, New York.

6.   Bjorklund, B., Bjorklund, V., Wiklund, B., Lundstrom, R.,Ekdahl, P. H., Hagbard, L., Kaijser, K., Eklund, G., and Luning, D. (1973): In: Immunological Techniques for detection of cancer, edited by Bjorklund B., p. 133. Bonniers, Stockholm.

7.   De Lellis, R.A., Ruie, A.H., Spiler, I., Nathanson, L., Tashjian, A.H., and Wolfe, H.J. (1978): Am. J. Clin. Pathol., 70: 587-594.

8.   Calmettes, C., Moukhtar, M.S., and Milhaud, G. (1978): Cancer Immunol Immunother., 4: 251-256.

9.   Hazard, J.B. (1977): Am. J. Pathol., 88: 214-249.

10. Iwanaga, T., T., Koyama, H., Uchiyama, S., Takahashi, Y.,Nakano, S. Itoh, T., Horai, T., Wada, A., and Tateishi, R. (1978): Cancer, 41: 1106-1112.

11. Krauss, S., Macy, S., and Ichiki, A.T. (1981): Cancer, 47: 2485-2492.

12   Lundstrom, R., Bjorklund, B., and Eklund, G. (1973): In: Immunological techniques for detection of cancer, edited by B. Bjorklund, p. 243. Bonniers, Stockholm.

13.   Luthgens, M., and Schelegel, G. (1981): Tumordiagnostik, 2: 179-188.

14.   Mariotti, S., Cupini, C., Giani, C., Lari, R., Rolleri, E, Falco, A., Marchisio, M., and Pinchera, A. (1982): Clin. Chim. Acta., 123: 347-356.

15.   Menendez-Botet, C.J., Oettgen, H.F., Pinsky, C.M., and Schwartz, M.K. (1978): Clin. Chem., 24: 868-872.

16.   Mross, K., Mross, D., Wolfrum, D.I., and Rauschecker, H. (1983): Klin. Wochenschr., 61: 461-468.

17.   Nemoto, T., Constantine, R., and Chu, T.M. (1979): J.N.C.I., 63: 1347-1350.

18.   Pacini, F., Pinchera, A., Giani, C., Doveri, F., and Baschieri, L. (1980): J. Endocrinol. Invest., 3: 283-292.

19.   Ruibal, A., Clotet, B., Pigrau, C., Duran-Bellido, P., Fraile, M. and Roca, I. (1982): Tumordiagnostik, 3: 40-44.

20.   Schlegel, G., Luthgens, M., Eklund, G., and Bjorklund, B. (1981): Tumordiagnostick, 2: 6-11.

21   Skrabanek, P., Cannon, D., Dempsey, J., Kirrane J., Neligan, M., and Powell, D. (1979): Experientia, 35: 1259.

22.   Van Herle, A.J., and Uller, R.P. (1975): J. Clin. Invest., 56: 272-277.

23.   Wolfrum, D.I., Mross, K., Mross, B., and Rauschecker, H. (1983) Verh. Dtsch. Krebs Ger., 4:861.

Progress in Cancer Research and Therapy,
Vol. 31, edited by F. Bresciani, et al.
Raven Press, New York © 1984.

Quality Control of Routine Steroid Hormone Receptor Assays

David T. Zava

Ludwig Institute for Cancer Research, 3010 Bern, Switzerland

Over the past several decades the measurement of tumor steroid hormone receptors has become commonplace in the clinical management of human breast cancer(1,5). Since it was recognized that the steroid hormone receptor assay would be a mainstay in the treatment of human breast cancer, interlaboratory quality control programs were initiated to critically evaluate the performance of the receptor assay among groups participating in common clinical studies (2,3,6,7). These periodic between-laboratory quality control programs proved very useful in helping some laboratories identify and eliminate some of the methodological differences that contributed to significant interlaboratory discordance in test results. External quality control programs of steroid hormone receptor assays, however, have proved to be somewhat limited in scope in that they provide no information on the performance of the results of the daily routine assay from which data for cooperative studies is actually compiled. Although there is an obvious need for an internal quality control mechanism to monitor the results of the daily routine steroid receptor assay the procedures for developing such an "in house" review mechanism have not been delineated. Thus, very few laboratories actually perform an internal control of their steroid hormone receptor assays, as is required by law for many other routine clinical tests.

In this report I will briefly summarize a series of two external quality control surveys carried out by the Ludwig Institute; an international study (2) and a national Swiss study (7), and then reveal in more detail the methods and results of an internal quality control program that we have successfully used to monitor the performance of our routine ER and PR assays.

I. SUMMARY OF INTERNATIONAL QUALITY CONTROL SURVEY

Our first external quality control study (2) was organized to evaluate the uniformity of ER and PR assay results among different laboratories participating in a common clinical breast cancer trial. Frozen calf uterus powders containing three different titers of ER and PR were prepared by a central coordinating laboratory and distributed among the participants. Enough tissue powder was distributed to allow 3-5 sequential analyses. The results are summarized in Table I.

Table 1. Oestrogen and progestin receptor analysis

Coded laboratory	(n)	Oestrogen receptor			(n)	Progestin receptor		
		11	12	13		11	12	13
C1	(12, 11, 11)	88 ± 7	227 ± 13	22 ± 4	(11, 7, 10)	422 ± 39	263 ± 12	34 ± 4
C2A	(1, 2, 2)	47	156, 195	11, 15	(1, 2, 2)	236	137, 138	27, 29
C2B	(6, 6, 5)	48 ± 5	170 ± 12	14 ± 1	(6, 6, 5)	218 ± 26	138 ± 11	28 ± 3
L1	(5)	57 ± 2	154 ± 6	6 ± 3	(5)	147 ± 38	222 ± 17	0
L2	(3)	46 ± 3	126 ± 8	7 ± 1	(3)	53 ± 7	52 ± 1	6 ± 1
L3	(3)	45 ± 4	130 ± 5	0	(2)	62 ± 10	60 ± 1	0
L4	(4)	47 ± 2	117 ± 3	10 ± 1	(4)	257 ± 53	143 ± 16	21 ± 1
L5	(3)	16 ± 1	43 ± 4	15 ± 1	(3)	41 ± 4	41 ± 8	14 ± 1
L6	(1)	17	137	6	(3)	207 ± 2	189 ± 2	17 ± 5
L7	(6)	63 ± 5	149 ± 18	6 ± 1	(6)	28 ± 9	33 ± 7	6 ± 2
L8	(6)	70 ± 4	175 ± 5	7 ± 2	(6)	85 ± 6	72 ± 6	8 ± 4
Total means*		51 ± 3	143 ± 7	8 ± 1		126 ± 16	109 ± 11	12 ± 2
(n)		(38)	(39)	(38)		(36)	(40)	(39)

Oestrogen and progestin receptors were assays in samples 11, 12, and 13 by the control centre in Louisville, KY before shipping to Berne for distribution (C1), after receiving samples returned from Berne (C2B) and after continuous storage in Louisville for a time period equal to the age of samples C2B (C2A). Assay values for oestrogen and progesterone receptors (mean ± S.E.M. fmol/mg cytosol protein) for samples 11, 12 and 13 are represented as L1–L8 for the coded participating laboratories. n represents the number of assays performed by each centre.
*The total means are calculated from C2A, C2B and L1–8, i.e. all the data collected after the dispatch of samples from Louisville (C1).

reproduced from ref 2

Although significant quantitative interlaboratory variations were observed in the tissue levels of ER and PR it was concluded that, with the exception of one outlier, all of the groups were able to categorize the samples into a range of low, medium and high ER and PR binding.

II. SUMMARY OF SWISS NATIONAL QUALITY CONTROL SURVEY

The second quality control study (7) was organized on a regional scale with the goal of trying to identify some of the methodological differences that contributed to inter- and intralaboratory variations in the ER and PR assay results seen in our first study (2). Tumor powders derived from the residual frozen stocks of preassayed human breast carcinomas were prepared for shipment to the various Swiss participants. Three types of tumor powders were prepared with less than 10, between 20 and 40, and greater than 100 fmoles ER and PR/mg cytosol protein. The samples were dispatched to the participating laboratories on solid CO_2. Samples were received by all laboratories within 24 hours. The laboratories were asked to prepare tissue extracts from half of each sample and save the remaining half of the frozen powder for shipment back to the coordinating center in Bern. From the tissue extract that was prepared by the participants half was assayed in-house and the remaining half snap frozen and shipped back to the coordinating center along with the frozen powder. Tissue powders and cytosols that were shipped back to the coordinating center were used to determine if: 1) receptors were destroyed during shipment (by comparing ER and PR in tissue shipped to participating centers with receptor values in tissue not shipped); 2) differences in methods and reagents used for preparing cytosols were responsible for any quantitative variations in binding sites (by comparing ER and PR values in cytosols prepared by participants but analyzed in the reference center); 3) interlaboratory assay results varied because of differences in the methods for determining the protein content of cytosols (by comparing protein values from cytosols assayed by the participating groups with protein values assayed by the reference center). A summary of these results is shown in Table 2.

TABLE 2. ER and PR for Reference (RL) and Participating (I-V) Laboratories

Category	Assay Laboratory	Estrogen Receptor Standard[a]			Progesterone Receptor Standard[a]		
		A	B	C	A	B	C
1	RL[b]	6±5	39±12	115±17	2±2	94±37	253±62
2	RL[b,c]	6±3	36±5	110±32	2±3	78±35	205±170
3	RL[b,d]	6±3	32±8	105±37	0	41±22	92±31
4	I[e]	4	115	281	41	134	168
	II	3	64	295	7	118	365
	III	5	26	75	5	75	227
	IV	5	25	105	0	76	109
	V	26	85	326	0	61	100
I-V Group Mean ± SD		9±9	63±35	216±105	11±15	93±28	192±93

a: fmoles/mg cytosol protein
b: mean values ± standard deviation for 5 assays (Category 1)
c: tumor powders returned by participants and then assayed by reference laboratory (Category 2)
d: tumor cytosols returned by participants and then assayed by reference laboratory (Category 3).
e: assayed by participating laboratories (Category 4).
with permission (ref. 7)

Within-laboratory Variability   In a comparison of the first three categories of binding values generated by the reference laboratory the low, medium and high concentrations of tumor ER, but not of PR, could be clearly distinguished whether the tissue remained in the reference laboratory (Category 1), was returned to the reference laboratory by the participants in the same frozen powder originally delivered to them (Category 2) or was returned to the reference laboratory in the form of cytosol prepared by the participants (Category 3). These results negate any possibility that group differences in receptor concentration could be due to the methods used for preparing cytosols (i.e., buffer, homogenization, centrifugation techniques, etc.) (Category 2), or that ER was destroyed in the frozen powders during transport (Category 3). Loss of PR was greater than that of ER during transport, especially in the form of frozen cytosols (Category 3), indicating its greater thermolability as reported previously (7).

Interlaboratory Variability   Although   there   was   only   minimal
within-laboratory variation of the ER and PR content of tumor powders
assayed in the reference laboratory (Category 1) five consecutive times
over a one-month period the between-laboratory concordance (Category 1
vs. Category 4) was not as uniform. The mean binding values of ER and
PR were either in close agreement with (Participants III and IV) or
higher than (Participants I, II and V) those reported by the reference
laboratory. There was not a definite consensus among the laboratories
about the quantitation of ER and PR binding sites in the tumor powders.
Nevertheless all groups (exceptions: Participant I, PR sample A, and
Participant V, ER sample A) were generally able to classify each tumor
into low-, medium- or high-range ER and PR. From a clinical point of
view perhaps the most important finding was that no laboratories
reported either false-positive or false-negative ER or PR values based
on a cutoff value of 10 fmoles/mg cytosol protein.

Comparison of Protein Content of Cytosols. We compared the protein
content of the tumor extracts prepared and analyzed by the
participating groups with the same extracts frozen and then shipped
back to and analyzed by the reference laboratory (Table 3).

TABLE 3   Protein Content of Standards Assayed by Reference Laboratory
          (RL) Compared with Participant's Laboratories (I-V)

Center	Protein Assay	Protein (mg/ml) A	B	C
RL/RL	Lowry	1.5/1.5	1.6/1.7	1.3/1.3
I/RL	Biorad	2.1/2.7	1.9/-	2.1/3.0
II/RL	Lowry	2.0/3.1	2.0/2.5	2.0/2.7
III/RL	Lowry	2.0/1.9	2.0/1.9	2.0/2.0
IV/RL	Lowry	2.0/1.7	2.0/1.6	2.0/1.6
V/RL	Turbidimetry	2.2/2.7	1.9/2.4	1.8/2.7

with permission (ref. 7)

The results reveal an obvious discrepancy in the protein values of
Laboratories I, II and V relative to the reference laboratory,
accounting in part for the higher receptor values reported by these
groups (Table 2).
    It was concluded from this national Swiss study that the differences
in ER and PR values reported by the group participants could not be
attributed to decay of receptors during transport from one laboratory
to another, to different methods of preparing tissue extracts, or to
differences in processing the laboratory data (data not shown-see ref
7). The results did indicate, however, that the source of error
leading to the quantitative discrepancies in the ER and PR binding
data between the laboratories were, in part, a consequence of
differences in the methods for quantitating the protein in the tissue
extracts and to differences in assay methodology.

INTERNAL QUALITY CONTROL PROGRAM

Although previous quality control studies were clearly useful for helping many laboratories identify and eliminate differences in methodology that led to significant variation in ER and PR binding values among groups participating in common clinical studies, it was obvious that these external quality control reviews were limited in scope because they were unable to pinpoint the inevitable errors incurred in the daily routine hormone receptor assay. For this reason, a third generation "in-house" quality control program was designed to serve as an adjunct to the periodic external quality control programs.

Methods for Preparing Internal Standards Receptor standards were prepared from the residual stocks of frozen (-70 C) breast tumors previously assayed (1-12 months). Tissue extracts were prepared from the breast tumors, as previously described (ref 7), and then pooled according to their preassayed ER and PR assay values. Three standards were prepared to yield ER and PR values that would mimic the wide range of ER and PR binding values that might be expected from routine steroid hormone receptor analyses of breast tumors. Standards contained, respectively, less than 10 (negative), between 10 and 30 (low positive), and greater than 100 fmol/mg protein (high positive) of ER and PR per sample. Tissue extracts from the various categories of receptor content were pooled, thoroughly mixed, aliquoted into 1.5-2 ml plastic vials with tight sealing caps, snap frozen in liquid nitrogen and then stored at -70°C until assayed. Cytosols were thawed at 0-4°C for 30 min and then assayed for ER and PR content by the dextran-coated charcoal method (2). The ER and PR content of each of the samples was first assessed by multiple dose (Scatchard) analysis to establish the binding constants and level of binding sites. Samples then were subsequently assayed each week using only a single-saturating dose of radioligand (7). The limits used to define the standards as negative, low-positive, or high-positive were based on the classical convention that ER and PR values less than 10 fmol/mg protein are negative, values 10-50 fmol/mg protein are low-positive and those greater than 50 fmol/mg protein are high-positive.

Interassay Reproducibility of Internal Quality Control Standards. The receptor binding values for the negative (A), low-positive (B) and high-positive (C) ER and PR standards assayed weekly over a four-month period (Figs 1A and1B) show that none of these standards deviated qualitatively from their respective categories even though there was a wide scatter of binding values for ER of Standard C. The much lower ER values of the last two assays of Month 12 could be accounted for by a decrease in protein concentration which was due to leakage of ice water during the thawing process into improperly sealed vials. In these isolated cases, both total ER binding and protein concentration decreased in parallel. The pattern of PR binding for Standards A, B and C were generally the same as for ER, with the exception that PR of Sample A quite often exceeded the 10 fmol/mg protein limits arbitrarily established as a cutoff value. PR samples B and C remained remarkably stable over this time course with one exception (Standard C, second assay-Month 3).

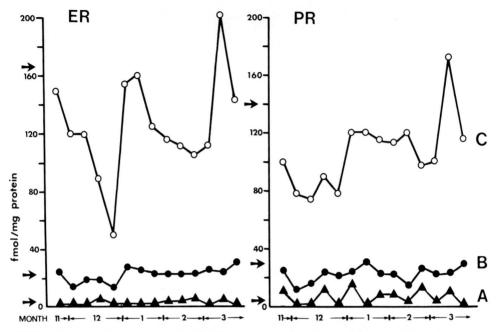

FIGS 1A and B Internal Quality Control Standards - Estrogen and Progesterone Receptors. The concentration of receptor binding sites derived from Scatchard plots are indicated by arrows.

Variation in Measurement of Protein Concentrations The protein concentrations of the three standards were measured by the method of Lowry (4). The individual values over the four-month period are illustrated in Figure 2. The protein values remained relatively constant, with the few exceptions already mentioned, caused by water leakage into the vials during the thawing process.

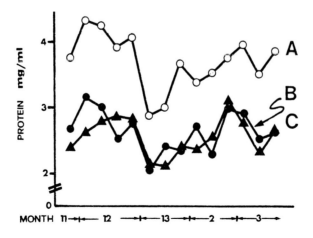

Fig 2. Protein Content of Internal Quality Control Standards

Use of Frozen Receptor Standards for External Quality Control of Peer Laboratories. In order for internal quality control samples to have significance within the framework of a cooperative study the samples must be analyzed by an external peer group to assure interlaboratory uniformity in receptor binding site concentrations. This requires that the standards remain stable during shipment to peer laboratories. Thus, the standards were shipped from our laboratory on solid CO_2 to another steroid hormone receptor laboratory for comparison of the quantitative values of our receptor standards against those of another laboratory. The results are presented in Table 4.

TABLE 4
Comparison Standards Assayed by an External Laboratory and by Bern.

Sample	Protein (mg/ml)		ER^1 (fmol/mg prot.)		PR^1 (fmol/mg prot.)	
	(E)	(B)	(E)	(B)	(E)	(B)
A	3.62	3.75	0	4	0	0
B	2.48	2.71	27	23	29	15
C	2.19	2.40	185	165	175	160

[1]Assayed by multiple dose (Scatchard) analysis.

Protein, ER and PR contents of Samples A, B and C are compared between our group and the peer laboratory. Receptor binding values, derived from Scatchard plots, protein concentrations, and ER and PR binding sites, were remarkably similar between laboratories despite the fact that the standards were in transit to the peer laboratory on solid CO_2 for over 24 hours. These results corroborate our second study demonstrating that frozen tumor cytosol standards can be shipped on solid CO_2 without appreciable loss of receptor binding sites. Therefore, such standards for use in internal quality control could be prepared by a central coordinating laboratory and distributed among participants of a common clinical study.

In conclusion, internal hormone receptor standards can easily be prepared from the residual stocks of preassayed frozen solid tumors. These standards, which fall within the usual range of ER and PR binding values normally observed in the routine measurement of breast tumors, can be used to monitor the performance of the daily routine hormonal receptor assay. The internal quality control standards can thus serve as a useful adjunct to external quality control surveys to help pinpoint the spurious errors in results that will inevitably occur in the daily routine hormone receptor assay.

REFERENCES

1. Allegra, J.C., Lippman, M.E., Thompson, E.B., Simon, R.T., Barlock, A., Green, L., Huff, K.K., Do, H.M.T., Aitken, S.C., and Warren, R.T. (1980) Eur. J. Cancer, 16:323-331.

2. Jordan, V.C., Zava, D.T., Eppenberger, U., Kiser, A., Sebek, S., Dowdle, E., Krozowski, Z., Bennett, R.C., Funder, J., Holdaway, I.M., and Wittliff, J.L. (1983) Eur. J. Cancer Clin. Oncol., 19:357-363.

3. King, R.J.B. (1980) Cancer, 46:2822-2824.

4. Lowry, D.H., Rosenbrough, W.J., Farr, A.L., and Randall, P.J. (1961) J. Biol. Chem., 193:265-275.

5. Osborne, C.K., Yochmowitz, M.G., Knight, W.A., and McGuire, W.L. (1980) Cancer, 46:2884-2888.

6. Raam, S., Gelman, R., Cohen, J.L., Bacharach, A., Fishchinger, A.J., Jacobson, H.I., Keshgegian, A.A., Konopka, S.J., and Wittliff, J.L. (1981) Eur J. Cancer, 17:643-649.

7. Zava, D.T., Wyler-Von Ballmoos, A., Goldhirsch, A., Roos, W., Takahashi, A., Eppenberger, U., Arrenbrecht, S., Martz, G., Losa, G., Gomez, F., Guelpa, C. (1982) Eur. J. Cancer Clin. Oncol., 18:713-721.

Progress in Cancer Research and Therapy,
Vol. 31, edited by F. Bresciani, et al.
Raven Press, New York © 1984.

Inter-Laboratory Variability in Estrogen and Progestin Receptor Assays[1]

A. Koenders and Th. Benraad

Department of Experimental and Chemical Endocrinology,
6525 GA Nijmegen, The Netherlands

The serious need for standardization and quality control of steroid receptor analyses has become increasingly clear (4,20). It may be noted that already in 1972 the EORTC Breast Cancer Cooperative Group agreed on certain methodological aspects of estrogen receptor assays in biopsies of human breast tumors (5). In 1979 these agreements were revised, the standardization was extended to progestin receptor assays and a quality control program was initiated for the laboratories of those centers taking part in multi-centre clinical trials organized by the EORTC Breast Cancer Cooperative Group (6). Thereafter, this EORTC Receptor Group has been enlarged with representatives from countries with their own national quality control program of steroid receptor analyses. At present, 15 laboratories from 7 countries (Belgium, Denmark, France, W.-Germany, Italy, the Netherlands and the United Kingdom) are represented in this EORTC Receptor Group. During all trials conducted so far, lyophilized samples were used as reference material because of the thermal stability of both estrogen and progestin receptor in this type of material (2,11). In addition, the EORTC Receptor Group announced in 1982 that lyophilized control samples are available twice yearly to all laboratories interested in validation of receptor assay results (13). Presently about 25 additional laboratories make use of this external quality control service program. A quality control assessment scheme very similar to the one organized by the EORTC Receptor Group is conducted in the Netherlands; it began in 1977, there are 18 participants and during the 10 trials conducted so far, more than 25 different lyophilized reference preparations have been analyzed (12).

The results of these quality control programs have been the subject of various reports (12,14,15). It is the purpose of this contribution to extend these reports with observations made during the most recent trials.

Preparation, distribution and analysis of lyophilized cytosols.

Most lyophilized cytosolic samples were prepared from uterine tissue (calf, pig, cow) obtained from local slaughtherhouses. Immediately upon removal from the animal the uterine tissue was placed on ice and trans-

---

[1]*Behalf of the EORTC Receptor Group and the laboratories and institutions participating in the quality control program of The Netherlands.*

ported to the laboratory. Uterine horns were cleaned of fat and adherent connective tissue and washed with cold (4°C) physiological saline solution. The uterine tissue was minced on ice with scissors and the small pieces of tissue were directly frozen in liquid nitrogen. Thereafter, these small pieces of tissue were pulverized, at the temperature of liquid nitrogen (-196°), to a fine powder by means of a Thermovac tissue pulverizer and a Microdismembrator. Tissue powder was thawed in an ice bath and stirred with phosphate buffer (0.02 M Na_2HPO_4/NaH_2PO_4, 1.5 mM EDTA, 3.0 mM NaN_3, pH 7.4) for 30 min at 4°C. In general a tissue weight/buffer volume ratio was chosen to give a cytosol protein concentration of about 4 mg/ml. The obtained tissue homogenate was centrifuged at 30,000 g for one hour at 2°C. Five ml aliquots of cytosolic supernatant were measured into glass vials, placed in liquid nitrogen and lyophilized for 48-72 hrs. The vials were sealed under vacuum while still in the lyophilization chamber and stored at 4°C until shipment.

The human breast tumor biopsies routinely analyzed show receptor values from zero to more than 1000 fmol/mg protein, while most cytosols prepared from animal uterine tissue have relatively high receptor values (> 100 fmol/mg protein). A few lyophilized control cytosols with low receptor concentrations could be prepared from selected residue specimens of human breast cancers and DMBA-induced rat mammary tumors, all of which had previously been assayed for steroid receptor content. In addition, it was investigated whether reference material with low receptor values could be prepared from calf uterine cytosol diluted with filler proteins. Cytosol prepared from receptor-negative breast tumors could be an ideal source but this material is not easy to obtain in sufficient quantities, Therefore, a number of other filler proteins were evaluated: human serum-albumin (HSA), human serum immunoglobulins, calf serum and heated, receptor-negative calf uterine cytosol. All these filler proteins were acceptable with regard to the preparation of control samples for the measurement of estrogen receptors, although dilution of receptor content in some cases resulted in a slight decrease of ER values. With regard to PgR analyses, the interference of these filler proteins was more pronounced and even precluded the detection of this receptor protein with the ligand R 5020, when excessive amounts of HSA (12) and calf serum (14) were added. Unfortunately, heat treatment of freshly prepared calf uterine cytosol, in order to decrease the concentration of active binding sites, resulted in poor agreement between single dose saturation assays and multipoint Scatchard analyses (both ER and PgR, 14). The use of normal calf muscle tissue as a filler protein is presently being studied.

All lyophilized control samples were distributed by mail without temperature control and on arrival the samples were to be stored at 4°C. The stability of the samples under these mailing conditions was studied by returning an extra set of samples to our laboratory in Nijmegen by one of the participants. The receptor content in these samples was assayed and found to be similar to vials continuously stored at 4°C. The participants received detailed instructions for the reconstitution of cytosol from the lyophilized material by the addition of ice cold water containing 10% glycerol.

In the quality control program conducted in the Netherlands each laboratory is allowed to use its own methods. Presently all participants use a dextran-coated charcoal technique for the separation of bound and free steroid and 14 out of 18 participants perform multipoint Scatchard analyses. Furthermore, all participants have received samples of the same batch of charcoal and the determination of non-specific binding has also been standardized, i.e. all laboratories use 10^{-6}M DES. About half of the participating laboratories perform progestin receptor assays and all use the same radioactive ligand (Org 2058). Finally, the standardization of protein determination according to the technique of Bradford (3, Coomassie Brilliant Blue), using human serum albumin standard, has decreased the inter-laboratory variation coefficient from more than 30% to less than 10%.

The EORTC Receptor Group has now published two reports containing recommendations concerning experimental procedures for the assessment of estrogen and progestin receptors in human breast cancer (5,6). During their most recent trials the participants agreed upon several assay conditions including the use of the charcoal technique combined with Scatchard analysis as a standard procedure. In addition it is now recommended that seven concentrations of radioactive ligand be used for the determination of specific binding and 3 determinations for non-specific binding. Chromatography of the radioactive ligands should be performed at least once for each batch used. All participants, without exception, now use ^{3}H Org 2058 for the determination of progestin receptors. The non-specific binding is determined with DES (ER) or Org 2058 (PgR). These competitors must be present at a final concentration of 10^{-6}M and should be added before or simultaneously with the labelled steroids. Incubation is performed overnight at 4°C. The final concentrations of dextran-coated charcoal (DCC) are 0.25% charcoal (Norit A sifted through nylon netting) and 0.025% dextran T70. The composition of this suspension with regard to adsorption of cytosol is currently under investigation. This suspension should be prepared 1 day prior to use. Finally, the determination of cytosol protein has been standardized (Coomassie Brilliant Blue and human serum albumin standard). All laboratories participating in the external program of the EORTC Receptor Group employ their own "in-house" methodologies.

Intra-laboratory Quality Control of routinely performed receptor assays.

Daily assessment of clinical assays performed under routine conditions is an absolute requirement. Lyophilized reference materials that are stable at 4°C for several months can be used for these purposes. Lyophilized human breast tumor cytosols have been analyzed concurrently with each series of human breast tumor assays in Nijmegen, in order to assess whether the performance of our routine dextran-coated charcoal technique is satisfactory. These control cytosols are prepared from a pool of many different breast tumor residue specimens which had previously been assayed for the presence of steroid receptor proteins. Four different control cytosols have been used and the results are summarized in table 1. The inter-assay coefficients of variation were, without one exeption (progestin receptor sample 2) all less than 13%. None of these lyophilized human breast tumor cytosols showed a systematic loss of ER binding sites, whereas two out of four samples displayed a very gradual decline of PgR binding sites. Samples 1 and 2 demonstrated a loss of PgR binding sites of about 25% and 40% respectively over a 9 month period. It may be noted that the calculated coefficient of variation of the PgR assays performed on sample 2 was considerably affected by this decline in receptor binding sites. Recently, Godolphin and Jacobson (8) compared four types of material for the control of routine assays of estrogen receptors in human breast tumors. It appeared that powdered and lyophilized human breast tumor tissue had excellent stability and could be analyzed with good precision (17%). This corresponds with our experience, using lyophilized material, for the daily clinical control of routine receptor measurements in human breast cancer. Despite strict quality control procedures, Raam et al.(19) observed coefficients of inter-assay variation for the estrogen receptor assay ranging from 21 to 44% (averaging $\pm$ 35%) for 6 different batches of pulverized calf uterine tissue powder stored as small aliquots at $-80^{\circ}C$. It appeared that the tissue homogenization step, that precedes cytosol preparation, contributed most significantly to this variation. Therefore, this type of preparation is less appropriate for the daily evaluation of receptor assay performance. It may be noted that lyophilized cytosols will be used during the forthcoming trial of the EORTC Receptor Group to examine long-term intra- and inter-laboratory variation of routine receptor analyses.

Table 1. Intra-laboratory quality control of routine estrogen and progestin receptor assays.

Sample[a]	period	n[b]	Estrogen Receptor mean	C.V.(%)	Progestin Receptor mean	C.V.(%)
1	3/81-12/81	46	69	8.9	117	9.2
2	11/81- 7/82	37	90	11.0	119	15.2
3	9/82- 2/83	25	49	12.8	78	8.3
4	3/83- 8/83	33	117	9.4	141	11.5

All receptor values are expressed as fmol/mg protein

[a] All four samples were prepared from human breast tumor specimens

[b] Number of receptor assays per time period

Selection of reference preparations for inter-laboratory quality control of steroid receptor assays.

Since 1978 quality control programs for estrogen and progestin receptor assays have been started in Australia (20), United Kingdom (10), Italy (7), USA (18,21), W.Germany (2), Switzerland (23) and the Netherlands (12). Moreover, the EORTC Breast Cancer Cooperative Group has initiated a standardization and quality control program for institutions participating in multi-centre clinical trials (6). Almost without exception, the quality control programs conducted so far, have made use of either pulverized frozen ($-70^{\circ}C$) tissue powders or of lyophilized cytosol preparations. Wittliff et. al. (22) states that "the advantage of a tissue powder over a reference cytosol or a lyophilized tissue is that it permits evaluation of the homogenising procedure". Raam et al.(19) found that fluctuations in receptor values are primarily an effect of tissue homogenization and concluded that for quality control, distribution of lyophilized cytosols should precede (lyophilized) tissue powders.

In 1983 the EORTC Receptor Group compared these two types of reference material i.e. fresh calf uterine tissue frozen in liquid nitrogen and dispatched on solid CO_2, and lyophilized cytosol prepared from the same tissue. Before freezing, the uterine tissue was mechanically minced in

order to assure homogeneity as much as possible. Each participant received five identical vials of each reference preparation, all of which were
to be analyzed within one week of arrival. Moreover, all ten vials (two
times five vials) were to be analyzed on the same day.

Fifteen laboratories participated in the trial. One participant did
not receive the frozen minced tissues, because they were held by customs
for several weeks. Furthermore, the results of one laboratory that was
participating for the first time were excluded due to use of incubation
conditions, tritiated ligands and a protein assay that differed from
those of all other participants. The results of the remaining 13 laboratories are summarized in tables 2 and 3.

Table 2. Summary of estrogen receptor results.
          EORTC Receptor Group 1983.

	Minced Calf Uterine Tissue	Lyophilized Calf Uterine Cytosol
Range	433-874	553-1020
Mean	602	712
S.D.	119	159
C.V.(%)	19.8	22.4

All receptor values are expressed as fmol/mg protein.

Table 3. Summary of progestin receptor results.
          EORTC Receptor Group 1983.

	Minced Calf Uterine Tissue	Lyophilized Calf Uterine Cytosol
Range	851-2383	883-2141
Mean	1419	1353
S.D.	447	384
C.V.(%)	31.5	28.4

All receptor values are expressed as fmol/mg protein.

Please notice that only the mean values of the assays performed on the
five identical vials are included in these tables. Comparison of receptor
results, expressed as fmol/mg protein, between frozen tissue and lyophilized cytosol demonstrates that, despite the large range of results reported for both ER (2.0 minced; 1.8 cytosol) and PgR (2.8 minced; 2.4 cytosol), the mean values of all participants were rather similar. Furthermore, the variation between laboratories is similar for frozen minced
tissue and lyophilized cytosol: ER about 20% and PgR about 30%. The DCC
receptor assay conditions for 10 of the 13 participants were in accord
with the previously described guidelines of this Receptor Study Group
(6,14). One laboratory reported results from agar gel electrophoresis,
while one participant employed single dose saturation analysis. The results

of these two laboratories remained within the range of estrogen receptor values reported by the 11 remaining laboratories conducting multipoint Scatchard analyses. However, both laboratories using the single point assay as well as one other laboratory that used ^{3}H R5020 instead of the recommended ligand ^{3}H Org 2058, reported relatively low PgR values, ranging from 851-1080 for the minced uterine tissue and from 883-1095 for the lyophilized cytosol. It should be mentioned that, with only the above noted exceptions, no obvious relation between the receptor methods employed and the receptor results obtained could be detected.

As reported before, the magnitude of intra-laboratory variation, i.e. the variation of the five assays performed on two sets of 5 identical vials, differed greatly (14). However,the intra-laboratory coefficients of variation were usually greater for minced tissue than for lyophilized cytosols. The median coefficient of variation of all participants was 12-13% for the minced specimen and 6-7% for the reference cytosol (Table 4).

Table 4. Intra-laboratory variation of estrogen and progestin receptor assays in two types of reference material. EORTC Receptor Group 1983.

Reference Material	Estrogen Receptor	Progestin Receptor
Minced Calf Uterine tissue frozen on dry ice	12.0%[a]	13.1%
Lyophilized Calf Uterine Cytosol	6.7%	6.2%

[a]Median value of all 13 participants.

This increase in variability may be attributed to: 1. heterogeneity of the minced tissue; 2. the procedure of tissue disruption; 3. extraction of receptor proteins. At this time, lyophilized cytosol is the reference material of choice to form the basis for inter-laboratory quality control studies. Some of the factors contributing to this choice are the ease of preparation and the possibility for distribution without temperature control. Furthermore, these samples can be stored for several months in the refrigerator thus contributing to its suitability for daily use as an intra-laboratory control preparation. In addition, it mimicks many of the binding characteristics of fresh or frozen material, including binding affinity, ligand binding specificity and behaviour during sucrose density gradient analysis (9). Lastly, it can be analyzed with good precision and shows an intra-laboratory variation that is considerably less than the variation obtained using the same material, which has been minced and frozen on dry ice.

Counting of radioactivity

Accuracy of the determination of radioactivity by liquid scintillation counting may contribute to the variability of receptor assay results. The accuracy of both counting and calculation by individual laboratories in the Netherlands has been checked with commercially available internal standard capsules (Lumac Systems AG, Basel). These ready-to-use capsules contain tritiated sucrose.

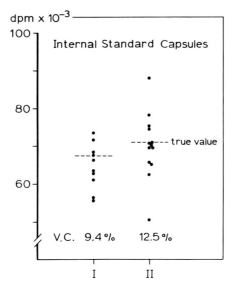

Fig. 1. Inter-laboratory variability of counting. Results of ready-to-use internal standard capsules containing calibrated amounts of tritiated sucrose (summary of two experiments).

Fig. 1 shows the appreciable variation in reported dpm's. In both trials, a wide range of dpm values, scattered around the true value given by the supplier, was observed with inter-laboratory coefficients of variation of around 10%.

In order to compare these results using the internal standard capsules with results using the ligand normally counted, the participants were requested to determine the amount of radioactivity (dpm) of a centrally provided lyophilized ^{3}H(estradiol)-BSA solution. Seventeen laboratories participated in this trial and several participants reported counting results from more than one liquid scintillation counter giving a total number of 25 observations. The values of the standard capsules varied between 141,600 and 225,800 dpm. The mean value of all participants was 174,300 ± 19,500 dpm with a variation coefficient of 11.2%. This mean value corresponds very well with the value of 173,000 dpm given by the supplier. No clear relation was found between the type of scintillation vials (glass, plastic), the type and volume of scintillation liquid or the volume of the quenched standards in relation to the volume of scintillation liquid added to the cytosol, and the final counting result.

The values of the ^{3}H-estradiol solution ranged from 29,300 to 46,200 dpm per 0,1 ml aliquot (Table 5). Fig. 2 shows the higly significant (P<0.001) correlation (r=0,9682) between the two counting results reported by the various participants. This implies that the accuracy of counting results was independent of the type of radioactive material. Therefore, the dpm's reported by each participant for the internal standard capsule can be used to recalculate the results observed for the ^{3}H(estradiol)-BSA solution. This is illustrated in Table 5. Correction of results by means of this internal standard reduced the inter-laboratory coefficient of variation from 11 to 2.8% (Table 5). It can be concluded that internal stan-

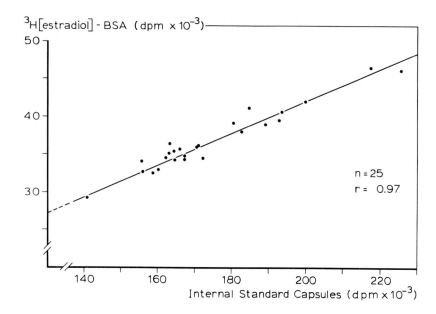

Fig. 2. Correlation between counting results of 17 laboratories for ready-to-use internal standard capsules and a lyophilized bovine serum albumin solution containing tritiated estradiol.

dardization presently is adequate for measuring the absolute counting efficiency in quality control programs of steroid receptor assays. This conclusion is in accord with the fact that the EORTC Receptor Group very recently has decided to employ internal standards for the estimation of liquid scintillation counting efficiency during their forthcoming trials.

Assignment of Estrogen Receptor Status.

   The characterization of a given human breast carcinoma as either ER-positive of ER-negative is one of the most important criteria in selecting patients with advanced breast cancer for endocrine therapy. Therefore, it is of utmost importance that participants in inter-laboratory quality control programs agree that a receptor positive reference preparation is indeed positive and that a receptor-negative sample is characterized as negative. Oxley et. al. (17) observed in a blind survey involving 47 unselected laboratories that 98% of participants concurred that a mid range ER-positive human breast carcinoma powder was positive. The median calculated value of all participants was about 25 fmol/mg protein. When a receptor-negative reference tissue powder was analyzed the rate of concurrence was 90%. Attention is drawn to the fact that participants used their own criteria for selecting a positive or negative-receptor result. In the quality control program of the Netherlands (15) the agreement on the presence or absence of estrogen receptor was more than 98% for lyophilized reference samples with high receptor content (>30 fmol/mg protein). For samples with a low receptor

Table 5. Summarized counting results of 17 laboratories obtained for a ^{3}H (estradiol) -BSA solution : Influence of internal standardization.

	Reported results (dpm/0.1 ml)	Corrected results [a] (dpm/0.1 ml)
Range	29,300-46,200	34,700-38,700
Mean	36,800	36,600
S.D.	4,060	1,020
C.V.(%)	11.0	2.8

[a]The reported dpm's were corrected by means of the results reported for the internal standard capsule:

$$\text{dpm's corrected=dpm's observed} \times \frac{173,000}{\text{dpm's capsule observed}}$$

value (10-30 fmol/mg protein) there was 85% agreement, while 12% of the assays performed on receptor-negative material were characterized as ER-positive. It appeared that at least some of the disagreements in receptor status were due to differences in the criteria applied by the individual laboratories. At that time of the study, the cut-off levels between receptor-positive and receptor-negative samples varied from 2 to 19 fmol/mg protein within the various institutes. This disturbing influence of the definitions employed by the individual laboratories for selecting a positive or negative result is illustrated in table 6. This table summarizes the results of 27 laboratories that analyzed two lyophilized reference samples with a very low receptor content. Both samples were analyzed in one assay. Sample A was prepared from calf uterine cytosol 10-fold diluted with a solution of human serum immunoglobulins, while sample B was prepared from numerous residue specimens of human breast tumor, all of which had previously been assayed in Nijmegen as ER-negative. The median value of all 27 participants was 13 and 8 fmol/mg protein for samples A and B, respectively. About 40% of the participants characterized the receptor-positive sample A as negative, while on the other hand 30% of participants classified the receptor-negative sample B as receptor-positive. Table 6 shows that only 1 out of 23 receptor (4%)

Table 6. Assignment of estrogen receptor status by individual laboratories in relation to the quantitative receptor result.

Reported value (fmol/mg protein)	No of assays in stated classification		
	Negative	Borderline	Positive
<5	9	–	1
5-10	13	–	–
10-15	3	4	4
15-20	1	2	13
>20	–	–	4

values below 10 fmol/mg protein was reported as ER-positive, while only one out of 20 (5%) assays above 15 fmol/mg protein was classified as negative. However, quantitative receptor assay results between 10 and 15 fmol/mg protein were characterized as receptor-negative, -borderline or -positive with approximately equal frequency. Therefore, the use of identical cut-off levels for discrimination between receptor-positive, -borderline or -negative breast tumor samples by institutions participating in multicentre clinical trials is highly recommended. Very recently, the EORTC Receptor Group observed 94% agreement of ER-positivity for a sample with a median value of 18, when a common cut-off limit of 10 fmol/mg protein was employed (14).

In the majority of laboratories protein is determined by the recommended Bradford technique (Coomassie Brilliant Blue) using human serum albumin (Kabi) as a standard, while a few participants still use a Lowry procedure with a bovine serum albumin standard. Using these two types of assays, results may be considerably different; e.g. sample A: Bradford 3.29 ± 0.28 (21 laboratories) and Lowry 6.56 ± 0.83 mg protein/ml cytosol (6 laboratories). Clearly problems can arise in assignment of receptor status with such great differences in protein determination techniques. The usefulness of protein standardization has been questioned in the light of observations that protein standardization or expressing the results as fmol/ml cytosol fails to significantly reduce the scatter in receptor results (17,18). Nevertheless, standardization of the type of protein assay and the standard employed is imperative in these quality control programs since the accuracy of the final receptor result (fmol/mg protein) and the characterization of receptor status both depend on the estimation of the protein concentration of the cytosol.

E.O.R.T.C. Receptor Group.

- Abteilung für Onkologische Biochemie, Dusseldorf, F.R.G.
  (H. Bojar);
- Antoni van Leeuwenhoekhuis, Amsterdam, the Netherlands
  (W. Nooyen);
- Cancerologie Expérimentale Laboratoire des Récepteurs Hormonaux,
  Faculté de Médicine de Marseille, Marseille, France
  (P. Martin);
- Centre Oscar Lambret, Laboratoire d' Endocrinologie Experimentale,
  Lille, France
  (J.P. Peyrat);
- Centro medico Oncologico, Ospedali Riuniti di Parma, Parma, Italy
  (C. Bozzetti, P. Mori);
- Department of Biochemistry, University of Glasgow, Glasgow, U.K.
  (R. Leake);
- Department of Experimental and Chemical Endocrinology, Sint Radboud Hospital, Nijmegen, the Netherlands
  (Th.J. Benraad, A. Koenders);
- The Fibiger Laboratory and the Finsen Institute, Copenhagen, Denmark
  (C. Rose and S. Thorpe);
- Frauenklinik der Freien Hansestadt Bremen, Onkologisches Labor,
  Bremen, F.R.G.
  (W. Jonat);
- Imperial Cancer Research Fund, Hormone Biochemistry Department,
  London, U.K.
  (R.J.B. King);

- Institut Jules Bordet, Bruxelles, Belgium
  (G. Leclercq);
- Istituto di Radiologia, University of Ferrara, Italy
  (D. Pelizzola, A. Piffanelli);
- Istituto di Ricerche Biomediche, "Antoine Marxer" (RBM),
  Ivrea, Italy
  (M. de Bortoli, S. Fumero);
- Max-Planck Institut für Experimentelle Endokrinologie,
  Hannover, F.R.G.
  (H.O. Hoppen, P.W. Jungblut);
- Rotterdamsch Radio-Therapeutisch Instituut, Rotterdam, the Netherlands
  (M.A. Blankenstein)

List of participating institutions in the Netherlands.

- Ziekenhuis "de Lichtenberg"	Amersfoort
- Antoni van Leeuwenhoekhuis	Amsterdam
- Stichting Medische Laboratoria	Breda
- Stichting Samenwerkende Delftse Ziekenhuizen	Delft
- Catharina Ziekenhuis	Eindhoven
- Sint Josef Ziekenhuis	Eindhoven
- Ziekenhuizen "de Stadsmaten" en "Ziekenzorg"	Enschede
- Sint Anna Ziekenhuis	Geldrop
- De Wever Ziekenhuis	Heerlen
- Laboratorium voor de Volksgezondheid in Friesland	Leeuwarden
- Academisch Ziekenhuis, Afdeling Pathologische Scheikunde	Leiden
- Sint Radboud Ziekenhuis, Afdeling Experimentele en Chemische Endocrinologie	Nijmegen
- Scientific Development, Group, Organon International B.V.	Oss
- Rotterdamsch-Radiotherapeutisch Instituut, Dr. Daniel den Hoed Kliniek	Rotterdam
- Stichting Onkologisch Instituut "Dr. Bernard Verbeeten"	Tilburg
- Academisch Ziekenhuis, afdeling Endocrinologie	Utrecht
- Laboratorium Nucleaire Geneeskunde "Voorburg"	Vught
- Sophia Ziekenhuis	Zwolle

ACKNOWLEDGMENT

A. Koenders and Th. Benraad present this work on behalf of the EORTC Receptor Group and the laboratories and institutions participating in the quality control program of the Netherlands.

REFERENCES

1. Benraad, Th., and Koenders, A. (1980): Cancer, 46:2762-2764.
2. Bojar, H., Staib, W., Beck, K., and Pilaski, J. (1980): Cancer, 46:2770-2774.
3. Bradford, M.M. (1976): Anal. Biochem., 72:248-254.
4. De Sombre, E.R., Carbone, P.P., Jensen, E.V., McGuire, W.L., Wells, S.A., Wittliff, J.L., and Lipsett, M.B. (1979): N. Eng. J. of Med., 301:1011-1012.
5. E.O.R.T.C. Breast Cancer Cooperative Group (1973): Eur. J. Cancer, 9:379-381.
6. E.O.R.T.C. Breast Cancer Cooperative Group (1980): Eur. J. Cancer, 16:1513-1515.
7. Fumero, S., and Piffanelli, A. (1981): Tumori, 67:301-306.
8. Godolphin, W., and Jacobson, B. (1980): J. of Immunoassay, 1(3):363-374.
9. Janes, G.R., Koenders, A.J., and Benraad, Th. (1982): J. Steroid Biochem., 17:387-394.
10. King, R.J.B. (1980): Cancer, 46:2822-2824.
11. Koenders, A., and Benraad, Th. (1981): Ligand Review, 3(4): 32-39.
12. Koenders, A., Geurts-Moespot, J., Hendriks, T., and Benraad, Th. (1981). In: Estrogen Receptor Assays in Breast Cancer, edited by G. Sarfaty, A.R. Nash and D.D. Keightley, pp. 69-82. Masson Publishing USA, Inc., New York.
13. Koenders, A., and Benraad, Th. (1982): Eur. J. Cancer Clin. Oncol., 18:608.
14. Koenders, A., and Thorpe, S.M. on behalf of the EORTC Receptor Group(1983): Eur. J. Cancer Clin. Oncol., 19:1221-1229 and 1467-1472.
15. Koenders, T., and Benraad Th.(1983): Breast Cancer Res. and Treatm., 3:255-266.
16. Nash, A.R., and Sarfaty, G.A., (1981). In: Estrogen Receptors Assays in Breast Cancer, edited by G. Sarfaty, A.R. Nash and D.D. Keightley, pp. 57-68. Masson Publishing USA, Inc., New York.
17. Oxley, D.K., Haven, G.T., Wittliff, J.L., and Gilbo, D. (1982): Am. J. Clin. Pathol., 78(4): 587-597.
18. Raam, S., Gelman, R., and Cohen, J.L. (1981): Eur. J. Cancer, 17: 643-649.
19. Raam, S., Gelman, R., Faulkner, J., White, G.M., and Cohen, J.L. (1982): Breast Cancer Res. and Treatm., 2:111-117.
20. Sarfaty. G.A., Nash, A.R., and Keightley, D.D. (eds) (1981): Estrogen Receptor Assays in Breast Cancer. Laboratory Discrepancies and Quality Assurance. Masson Publishing USA, Inc., New York.
21. Wittliff, J.L. (1980): Cancer, 46:2953-2960.
22. Wittliff, J.L., Wiehle, S.A., Eckman, J.B., Smalley, R.V., Bartolucci, A.A., and Durant, J.R. (1981). In: Estrogen Receptor Assays in Breast Cancer, edited by G. Sarfaty, A.R. Nash and D.D. Keightley, pp. 105-125. Masson Publishing USA, Inc., New York.
23. Zava, D.T., and Guelpa, C. (1982): Eur. J. Cancer Clin. Oncol., 18:713-721.

Progress in Cancer Research and Therapy,
Vol. 31, edited by F. Bresciani, et al.
Raven Press, New York © 1984.

Coevaluation of Steroid Receptors in Microsamples of Breast Cancer Tissue

J.L. Moll, G. Milano, J.L. Formento, M. Francoual, B.P. Krebs,
C.M. Lalanne, J.L. Boublil, and M. Namer

Centre Antoine-Lacassagne, 06054 Nice Cedex, France

SUMMARY

Oestradiol (ER) and progesterone (PR) receptor levels were measured in 26 tumor fragments (200-500 mg) from breast cancer patients. After tissue pulverization, one part was analyzed by the routine DCC method; the other part was analyzed by the following micromethod: (i) cytosol incubation using the DCC procedure but in the simultaneous presence of ^{3}HR 5020; (ii) extraction of steroids bound to the receptor by precipitation with ethanol:TCA; (iii) HPLC on a modular system, with a C_{18} 5 μm column and elution with a methanol/water mixture (4 vol:1 vol). Fractions were collected and the ^{3}H radioactivity counted.

Separation of oestradiol from R 5020 was rapid and complete. A very satisfactory correlation was obtained between the two methods: ER r = 0.996, p <0.001; PR r = 0.975, p <0.001. This implies that the thresholds of positivity, i.e. for therapeutic decisions, remain unchanged. Simultaneous measurement of ER and PR in a single needle biopsy is thus possible with this micromethod.

INTRODUCTION

The measurement of steroid hormone receptors is now a well-recognized common laboratory procedure (11). The value of this procedure results from the fact that breast cancer patients whose tumor contains both oestradiol (ER) and progesterone (PR) receptors are likely to respond to endocrine treatments in 75% of cases; this proportion drops to only 10% for patients whose tumors do not contain such receptors (11).

The most common measurement technique, involving the use of Dextran-coated charcoal (DCC) (12), has certain intrinsic limits: a separate cytosol fraction is required for each of the receptors to be measured (1). This necessitates a relatively large amount of biological material that can only be obtained from a tumor fragment taken from the surgical specimen. This constraint considerably limits the applicability of receptor measurement, especially for tumors in situ, despite the fact that the cellular heterogeneity of breast cancer tumors is well-recognized (6). Although several authors have described the measurement of steroid receptors in needle biopsy samples, it seems difficult to evaluate

several receptors in a single sample (3,16). A recent method has been
described for the simultaneous measurement of both ER and PR using different radioelements ([125] I-oestradiol and [3]HR 5020). The inherent problem with this method, however, is the emission of beta rays by the ^{125}I,
which renders this procedure difficult to use on a routine basis (18).
A combination of the DCC technique and high pressure liquid chromatography has also been reported on (10). We adopted this last technique
and attempted to determine its validity based on correlation with the
routine DCC procedure and evaluation of its reproducibility.

MATERIALS AND METHODS

Collection of samples

The present study is based on the analysis of ER and PR measurements
obtained by two methods: the method developed by us and the classical
DCC method (12) used on a routine basis. Following extemporaneous
anatomopathological study, fragments of the tumors were divided into two
parts. One part was used for measurement of the ER and PR concentrations
so as to provide an immediate result to the clinician; the other part
(200-500 mg) was rapidly placed in liquid nitrogen for later use in the
comparative study.
Samples were selected on the basis of initial results in order to
obtain objective coverage of the entire range of values generally observed. The comparative study thus included tumors from 26 patients. At
the time of assay, the tumor fragments were assessed by two methods:
the classical method used previously (in order to avoid a bias in results
caused by freezing/thawing) and the micromethod described herein.

Materials

Steroids: [3]H oestradiol (specific activity 111 Ci/mmol), [3]HR5020
(specific activity 87 Ci/mmol) and unlabelled R5020 were purchased
from New England Nuclear (NEN, Boston, Mass.). Diethylstilboestrol
(DES) was purchased from SIGMA Chemical Co. (St. Louis, Mo.).
Buffer solution: buffer R consisted of Tris/HCl 10^{-2} M, EDTA 10^{-3} M,
dithiothreitol (DTT) 0.5 10^{-3} M, glycerol 10% (vol/vol); pH 7.4
Dextran-coated charcoal solutions: in Tris 10^{-2} M (pH 8.0): 0.5% Norit
charcoal and 0.05% Dextran T 70 (DCC-A) or 2.5% Norit charcoal and
0.25% Dextran T 70 (DCC-B).
Cytosol preparation by the usual method (cytosol A): The tumor fragment stored in liquid nitrogen was ground and pulverized with a
THERMOVAC pulverizer (IND Corp., Copiague, New York, USA). The fine
powder obtained was then placed in 10 volumes of buffer R. This solution was homogeneized using a Polytron PT 10-20 homogenizer (Brinkman
Instrument, Inc., Lucerne, Switzerland) at a speed setting of 6 for
3 x 5 second intervals in an ice bath. The homogenate was then centrifuged for 40 minutes at 105,000 x g at 2° C (Kontron Ultracentrifuge Unit, France).
Cytosol preparation for the micromethod (cytosol B): After pulverization with the THERMOVAC pulverizer, the fine powder (30 mg) was homogeneized in 300 μl of buffer R with a glass-glass Potter in an ice
bath. The homogenate was then centrifuged for 40 minutes at 105,000
x g at 2° C.

Methods

Usual assay procedure for ER and PR.
For each receptor assay, 100 µl of cytosol A were incubated, in duplicates, in the presence of 100 µl of a solution of a tritiated hormone in buffer R. Final concentrations were:
- ^{3}H oestradiol: 10 nM, 5 nM, 1 nM
- ^{3}HR 5020: 20 nM, 12 nM, 3 nM

The same incubation was repeated for each hormone in the presence of an excess of the unlabelled hormone expressed as dry extract (evaluation of nonspecific binding). Thus, for oestradiol, 100 times more DES was used for each concentration; for R 5020, 200 times more unlabelled R 5020 was used for each concentration. Each test was performed twice. Incubation lasted 16 hours at 2° C for ER and 2 hours at 2° C followed by 2 hours at 2° C in the presence of 100 µl of a glycerol/buffer R solution (60:40, vol/vol) for PR. Upon completion of incubation, 500 µl of DCC-A solution prepared 24 hours earlier were added to each tube. For ER, incubation lasted 30 min. at 2° C; for PR, 15 min. at 2° C during vigorous shaking. Tubes were centrifuged for 20 min. at 2800 x g at 2° C and 500 µl of supernatant were counted for radioactivity with 4.5 ml of Picofluor 30 (Packard). 50 µl of cytosol were utilized to measure proteins by the method of Lowry (9). Calculation of specific binding: the specific binding for each hormone was determined by subtracting the nonspecific bound from the total bound. The ER level considered was the mean of the two specific bound values obtained at the two saturating concentrations (5 nm and 10 nM). Determination of PR levels at the two saturating concentrations (12 nM and 20 nM) was performed in the same manner.

Micromeasurement for ER and PR.
Three successive steps were performed: (1) incubation of cytosol B and separation of the free hormones by DCC; (2) precipitation of the proteins and extraction of the hormones bound to the receptors; (3) separation of hormones by HPLC and measurement of the radioactivity of the various fractions eluted.
- Step 1: cytosol incubation was identical to the reference method except that ^{3}H oestradiol and the 3HR 5020 were coincubated in the same 100 µl aliquot of cytosol. Only one concentration of labelled hormone was utilized, i.e. ^{3}H oestradiol 7.5 nM (final concentration) and ^{3}HR 5020 15 nM (final concentration). The nonspecific binding was evaluated on another 100 µl aliquot by repeating incubation in the presence of dry extract of unlabelled hormone: 100 times more DES and 200 times more R5020. Incubation was carried out for 16 hours at 2° C, after which 100 µl of solution DCC-B were added. Following 15 minutes of incubation at 2° C, centrifugation was performed for 20 minutes at 2800 x g at 2° C.
- Step 2: To 200 µl of supernatant were added 200 µl of pure ethanol and 20 µl of an aqueous solution of 5% trichloracetic acid. The tubes were placed on an agitator for 2 hours at 2°C, then centrifuged for 20 minutes at 2800 x g at 2° C; the final supernatant was then available for separation by HPLC.
- Step 3: The HPLC system consisted of a 6000 A pump (Waters Assoc., Milford, Mass., USA), a U6K injector (Waters), a Model 440 absorbance detector (Waters) fitted with a 254 nm interferential filter and a Data Module Integrator (Waters). Chromotographic separation of the

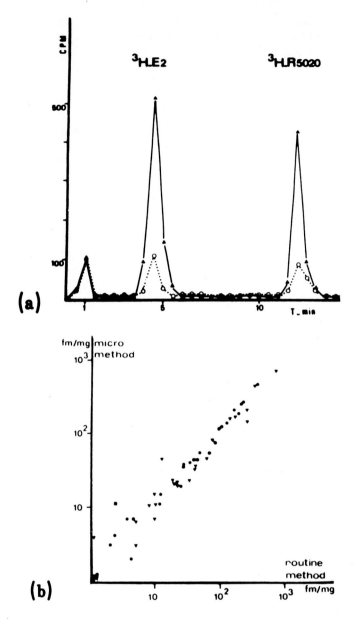

Fig.1(a)   HPLC PROFILE OF EXTRACTED CYTOSOLS: —— TOTAL BOUND;
--- NONSPECIFIC BOUND. Fig.1(b)   CORRELATION BETWEEN THE TWO METHODS
(26 cases) : ● ER; ▼PR

steroids was performed with a radial compression system (RCM 100,
Waters) using Rad-Pak cartridges filled with 10 μm microparticles of
reversed phase C_{18} (Waters). Elution was performed with a methanol/
water mixture: 75:25 (vol/vol). The flow rate was 2.5 ml/min.
100 μl of unlabelled solutiots of oestradiol (10^{-4}M) and R 5020
(5 . 10^{-5}M) were first injected to identify the respective retention
times of these steroids at 254 nm. The UV detector and the recorder

were then disconnected, and 100 µl of supernatant from the extraction phase were injected. 625 µl fractions were collected at the column outlet (one fraction every 15 seconds at a flow rate of 2.5 ml/min.). 4.5 ml of Picofluor scintillating fluid were added, the tubes were mixed well, and the radioactivity was measured on a Packard LS Spectrometer.

Calculation of specific binding: For every peak corresponding to the retention time of each steroid, the specific binding was calculated by subtracting the peak for incubation in the presence of labelled hormone and an excess of unlabelled hormone (nonspecific bound) from the peak for incubation in the presence of labelled hormone only (total bound). Results were expressed in fmol/mg protein.

RESULTS

Figure 1(a) represents an HPLC profile allowing quantification of ER and PR after incubation of a cytosol from a tumor specimen. The comparison of results obtained for our 26 patients using the reference method and our micromethod is illustrated in Figure 1(b). Correlations were $r = 0.996$ for ER and $r = 0.975$ for PR, with $p < 0.001$. Microassay reproducibility was assessed by measuring 5 aliquots of the same cytosol: the coefficient of variation was 5.2% for ER, 9.5% for PR.

DISCUSSION

The original method described herein allows simultaneous measurement of steroid receptors in a very small volume of cytosol, progress made possible by associating the classical DCC technique with HPLC. The two additional steps introduced are relatively rapid: three hours suffice for extraction of the steroids bound to the receptors, their separation by HPLC, their collection and quantification.

This work represents a new application of HPLC, which appears at present to be one of the most valuable techniques in clinical biochemistry (4). HPLC is a procedure particularly well adapted for the separation and quantification of steroid hormones . This study was centered on the two main receptors ER and PR since their evaluation has been proven useful in clinical oncology for patients with breast cancer (17). The chromatographic conditions defined also permit correct separation of dexamethasone from the other two hormones, thereby increasing the technique's potential range of applications (unshown result). Inclusion of androgen receptor measurements in this system involves a problem since metribolone (R1881) has a nearly identical affinity for androgen and progesterone receptors (13).

The highly satisfactory correlation observed between the microassay and the reference DCC method implies that the thresholds of positivity established on the basis of the DCC method are not susceptible to be modified by the microassay, and thus should not change the criteria used by clinicians in decision-making. Reproducibility tests gave coefficients of variation close to 10%, indicating that the microassay is reliable, and thus obviating the need for replicate measurements. Thus, with as little as 300 µl of cytosol, the protein concentration (50 µl) and the concentration of steroid receptors (2 x 100 µl) can be determined simultaneously. It is generally admitted that the lower limit for the protein concentration in cytosol is 1 mg/ml if the DCC technique is to be successful (16,8). On this basis, samples of approx. 20-30 mg could be analyzed by the microassay described above. This weight corresponds to the amount of tissue obtained by needle biopsy (3). This method is now employed for the simultaneous coevaluation of ER and PR in biopsy specimens from in situ breast cancer tumors. To date, 70 biopsy samples have been tested in our laboratory. Automatization of the procedure can be envisaged by adding a continuous flux radioactivity detector, but for the time being the sensitivity of such apparatus is not compatible with the activities measured (beginning at 50 dpm).

The heterogeneity of steroid receptors within a mammary tumor is a well-established fact (6,15), which can probably be explained by the histological disparity of mammary tumors themselves (5). It is thus advisable to couple each quantification of steroid receptors in a biopsy specimen with anatomopathological study of a biopsy sample from a nearby site.

In the case of advanced breast cancer, there is a current consensus among clincians that surgical tumor exeresis should be preceded by a therapeutic protocol associating radiotherapy and chemotherapy (2). Consequently, the biochemical characteristics of cancer cells removed during surgery are in theory no longer representative of the primary tumor prior to treatment. It is thus preferable to measure ER and PR in a biopsy sample before any treatment is given in order to validly evaluate the degree of hormone dependence. Certain studies suggest that ER status in any given patient changes as the tumor progresses (14); other reports indicate that the discordance rate was specifically related to treatment by tamoxifen during the intervals between biopsies (7). To confirm and complete these studies, it would undoubtedly be interesting to conduct a sequential study based on ER and PR receptor measurements in repeat biopsies of accessible lesions. The microassay described above is susceptible to constitute the analytical basis for such a program.

REFERENCES

1. Allegra, J.C., Lippman, M.E., Thomson, E.B., Simon, R., Barloock,A., Green, H., Huff, K.K., Do, H.M.T., and Aitken, S.S. (1979): Cancer Res., 39: 1447-1454.
2. Bruckmann, J.E., Harris, J.R., Levene, M.B., Chaffey, J.T., and Hellman, S. (1979): Cancer, 43: 985-993.
3. Delarue, J.L., Mouriesse, H., Contesso, G., May-Levin, F., and Sancho-Garnier, H. (1981): Biomedecine, 34: 153-160.
4. Elin, R.J. (1980): Science, 210: 286-289.
5. Gairard, B., Calderoli, H., Keiling, R., Renaud, R., Bellocq, J.P., and Koehl, C. (1981): Lancet, 8260/61: 1419.
6. Hawkins, R.A., Hill, A., Freedman, B., Gore, S.M., Roberts, M.M., and Forrest, A.P.M. (1977): Br. J. Cancer, 36: 355-359.
7. Hull III, D.F., Clark, G.M., Osborne, C.K., Chamness, G.C., Knight III, W.A., and McGuire, W.L. (1983): Cancer Res., 43: 413-416.
8. Leclercq, G., Heuson, J., Schoenfeld, R., Mattheim, W.H., and Tagnon, H.J. (1973): Eur. J. Cancer, 9: 665.
9. Lowry, O.H., Rosebrough, N.J., Farr, A.L., and Randall, R.J. (1951): J. Biol. Chem., 193: 365-269.
10. Magdalenat, H. (1979): Cancer Treatment Reports, 7: 1147.
11. McGuire, W.L. (1980): Rec. Prof. Horm. Res., 36: 135-156.
12. McGuire, W.L., De la Garza, M., and Chamness, G.C. (1977): Cancer Res., 37: 637-639.
13. Ojasoo, T., and Raynaud, J.P. (1978): Cancer Res., 38: 4186-4198.

14. Osborne, C.K., and McGuire, W.L. (1979): Bull. Cancer, 66: 203-210.
15. Poulsen, H.S. (1981): Eur. J. Cancer, 17: 494-501.
16. Poulsen, H.S., Schultz, H., and Bichel, P. (1979): Eur. J. Cancer, 15: 1431-1438.
17. Saez, S. (1981): Ann. Endocrinol., 42: 306-314.
18. Thibodeau, S.N., Freeman, L., and Jiang, N.S. (1981): Clin. Chem., 27 (5): 687-691.

Progress in Cancer Research and Therapy,
Vol. 31, edited by F. Bresciani, et al.
Raven Press, New York © 1984.

Comparison of Biochemical Receptor Estimation and Histochemical Staining with Fluorescent Steroid Hormone Derivatives, in Receptor-Positive and Receptor-Negative Human Tumour Cell Lines

*Els M.J.J. Berns, *Eppo Mulder, **Rien A. Blankenstein,
*Focko F.G. Rommerts, and *Henk J. van der Molen

*Department of Biochemistry (Division of Chemical Endocrinology), Medical
Faculty, Erasmus University, 3000 DR Rotterdam; and **Department of Biochemistry,
Rotterdam Radio-Therapeutic Institute, Dr. Daniel den Hoed Clinic,
Rotterdam, The Netherlands*

Fluorescent labelled steroids could be of great value as reagents for assessing steroid hormone receptors in both mammary tumors and in prostatic carcinoma, especially when only limited amounts of tissue are available. Histochemical methods for the visualization of the receptor might be faster and cheaper, they would permit more precise, cell-by-cell analysis and they might be applied to small amounts of tissue, or even aspirated cells. Histochemical methods depend on either immunochemical localization of the receptor (a procedure still in development, 8) or on direct visualization of the receptor–bound steroid–fluorescein conjugates (e.g. 1,11,17,20,21). Contradictory results, however, with respect to the usefulness of fluorescent steroid conjugates for the detection of steroid hormone receptors in cells or in tissues have been published. Variability in results may have arisen from ill-defined tissue preparations and incubation techniques or impure preparations of steroid conjugates. Tissue sections contain a variety of intact cells, damaged cells and dead cells and during fixation and incubation denaturation and diffusion of proteins may occur. Therefore the experiments in this investigation were performed with intact cultured cells or with cells which were reproducably damaged by a standard procedure. For a reliable localization of steroid receptors with fluorescent conjugated steroids several criteria should be fulfilled (Table 1).

It has been suggested that fluorescent conjugates bind predominantly to a type of binding sites with lower affinity and present in higher concentration than the true receptors (7,19). A histochemical method would remain valuable when the fluorescent–labelled steroids permit the identification of receptor-positive and -negative cells. It is therefore necessary that a good correlation exists between staining intensity and receptor content.

The present report describes our attempts to use oestrogens and

TABLE 1. Criteria for fluorescent conjugated steroids
which bind to receptors

───

1. Competition with natural ligand
2. High relative binding affinity
3. Low non-specific binding
4. Saturable binding
5. Concentration of binding sites must be in agreement
   with biochemically measured concentration

───

androgens coupled through either BSA or a hemisuccinate bridge to the
fluorescent ligands and coumestrol, in a histochemical assay for
detection of binding proteins in receptor-positive and -negative cells.
For these studies we used cell lines with biochemically characterized
oestrogens and androgen receptor content.

EXPERIMENTAL

Cell lines

- MCF-7, a human breast cancer cell line, provided by the Breast Cancer
  Animal and Human Tumour and Human Cell Culture Bank, National Cancer
  Institute, National Institutes of Health, Bethesda, MD, U.S.A.
- NHIK-3025, originally provided by Norsk Hydro's Institute for Cancer
  Research, Oslo, Norway), is derived from an early stage of a carcinoma
  of the human uterine cervix (15,18).
- PC-93 and EB-33, permanent human tumour cell lines, both initiated
  from a human prostate adenocarcinoma and shown to be hormone-
  independent, were provided by the Department of Urology, Erasmus
  University, Rotterdam, The Netherlands (6,22).

Fluorescent ligands

- E_2-6-CMO-BSA-FITC: 17β-oestradiol-6-carboxymethyloxime-bovine serum
  albumin-fluorescein-isothiocyanate
- E_2-HS-FA: 17β-oestradiol-17-hemisuccinate-fluoresceinamine
- Coumestrol: [1-(2,4-dihydroxyphenyl)-6-hydroxy-3-benzofuran
  carboxylic acid lactone]
- T-17-HS-BSA-FITC: testosterone-17β-hemisuccinate-bovine serum albumin
  -fluorescein-isothiocyanate
- T-HS-FA: testosterone-17β-hemisuccinate-fluoresceinamine
- DHT-HS-FA: dihydrotestosterone-17β-hemisuccinate-fluorescein-
  amine

Biochemical procedures

a) Receptor isolation and sucrose gradient centrifugation
   Receptors were isolated from nuclei or cytoplasm as described earlier
   (15) and sucrose gradient centrifugation of nuclear extracts was
   performed in 5-20% sucrose gradients with the addition of 0.4 M KCl
   (24).

b) Receptor assay
Receptors were estimated essentially as described by Chamness et al. (3) with addition of 10 mM pyridoxal phosphate (final concentration) (16). The KCl concentration during precipitation was below 0.04 M.

c) Determination of the relative binding affinity (RBA)
The RBA of the oestrogen derivatives was estimated as described by Van Beurden-Lamers et al. (24). The RBA of the androgen derivatives was estimated as described by Bonne & Raynaud (2).

Histochemical procedures

Staining of intact cells:
Cells were:
1) washed twice with Dulbecco's phosphate-buffered saline (PBS, Gibco).
2) incubated in 1 ml RPMI-medium (Gibco) without foetal calf serum (FCS, Gibco) with the ligand for 1 h at 37°C.
3) washed four times with PBS-buffer (buffer was changed every 15 min).

Staining of "freeze-damaged" cells:
Cells were:
1) washed twice with PBS.
2) "freeze-damaged", to simulate the freeze/thaw sequence in the preparation of frozen sections (23) (cells were covered with 2.6% (w/v) Ficoll, immersed for 30 sec in liquid nitrogen and thawed at room temperature).
3) air-dried, 1 h at 4°C.
4) incubated with the ligand for 1 h at 20°C.
5) washed four times with PBS buffer (buffer was changed every 15 min).

Microscopy

Cells were immediately examined under a fluorescence microscope (Leitz Orthoplan, with epifluorescence equiped with a 100-Watt mercury bulb and a Orthomat). For coumestrol the cells were excited at 340 nm and viewed at 410 nm; for FITC excited at 485 nm and viewed at 510 nm. The pattern and intensity of staining of the cells were evaluated, and recorded on Kodak Ectachrome 160 film.

RESULTS AND DISCUSSION

Biochemical studies

Oestrogen receptor content of MCF-7 and PC-93 cells
Oestrogen receptor content in nuclei and cytoplasm was determined in MCF-7 and PC-93 cell lines. Figure 1 shows sucrose sedimentation profiles of nuclear extracts from MCF-7 cells and PC-93 cells. A peak of [^{3}H]oestradiol sedimenting at 4.1 S was observed for MCF-7 cells. In nuclear extracts from PC-93 cells, no binding of [^{3}H]oestradiol was observed. By protamine sulphate precipitation assay 175 fmol receptor/mg protein was measured in nuclear extracts of MCF-7 cells, while specific oestradiol binding was not detectable in the nuclear extract of PC-93 cells.
Similar results were obtained for the cytoplasmic receptors by Scatchard binding analysis. Cytoplasmic oestrogen receptor content in the

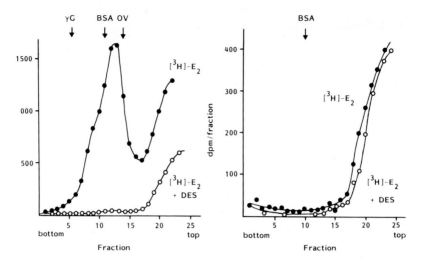

FIG. 1. Sucrose gradient sedimentation profiles of oestrogen receptors exracted with 0.4 M KCl from nuclei of MCF-7 cells (left panel) and PC-93 cells (right panel). The cells were incubated for 1 h at 37°C with 10 nM [^{3}H]oestradiol (E_2) in the absence (closed circles) or presence of a 100-fold molar excess of diethylstilboestrol (DES, open circles).
The sucrose gradients contained 0.4 M KCl. Gamma globulin (γ-G, 7.2 S), bovine serum albumin (BSA, 4.6 S) and ovalbumin (OV, 3.6 S) were used as sedimentation markers.

MCF-7 cells was 65 and 84 fmol receptor/mg cytosol protein (Kd = 0,31 nM) in two separate experiments. Oestrogen receptors were absent from the PC-93 cells.

Androgen receptor content of PC-93, NHIK-3025 and EB-33 cells
    The androgen receptor content of the tumour cell lines PC-93, NHIK 3025 and EB-33 was determined in the nuclear extracts. A peak of radioactivity sedimenting at 4.6-4.8 S was observed for both PC-93 and NHIK-3025 cells. A 100-fold molar excess of either T, DHT or R1881 caused a complete displacement of [^{3}H]testosterone, indicating the limited capacity of this binding system. No incorporation of label was observed

TABLE 2. Receptor content of cell lines

Cell line	receptors for oestrogens	androgens
MCF-7	+	+
PC-93	−	+
NHIK-3025	−	+
EB-33	−	−

TABLE 3. <u>Relative binding affinities (RBA) of the fluorescent ligands</u>

Oestrogenic ligands	RBA (%)	Androgenic ligands	RBA (%)
Oestradiol (E_2)	100	Methyltrienolone	100
E_2-6-CMO-BSA-FITC*)	4.3	T-17β-HS-BSA-FITC	0.1
E_2-6-CMO-BSA-FITC**)	1.8	T-17β-HS-FA	0.1
E_2-17β-HS-FA	0.1	DHT-17β-HS-FA	4
Coumestrol	1.4		

* Commercial preparation, used without purification.
** Free oestradiol partially removed.

in the nuclear extracts from EB-33 cells incubated either with [3H]testosterone, [3H]DHT or [3H]methyltrienolone. The receptor content of the nuclear extracts was also measured with a protamine sulphate precipitation assay. Amounts of 49, 57 and 8 fmole receptor/mg DNA were measured for PC-93, NHIK-3025 and EB-33 cells respectively. The presence of low amounts of labelled steroid receptor complexes in the nuclear extracts of EB-33 cells could either indicate the absence of receptors or a defective nuclear translocation mechanism of the androgen receptor in these cells. Therefore we have also measured the androgen receptor content in the cytosol fraction of the EB-33 cells, and again very low amounts of androgen receptor were measured (less than 2 fmole receptor/mg cytosol protein).

The results from our study and previous reports (12,15,18) are summarized in Table 2.

Relative binding affinities of the fluorescent ligands

The relative binding affinities of the fluorescent ligands for the oestrogen receptors in the cytosol of the uterus from an ovariectomized rat were calculated as the ratio of concentration of E_2 and the fluorescent ligands required to reduce 3H-E_2 specific binding by 50% (Table 3). The relative binding affinities of the fluorescent ligands for the androgen receptors in the cytosol of the prostate from a castrated rat were calculated as the ratio of concentration of methyltrienolone and the fluorescent ligands required to reduce 3H-methyltrienolone specific binding by 50%. The fluorescent ligands show low relative binding affinities.

Histochemical studies

Fluorescent staining of intact and "freeze-damaged" cells

Intact cells were stained with 10^{-5} M, 10^{-7} M and 10^{-9} M of the fluorescent ligand. No difference in fluorescent staining was observed between steroid hormone receptor-positive and -negative cells, after addition of the hemisuccinate conjugated derivatives (examples in Fig. 2 a/b) or coumesterol. Addition of the native ligand at a concentration of

TABLE 4.   Results histochemical assay.
           For all cell-lines used in this study.

Intact cells:	– Non protein conjugates:
	    cytoplasmic fluorescence
	– BSA-derivatives:
	    no fluorescence

"Freeze–damaged" cells:	– Non protein conjugates:
	    cytoplasmic fluorescence
	– BSA-derivatives:
	    nuclear fluorescence
	    predominates

1) Staining is independent of the presence of receptors
2) Staining is not suppressed with excess native ligand
   (oestrogen or androgen)

10^{-7} M (e.g. oestradiol to the oestrogen receptor-containing cells) to the staining solution, produced no decrease in intensity and again no difference in fluorescent cytoplasmic staining between receptor-positive and -negative cells was observed. No fluorescence was observed with the BSA-linked derivatives, which is due to the impermeability of the cell membrane for the albumin derivative. Pretreatment of intact cells for 24 h prior to staining in steroid hormone-free medium, did not affect the fluorescence. Addition of FITC, the fluorescent moiety of the albumin steroid complex, also resulted in a fluorescent staining of the cells. This green stain differs in colour shade from the E_2-6-CMO-BSA-FITC or T-17-HS-BSA-FITC stain, which is bright apple-green. Addition of fluorescein amine, the reagent used for synthesis of E_2-HS-FA, T-HS-FA or DHT-HS-FA to the intact cells, did not reveal any fluorescence (see Table 4).

"Freeze-damaged" cells were also stained with 10^{-5} M, 10^{-7} M and 10^{-9} M of the fluorescent ligand. Again no difference in fluorescent staining was observed between the receptor-positive and -negative cells. All cell types stained with the HS-linked derivative showed a cytoplasmic fluorescence. When stained with the BSA-linked derivative, all cell lines revealed cytoplasmic and more intense nuclear fluorescence (e.g. examples in Fig. 2 c/d), whereas with coumestrol no fluorescence was observed at all. Addition of the native ligand at a concentration of 10^{-7} M did not affect the staining pattern. With unconjugated FITC and FA, results with damaged cells were the same as for the intact cells (see Table 4).

From these experiments it can be concluded, that the staining patterns observed for the fluorescent ligands, under different experimental conditions, showed no relation to the oestrogen or androgen receptors estimated by biochemical methods. These results are in agreement with recently published observations, some which were obtained with tissue sections of tumours (McCarty et al. (14), Chamness et al. (4), Joyce et al. (9) and Lämmel et al. (10)).

For example, Joyce et al. (9) showed for oestrogen-labelled fluorescent conjugates (oestrogens coupled through a variety of short spacers) that these compounds did not bind to the classical oestrogen

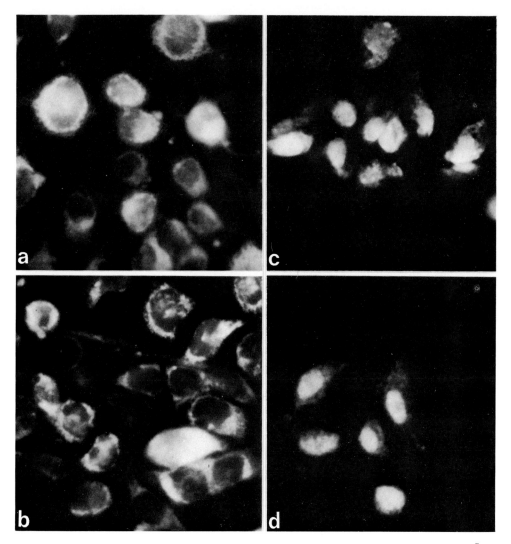

FIG. 2. In intact MCF-7 cells (a) and PC-93 cells (b) stained with 10^{-5} M E_2-HS-FA for 1 h, as described in the experimental section, only cytoplasmic staining was observed. In "freeze-damaged" MCF-7 cells (c) and PC-93 cells (d) stained with 10^{-5} M E_2-6-CMO-BSA-FITC for 1 h, as described in the experimental section, besides cytoplasmic staining mainly nuclear staining was observed. Magnification 400x.

receptors in thin sections of breast tumour tissue. Moreover, Lämmel et al. (10) reported for dihydrotestosterone-labelled FITC conjugates with a variety of short spacers, that it was not possible to demonstrate androgen receptors in tissue slices obtained from human prostatic carcinomas and human benign prostatic hyperplasia.

Clark et al. (7) and Panko et al. (19) claimed that 2-10 times more so-called "type II binding sites" may be present in breast carcinomas. However, with standard fluorescence microscopy one would probably neither detect the 10,000 true receptor molecules nor the 100,000 type II binding sites in a cell, because these concentrations of these sites are below the limit of detection of fluorescein molecules in a cell (5). The fluorescence observed in the cells used in the present study must therefore be due to binding of the ligands to low affinity binding sites present in higher concentration than the type II binding sites. From the results of this study it appears also that the concentration of these low affinity binding sites, estimated with fluorescent ligands, is not correlated with the concentration of true receptors and therefore cannot be used as a basis for discrimination between oestrogen or androgen receptor-positive and -negative cells. Future studies should concentrate on both the development of compounds with a high affinity for the receptor and on intensifier systems, permitting the detection of low concentrations of fluorescent molecules (13). In addition, immunohistochemical methods (receptor antibodies) may open new perspectives (8).

CONCLUSIONS

From the results presented in this study we conclude that:
1. Oestrogen or androgen receptor-positive as well as -receptor-negative cells are stained with the fluorescent ligands.
2. Receptors, both for oestrogens and androgens, cannot be visualized with these low affinity fluorescent ligands.
3. Fluorescence of the cells is probably due to binding to low affinity binding sites.
4. The presence of these low affinity binding sites appears not to be related to the presence or absence of the oestrogen or androgen receptors.

ACKNOWLEDGEMENTS

The excellent advices and excellent technical assistance of Joan Bolt-de Vries and Ed de Graaf are greatly appreciated.
The authors wish to thank Dr. Ton F.P.M. de Goeij (State University Limburg, Maastricht, The Neterlands) for the preparation and purification of the fluorescent androgen derivatives.
This study was supported by the Dutch Cancer Society (Koningin Wilhelmina Fonds) through a grant No. IKR: 82-4.

REFERENCES

1. Barrows, G.H., Stroupe, S.B., and Riehm, J.D. (1980): Am. J. Clin. Pathol., 73:330-339.
2. Bonne, C., and Raynaud, J.P. (1976): Steroids, 27:497-507.
3. Chamness, G.C., Huff, K., and Mcguire, W.L. (1975): Steroids, 25:627-635.
4. Chamness, G.C., Mercer, W.D., and McGuire, W.L. (1980): J. Histochem. Cytochem., 28:792-798.
5. Chamness, G.C., and McGuire, W.L. (198?): Arch Pathol Lab Med, 106:53-54.
6. Claas, F.H.J., and van Steenbrugge, G.J. (1983): Tissue Antigens, 21:227-232.
7. Clark, J.H., Hardin, J.W., Upchurch, S., and Eriksson, H. (1978): J. Biol. CHem., 253:7630-7634.
8. Greene, G.L., Nolan, C., Engler, J.P., and Jensen, E.V. (1980): Proc. Natl. Acad. Sci. USA, 77:5115-5119.

9. Joyce, B.G., Nicholson, R.I., Morton, M.S., and Griffiths, K. (1982): Eur. J. Cancer Clin. Oncol., 18: 1147-1155.
10. Lämmel, A., Krieg, M., and Klötzl, G. (1983): The Prostate, 4:271-282.
11. Lee, S.H. (1981): Histochemistry, 71:491-500.
12. Lipman, M.E., and Huff, K. (1976): Cancer, 38:868-874.
13. Martin, P.M., Benyahia, B., Magdelenat, H., and Katzenellenbogen, J.A. (1982): J. Steroid Biochem., 17: xl.
14. McCarty, K.S. Jr., Woodard, B.H., Nicols, D.E., Wilkinson, W., and McCarty, K.S. Sr. (1980): Cancer, 46:2842-2845.
15. Mulder, E., Peters, M.J., de Vries, J., van der Molen, H.J., Østgaard, K., Eik-Nes, k.B., and Oftebro, R. (1978): Molec. Cell. Endocr., 11:309-323.
16. Mulder, E., Vrij, L., and Foekens, J.A. (1981): Molec. Cell. Endocr., 23:283-296.
17. Nenci, I., Dandliker, W.B., Meyers, C.Y., Marchetti, E. Marzola, A. and Fabris, C. (1980): J. Histochem. Cytochem., 28:1081-1088.
18. Oftebro, R., and Nordbye, K. (1969): Exp. Cell Res., 58:439-460.
19. Panko, W.B., Mattioli, C.A., and Wheeler, T.M. (1982): Cancer, 49:2148-2152.
20. Pertschuk, L.P., Tobin, E.H., Gaetjens, E., Carter, A.C., Degenshein, G.A., Bloom, N.D., and Brigati, D.J. (1980): Cancer, 46:2896-2901.
21. Pertschuk, L.P., Tobin, E.H., Tanapat, P., Gaetjens, E., Carter, A.C., Bloom, N.D., Macchia, R.J., and Eisenberg, K.B. (1980): J. Histochem. Cytochem., 28:779-810.
22. Schröder, F.H., and Jellinghaus, W. (1978): Natl. Cancer Inst. Monogr., 49:41-46.
23. Underwood, J.C.E., Sher, E., Reed, M., Eisman, J.A., and Martin, T.J. (1982): J. Clin. Pathol., 35:401-406.
24. Van Beurden-Lamers, W.M.O., Brinkmann, A.O., Mulder, E., and van der Molen, H.J. (1974): Biochem. J., 140:495-502.

Subject Index[1]

---

[1]British and American spellings are used in text. For consistency this index uses American spellings only.